Cognitive Enhancement

Pharmacologic, Environmental and Genetic Factors

Cognitive Enhancement
Pharmacologic, Environmental and Genetic Factors

Edited by

Shira Knafo
Unidad de Biofísica CSIC, UPV/EHU,
Campus Universidad del País Vasco, and
IkerBasque, Basque Foundation for Science,
Basque Country, Spain

César Venero
Psychobiology Department,
Faculty of Psychology,
Universidad Nacional de Educación a Distancia (UNED),
Madrid, Spain

AMSTERDAM • BOSTON • HEIDELBERG • LONDON
NEW YORK • OXFORD • PARIS • SAN DIEGO
SAN FRANCISCO • SINGAPORE • SYDNEY • TOKYO

Academic Press is an imprint of Elsevier

Academic Press is an imprint of Elsevier
32 Jamestown Road, London NW1 7BY, UK
525 B Street, Suite 1800, San Diego, CA 92101-4495, USA
225 Wyman Street, Waltham, MA 02451, USA
The Boulevard, Langford Lane, Kidlington, Oxford OX5 1GB, UK

ISBN: 978-0-12-417042-1

British Library Cataloguing in Publication Data
A catalogue record for this book is available from the British Library

Library of Congress Cataloging in Publication Data
A catalog record for this book is available from the Library of Congress

For information on all Academic Press publications
visit our website at http://store.elsevier.com/

Typeset by TNQ Books and Journals
www.tnq.co.in

Printed and bound in the United States of America

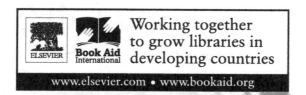

Dedication

This book is dedicated to the memory of my dear sister
Naama Ruth Yemini (Knafo), who loved life, but passed
away in 2014 at 47.

The editors dedicate this book to their families and to
patients suffering from cognitive impairment and
their families, in the hope that the continued advance of
research will soon produce a remedy to their suffering.

Contents

3. Molecular Mechanisms of Drug-Induced Cognitive Enhancement

Shira Knafo and Jose A. Esteban

4. Role of Environment, Epigenetics, and Synapses in Cognitive Enhancement

Ciaran M. Regan

8.   Can Stem Cells Be Used to Enhance Cognition?

Natalie R.S. Goldberg and Mathew Blurton-Jones

9.   Alzheimer's Disease and Mechanism-Based Attempts to Enhance Cognition

Jonathan E. Draffin, Shira Knafo and Michael T. Heneka

10. Pharmacological Treatment of Cognitive Dysfunction in Neuropsychiatric Disorders

César Venero

Contributors

Daniel L. Alkon Blanchette Rockefeller Neurosciences Institute, Rockville, MD, USA

Mathew Blurton-Jones Department of Neurobiology & Behavior, University of California Irvine, Irvine, CA, USA; Sue and Bill Gross Stem Cell Research Center, University of California Irvine, Irvine, CA, USA; Institute for Memory Impairments and Neurological Disorders, University of California Irvine, Irvine, CA, USA

Roi Cohen Kadosh Department of Experimental Psychology, University of Oxford, Oxford, United Kingdom

Jonathan E. Draffin Centro de Biología Molecular Severo Ochoa, Consejo Superior de Investigaciones Científicas/Universidad Autónoma de Madrid, Madrid, Spain

Martin Dresler Max Planck Institute of Psychiatry, Munich, Germany; Donders Institute for Brain, Cognition and Behaviour, Radboud University Medical Centre, Nijmegen, Netherlands

Veljko Dubljević Neuroethics Research Unit, Institut de Recherches Cliniques de Montréal (IRCM); Department of Neurology and Neurosurgery, McGill University, Montréal, QC, Canada; International Centre for Ethics in the Sciences and Humanities, University of Tübingen, Germany

Jose A. Esteban Centro de Biología Molecular Severo Ochoa, Consejo Superior de Investigaciones Científicas/Universidad Autónoma de Madrid, Spain

Natalie R.S. Goldberg Department of Neurobiology & Behavior, University of California Irvine, Irvine, CA, USA

Inbal Goshen Edmond and Lily Safra Center for Brain Sciences, The Hebrew University, Jerusalem, Israel

Michael T. Heneka Department of Neurology, Clinical Neuroscience Unit, Universitätsklinikum Bonn, Bonn, Germany; German Center for Neurodegenerative Disease (DZNE), Bonn, Germany

Tsuneya Ikezu Laboratory of Molecular NeuroTherapeutics, Departments of Pharmacology & Experimental Therapeutics and Neurology, Boston University School of Medicine, Boston, MA, USA

Shira Knafo Unidad de Biofísica, CSIC, UPV/EHU, Universidad del País Vasco, Ikerbasque, The Basque Foundation for Science, Leioa, Spain

Yong-Seok Lee Department of Life Science, College of Natural Science, Chung-Ang University, Seoul, Republic of Korea

Chung Yen Looi Department of Experimental Psychology, University of Oxford, Oxford, United Kingdom

Yanir Mor Edmond and Lily Safra Center for Brain Sciences, The Hebrew University, Jerusalem, Israel

Thomas J. Nelson Blanchette Rockefeller Neurosciences Institute, Morgantown, WV, USA

Ciaran M. Regan School of Biomolecular and Biomedical Science, UCD Conway Institute, University College Dublin, Belfield, Dublin, Ireland

Dimitris Repantis Charité Universitätsmedizin, Department of Psychiatry, Berlin, Germany

Anat Shapir Edmond and Lily Safra Center for Brain Sciences, The Hebrew University, Jerusalem, Israel

Miao-Kun Sun Blanchette Rockefeller Neurosciences Institute, Morgantown, WV, USA

César Venero Faculty of Psychology, Universidad Nacional de Educación a Distancia (UNED), Madrid, Spain

Chapter 1

What Is Cognitive Enhancement?

Veljko Dubljević,[1,2,3] César Venero[4] and Shira Knafo[5]

[1]Neuroethics Research Unit, Institut de Recherches Cliniques de Montréal (IRCM), Montréal, Canada; [2]Department of Neurology and Neurosurgery, McGill University, Montreal, Canada; [3]International Centre for Ethics in the Sciences and Humanities, University of Tübingen, Germany; [4]Faculty of Psychology, Universidad Nacional de Educación a Distancia (UNED), Madrid, Spain; [5]IKERBASQUE, Molecular Cognition Laboratory, Unidad de Biofísica CSIC-UPV/EHU, Campus Universidad del País Vasco, Leioa, Spain

GENERAL DEFINITION OF COGNITIVE ENHANCEMENT

The term "cognitive enhancement" is currently associated with a wide range of existing, emerging, and visionary biomedical technologies that intend to improve the cognitive status of animals and human beings. As such, it offers the promise (or threat) of drastically changing the lives of citizens. Among the technologies proposed for use in humans are drugs that boost "brain power," neuroimplants that may interface with computers or artificial means of augmenting cognition, new brain stimulation technologies to alleviate pain and control mental focus, and highly sophisticated prosthetic applications to provide specialized sensory input or mechanical output (e.g., STOA, 2009). Most of these technologies have either been established in animal models (e.g., Warwick, 2008) or they have already been used in humans (e.g., Dubljevic, 2013a). In this chapter, we will clarify what is meant by the term "cognitive enhancement" as it is currently used in the academic literature and provide an overview of the different issues addressed in this book.

In the most general sense, cognitive enhancement can be considered as the improvement in performance related to cognitive tasks. The term "cognitive enhancement" is usually used without clarifying any of the nuances associated with its meaning, yet it refers to a wide range of practices and assumptions that impinge on other concepts. Indeed, this term is often defined distinctly in different spheres, and for example, public health and epidemiological studies usually describe the use of drugs for cognitive enhancement as the "nonmedical use of prescription drugs," "drug misuse," or even "drug abuse" (e.g., De Santis et al., 2008; Franke et al., 2010). On the other hand, contributions in the interdisciplinary bioethics literature regarding cognitive enhancement (e.g., Harris, 2011), as well as in neuroscientific (e.g., Greely et al., 2008) and clinical

Cognitive Enhancement. http://dx.doi.org/10.1016/B978-0-12-417042-1.00001-2

journals (Larriviere et al., 2009), generally have a more positive attitude toward the effects of cognitive enhancers, as reflected in their preferred examples (coffee, education, etc.).

DIFFERENT CLASSES OF COGNITIVE ENHANCEMENT

The general definition of cognitive enhancement is usually articulated by its proponents, and although chiefly considered through the application of medical tools, it may involve a wider range of approaches (e.g., computer technology, education, etc.). For example, "cognitive enhancement" is commonly considered to be applied in healthy individuals, although this term has also been used historically in Alzheimer's research (see Chapter 9) and in research into neuropsychiatric illnesses involving cognitive impairment, such as schizophrenia and depression (see Chapter 10). In these pathologies, cognitive enhancement clearly refers to possible *therapeutic* interventions to improve the memory or cognitive function of patients. Thus, it is a term that is often used nonspecifically and, sometimes, academic contributions consider both contexts together. This makes the normative implications harder to define and, to some extent, may confuse the specific scientific questions underlying both these contexts. That is why "general improvement in cognitive performance" is sometimes differentiated from "maintenance of cognitive performance" and from "augmented cognitive performance."

LIFESTYLE USE VERSUS THERAPEUTIC USE OF COGNITIVE ENHANCERS

In a more technical sense, cognitive enhancement could be defined as the use of pharmaceutical drugs (see Chapters 3 and 11) or devices (see Chapters 11 and 12) for non–health-related improvement of cognition. This definition has the virtue of dissociating contexts that are socially encouraged from those that are legitimately discouraged or even prohibited. The preventive, curative, rehabilitative, and compensatory uses of pharmaceutical drugs and devices are important elements in meeting health needs. By contrast, the use of medical means to gain competitive advantage is an issue that might cause social problems (please refer to Chapter 13 in which ethical issues are discussed) and, as such, the distinction between therapy and enhancement is largely context dependent.

The concept of therapy was taken to be fairly unproblematic for a long time, yet once people realized the potential of certain technologies, they began to consider the conceptual differences between, say, vaccination and enhancement. That is not to say that new technologies have blurred the boundary themselves; rather, our attitude has shifted from taken-for-granted to the need to explain. This is why it is useful to set apart the concept of enhancement that explicitly excludes medical needs from the *therapeutic* uses of the same technology (i.e., preventive, curative, rehabilitative, and compensatory). In this sense, it is also useful to clarify the extent of moral unease felt about enhancement and the appropriate regulatory response of the state (see Dubljevic, 2012a,b for a longer argument). For example, when a given technology or social practice is not yet proved to be detrimental per se but it might cause social problems if unregulated, the appropriate response is some form of discouragement (see Dubljevic, 2013a,b).

However, notions other than cognitive enhancement have also been used to capture the concept of nonmedical drug use to improve performance. For example, "lifestyle use" of drugs may in part reflect pharmaceutical drug use that does not correspond to a medical condition or need in the traditional sense of the term but rather, to the demand for greater performance or a modified lifestyle. It may be claimed that references to the use of cognitive enhancement in the scientific literature obscure a longer history of nonmedical drug use to enhance performance. Indeed, a group of Australian authors (Bell et al., 2012) argued that the use of drugs for enhancement may even cross the border of illegal drug use (e.g., cocaine and amphetamines). This consideration adds normative implications as prohibition would be the assumed regulatory response, which might not be fully justifiable on judicial grounds. For this reason, the use of medical drugs to enhance cognitive function by healthy adults, such as Adderall (amphetamine) and Ritalin (methylphenidate, see Chapter 11), or devices such those involving transcranial direct current stimulation (tDCS, see Chapter 12), has to be dissociated from both the therapeutic drug use and the leisure use of illegal substances.

THE ASPECTS OF COGNITION BEING ENHANCED

A further issue is to understand exactly what is improved by cognitive enhancement (i.e., what capacity). The naive and undifferentiated term "cognitive enhancement" (as well as more popular terms for such enhancers, such as "smart drugs") suggests that the use of said stimulants generally improves cognition, or even IQ. However, it is important to note that current evidence is contradictory with respect to the possible "enhancement" caused by currently available cognitive enhancers (see, e.g., Ilieva et al., 2013). This has led some to conclude that the label "cognitive enhancement" may be a misnomer (see Vrecko, 2013). Accordingly, much like a drug undergoing clinical trials cannot properly be called a "treatment" or "therapy" before its effectiveness has been proved, prescription stimulants should not be called "cognitive enhancers" until there is scientific proof that they actually increase cognitive function or IQ. Many of the "smart drugs" have not been tested in the same way or with the same rigor for enhancement as they were for the original therapeutic applications (see Chapters 9, 10, and 11), and recent reviews have highlighted the limited evidence supporting claims of enhancement (see, e.g., Repantis et al., 2010). Obviously, we need a stricter definition of specific aspects of cognitive enhancement. Improved cognitive function (such as IQ, working memory, etc.), for which there is currently insufficient evidence, should be referred to as "augmented cognitive performance" and, as such, distinguished from "maintained cognitive performance." "Maintained cognitive performance" refers to the prolongation of normal cognitive activity and a dampening of the effects of fatigue and sleep deprivation, for which there is strong evidence (see, e.g., Estrada et al., 2012; Lagarde, 1995).

"General improved performance" has been analyzed as a descriptive that can be applied to cognitive enhancement, and it has been rejected as unspecific, since it does not distinguish even the therapeutic use of drugs and devices. On the one hand, "augmented cognitive performance" can be applied to healthy adults using drugs or devices to improve general IQ, working memory, or accuracy of recall, thereby achieving significantly better levels of cognitive functioning. On the other hand, "maintained cognitive performance" refers to the use of drugs or devices that serve to maintain normal levels of cognitive activity for longer periods of time, while reducing the impairment associated with fatigue and sleep deprivation. While the evidence supporting the former remains somewhat controversial, current "cognitive enhancers" undoubtedly provide such maintenance effects, although some issues regarding safety remain unclear.

ARE TODAY'S "COGNITIVE ENHANCERS" TRULY EFFICIENT?

It is currently not easy to define improvement in cognition. For an individual interested in enhancement, the effect depends on the expectations of a subjective improvement in performance in real-life settings, whereas a regulatory review body usually requires controlled laboratory settings to assess claims of improved cognition. Since the benefits of cognitive enhancers should by definition not involve the response to a clear pathology, lesion, or identified behavioral or mental health problem, establishing the basal measures to evaluate the effects of enhancement is likely to be somewhat controversial. The studies carried out to date have examined the enhancement of extant neuropharmaceuticals (see Ilieva et al., 2013; Repantis et al., 2010) and brain stimulation techniques, such as transcranial magnetic stimulation (Luber and Lisanby, 2013) and tDCS (Dockery et al., 2009; see Chapter 12), through the performance of specific tasks in controlled laboratory settings. However, critics point out that these tasks do not fully capture the effects on the more general capacities underlying them or on other tasks (see Iuculcano and Cohen Kadosh, 2013; Ranisch et al., 2013; Vrecko, 2013) and that cognitive enhancers should (also) be examined in the context of real-world performance.

POSSIBLE RISKS IN THE USE OF COGNITIVE ENHANCERS

The nonspecific term "cognitive enhancement" has an in-built positive connotation that diverts attention from the possible short-term and long-term risks or the side effects associated with using drugs or devices to stimulate the brain for non-medical reasons and without any relevant knowledge or supervision. Drugs such as ampakines (see Chapter 3) might augment cognitive performance in the sense of increasing general IQ, working memory or more accurate recall, yet perhaps they will not work in humans (Goff et al., 2008). Furthermore, these drugs might produce some side effects, or they may be harmless (Goff et al., 2008). Indeed, even "maintained cognitive performance" raises important ethical issues, depending on the potential side effects of the substances (or devices) used (see Dubljevic, 2012b; Ranisch et al., 2013; and Chapter 13). The issue of whether new "cognitive enhancers" are harmless like coffee or dangerous like amphetamines can only be resolved once research into the effects of new drugs (or devices) has delivered robust and reliable findings, something to which this book will contribute.

A JOURNEY THROUGH THIS BOOK

After defining the possible meanings of cognitive enhancement in its multiple forms, this book looks in depth at a number of the traditional and cutting-edge technologies that are currently studied and employed in experimental animals and sometimes, in humans. Unlike traditional approaches (e.g., enriched environment, Chapter 4), most of the innovative approaches are invasive and they are therefore unlikely to be tested on human beings. Nevertheless, they provide precious insight into the avenues of current research that may lead to future modes of enhancement.

As described in Chapter 2, one of the most common approaches to develop new cognitive enhancers is to identify the pathways involved in learning and memory, and to test activators specific to these pathways. In a second, often used approach, pathways leading to synaptic loss or cell death are identified and inhibited. A third approach described in this chapter relies on the activation of normal cell repair mechanisms to restore lost synapses.

Having understood the signaling pathways that globally modulate learning and memory, it is essential to uncover the specific molecular and synaptic events mediating cognitive function. Accordingly, sophisticated molecular and electrophysiological tools are described in Chapter 3 based on the idea that facilitating synaptic plasticity may eventually lead to better cognitive function, a result that can be achieved by manipulating the activity of neurotransmitter receptors. This chapter also describes how synthetic compounds specifically engineered to boost synaptic transmission and plasticity positively affect cognitive capacity in a variety of experimental paradigms. Although the routine use of these drugs in humans is still a long way off, experiments in animals are encouraging and represent the first essential step for the selection of drugs for clinical trials. Together, Chapters 2 and 3 provide valuable insights into the molecular mechanisms believed to induce cognitive enhancement and how this knowledge can be used to develop new, mechanism-based drugs for use in healthy humans or in individuals suffering from cognitive impairment. Nonetheless, drugs are not necessarily the optimal approach to enhance cognitive function.

Chapter 4 describes how control over the environment may represent a more physiological approach to cognitive enhancement, focusing on how the incredible plasticity of the brain is used to evolve behaviors that accommodate the inherent uncertainty and probabilistic nature of the environment. This plasticity requires a constant interaction between the genome and the environment, whereby the latter regulates the cell signals and functions that control gene expression. Such epigenetic mechanisms represent ideal devices, as many transcription factors control neuronal structure and function, supporting the interplay between hippocampal and neocortical assemblies necessary for the formation and modification of new and existing representations.

Moving on to an approach that is only possible in rodents, Chapter 5 describes genetic engineering technologies to produce transgenic mice. This is a commonly used method to study cognitive function at distinct levels, ranging from molecules to behaviors. This chapter analyzes how negative genetic manipulations cause behavioral deficits in mutant animals, while cognitive functions are enhanced in some such transgenic mice. The phenotype of these mice is summarized, along with the signaling pathways affected by the genetic manipulation. This overview of "smart" transgenic mice reveals that cognitive enhancement can be achieved by altering the regulation of molecules involved in cell signaling events, shifting this from the receptors at the cell surface to the transcription factors in the nucleus of neurons. Understanding the mechanisms of memory enhancement is therefore an important tool to elucidate the basic mechanisms underlying learning and memory, as well as to develop treatments for cognitive disorders.

This book also contains three chapters describing cutting-edge experimental technologies that are currently being employed to enhance cognitive functions in rodents. Chapter 6 describes how recovering cognitive function through viral gene therapy has become feasible in the last decade. This approach involves delivering genes of interest into the specific brain region to either protect neurons or to enhance neural regeneration, thereby promoting cognitive function. The chapter focuses on adeno-associated virus (AAV) vectors, those most widely used in basic research and that are currently being tested in clinical trials to treat neurodegenerative disorders. This chapter delves into the background of the AAV vector system, as well as analyzing successful candidate transgenes to enhance neurogenesis and hippocampal function, and it describes their application in cognitive enhancement.

Chapter 7 describes another innovative approach that has become popular in the past decade. Optogenetics is a method that permits real-time control of genetically defined neuronal populations using light-sensitive proteins. This chapter shows how optogenetic tools can be used to gain new insights into the way in which memories are formed, saved, and extracted. The incorporation of optogenetic tools into the field of learning and memory has led to an important increase in our understanding of the networks underlying complex cognitive processes. Hence, this chapter focuses on how optogenetics can be used for memory generation and cognitive enhancement.

Chapter 8 describes another cutting-edge technology, to date used only in a laboratory setting. It explains how multipotent stem cells within the adult brain play a critical role in cognition and the strategies to favor neural stem cell populations within key brain regions that are being developed to enhance cognition in rodents. The relationship between neural stem cells and cognition in the healthy, aging, and pathological brain and the molecular mechanisms by which stem cells may exert their effects on learning and memory are also addressed. Moreover, the brain's capacity for plasticity and regeneration is reviewed, along with the potential role of endogenous neurogenesis and stem cell transplantation to augment this capacity.

Chapter 9 describes the cognition-enhancing manipulations overcoming the cognitive deficits related to Alzheimer's disease. Unfortunately, in most cases the strategies that have proved successful in rodents tend to fail in human beings. Examples of manipulations are described, and the possible causes of failure are analyzed. A significant part of this chapter is dedicated to clinical trials in Alzheimer's patients that failed to recapitulate the positive effects found in rodents. In some cases, the failure of the treatment can be easily traced, as when the treatment produced significant side effects. However, in most cases, there is no ready explanation for failure.

Chapter 10 reviews different pharmaceutical treatments approved by the Food and Drug Administration to reverse or ameliorate neurocognitive deficits frequently found in several neuropsychiatric disorders or those being tested in clinical trials. Crucially, cognitive deficits are at times a core feature of such disorders. The chapter focuses on pharmacological treatments that effectively improve some aspects of cognition in certain neuropsychiatric illnesses, including attention-deficit/hyperactive disorder, schizophrenia, bipolar disorder, posttraumatic stress disorder, and depression.

Chapter 11 summarizes empirical data on the approaches to enhance cognitive capabilities in humans using pharmaceuticals, nutrition, physical exercise, sleep, meditation, mnemonic strategies, computer training, and brain stimulation. This chapter also describes the drugs that are currently being used in patients suffering from Alzheimer's disease. Unfortunately, antidementia drugs offer only minor benefits in cognitive function and none of them seem to have disease-modifying properties. The mixed evidence for the efficacy of many pharmaceutical drugs currently used for cognitive enhancement is summarized, while a growing body of evidence for several nonpharmacological interventions indicates reliable cognition-enhancing effects. In this respect, Chapter 12 provides valuable data on the use of noninvasive brain stimulation for cognitive enhancement, such as tDCS. The evidence of the safety, beneficial impacts, and cost-benefit ratio of these techniques at the individual and societal level are discussed in detail, along with the mechanisms and physiological effects of tDCS and its effects on human cognition.

The final chapter of this book (Chapter 13) summarizes the ethical issues that may arise once efficient cognitive enhancers are developed for human use.

It starts by describing possible scenarios that may currently sound unrealistic yet that serve to reflect on the danger of unregulated use of cognitive enhancers. This chapter explains why and how authorities should strictly control the prescription of cognitive enhancers, adapting state laws to these new technologies.

To summarize, this book contains a vast amount of information regarding traditional and modern strategies aimed at enhancing cognitive function, both in animals and humans. The editors made an effort to make this book accessible to the general public, although some of the chapters may be more scientifically oriented than others. Nevertheless, the general goal of this book is to bring together the bulk of information available in this field, in the hope that this will eventually help scientists to develop new, more efficient approaches to treat cognitive impairment.

REFERENCES

Bell, S.K., Lucke, J., Hall, W., 2012. Lessons for enhancement from the history of cocaine and amphetamine use. Am. J. Bioeth. Neurosci. 3 (2), 24–29.

De Santis, A.D., Webb, E.M., Noar, S.M., 2008. Illicit use of prescription ADHD medications on a college campus: a multimethodological approach. J. Am. Coll. Health 57 (3), 315–324.

Dockery, C.A., Hueckel-Weng, R., Birbaumer, N., Plewnia, C., 2009. Enhancement of planning ability by transcranial direct current stimulation. J. Neurosci. 29 (22), 7271–7277.

Dubljević, V., 2012a. Principles of justice as the basis for public policy on psychopharmacological cognitive enhancement. Law Innovation Technol. 4 (1), 67–83.

Dubljević, V., 2012b. Toward a legitimate public policy on cognition enhancement drugs. Am. J. Bioeth. Neurosci. 3 (3), 29–33.

Dubljević, V., 2013a. Prohibition or coffee-shops: regulation of amphetamine and methylphenidate for enhancement use by healthy adults. Am. J. Bioeth. 13 (7), 23–33.

Dubljević, V., 2013b. Cognitive enhancement, rational choice and justification. Neuroethics 6 (1), 179–187.

Estrada, A., Kelley, A.M., Webb, C.M., Athy, J.R., Crowley, J.S., 2012. Modafinil as a replacement for dextroamphetamine for sustaining alertness in military helicopter pilots. Aviat. Space Environ. Med. 83 (6), 556–564.

Franke, A.G., Bonertz, C., Christmann, M., Huss, M., Fellgiebel, A., Hildt, E., et al., 2010. Non-medical use of prescription stimulants and illicit use of stimulants for cognitive enhancement in pupils and students in Germany. Pharmacopsychiatry 44 (2), 60–66.

Goff, D.C., Lamberti, J.S., et al., 2008. A placebo-controlled add-on trial of the Ampakine, CX516, for cognitive deficits in schizophrenia. Neuropsychopharmacology 33 (3), 465–472.

Greely, H., Sahakian, B., Harris, J., Kessler, R.C., Gazzaniga, M., Campbell, P., et al., 2008. Towards responsible use of cognitive-enhancing drugs by the healthy. Nature 456 (7224), 702–705.

Harris, J., 2011. Chemical cognitive enhancement: Is it unfair, unjust, discriminatory, or cheating for healthy adults to use smart drugs. In: Illes, J., Sahakian, B. (Eds.), Oxford handbook of Neuroethics. Oxford University Press, Oxford, UK, pp. 265–272.

Ilieva, I., Boland, J., Farah, M.J., 2013. Objective and subjective cognitive enhancing effects of mixed amphetamine salts in healthy people. Neuropharmacology 64 (1), 496–505.

Iuculcano, T., Cohen Kadosh, R., 2013. The mental cost of cognitive enhancement. J.Neurosci. 33 (10), 4482–4486.

Larriviere, D., Williams, M.A., Rizzo, M., Bonnie, R.J., 2009. Responding to requests from adult patients for neuroenhancements: guidance of the ethics, law and humanities committee. Neurology 73 (17), 1406–1412.

Lagarde, D., Batejet, D., Van Beers, P., Sarafian, D., Pradella, S., 1995. Interest of modafinil, a new psychostimulant, during a sixty-hour sleep deprivation experiment. Fundam. Clin. Pharmacol. 9 (3), 271–279.

Luber, B., Lisanby, S.H., 2013. Enhancement of human cognitive performance using transcranial magnetic stimulation (TMS). Neuroimage. http://dx.doi.org/10.1016/j.neuroimage.2013.06.007 (Epub ahead of print) June 13th, 2013.

Ranisch, R., Garofoli, D., Dubljević, V., 2013. 'Clock shock', motivational enhancement and performance maintenance in Adderall use. Am. J. Bioeth. Neurosci. 4 (1), 13–14.

Repantis, D., Schlattmann, P., Laisney, O., Heuser, I., 2010. Modafinil and methylphenidate for neuroenhancement in healthy individuals: a systematic review. Pharmacol. Res. 62 (3), 187.

Science and Technology Options Assessment [STOA], 2009. Human Enhancement Study. Rathenau Institute, The Hague, The Netherlands.

Vrecko, S., 2013. Just how cognitive is 'cognitive enhancement'? Am. J. Bioeth. Neurosci. 4 (1), 4–12.

Warwick, K., 2008. Cybernetic enhancements. In: Zonneveld, L., Dijstelbloem, H., Ringoir, D. (Eds.), Reshaping the Human Condition. Exploring Human Enhancement. Rathenau Institute, The Hague, The Netherlands, pp. 123–131.

Chapter 2

Signaling Pathways Involved in Cognitive Enhancement

Thomas J. Nelson,[1] Miao-Kun Sun[1] and Daniel L. Alkon[2]

[1]*Blanchette Rockefeller Neurosciences Institute, Morgantown, WV, USA;* [2]*Blanchette Rockefeller Neurosciences Institute, Rockville, MD, USA*

INTRODUCTION

Cognitive enhancement is a general strategy for treating the effects of conditions involving cognitive impairment such as traumatic brain injury, Down syndrome, and neurodegenerative diseases (e.g., Alzheimer's disease). The goal of cognitive enhancement therapy is to develop treatments that, while not necessarily effecting a cure, can improve the quality of life for patients suffering such conditions. In a broad sense, however, cognitive enhancement also includes pharmacological and other means for increasing memory and cognitive capacity, targeting both cognitive disorders and normal mentation. Such drugs would be valuable even if effective treatments for specific disorders are eventually found, because arresting disease progression at a late stage of a neurodegenerative disease would be of marginal value without some way of enhancing normal cognitive function and repairing the accumulated injuries to synaptic pathways and networks.

One approach to finding cognitive enhancers is to identify the molecular signaling pathways of learning and memory and search for compounds that activate the relevant components of the pathway. These targets could include protein kinases, cell surface receptors, neural signaling mechanisms, components of synaptic transmission, or enzymes anywhere along the signaling pathway. This approach could also involve stimulating enzymes involved in neurotransmitter synthesis, enhancing the contacts between pre- and post-synaptic proteins, or inducing the maturation of synapses.

A second approach is to activate normal neuronal repair mechanisms in order to restore synaptic pathways that have been lost. Again, this depends on understanding the signaling pathways and how they interact. An example would be a drug that induces the formation of new synapses. This approach is potentially more powerful, because it can be directed toward reversing the underlying neurodegeneration rather than simply stimulating a signaling pathway.

Cognitive Enhancement. http://dx.doi.org/10.1016/B978-0-12-417042-1.00002-4

In this chapter, we will review the signaling pathways involved in these two approaches. For each approach, we will consider potential therapeutic agents that act on these pathways, mainly small molecule drugs, along with their potential benefits and drawbacks.

STRESS AS A COGNITIVE ENHANCER

One challenge in classifying cognitive enhancers is to discriminate between substances that directly activate mechanisms of memory and cognition and those that act indirectly by affecting performance or by activating stress mechanisms. Acute stress produces a generalized activation of neuronal activity and profound biochemical changes that can enhance (McGaugh and Roozendaal, 2002) or impair (Wang et al., 2013; Eagle et al., 2013; Lee et al., 2013) memory encoding and formation. Thus, stress, and agents that induce stress, may be thought of in certain contexts as cognitive enhancers. For example, fear stress activates the basolateral complex in the amygdala, which is critically involved in the storage of conditioned fear memories, but not spatial or declarative memories. Animals subjected to threatening stimuli show increases in phospho-ERK2 (extracellular signal-related kinase 2) in the amygdala, which is associated with reduced inhibitory control of GABAergic interneurons, resulting in increased neuronal excitability (Martijena and Molina, 2012).

Although not completely understood, in general, the release of catecholamines and glucocorticoids following sympathetic nervous system activation enhances memory consolidation through a variety of mechanisms, while at the same time interfering with memory retrieval. Catecholamines such as norepinephrine influence the amygdala via the β-adrenoreceptor, which is coupled to adenylate cyclase and cyclic adenosine monophosphate (cAMP) synthesis. cAMP acts through cAMP-responsive element-binding protein (CREB) and induces the synthesis of a number of genes, including brain-derived neurotrophic factor (BDNF) and c-fos, and promotes synaptic growth. Because of this, a large industry has arisen to search for drug compounds that can activate the CREB pathway (Scott et al., 2002).

Glucocorticoid receptor agonists administered to the medial prefrontal cortex also enhance memory by effects on the noradrenergic system via G-protein coupled receptors that do not involve changes in DNA synthesis (Barsegyan et al., 2010). As with catecholamines, cAMP-dependent protein kinase is the proximate biochemical mediator of stress signaling (Schwabe et al., 2012). Although the amygdala is not a storage site for spatial or declarative memories, glucocorticoid receptor stimulation in the basolateral amygdala can affect spatial memory via its neuronal projections to the hippocampus. The cognitive enhancement effect of stress may also be due in part to increased exclusion of unrelated information (Henckens et al., 2009). It is important to mention, though, that stress reduces glutamatergic transmission and glutamate receptor surface expression in the prefrontal pyramidal neurons (Wei et al., 2013), and also alters the production and survival of new neurons in the hippocampus (Schoenfeld and Gould, 2012). Stress also reduces levels of BDNF (Masi and Brovedani, 2011), leading to a reduction of synaptic growth. These findings imply that stress has numerous detrimental effects and must be regarded with caution.

BIOCHEMICAL SIGNALING PATHWAYS IN LEARNING

A fundamental property of cognitive enhancers is the ability to facilitate learning. It has long been known that calcium and other cations are involved in the signaling pathways of learning. Alkon and Rasmussen (1988) proposed a cellular model of cell activation that involved spatially discrete responses to a stimulus mediated by calcium. Alkon et al. (1982) also identified changes in membrane potassium currents during the retention of associative learning in the marine invertebrate *Hermissenda crassicornis*. From these and many other experiments, it was clear that ion channels were critically involved in learning. One protein that affects ion channels is protein kinase C (PKC).

Protein Kinase C

Early research with marine invertebrates identified PKC as a central component of learning and memory. Bank et al. (1988) identified an increase in PKC in crude membrane fractions of CA1 hippocampus prepared from rabbits subjected to rabbit classical eyelid conditioning. This was correlated with focal increments of [^{3}H]phorbol-12,13-dibutyrate binding (Olds et al., 1989). Increased phosphorylation of PKC substrates was found following associative learning in *Hermissenda* (Neary et al., 1981; Nelson et al., 1990). PKC was also found to regulate A-type potassium channels, which had previously been associated with classical conditioning in *Hermissenda* (Alkon et al., 1982) and rabbits (Alkon et al., 1988; Etcheberrigaray et al., 1992). Activation of PKC with bryostatin 1 enhances learning and memory, while at the same time increasing the numbers of mushroom spines, perforated postsynaptic densities, and double-synapse presynaptic boutons associated with spines. Ro 31-8220, an inhibitor of PKC, prevents these effects (Hongpaisan and Alkon, 2007). PKC activation was found to induce the synthesis of other proteins when given several days before training (Alkon et al., 2005). This protein synthesis greatly decreased the number of training events required for memory acquisition in *Hermissenda* and prolonged retention from 7 min to over 1 week, indicating a markedly reduced threshold for long-term consolidation.

Indeed, protein synthesis had long been recognized as essential for long-term memory acquisition. Much of the protein synthesis that occurs during learning occurs locally in neuronal dendrites, which confer specificity to associative memories (Jiang and Schuman, 2002; Govindarajan et al., 2011).

Bryostatin, phorbol esters, and similar PKC activators, such as ingenol and picologs, bind to the C1A and C1B domains on PKC (DeChristopher et al., 2012; Nelson and Alkon, 2009). The natural ligand for C1 domains is 1,2-diacylglycerol (Blumberg et al., 2008). Conventional PKC isoforms (α, βI, βII, and γ), and novel PKC isoforms (δ, ϵ, η, and θ) also possess a C2 domain, which binds phosphatidic acid and phosphatidylserine (Corbalán-Garcia et al., 2003; Conesa-Zamora et al., 2001). These lipids have been implicated in neurite outgrowth and spine formation (Ammar et al., 2013; Shirai et al., 2010), and artificial ligands of the PKC C2 domain, such as DCP-LA, have been shown to restore mature mushroom spine synapses and prevent memory loss in aging rats (Hongpaisan et al., 2013).

In conventional PKC isoforms, the C2 domain participates in calcium binding (Steinberg, 2008). As with the C1 domain, the C2 domain is not unique to PKC but is also found in many other proteins (Kim et al., 2003), including proteins involved in synaptic vesicle exocytosis, such as synaptotagmins (Martens, 2010; Südhof and Rizo, 1996). C1- and C2-like domains are found in the sequences of many proteins involved in synaptic enhancement or neurotransmitter release. Thus, both classes of PKC activators may also have strong non-PKC effects on synaptic vesicle release and, hence, produce cognitive enhancement.

Other C1-Domain Proteins

PKC is not the only protein that possesses a C1 domain. Many other proteins bind 1,2-diacylglycerol and possess homologous domains, including Rat sarcoma guanyl releasing protein 1 (Lorenzo et al., 2000) and the Mammalian Uncoordinated (Munc)-13 family proteins (Wojcik and Brose, 2007). These proteins are all located in neurons and participate in dendritic growth and synaptic vesicle release, and thus cannot be overlooked as potential neurological targets for bryostatin and similar cognitive enhancers.

Bryostatin 1 and phorbol ester (phorbol-12-myristate-13-acetate, PMA)

Like PKC, Munc13 has multiple isoforms. The Munc13-3 isoform is found primarily in the cerebellum granule and Purkinje cells, where it regulates motor learning. The more abundant Munc13-1 isoform, which is expressed throughout the brain, is particularly interesting as a potential target for cognitive enhancers, because it is a synaptic vesicle c, colocalizing with the presynaptic marker synaptophysin (Augustin et al., 2001), and thus is well positioned to change synaptic efficiency. Basu et al. (2007) found that phorbol dibutyrate binding to Munc 13 lowers the energy barrier for synaptic vesicle fusion. Diacylglycerol and phorbol esters augment neurotransmitter release in hippocampal neurons; Munc13, and not PKC, is the protein responsible for this effect (Rhee et al., 2002).

Whichever protein is responsible, C2-domain activators such as DCP-LA and DCP-LA methyl ester produce beneficial morphological and behavioral effects, indicating potential value as cognitive enhancers (Hongpaisan et al., 2011, 2013). In Tg2576 and 5XFAD transgenic mice, often used as models for familial Alzheimer's disease, DCP-LA prevents synaptic loss and cognitive deficits (Hongpaisan et al., 2011). Bryostatin has similar effects (Hongpaisan et al., 2011, 2013; Sun and Alkon, 2005).

PKC Substrates

Many PKC substrates are also involved in cognitive and learning pathways. One is Myristoylated Alanine-Rich C-Kinase Substrate (MARCKS), an acidic membrane-bound protein. Phosphorylation of MARCKS by PKC inhibits its association with actin and with the plasma membrane, reducing its ability to crosslink F-actin, and triggering dendritic spine destabilization (Calabrese and Halpain, 2005). PKC-induced spine destabilization can be prevented by creating a nonphosphorylatable MARCKS mutant. Dendritic spines are highly dynamic; over 80% of the F-actin in spines turns over every minute (Koleske, 2013). Thus, PKC, in conjunction with signaling molecules that promote stabilization, may be preferentially involved in the early stages of dendritic restructuring during development, or during adulthood when dendritic spines have largely stabilized.

Another PKC substrate important in cognitive function is GAP-43, a growth cone-associated protein that is essential for neurite outgrowth. Like MARCKS, GAP-43 interacts with actin filaments. After phosphorylation by PKC, GAP-43 promotes the stabilization of long filaments (He et al., 1997). PKC activation increases the level of autophosphorylated CaMKII and promoted association with NMDA receptors, possibly through phosphorylation of calmodulin-binding proteins such as neuromodulin (Yan et al., 2011), indicating overlap of their signaling pathways, but there is little evidence of any physiological direct phosphorylation. Although not fully understood, these interactions between signaling kinases such as CaMKII and PKC and cytoskeletal proteins such as actin modify the geometry of dendritic spines, and thereby directly change the function and connectivity of the neuronal networks responsible for cognition.

Structural Proteins

Dendritic spines are the primary site of excitatory input on most principal neurons. Their sizes, shapes, and numbers change during aging, memory formation, and neurodegenerative disease progression. The mature so-called mushroom spines are formed from an enlargement of thin spines during synaptic enhancement. The stability of these spines suggests, to many investigators, their involvement in long-term memory (Bourne and Harris, 2007). If so, an effective memory therapy should restore the brain's capacity to form mushroom spines.

As mentioned above, changes in structural proteins, particularly actin, play an important role in cognitive enhancement. A cytoskeletal change in dendritic spines is the most well established candidate for the biochemical localization of memory (Hotulainen and Hoogenraad, 2010; Kasai et al., 2010). The rearrangement of the actin cytoskeleton is instrumental in synaptic maturation and memory (Hotulainen and Hoogenraad, 2010). Spine length and morphology are modified by learning and profoundly affect synaptic transmission. Defects in dendritic spine cytoskeleton are observed in patients with mental retardation (Newey et al., 2005), traumatic brain injury (TBI) (Gao et al., 2011), and Alzheimer's disease (Perez-Cruz et al., 2011). Thus, it is no surprise that many cognitive enhancers modify the actin cytoskeleton either directly or indirectly.

Rho GTPases

Reorganization of structural proteins is effected in part by small GTP-binding proteins, which bind and hydrolyze GTP. Perhaps the most important of these are the Rho GTPases. Rho is the name for a family of small GTPases that regulate the actin cytoskeleton, including RhoA, Rac1, and Cdc42 (Ridley, 2006). Rac1 and Cdc42 are important for spine formation and growth, whereas RhoA is important for spine loss (Newey et al., 2005). Rho proteins are therefore instrumental in regulating synaptogenesis (Tolias et al., 2011).

The activity of Rho family proteins is modulated by a number of proteins called guanine nucleotide exchange factors (GEFs), which promote GDP–GTP exchange, and GTPase-activating proteins (GAPs), which promote GTP hydrolysis (Rossman et al., 2005). Specificity of action among Rho family proteins is determined by specific GEFs and GAPs. For example, Rac GAPs include α1-, α2-, β1-, and β2-chimaerin, all of which possess a bryostatin-binding C1 site (Sosa et al., 2009). α1-Chimaerin is a brain-specific Rac GAP, found in dendritic spines (Buttery et al., 2006). Binding of phorbol ester or diacylglycerol causes recruitment of α1-chimaerin to the membrane and pruning of the dendritic arbor (Buttery et al., 2006). In the presence of phorbol ester, α1-chimaerin binds to the N2A subunit of the NMDA receptor, causing inactivation of Rac and inhibition of its dendrite-pruning activity (Van de Ven et al., 2005) (Figure 2.1).

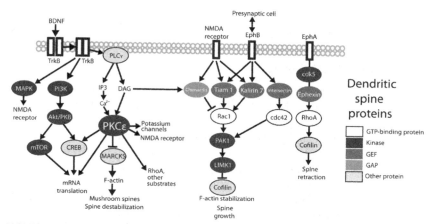

FIGURE 2.1   Signaling pathways involved in dendritic spine growth. Dendritic spine growth is a highly dynamic process that is mediated by rearrangement of the actin cytoskeleton. Postsynaptic receptors including TrkB, NMDA receptors, and EphA and B initiate signaling cascades that involve small GTP-binding proteins (particularly Rac1 and cdc42), protein kinases (such as PAK1, Akt/PKB, and PKC), guanine nucleotide exchange factors (GEF), and GTPase activating proteins (GAP). These pathways converge on cofilin, a protease that disassembles actin filaments. Inhibition of cofilin produces F-actin stabilization, whereas the activation of cofilin produces spine retraction. There is evidence that both processes play important roles in synaptic plasticity.

In contrast to protein kinase C, which is activated and then rapidly down-regulated by phorbol esters, α1-chimaerin is rapidly ubiquitinated and degraded under basal conditions, but is stabilized by C1 binding molecules such as 1,2-diacylglycerols or phorbol esters (Marland et al., 2011). Overexpression of a constitutively active Rac1 mutant causes phospholipase C, the enzyme that produces 1,2-diacylglycerol from phospholipids, to increase α1-chimaerin levels in cultured rat hippocampal neurons (Marland et al., 2011).

Rac GEFs include Tiam1, Kalirin 7, Kalirin, and Trio (Buttery et al., 2006). Kalirin 7 is the most well studied of these, and has been shown to localize in dendritic spines and postsynaptic densities. Rac GEFs such as Kalirin 7 are essential for the activity of EphA receptors, which are large tyrosine kinases that control dendritic spine maturation (Penzes and Jones, 2008). Tiam1 is located in the postsynaptic density and binds to the NMDA receptor, where it participates in dendritic arborization (Tolias et al., 2005). Kalirin 7 is phosphorylated in mouse brain by CaMKII, cAMP-dependent protein kinase, and PKC (Kiraly et al., 2011).

Identifying the optimal site for development of drugs to modulate Rho and related proteins awaits a fuller understanding of these biochemical pathways leading to dendritic outgrowth. It is already clear, however, that signaling proteins such as the small GTP-binding proteins and NMDA receptors are promising starting points in the search for cognitive enhancers. NMDA receptor antagonists, including memantine, amantidine, dextromethorphan, and

nitromemantines, are under consideration for treatment of glutamate excitotoxicity, and may prove beneficial as neuroprotective agents (Lopes et al., 2013).

Ephrins and NMDA Receptors

Although the small GTPases are the messenger proteins in activating synaptic
actin reorganization, it is the NMDA and Eph receptors that are the principal
effectors in regulating synaptogenesis during development, and it is the proteases,
members of the cofilin family, that do the proximate work. EphA activates cofilin,
a member of the actin-depolymerizing-factor (ADF/cofilin) family, to promote
spine retraction (Zhou et al., 2012). It is hypothesized that the function of retraction is to prevent unlimited growth of spines during development, and preserve
the capacity for spine remodeling in the mature brain (Murai et al., 2003). EphB
activates Cdc42 and Rac via their respective GEFs (intersectin and Tiam1 + Kali-
nin) to promote spine maturation by inhibiting cofilin (Tolias et al., 2007). EphB
receptor activation induces phosphorylation of the NMDA receptor, modifying
calcium influx (Dalva et al., 2000), which is an intrinsic part of synaptic plasticity.
In early development, Rac also activates PAK1 (p21 protein activated kinase 1),
which promotes spine and synapse formation (Zhang et al., 2005).

As predicted more than 64 years ago by Hebb, synapse formation involves
both forward (presynaptic to postsynaptic) and reverse (postsynaptic to presynaptic) signaling (Lim et al., 2008). Both forward and reverse signaling use
EphB. Ephrin-EphB signaling acts at two stages: in the early stage by increasing neurotransmitter release, and then later by enhancing postsynaptic glutamate responsiveness (Murai and Pasquale, 2011; Hruska and Dalva, 2012). This
implies that the retrograde signaling occurs first, with ephrin-B signaling promoting presynaptic maturation, and the anterograde signaling and postsynaptic maturation occurring later. As the synapse matures, the relative importance
of α-amino-3-hydroxy-5-methyl-4-isoxazolepropionic acid receptor (AMPA)
receptors versus NMDA receptors increases (Wu et al., 1996; Hall and Ghosh,
2008). The increased AMPAR/NMDAR ratio is associated with rapid dendritic
spine enlargement (beginning within 10s), which requires calcium-calmodulin-
dependent protein phosphorylation to become long-lasting (Matsuzaki et al.,
2004). Long-lasting enlargement can be blocked by latrunculin A, an inhibitor
of actin polymerization, indicating that cytoskeletal arrangements are a critical
step in activity-induced synaptic potentiation (Matsuzaki et al., 2004).

The cytoskeleton rearrangement pathways involved in dendritic growth are
shown in Figure 2.1.

Calmodulin-Dependent Kinase II

Calmodulin-dependent protein kinase II (CaMKII) is an abundant protein that
is essential for synaptic plasticity and learning. Recently, it has been shown to
be important for synaptic organization (Hell, 2014). Thus, activators of CaMKII

would be expected to behave as cognitive enhancers. One such compound, CNB-001, has been reported to enhance memory in object recognition tasks in the rat (Maher et al., 2010). Another possibility is the antidepressant tianeptine (7-[3-chloro-6-methyl-5,5-dioxo-6,11-dihydro-(c,f)-dibenzo-(1,2-thiazepine)-11-yl-amino]-heptanoic acid, sodium salt), a selective serotonin reuptake enhancer (SSRE) that is reported to increase BDNF levels (Della et al., 2012) and increase the phosphorylation state of AMPA receptors by activating CaMKII (Zhang et al., 2013). Another CaMKII activator is the polyphenol tetrahydroxystilbene (Wang et al., 2011).

Neurosteroids

Estrogens such as 17β-estradiol can function as cognitive enhancers, and improve learning performance in Morris water maze tasks (Li et al., 2004; Sandstrom and Williams, 2001) and inhibitory avoidance (Frye and Rhodes, 2002). Just as with insulin (see below), the estrogen receptor in the brain serves an entirely different function in the brain from its function in the periphery. Activation of the estrogen receptor ERβ with 17β-estradiol facilitates long-term potentiation in rat hippocampal slices (Kramár et al., 2009), increases hippocampal synapse density (Woolley and McEwen, 1992), and also increases the surface expression of AMPA-type glutamate receptors (Liu et al., 2008).

WAY-200070 and 17β-estradiol

CNS-derived estradiol is synthesized by aromatization of testosterone, and not only acts on the nuclear estrogen receptor, but also acts directly on neuronal membranes (Murphy et al., 1998). The level of aromatase is significantly higher in the prefrontal cortex of young female rats than their age-matched males. This may be responsible for the sex-dependent difference in responding to repeated stress (Wei et al., 2013). Aromatase is strongly inhibited by calcium-dependent phosphorylation by PKC and by cAMP-dependent protein kinase (Balthazart and Ball, 2006). At least some of the effects of estradiol are mediated by PKC/ERK pathways (Keshamouni et al., 2002).

Estradiol increases CREB phosphorylation in vivo (Liu et al., 2008) and increases dendritic branching and spine number (Liu et al., 2008; Li et al., 2004) and number of mushroom spines (Liu et al., 2008) as well as levels of AMPA receptors, which are involved in hippocampal long-term potentiation. In the case of estradiol, the effect is attributed to the activation of the small GTPase RhoA and the phosphorylation and inactivation of cofilin, a protease that cleaves actin. Activation of ERβ protects brains from ischemic damage (Raval et al., 2013) and may be responsible for neural protection against vascular dementia in females. Activation of estrogen receptors using ERβ-specific agonists such as WAY-200070 or WAY-202779, which readily cross the blood–brain barrier, increases the density of mushroom spines and improves performance in spatial learning tasks (Murphy et al., 1998). Estradiol also downregulates BDNF levels in GABAergic inhibitory interneurons, leading to increased excitability and activity-dependent formation of dendritic spines in hippocampal neurons (Balthazart and Ball, 2006).

Unlike the parent molecule cholesterol, neurosteroids such as 17β-estradiol are said to have little difficulty crossing the blood–brain barrier (Lee et al., 2013), but they are also synthesized in the principal neurons and a subpopulation of astrocytes. Despite this, physiological levels of estradiol derived from the periphery (10^{-12} M in males and 10^{-10} M in females) are unable to compensate for a decrease in hippocampal estradiol caused by local application of the aromatase inhibitor letrozole, suggesting that the central and peripheral compartments are strictly segregated (Kretz et al., 2004).

BIOCHEMICAL SIGNALING PATHWAYS IN NEURONAL REPAIR

A complementary approach for cognitive enhancement is inhibiting synaptic and cellular loss that may occur concomitant to injury and disease. Cognitive enhancers that inhibit synaptic loss would have the advantage of treating neurodegenerative diseases and head injury, while having little effect on healthy individuals. This class would therefore be more disease-specific and have a lower potential for abuse than general cognitive enhancers, which is an important concern for pharmaceutical companies.

Neurotrophins

Neurotrophins (NTs) are hormone-like peptides that have a multitude of effects on neuronal survival. The first NT to be discovered was nerve growth factor (NGF), which was discovered in the 1950s by Levi-Montalcini and Cohen. Thirty years later, BDNF was discovered, followed by NT-3, NT-4, ciliary neurotrophic factor, and members of the glial cell-line neurotrophic factor family. The NT most widely studied with respect to synaptic restoration is BDNF.

Both BDNF mRNA and BDNF itself are decreased in aging (Calabrese et al., 2013) and in Alzheimer's disease (Murray et al., 1994; Phillips et al., 1991; Connor et al., 1997). Phosphorylation of the high-affinity receptor for BDNF, TrkB, is also decreased in aged rats (Calabrese et al., 2013). PKC phosphorylation of CARM1, a protein that methylates the RNA-binding protein HuD (ELAV, embryonic lethal abnormal vision protein 4), increases the stability and expression of BDNF, NGF, and NT-3 mRNA. This has been shown to enhance dendritic maturation of hippocampal neurons in culture (Lim and Alkon, 2012). Thus, it may be possible to increase BDNF, and thereby enhance cognition, by pharmacological modulation of NT receptors and NT messenger RNA.

Although BDNF synthesis is regulated by PKC, the actions of BDNF and TrkB receptors appear to rely primarily on the phosphatidylinositol-3 kinase (PI3K)/Akt pathways, ERK/Ras, and phospholipase Cγ pathways (Xia et al., 2010; Leal et al., 2014). Akt (formerly known as protein kinase B) is a kinase involved in a variety of apoptosis-inhibiting pathways. Environmental enrichment increases Akt, BDNF levels, and the number of dendritic spines in mouse hippocampus, producing cognitive enhancement and neurogenesis (Ramírez-Rodríguez et al., 2014).

Since BDNF is involved in both short-term synaptic function and activity-dependent synaptic maturation, impairment of which is one of the earliest changes in Alzheimer's disease, BDNF would be highly effective as a cognitive enhancer, and finding ways to increase brain levels of BDNF has been a topic of major interest. Unfortunately, BDNF, like other NTs, is unable to cross the blood–brain barrier (Pardridge et al., 1998). Thus, most emphasis has been on small molecule agonists of Trk receptors and small molecules that induce the synthesis of NTs. One such molecule, 4-methylcatechol, was reported to induce NGF synthesis (Kaechi et al., 1993, 1995) and to increase BDNF mRNA and BDNF-like immunoreactivity by about 50% in cerebral cortex when administered peripherally to ten-day-old rats (Fukumitsu et al., 1999), but not adult rats (Nitta et al., 1999). When administered intracerebroventricularly, 4-methylcatechol was reported to enhance spatial learning and memory in rats and produce an antidepressant effect (Sun and Alkon, 2008). The mechanism by which it induces BDNF is unknown, but in general BDNF can be induced by a variety of transcription factors, including CREB, calcium-response factor, and Neuronal Per Arnt Sim domain protein 4 (NPAS4) (Calabrese et al., 2013). There is also some evidence that 4-methylcatechol directly stimulates Trk family NT receptors and MAP kinases (Sometani et al., 2002).

Methylcatechol and 7,8-dihydroxyflavone

BDNF can also be induced by physical exercise and environmental enrichment (Ambrogini et al., 2013) and by TBI (Grundy et al., 2000) or excitotoxic damage induced by peripheral kainic acid (Goutan et al., 1998), which is consistent with the idea that NT release is important in neuronal repair.

NT Receptor Activators

Although 4-methylcatechol is only able to cross the blood–brain barrier of juvenile rats (Fukumitsu et al., 1999; Fukuhara et al., 2012), another TrkB activator, 7,8-dihydroxyflavone, is reported to cross the blood–brain barrier and influence emotional learning in the amygdala (Andero et al., 2011; Zeng et al., 2012). Although the affinity and specificity of this particular compound are not particularly high, it could be a reasonable starting point for drug development.

An alternative approach is to activate pathways downstream of TrkB. The advantage of this would be enhanced specificity. TrkB activates three pathways that play important roles in synaptic growth and memory (Yamada and Nabeshima, 2003):

1. **Mitogen-activated protein kinase signaling**.
2. **NMDA signaling**. Activation of TrkB receptors results in phosphorylation of the NR1 and NR2B subunits of NMDA receptors, and results in enhanced glutamate release.
3. **Akt/PKB**. In the Akt pathway, TrkB acts through a series of phosphorylation steps involving PI3K, Akt, and mammalian target of rapamycin, which is a regulator of mRNA translation. This pathway involves phospholipase Cγ (PLCγ), which cleaves phospholipids at the phosphate site, producing inositol 1,4,5-trisphosphate (IP3) and 1,2-diacylglycerol. IP3 in turn is an important messenger for the IP3 receptor on the endoplasmic reticulum, which is a major component of calcium-induced calcium release, along with the ryanodine receptor (RyR).

Synaptogenesis and Apolipoprotein E

Synaptogenesis is the creation of new synapses. Although often thought of as occurring during embryogenesis, new synapses are also formed during learning and synaptic repair. The signaling pathways involved in synaptogenesis thus may suggest novel treatment possibilities for cognitive enhancement in patients with neurodegenerative diseases such as Alzheimer's disease, for which synapse loss is a major pathophysiological hallmark (Terry et al., 1991; Lu et al., 2013; see Chapter 9), or in patients with major depression, in which synaptic function is impaired (Timmermans et al., 2013).

Cholesterol released from astrocytes in the form of a complex with the cholesterol transport protein apolipoprotein E (ApoE) is an important signal for synaptogenesis (Mauch et al., 2001; Fester et al., 2009; Goritz et al., 2005). Sen et al. (2012) found that the cholesterol-ApoE3 complex, acting through LDL receptor-related protein 1 (LRP1) and PKCε, also protects against synaptic loss induced by β-amyloid (Figure 2.2). ApoE receptors, such as LRP1, can also mediate clearance of β-amyloid from the CNS (Zlokovic et al., 2010; Deane et al., 2004), making them potential targets for antiamyloid therapies as well as cognitive enhancers. The activation of PKCε also protects against synapse

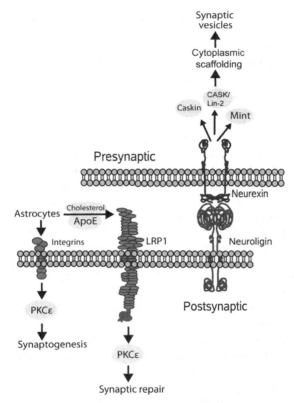

FIGURE 2.2   Structural pathways in synaptogenesis. Astrocytes stimulate synaptogenesis directly through astrocyte-neuron contact via integrin receptors, and indirectly through secreted factors such as cholesterol-apolipoprotein E (ApoE) complex. The low-density lipoprotein receptor-related protein 1 (LRP1), a receptor for the cholesterol-ApoE complex, induces protein kinase C (PKC) synthesis. PKC is also activated by arachidonic acid released after integrin receptor activation. Interactions between the postsynaptic adhesion protein neuroligin and the presynaptic protein neurexin strengthen the synaptic connection and induce presynaptic differentiation via calcium/calmodulin-dependent serine protein kinase (CASK), Caskin, and Mint1, a Munc18 interacting protein. This multiprotein complex may be important in synaptic vesicle exocytosis. Other secreted factors, including Wnt protein and thrombospondins, are also involved in synaptogenesis.

loss in TBI (Zohar et al., 2011), confirming that PKCε plays an important role in neurorepair and neuroprotection. ApoE is also important in maintaining the adult dentate gyrus neural progenitor pool (Yang et al., 2011). These data support the hypotheses that the ApoE-PKCε pathway is a neurorepair mechanism and that ApoE signaling pathways through LRP1 and PKCε are activated after TBI to induce synaptic repair. If so, therapeutic agents that augment the production of cholesterol-ApoE complexes could be valuable as cognitive enhancers.

The repair response after TBI is characterized by large increases in ApoE (Chen et al., 1997), NTs such as BDNF (Grundy et al., 2000), thrombospondins (Christopherson et al., 2005), and amyloid precursor protein (Van Den Heuvel et al., 1999). TBI also markedly increases the production of β-amyloid (Olsson et al., 2004); even a single brain injury can produce β-amyloid plaque deposition similar to that observed in Alzheimer's disease patients (Johnson et al., 2011). These proteins may constitute the brain's synaptic repair response.

ApoE4, the variant associated with Alzheimer's disease (Jellinger et al., 2001; Corder et al., 1993; Schmechel et al., 1993), has a markedly different lipid specificity than ApoE3 (Hauser et al., 2011). ApoE4 also correlates with poorer outcome after TBI (Lichtman et al., 2000; Teasdale et al., 1997; Chamelian et al., 2004). ApoE4 produces deficiencies in neuronal repair (Mahley et al., 2007; Ji et al., 2003). ApoE4 is also associated with ischemic stroke (McCarron et al., 1999), subarachnoid hemorrhage (Lanterna and Biroli, 2009), multiple sclerosis (Chapman et al., 2001; Fazekas et al., 2001), and frontotemporal dementia (Agosta et al., 2009), consistent with the idea of ApoE as a general repair molecule. Although some evidence suggests that ApoE4 may itself be toxic (Mahley and Huang, 2012), and may participate in β-amyloid oligomerization (Hashimoto et al., 2012; Holtzman and Hyman, 2012) or stabilize β-amyloid oligomers (Cerf et al., 2011), the evidence so far is also consistent with its primary effect being competition with ApoE3 and impairment of the growth and repair functions of ApoE3.

Thus, in addition to the well-known role of ApoE in cholesterol transport, it is now clear that ApoE also participates in cell signaling, learning, and neurorepair. Pharmacological modification of ApoE signaling via receptor agonists is therefore a potential route to cognitive enhancement. However, the mechanism by which ApoE mediates the neurorepair response is still incompletely understood.

Synaptic Assembly

Astrocytes also induce synaptogenesis via direct local contact. Activation of neuronal integrin receptors by astrocytic contact releases arachidonic acid, which then activates PKC and induces synaptogenesis (Hama et al., 2004). Synaptic assembly is strengthened by adhesion proteins neurexin and neuroligin. Dimerization of specific neurexins and neuroligins induces presynaptic differentiation (Shipman and Nicoll, 2012). This is mediated by calcium/calmodulin-dependent serine protein kinase (CASK), a presynaptic scaffolding protein that forms a tripartite complex with Caskin, and Mint1, a Munc-18 interacting protein (Stafford et al., 2011; Tabuchi et al., 2002). CASK also interacts with rabphilin3a, a synaptic vesicle protein involved in synaptic vesicle exocytosis (Zhang et al., 2001) (Figure 2.2). Other secreted factors, including Wnt protein and thrombospondins, are also involved in synaptogenesis. Thus, a promising route to cognitive enhancers might be to stimulate the release of synaptogenic factors from astrocytes.

Apoptosis Inhibitors

If a neuron is injured or stressed, it may undergo apoptosis. Apoptosis can be intrinsic, involving mitochondria and the endoplasmic reticulum, or extrinsic, initiated by the activation of cell surface receptors. Apoptosis is triggered by either DNA damage or loss of cell-survival factors, which cause proapoptotic proteins from the mitochondria to activate caspase proteases and thus caspase-activated DNase. Alternatively, apoptosis can be triggered by Apoptosis-Inducing Factor, a mitochondrial intermembrane flavoprotein, in a caspase-independent fashion. Activation of PKCε has been found to attenuate induced apoptosis in the hippocampus. Thus, it is has been suggested (Sun et al., 2009) that PKCε activators may act to inhibit apoptosis, thereby enhancing their usefulness as cognitive enhancers that act specifically on patients with brain injury or stroke. Apoptosis inhibitors might also benefit other conditions associated with apoptosis, such as acute radiation sickness.

There is also evidence that CREB inhibits apoptosis (Walton and Dragunow, 2000), and CREB phosphorylation is increased after ischemic stress (Kitagawa, 2007), leading to the suggestion that it may also be a survival factor. However, so far most research has been oriented toward enhancing apoptosis. For example, antisense oligonucleotide inhibitors of X-linked Inhibitor of Apoptosis Protein are undergoing clinical trials as potential anticancer agents. Several apoptosis inhibitors are known, but inhibiting apoptosis is problematic and none has yet been approved for clinical use.

PKC Activators as Neuroprotective Agents

However, the idea of using apoptosis inhibitors as cognitive enhancers is not yet dead. As mentioned above, PKCε is reported to have antiapoptotic activity (Basu and Sivaprasad, 2007; Ding et al., 2002; Gillespie et al., 2005; Okhrimenko et al., 2005; Sivaprasad et al., 2007). This raises the prospect of using PKCε activators such as DCP-LA as CNS apoptosis inhibitors. Other isozymes can also participate; for example, PKCα, β, βII, and γ are transiently overexpressed in cochlear hair cells during the regenerative phase after injury by the glutamate analog AMPA (Lerner-Natoli et al., 1997). However, among PKC isozymes, the two biggest players in the life-and-death struggle between growth and apoptosis seem to be PKCε and δ.

The interactions of PKC isozymes with apoptosis pathways are complex. Although PKCδ is sometimes regarded as the apoptosis isozyme, PKCδ inhibits apoptosis induced by oxidized low-density lipoproteins (Larroque-Cardoso et al., 2013) or irradiation (Bluwstein et al., 2013). However, downregulation of PKCε, which is generally antagonistic to PKCδ, enhances apoptosis by interfering with PKCε's ability to downregulate the antiapoptotic factor BCL2 (Körner et al., 2013). Moreover, caspases can proteolytically cleave PKCδ, ε, θ, and ζ (Basu and Sivaprasad, 2007; Mizuno et al., 1997; Datta et al., 1997; Smith et al., 2000). Thus, more research is needed to determine how much of PKC's neuroprotective activity depends on its effect on apoptosis.

Tianeptine and FK506

Cocaine

Although not commonly regarded as a general cognitive enhancer, cocaine enhances addiction pathways by increasing the number of dendritic spines in the nucleus accumbens, a part of the brain's underlying reward mechanisms, through a mechanism involving activation of cAMP-dependent kinase, which inhibits the protein phosphatase calcineurin. This reduces the activity of myocyte enhancer factor 2 (MEF2), a transcription factor that is inhibited by phosphory-lation (Pulipparacharuvil et al., 2008). MEF2 activity promotes elimination of existing excitatory synapses, so inhibition of MEF2 results in an increase in spine density. This increase could be a homeostatic adaptation to cocaine.

Calcineurin Inhibitors

Because the activation of cAMP-dependent kinase inhibits calcineurin, one would expect calcineurin inhibitors to be candidates for cognitive enhanc-ers. Indeed, the most well-known calcineurin inhibitor, FK506, which is used as an immunosuppressant, is reported to rescue synaptic plasticity defects in Swedish mutation Alzheimer's disease model mice (Cavallucci et al., 2013; Rozkalne et al., 2011). FK506 also blocks the loss of synaptic spines pro-duced by TBI (Campbell et al., 2012). However, some studies show the oppo-site effect. One report found that FK506 inhibited synaptic transmission and induction of hippocampal long-term potentiation (Lu et al., 1997), so the picture is still unclear.

FK506 is also relevant in another aspect. Several FK506 binding proteins, including FKBP12 and FKBP12.6, regulate the ryanodine receptor, a large ion channel located in the endoplasmic reticulum and sarcoplasmic reticulum that is involved in calcium-induced calcium release. RyRs amplify intracellular calcium signaling and are thus important in memory formation (Adasme et al., 2011). Their dysfunction may also underlie many memory disorders. The type 2 RyR (RyR2) is abundant in the brain, and restraint stress has been found to result in depletion of FKBP12.6 from the channel complex, causing intracellular calcium leak and cognitive dysfunction (Liu et al., 2012). Spatial learning increases the expression of the type 2 ryanodine receptor in rat hippocampus (Zhao et al., 2000; Alkon et al., 1998). Blocking RyRs has been found to reduce β-amyloid load and memory impairment in the Tg2576 mouse model of Alzheimer's disease (Oulès et al., 2012). The ryanodine receptor can be activated by suramin, the signaling molecule cyclic ADP-ribose, FKBP12, and caffeine, and blocked by FKBP12.6. Given the immense significance of calcium in neuronal response, RyR modulators in general, and FKBPs in particular, would appear to be ideal candidates for cognitive enhancers.

Antidepressants

Antidepressants are, almost by definition, cognitive enhancers. The antidepressant action of drugs such as tianeptine is increasingly recognized as being mediated in part by promotion of synaptic plasticity and growth (Zhang et al., 2013). This is supported by a strong association between depression and Alzheimer's disease, for which the earliest effect is a loss of synapses. Depression is also associated with a loss of synapses (Hajszan et al., 2009; Masi and Brovedani, 2011), and some antidepressants induce synaptogenesis (Duman and Aghajanian, 2012). Conversely, the synaptogenic compound bryostatin 1 also shows antidepressant activity, at least when administered intracebroventricularly (Sun and Alkon, 2005). Thus, antidepressants might be useful in reversing the loss of synapses that occurs in dementia, and may be thought of as cognitive enhancers. Increased synaptic activity can also suppress apoptosis by itself (Léveillé et al., 2010), suggesting that antidepressants could potentially even protect against neuronal loss.

Other molecules proposed as synaptic enhancers include cholinergic stimulants (Pa et al., 2013; Lieberman et al., 2013; Evans et al., 2013; Chambon et al., 2012), estrogens (Frick, 2013), monoaminergic agents (Mereu et al., 2013), some neurotrophic factors and their enhancers (Lee et al., 2013; Sun et al., 2008), agents that facilitate AMPAR synaptic delivery and activity (Kessels and Malinow, 2009; Henley et al., 2011), agents that enhance the expression or activity of the neural cell adhesion molecule histone deacetylase inhibitors (Gräff and Tsai, 2013; Hawk et al., 2012), and some polyphenols (Bhullar and Rupasinghe, 2013; Pasinetti, 2012; Schaffer et al., 2012).

Insulin

Animals with artificial diabetes induced by streptozotocin exhibit memory deficiencies (Mayer et al., 1990). Although insulin is usually thought of as a pancreatic hormone, insulin and insulin-related peptides appear to be segregated and synthesized independently in the brain (Zhao et al., 1999), primarily in the hypothalamus, hippocampus, olfactory bulb, and cerebellum. Insulin also crosses the blood–brain barrier through a saturable transporter specific for insulin (Banks, 2004).

Insulin may have a different function in the brain than in the periphery, although many of the brain effects of insulin and insulin-like peptides are important behavioral adaptations to energy availability, such as the ability to sense nutrients and evaluate the possibilities of obtaining valuable food. This has led to the hypothesis that insulin and insulin-like growth factor-1 (IGF-1) may be useful as potent synaptic enhancers (Derakhshan and Toth, 2013). However, as with neurosteroids, these peptides have strong nonneuronal effects in the periphery that make behavioral testing of systemically administered drugs challenging.

Acute intranasal administration of insulin was reported to enhance verbal memory in Alzheimer's disease patients and older patients with mild cognitive impairment (Reger et al., 2006, 2008). Insulin stimulates neurite growth, possibly by acting on pathways downstream of NGF (Recio-Pinto et al., 1984). IGF-1 and insulin also protect cells against apoptosis (Tanaka et al., 1998; Ghasemi et al., 2013).

Rosiglitazone is an antidiabetic drug formerly marketed as Avandia by GlaxoSmithKline. It binds to the peroxisome proliferator-activated receptor γ and regulates the expression of genes related to glucose uptake and disposal (Derosa and Maffioli, 2012). Because they were thought to possess anti-inflammatory activity and reduce insulin sensitivity, rosiglitazone and pioglitazone were subjected to clinical trials in Alzheimer's disease patients, but have thus far been found to be ineffective (Miller et al., 2011). However, some reports show that rosiglitazone can improve synaptic plasticity in dentate gyrus of aged rats, possibly by improving glucose utilization (Derakhshan and Toth, 2013). Thus, rosiglitazone or some derivative of it may yet find use as a general cognitive enhancer.

Rosiglitazone and streptozotocin

DISADVANTAGES OF COGNITIVE ENHANCERS

Not all synaptic enhancement is desirable. Addiction is a form of synaptic plasticity that is considered undesirable: a form of "aberrant" learning. The connection between cocaine addiction and synaptic enhancers was mentioned above. In this context, it is worth mentioning that there is evidence for a role of PKCε in preventing addiction. Deletion of PKCε increases the addiction sensitivity to morphine (Newton et al., 2007), cannabinoids (Wallace et al., 2009), ethyl alcohol (Lesscher et al., 2009), and benzodiazepines (Hodge et al., 1999). A recent review (Olive and Newton, 2010) discusses various PKC isozymes involved in mediating biological responses to drugs of abuse.

The effect of addiction on dendritic spines is specific to the nucleus accumbens. For example, nicotine relapse produces long-term increases in the head diameter and AMPA/NMDA ratio in dendritic spines in the nucleus accumbens (Gipson et al., 2013). The onset of reward from low-dose amphetamine produces similar effects, which are tied to ΔFosB and the D1 dopaminergic receptor (Pitchers et al., 2013).

In other brain regions, drugs of abuse appear to act through diverse pathways, depending on their mode of action. Psychostimulants and opioids induce Fos and Npas4 genes, whereas ethanol and opioids strongly induce an overlapping but separate set of genes including Fkbp5 and S3-12 (Piechota et al., 2010). Chronic intake of ethanol, the classic cognitive diminisher, reduces the overall number of dendritic spines in cultured neurons related to glutamatergic neurotransmission (Romero et al., 2013).

CHALLENGES IN DEVELOPING COGNITIVE ENHANCERS

The only drugs that have so far been approved in the United States specifically as cognitive enhancers are drugs like donepezil, rivastigmine, and galantamine, which provide some symptomatic treatment of Alzheimer's disease. However, many drugs with cognitive enhancing activity, such as the stimulants modafinil and methylphenidate and the AMPA receptor agonist piracetam, which is not yet approved in the United States, are often used off-label. There are two major challenges in measuring behavioral effects of cognitive enhancers. As mentioned above, many enhancers, such as insulin and neurosteroid hormones, have profound physiological effects on peripheral cells. Substances that affect synaptic growth often have strong effects on performance. High-cholesterol diets, commonly used in testing the effects of cholesterol on memory, cause weight gain, increased insulation from cold, and increased buoyancy, all of which can compromise comparisons with control rats in tests such as the Morris water maze. Moreover, high cholesterol can increase circulating levels of hormones such as leptin, which can be transported across the blood–brain barrier and may itself be a cognitive enhancer (Valladolid-Acebes et al., 2013). Any cognitive enhancer that affects food intake would have similar effects.

Secondly, the behavioral models are imperfect. Although associative learning can be measured reasonably rigorously with the standard three-group (paired, unpaired, and naïve) protocol, testing cognitive enhancers for conditions such as depression and post-traumatic stress disorder presents greater challenges. For example, how does one determine whether a rat is feeling depressed? Rodent depression produces a number of measurable changes, including a lack of grooming and apathy regarding swim tasks and maze choices. The most commonly used test for depression in rodents is the learned helplessness model (Pryce et al., 2011), exemplified by behavioral tests such as the forced swim test (Pollak et al., 2010). According to this model, depression is a learned response that must be unlearned. Thus, one might think that memory enhancers, instead of combating depression through their synaptogenic properties, might prolong or deepen depression, and that such patients might benefit more from memory-*inhibiting* drugs. However, it should be remembered that unlearning (i.e., extinction) is not simply passive forgetting, but is itself a form of learning (Robleto et al., 2004). Thus, enhancers of synaptic plasticity may also be useful in these situations as well.

REFERENCES

Adasme, T., Haeger, P., Paula-Lima, A.C., Espinoza, I., Casas-Alarcón, M.M., Carrasco, M.A., et al., 2011. Involvement of ryanodine receptors in neurotrophin-induced hippocampal synaptic plasticity and spatial memory formation. Proc. Natl. Acad. Sci. U.S.A. 108, 3029–3034.

Agosta, F., Vossel, K.A., Miller, B.L., Migliaccio, R., Bonasera, S.J., Filippi, M., et al., 2009. Apolipoprotein E ε4 is associated with disease-specific effects on brain atrophy in Alzheimer's disease and frontotemporal dementia. Proc. Natl. Acad. Sci. U.S.A. 106, 2018–2022.

Alkon, D.L., Lederhendler, I., Shoukimas, J.J., 1982. Primary changes of membrane currents during retention of associative learning. Science 215, 693–695.

Alkon, D.L., Rasmussen, H., 1988. A spatial-temporal model of cell activation. Science 239, 998–1005.

Alkon, D.L., Naito, S., Kubota, M., Chen, C., Bank, B., Smallwood, J., et al., 1988. Regulation of Hermissenda K+ channels by cytoplasmic and membrane-associated C-kinase. J. Neurochem. 51, 903–917.

Alkon, D.L., Nelson, T.J., Zhao, W., Cavallaro, S., 1998. Time domains of neuronal Ca^{2+} signaling and associative memory: steps through a calexcitin, ryanodine receptor, K+ channel cascade. Trends Neurosci. 21, 529–537.

Alkon, D.L., Epstein, H., Kuzirian, A., Bennett, M.C., Nelson, T.J., 2005. Protein synthesis required for long-term memory is induced by PKC activation on days before associative learning. Proc. Natl. Acad. Sci. U.S.A. 102, 16432–16437.

Ambrogini, P., Lattanzi, D., Ciuffoli, S., Betti, M., Fanelli, M., Cuppini, R., 2013. Physical exercise and environment exploration affect synaptogenesis in adult-generated neurons in the rat dentate gyrus: possible role of BDNF. Brain Res. 1534, 1–12.

Ammar, M.R., Humeau, Y., Hanauer, A., Nieswandt, B., Bader, M.F., Vitale, N., 2013. The Coffin-Lowry syndrome-associated protein RSK2 regulates neurite outgrowth through phosphorylation of phospholipase D1 (PLD1) and synthesis of phosphatidic acid. J. Neurosci. 33, 19470–19479.

Andero, R., Heldt, S.A., Ye, K., Liu, X., Armario, A., Ressler, K.J., 2011. Effect of 7,8-dihydroxyflavone, a small-molecule TrkB agonist, on emotional learning. Am. J. Psychiatry 168, 163–172.

Augustin, I., Korte, S., Rickmann, M., Kretzschmar, H.A., Südhof, T.C., Herms, J.W., Brose, N., 2001. The cerebellum-specific Munc13 isoform Munc13-3 regulates cerebellar synaptic transmission and motor learning in mice. J. Neurosci. 21, 10–17.

Balthazart, J., Ball, G.F., 2006. Is brain estradiol a hormone or a neurotransmitter? Trends Neurosci. 29, 241–249.

Bank, B., DeWeer, A., Kuzirian, A.M., Rasmussen, H., Alkon, D.L., 1988. Classical conditioning induces long-term translocation of protein kinase C in rabbit hippocampal CA1 cells. Proc. Natl. Acad. Sci. U.S.A. 85, 1988–1992.

Banks, W.A., 2004. The source of cerebral insulin. Eur. J. Pharmacol. 490, 5–12.

Barsegyan, A., Mackenzie, S.M., Kurose, B.D., McGaugh, J.L., Roozendaal, B., 2010. Glucocorticoids in the prefrontal cortex enhance memory consolidation and impair working memory by a common neural mechanism. Proc. Natl. Acad. Sci. U.S.A. 107, 16655–16660.

Basu, A., Sivaprasad, U., 2007. Protein kinase C epsilon makes the life and death decision. Cell Signal 19, 1633–1642.

Basu, J., Betz, A., Brose, N., Rosenmund, C., 2007. Munc13-1 C1 domain activation lowers the energy barrier for synaptic vesicle fusion. J. Neurosci. 27, 1200–1210.

Bhullar, K.S., Rupasinghe, H.P., 2013. Polyphenols: multipotent therapeutic agents in neurodegenerative diseases. Oxid. Med. Cell. Longev, Article 891748, 18 pages.

Blumberg, P.M., Kedei, N., Lewin, N.E., Yang, D., Czifra, G., Pu, Y., et al., 2008. Wealth of opportunity – the C1 domain as a target for drug development. Curr. Drug Targets 9, 641–652.

Bluwstein, A., Kumar, N., Léger, K., Traenkle, J., Oostrum, J., Rehrauer, H., et al., 2013. PKC signaling prevents irradiation-induced apoptosis of primary human fibroblasts. Cell Death Dis. 4, e498.

Bourne, J., Harris, K.M., 2007. Do thin spines learn to be mushroom spines that remember? Curr. Opin. Neurobiol. 17, 381–386.

Buttery, P., Beg, A.A., Chih, B., Broder, A., Mason, C.A., Scheiffele, P., 2006. The diacylglycerol-binding protein alpha1-chimaerin regulates dendritic morphology. Proc. Natl. Acad. Sci. U.S.A. 103, 1924–1929.

Calabrese, B., Halpain, S., 2005. Essential role for the PKC target MARCKS in maintaining dendritic spine morphology. Neuron 48, 77–90.

Calabrese, F., Guidotti, G., Racagni, G., Riva, M.A., 2013. Reduced neuroplasticity in aged rats: a role for the neurotrophin brain-derived neurotrophic factor. Neurobiol. Aging 34, 2768–2776.

Campbell, J.N., Register, D., Churn, S.B., 2012. Traumatic brain injury causes an FK506-sensitive loss and an overgrowth of dendritic spines in rat forebrain. J. Neurotrauma 29, 201–317.

Cavallucci, V., Berretta, N., Nobili, A., Nisticò, R., Mercuri, N.B., D'Amelio, M., 2013. Calcineurin inhibition rescues early synaptic plasticity deficits in a mouse model of Alzheimer's disease. Neuromolecular Med. 15, 541–548.

Cerf, E., Gustot, A., Goormaghtigh, E., Ruysschaert, J.M., Raussens, V., 2011. High ability of apolipoprotein E4 to stabilize amyloid-β peptide oligomers, the pathological entities responsible for Alzheimer's disease. FASEB J. 25, 1585–1595.

Chambon, C., Jatzke, C., Wegener, N., Gravius, A., Danysz, W., 2012. Using cholinergic M1 receptor positive allosteric modulators to improve memory via enhancement of brain cholinergic communication. Eur. J. Pharmacol. 697, 73–80.

Chamelian, L., Reis, M., Feinstein, A., 2004. Six-month recovery from mild to moderate traumatic brain injury: the role of APOE-ε4 allele. Brain 127, 2621–2628.

Chapman, J., Vinokurov, S., Achiron, A., Karussis, D.M., Mitosek-Szewczyk, K., Birnbaum, M., et al., 2001. APOE genotype is a major predictor of long-term progression of disability in MS. Neurology 56, 312–316.

Chen, Y., Lomnitski, L., Michaelson, D.M., Shohami, E., 1997. Motor and cognitive deficits in apolipoprotein E-deficient mice after closed head injury. Neuroscience 80, 1255–1262.

Christopherson, K.S., Ullian, E.M., Stokes, C.C., Mullowney, C.E., Hell, J.W., Agah, A., et al., 2005. Thrombospondins are astrocyte-secreted proteins that promote CNS synaptogenesis. Cell 120, 421–433.

Conesa-Zamora, P., Lopez-Andreo, M.J., Gómez-Fernández, J.C., Corbalán-García, S., 2001. Identification of the phosphatidylserine binding site in the C2 domain that is important for PKC α activation and in vivo cell localization. Biochemistry 40, 13898–13905.

Connor, B., Young, D., Yan, Q., Faull, R.L., Synek, B., Dragunow, M., 1997. Brain-derived neurotrophic factor is reduced in Alzheimer's disease. Brain Res. Mol. Brain Res. 49, 71–81.

Corbalán-Garcia, S., Sánchez-Carrillo, S., García-García, J., Gómez-Fernández, J.C., 2003. Characterization of the membrane binding mode of the C2 domain of PKCε. Biochemistry 42, 11661–11668.

Corder, E.H., Saunders, A.M., Strittmatter, W.J., Schmechel, D.E., Gaskell, P.C., Small, G.W., et al., 1993. Gene dose of apolipoprotein E type 4 allele and the risk of Alzheimer's disease in late onset families. Science 261, 921–923.

Dalva, M.B., Takasu, M.A., Lin, M.Z., Shamah, S.M., Hu, L., Gale, N.W., Greenberg, M.E., 2000. EphB receptors interact with NMDA receptors and regulate excitatory synapse formation. Cell 103, 945–956.

Datta, R., Kojima, H., Yoshida, K., Kufe, D.J., 1997. Caspase-3-mediated cleavage of protein kinase C theta in induction of apoptosis. J. Biol. Chem. 272, 20317–20320.

Deane, R., Wu, Z., Sagare, A., Davis, J., Du Yan, S., Hamm, K., et al., 2004. LRP/amyloid beta-peptide interaction mediates differential brain efflux of Aβ isoforms. Neuron 43, 333–344.

DeChristopher, B.A., Fan, A.C., Felsher, D.W., Wender, P.A., 2012. "Picolog," a synthetically-available bryostatin analog, inhibits growth of MYC-induced lymphoma in vivo. Oncotarget 3, 58–66.

Della, F.P., Abelaira, H.M., Réus, G.Z., Ribeiro, K.F., Antunes, A.R., Scaini, G., et al., 2012. Tianeptine treatment induces antidepressive-like effects and alters BDNF and energy metabolism in the brain of rats. Behav. Brain Res. 233, 526–535.

Derakhshan, F., Toth, C., 2013. Insulin and the brain. Curr. Diabetes Rev. 9, 102–116.

Derosa, G., Maffioli, P., 2012. Peroxisome proliferator-activated receptor-γ (PPAR-γ) agonists on glycemic control, lipid profile and cardiovascular risk. Curr. Mol. Pharmacol. 5, 272–281.

Ding, L., Wang, H., Lang, W., Xiao, L., 2002. Protein kinase C-epsilon promotes survival of lung cancer cells by suppressing apoptosis through dysregulation of the mitochondrial caspase pathway. J. Biol. Chem. 277, 35305–35313.

Duman, R.S., Aghajanian, G.K., 2012. Synaptic dysfunction in depression: potential therapeutic targets. Science 338, 68–72.

Eagle, A.L., Fitzpatrick, C.J., Perrine, S.A., 2013. Single prolonged stress impairs social and object novelty recognition in rats. Behav. Brain Res. 256, 591–597.

Etcheberrigaray, R., Matzel, L.D., Lederhendler, I.I., Alkon, D.L., 1992. Classical conditioning and protein kinase C activation regulate the same single potassium channel in *Hermissenda crassicornis* photoreceptors. Proc. Natl. Acad. Sci. U.S.A. 89, 7184–7188.

Evans, S., Gray, M.A., Dowell, N.G., Tabet, N., Tofts, P.S., King, S.L., Rusted, J.M., 2013. APOE E4 carriers show prospective memory enhancement under nicotine, and evidence for specialisation within medial BA10. Neuropsychopharmacology 38, 655–663.

Fazekas, F., Strasser-Fuchs, S., Kollegger, H., Berger, T., Kristoferitsch, W., Schmidt, H., et al., 2001. Apolipoprotein E ε4 is associated with rapid progression of multiple sclerosis. Neurology 57, 853–857.

Fester, L., Zhou, L., Butow, A., Huber, C., von Lossow, R., Prange-Kiel, J., et al., 2009. Cholesterol-promoted synaptogenesis requires the conversion of cholesterol to estradiol in the hippocampus. Hippocampus 19, 692–705.

Frick, K.M., 2013. Epigenetics, estradiol, and hippocampal memory consolidation. J. Neuroendocrinol. 25, 1151–1162.

Frye, C.A., Rhodes, M.E., 2002. Enhancing effects of estrogen on inhibitory avoidance performance may be in part independent of intracellular estrogen receptors in the hippocampus. Brain Res. 956, 285–293.

Fukuhara, K., Ishikawa, K., Yasuda, S., Kishishita, Y., Kim, H.K., Kakeda, T., et al., 2012. Intracerebroventricular 4-methylcatechol (4-MC) ameliorates chronic pain associated with depression-like behavior via induction of brain-derived neurotrophic factor (BDNF). Cell Mol. Neurobiol. 32, 971–977.

Fukumitsu, H., Sometani, A., Ohmiya, M., Nitta, A., Nomoto, H., Furukawa, Y., Furukawa, S., 1999. Induction of a physiologically active brain-derived neurotrophic factor in the infant rat brain by peripheral administration of 4-methylcatechol. Neurosci. Lett. 274, 115–118.

Gao, X., Deng, P., Xu, Z.C., Chen, J., 2011. Moderate traumatic brain injury causes acute dendritic and synaptic degeneration in the hippocampal dentate gyrus. PLoS One 6, e24566.

Ghasemi, R., Haeri, A., Dargahi, L., Mohamed, Z., Ahmadiani, A., 2013. Insulin in the brain: sources, localization and functions. Mol. Neurobiol. 47, 145–171.

Gillespie, S., Zhang, X.D., Hersey, P., 2005. Variable expression of protein kinase C epsilon in human melanoma cells regulates sensitivity to TRAIL-induced apoptosis. Mol. Cancer Ther. 4, 668–676.

Gipson, C.D., Reissner, K.J., Kupchik, Y.M., Smith, A.C., Stankeviciute, N., Hensley-Simon, M.E., Kalivas, P.W., 2013. Reinstatement of nicotine seeking is mediated by glutamatergic plasticity. Proc. Natl. Acad. Sci. U.S.A. 110, 9124–9129.

Goritz, C., Mauch, D.H., Pfrieger, F.W., 2005. Multiple mechanisms mediate cholesterol-induced synaptogenesis in a CNS neuron. Mol. Cell. Neurosci. 29, 190–201.

Goutan, E., Martí, E., Ferrer, I., 1998. BDNF, and full length and truncated TrkB expression in the hippocampus of the rat following kainic acid excitotoxic damage. Evidence of complex time-dependent and cell-specific responses. Brain Res. Mol. Brain Res. 59, 154–164.

Govindarajan, A., Israely, I., Huang, S.Y., Tonegawa, S., 2011. The dendritic branch is the preferred integrative unit for protein synthesis-dependent LTP. Neuron 69, 132–146.

Gräff, J., Tsai, L.H., 2013. The potential of HDAC inhibitors as cognitive enhancers. Annu. Rev. Pharmacol. Toxicol. 53, 311–330.

Grundy, P.L., Patel, N., Harbuz, M.S., Lightman, S.L., Sharples, P.M., 2000. Glucocorticoids modulate BDNF mRNA expression in the rat hippocampus after traumatic brain injury. Neuroreport 11, 3381–3384.

Hajszan, T., Dow, A., Warner-Schmidt, J.L., Szigeti-Buck, K., Sallam, N.L., Parducz, A., et al., 2009. Remodeling of hippocampal spine synapses in the rat learned helplessness model of depression. Biol. Psychiatry 65, 392–400.

Hall, B.J., Ghosh, A., 2008. Regulation of AMPA receptor recruitment at developing synapses. Trends Neurosci. 31, 82–89.

Hama, H., Hara, C., Yamaguchi, K., Miyawaki, A., 2004. PKC signaling mediates global enhancement of excitatory synaptogenesis in neurons triggered by local contact with astrocytes. Neuron 41, 405–415.

He, Q., Dent, E.W., Meiri, K.F., 1997. Modulation of actin filament behavior by GAP-43 (neuro-modulin) is dependent on the phosphorylation status of serine 41, the protein kinase C site. J. Neurosci. 17, 3515–3524.

Hell, J.W., 2014. CaMKII: claiming center stage in postsynaptic function and organization. Neuron 81, 249–265.

Hashimoto, T., Serrano-Pozo, A., Hori, Y., Adams, K.W., Takeda, S., Banerji, A.O., et al., 2012. Apolipoprotein E, especially apolipoprotein E4, increases the oligomerization of amyloid beta peptide. J. Neurosci. 32, 15181–15192.

Hauser, P.S., Narayanaswami, V., Ryan, R.O., 2011. Apolipoprotein E: from lipid transport to neurobiology. Prog. Lipid Res. 50, 62–74.

Holtzman, D.M., Hyman, B.T., 2012. Apolipoprotein E, especially apolipoprotein E4, increases the oligomerization of amyloid β peptide. J. Neurosci. 32, 15181–15192.

Hawk, J.D., Bookout, A.L., Poplawski, S.G., Bridi, M., Rao, A.J., Sulewski, M.E., et al., 2012. NR4A nuclear receptors support memory enhancement by histone deacetylase inhibitors. J. Clin. Invest. 122, 3593–3602.

Henckens, M., Hermans, E.J., Pu, Z., Joels, M., Fernandez, G., 2009. Stressed memories: how acute stress affects memory formation in humans. J. Neurosci. 29, 10111–10119.

Henley, J.M., Barker, E.A., Glebov, O.O., 2011. Routes, destinations and delays: recent advances in AMPA receptor trafficking. Trends Neurosci. 34, 258–268.

Hodge, C.W., Mehmert, K.K., Kelley, S.P., McMahon, T., Haywood, A., Olive, M.F., et al., 1999. Supersensitivity to allosteric GABA(A) receptor modulators and alcohol in mice lacking PKCε. Nat. Neurosci. 2, 997–1002.

Hongpaisan, J., Alkon, D.L., 2007. A structural basis for enhancement of long-term associative memory in single dendritic spines regulated by PKC. Proc. Natl. Acad. Sci. U.S.A. 104, 19571–19576.

Hongpaisan, J., Sun, M.K., Alkon, D.L., 2011. PKC ε activation prevents synaptic loss, Aβ elevation, and cognitive deficits in Alzheimer's disease transgenic mice. J. Neurosci. 31, 630–643.

Hongpaisan, J., Xu, C., Sen, A., Nelson, T.J., Alkon, D.L., 2013. PKC activation during training restores mushroom spine synapses and memory in the aged rat. Neurobiol. Dis. 55, 44–62.

Hotulainen, P., Hoogenraad, C.C., 2010. Actin in dendritic spines: connecting dynamics to function. J. Cell Biol. 189, 619–629.

Hruska, M., Dalva, M.B., 2012. Ephrin regulation of synapse formation, function and plasticity. Mol. Cell. Neurosci. 50, 35–44.

Jellinger, K.A., Paulus, W., Wrocklage, C., Litvan, I., 2001. Traumatic brain injury as a risk factor for Alzheimer disease. Comparison of two retrospective autopsy cohorts with evaluation of ApoE genotype. BMC Neurol. 1, 3.

Ji, Y., Gong, Y., Gan, W., Beach, T., Holtzman, D.M., Wisniewski, T., 2003. Apolipoprotein E isoform-specific regulation of dendritic spine morphology in apolipoprotein E transgenic mice and Alzheimer's disease patients. Neuroscience 122, 305–315.

Jiang, C., Schuman, E.M., 2002. Regulation and function of local protein synthesis in neuronal dendrites. Trends Biochem. Sci. 27, 506–513.

Johnson, V.E., Stewart, W., Smith, D.H., 2011. Widespread Tau and amyloid-beta pathology many years after a single traumatic brain injury in humans. Brain Pathol. 22, 142–149.

Kaechi, K., Furukawa, Y., Ikegami, R., Nakamura, N., Omae, F., Hashimoto, Y., et al., 1993. Pharmacological induction of physiologically active nerve growth factor in rat peripheral nervous system. J. Pharmacol. Exp. Ther. 264, 321–326.

Kaechi, K., Ikegami, R., Nakamura, N., Nakajima, M., Furukawa, Y., Furukawa, S., 1995. 4-Methylcatechol, an inducer of NGF synthesis, enhances peripheral nerve regeneration across nerve gaps. J. Pharmacol. Exp. Ther. 272, 1300–1304.

Kasai, H., Fukuda, M., Watanabe, S., Hayashi-Takagi, A., Noguchi, J., 2010. Structural dynamics of dendritic spines in memory and cognition. Trends Neurosci. 33, 121–129.

Keshamouni, V.G., Mattingly, R.R., Reddy, K.B., 2002. Mechanism of 17-β-estradiol-induced Erk1/2 activation in breast cancer cells. A role for HER2 and PKC-δ. J. Biol. Chem. 277, 22558–22565.

Kessels, H.W., Malinow, R., 2009. Synaptic AMPA receptor plasticity and behavior. Neuron 61, 340–350.

Kim, C.Y., Koo, Y.D., Jin, J.B., Moon, B.C., Kang, C.H., Kim, S.T., et al., 2003. Rice C2-domain proteins are induced and translocated to the plasma membrane in response to a fungal elicitor. Biochemistry 42, 11625–11633.

Kiraly, D.D., Stone, K.L., Colangelo, C.M., Abbott, T., Wang, Y., Mains, R.E., Eipper, B.A., 2011. Identification of kalirin-7 as a potential post-synaptic density signaling hub. J. Proteome Res. 10, 2828–2841.

Kitagawa, K., 2007. CREB and cAMP response element-mediated gene expression in the ischemic brain. FEBS J. 274, 3210–3217.

Koleske, A.J., 2013. Molecular mechanisms of dendrite stability. Nat. Rev. Neurosci. 14, 536–550.

Körner, C., Keklikoglou, I., Bender, C., Wörner, A., Münstermann, E., Wiemann, S., 2013. MicroRNA-31 sensitizes human breast cells to apoptosis by direct targeting of protein kinase C epsilon (PKCε). J. Biol. Chem. 288, 8750–8761.

Kramár, E.A., Chen, L.Y., Brandon, N.J., Rex, C.S., Liu, F., Gall, C.M., Lynch, G., 2009. Cyto-skeletal changes underlie estrogen's acute effects on synaptic transmission and plasticity. J. Neurosci. 29, 12982–12993.

Kretz, O., Fester, L., Wehrenberg, U., Zhou, L., Brauckmann, S., Zhao, S., et al., 2004. Hippocampal synapses depend on hippocampal estrogen synthesis. J. Neurosci. 24, 5913–5921.

Lanterna, L.A., Biroli, F., 2009. Significance of apolipoprotein E in subarachnoid hemorrhage: neuronal injury, repair, and therapeutic perspectives–a review. J. Stroke Cerebrovasc. Dis. 18, 116–123.

Larroque-Cardoso, P., Swiader, A., Ingueneau, C., Nègre-Salvayre, A., Elbaz, M., Reyland, M.E., et al., 2013. Role of protein kinase C δ in ER stress and apoptosis induced by oxidized LDL in human vascular smooth muscle cells. Cell Death Dis. 4, e520.

Leal, G., Comprido, D., Duarte, C.B., 2014. BDNF-induced local protein synthesis and synaptic plasticity. Neuropharmacology 76 (Pt C), 639–656.

Lee, B., Sur, B., Shim, I., Lee, H., Hahm, D.H., 2013. Baicalin improves chronic corticosterone-induced learning and memory deficits via the enhancement of impaired hippocampal brain-derived neurotrophic factor and cAMP response element-binding protein expression in the rat. J. Nat. Med. 68, 132–143.

Lerner-Natoli, M., Ladrech, S., Renard, N., Puel, J.L., Eybalin, M., Pujol, R., 1997. Protein kinase C may be involved in synaptic repair of auditory neuron dendrites after AMPA injury in the cochlea. Brain Res. 749, 109–119.

Lesscher, H.M., Wallace, M.J., Zeng, L., Wang, V., Deitchman, J.K., McMahon, T., et al., 2009. Amygdala protein kinase C epsilon controls alcohol consumption. Genes Brain Behav. 8, 493–499.

Léveillé, F., Papadia, S., Fricker, M., Bell, K.F., Soriano, F.X., Martel, M.A., et al., 2010. Suppression of the intrinsic apoptosis pathway by synaptic activity. J. Neurosci. 30, 2623–2635.

Li, C., Brake, W.G., Romeo, R.D., Dunlop, J.C., Gordon, M., Buzescu, R., et al., 2004. Estrogen alters hippocampal dendritic spine shape and enhances synaptic protein immunoreactivity and spatial memory in female mice. Proc. Natl. Acad. Sci. U.S.A. 101, 2185–2190.

Lichtman, S.W., Seliger, G., Tycko, B., Marder, K., 2000. Apolipoprotein E and functional recovery from brain injury following post acute rehabilitation. Neurology 55, 1536–1539.

Lieberman, J.A., Dunbar, G., Segreti, A.C., Girgis, R.R., Seoane, F., Beaver, J.S., et al., 2013. A randomized exploratory trial of an α-7 nicotinic receptor agonist (TC-5619) for cognitive enhancement in schizophrenia. Neuropsychopharmacology 38, 968–975.

Lim, B.K., Matsuda, N., Poo, M.M., 2008. Ephrin-B reverse signaling promotes structural and functional synaptic maturation in vivo. Nat. Neurosci. 11, 160–169.

Lim, C.S., Alkon, D.L., 2012. Protein kinase C stimulates HuD-mediated mRNA stability and protein expression of neurotrophic factors and enhances dendritic maturation of hippocampal neurons in culture. Hippocampus 22, 2303–2319.

Liu, F., Day, M., Muñiz, L.C., Bitran, D., Arias, R., Revilla-Sanchez, R., et al., 2008. Activation of estrogen receptor-beta regulates hippocampal synaptic plasticity and improves memory. Nat. Neurosci. 11, 334–343.

Liu, X., Betzenhauser, M.J., Reiken, S., Meli, A.C., Xie, W., Chen, B.X., et al., 2012. Role of leaky neuronal ryanodine receptors in stress-induced cognitive dysfunction. Cell 150, 1055–1067.

Lopes, J.P., Tarozzo, G., Reggiani, A., Piomelli, D., Cavalli, A., 2013. Galantamine potentiates the neuroprotective effect of memantine against NMDA-induced excitotoxicity. Brain Behav. 3, 67–74.

Lorenzo, P.S., Beheshti, M., Pettit, G.R., Stone, J.C., Blumberg, P.M., 2000. The guanine nucleotide exchange factor RasGRP is a high-affinity target for diacylglycerol and phorbol esters. Mol. Pharmacol. 57, 840–846.

Lu, B., Nagappan, G., Guan, X., Nathan, P.J., Wren, P., 2013. BDNF-based synaptic repair as a disease-modifying strategy for neurodegenerative diseases. Nat. Rev. Neurosci. 14, 401–416.

Lu, Z., Hornia, A., Jiang, Y.W., Zang, Q., Ohno, S., Foster, D.A., 1997. Tumor promotion by depleting cells of protein kinase C delta. Mol. Cell Biol. 17, 3418–3428.

Maher, P., Akaishi, T., Schubert, D., Abe, K., 2010. A pyrazole derivative of curcumin enhances memory. Neurobiol. Aging 31, 706–709.

Mahley, R.W., Huang, Y., Weisgraber, K.H., 2007. Detrimental effects of apolipoprotein E4: potential therapeutic targets in Alzheimer's disease. Curr. Alzheimer Res. 4, 537–540.

Mahley, R.W., Huang, Y., 2012. Apolipoprotein E sets the stage: response to injury triggers neuropathology. Neuron 76, 871–885.

Marland, J.R., Pan, D., Buttery, P.C., 2011. Rac GTPase-activating protein (Rac GAP) α1-Chimaerin undergoes proteasomal degradation and is stabilized by diacylglycerol signaling in neurons. J. Biol. Chem. 286, 199–207.

Martens, S., 2010. Role of C2 domain proteins during synaptic vesicle exocytosis. Biochem. Soc. Trans. 38 (Pt 1), 213–216.

Martijena, I.D., Molina, V.A., 2012. The influence of stress on fear memory processes. Braz. J. Med. Biol. Res. 45, 308–313.

Masi, G., Brovedani, P., 2011. The hippocampus, neurotrophic factors and depression: possible implications for the pharmacology of depression. CNS Drugs 25, 913–931.

Matsuzaki, M., Honkura, N., Ellis-Davies, G.C., Kasai, H., 2004. Structural basis of long-term potentiation in single dendritic spines. Nature 429, 761–766.

Mauch, D.H., Nagler, K., Schumacher, S., Goritz, C., Muller, E., Otto, A., Pfreiger, F., 2001. CNS synaptogenesis promoted by glia-derived cholesterol. Science 294, 1354–1357.

Mayer, G., Nitsch, R., Hoyer, S., 1990. Effects of changes in peripheral and cerebral glucose metabolism on locomotor activity, learning and memory in adult male rats. Brain Res. 532, 95–100.

McCarron, M.O., Delong, D., Alberts, M.J., 1999. APOE genotype as a risk factor for ischemic cerebrovascular disease: a meta-analysis. Neurology 53, 1308–1311.

McGaugh, J.L., Roozendaal, B., 2002. Role of adrenal stress hormones in forming lasting memories in the brain. Curr. Opin. Neurobiol. 12, 205–210.

Mereu, M., Bonci, A., Newman, A.H., Tanda, G., 2013. The neurobiology of modafinil as an enhancer of cognitive performance and a potential treatment for substance use disorders. Psychopharmacology (Berl) 229, 415–434.

Miller, B.W., Willett, K.C., Desilets, A.R., 2011. Rosiglitazone and pioglitazone for the treatment of Alzheimer's disease. Ann. Pharmacother. 45, 1416–1424.

Mizuno, K., Noda, K., Araki, T., Imaoka, T., Kobayashi, Y., Akita, Y., et al., 1997. The proteolytic cleavage of protein kinase C isotypes, which generates kinase and regulatory fragments, correlates with Fas-mediated and 12-O-tetradecanoyl-phorbol-13-acetate-induced apoptosis. Eur. J. Biochem. 250, 7–18.

Murai, K.K., Nguyen, L.N., Irie, F., Yamaguchi, Y., Pasquale, E.B., 2003. Control of hippocampal dendritic spine morphology through ephrin-A3/EphA4 signaling. Nat. Neurosci. 6, 153–160.

Murai, K.K., Pasquale, E.B., 2011. Eph receptors and ephrins in neuron-astrocyte communication at synapses. Glia 59, 1567–1578.

Murphy, D.D., Cole, N.B., Segal, M., 1998. Brain-derived neurotrophic factor mediates estradiol-induced dendritic spine formation in hippocampal neurons. Proc. Natl. Acad. Sci. U.S.A. 95, 11412–11417.

Murray, K.D., Gall, C.M., Jones, E.G., Isackson, P.J., 1994. Differential regulation of brain-derived neurotrophic factor and type II calcium/calmodulin-dependent protein kinase messenger RNA expression in Alzheimer's disease. Neuroscience 60, 37–48.

Neary, J.T., Crow, T., Alkon, D.L., 1981. Change in a specific phosphoprotein band following associative learning in Hermissenda. Nature 293, 658–660.

Nelson, T.J., Collin, C., Alkon, D.L., 1990. Isolation of a G protein that is modified by learning and reduces potassium currents in Hermissenda. Science 247, 1479–1483.

Nelson, T.J., Alkon, D.L., 2009. Neuroprotective versus tumorigenic protein kinase C activators. Trends Biochem. Sci. 34, 136–145.

Newey, S.E., Velamoor, V., Govek, E.E., Van Aelst, L., 2005. Rho GTPases, dendritic structure, and mental retardation. J. Neurobiol. 64, 58–74.

Newton, P.M., Kim, J.A., McGeehan, A.J., Paredes, J.P., Chu, K., Wallace, M.J., et al., 2007. Increased response to morphine in mice lacking protein kinase C epsilon. Genes Brain Behav. 6, 329–338.

Nitta, A., Ito, M., Fukumitsu, H., Ohmiya, M., Ito, H., Sometani, A., et al., 1999. 4-methylcatechol increases brain-derived neurotrophic factor content and mRNA expression in cultured brain cells and in rat brain in vivo. J. Pharmacol. Exp. Ther. 291, 1276–1283.

Okhrimenko, H., Lu, W., Xiang, C., Hamburger, N., Kazimirsky, G., Brodie, C., 2005. Protein kinase C-epsilon regulates the apoptosis and survival of glioma cells. Cancer Res. 65, 7301–7309.

Olds, J.L., Anderson, M.L., McPhie, D.L., Staten, L.D., Alkon, D.L., 1989. Imaging of memory-specific changes in the distribution of protein kinase C in the hippocampus. Science 245, 866–869.

Olive, M.F., Newton, P.M., 2010. Protein kinase C isozymes as regulators of sensitivity to and self-administration of drugs of abuse-studies with genetically modified mice. Behav. Pharmacol. 21, 493–499.

Olsson, A., Csajbok, L., Ost, M., Höglund, K., Nylén, K., Rosengren, L., et al., 2004. Marked increase of beta-amyloid(1-42) and amyloid precursor protein in ventricular cerebrospinal fluid after severe traumatic brain injury. J. Neurol. 251, 870–876.

Oulès, B., Del Prete, D., Greco, B., Zhang, X., Lauritzen, I., Sevalle, J., et al., 2012. Ryanodine receptor blockade reduces amyloid-β load and memory impairments in Tg2576 mouse model of Alzheimer disease. J. Neurosci. 32, 11820–11834.

Pa, J., Berry, A.S., Compagnone, M., Boccanfuso, J., Greenhouse, I., Rubens, M.T., et al., 2013. Cholinergic enhancement of functional networks in older adults with mild cognitive impairment. Ann. Neurol. 73, 762–773.

Pardridge, W.M., Wu, D., Sakane, T., 1998. Combined use of carboxyl-directed protein pegylation and vector-mediated blood-brain barrier drug delivery system optimizes brain uptake of brain-derived neurotrophic factor following intravenous administration. Pharmacol. Res. 15, 576–582.

Pasinetti, G.M., 2012. Novel role of red wine-derived polyphenols in the prevention of Alzheimer's disease dementia and brain pathology: experimental approaches and clinical implications. Planta Med. 78, 1614–1619.

Penzes, P., Jones, K.A., 2008. Dendritic spine dynamics—a key role for kalirin-7. Trends Neurosci. 31, 419–427.

Perez-Cruz, C., Nolte, M.W., van Gaalen, M.M., Rustay, N.R., Termont, A., Tanghe, A., et al., 2011. Reduced spine density in specific regions of CA1 pyramidal neurons in two transgenic mouse models of Alzheimer's disease. J. Neurosci. 31, 3926–3934.

Phillips, H.S., Hains, H.S., Armanini, M., Laramee, G.R., Johnson, S.A., Winslow, J.W., 1991. BDNF mRNA is decreased in the hippocampus of individuals with Alzheimer's disease. Neuron 7, 695–702.

Piechota, M., Korostynski, M., Solecki, W., Gieryk, A., Slezak, M., Bilecki, W., et al., 2010. The dissection of transcriptional modules regulated by various drugs of abuse in the mouse striatum. Genome Biol. 11, R48.

Pitchers, K.K., Vialou, V., Nestler, E.J., Laviolette, S.R., Lehman, M.N., Coolen, L.M., 2013. Natural and drug rewards act on common neural plasticity mechanisms with ΔFosB as a key mediator. J. Neurosci. 33, 3434–3442.

Pollak, D.D., Rey, C.E., Monje, F.J., 2010. Rodent models in depression research: classical strategies and new directions. Ann. Med. 42, 252–264.

Pryce, C.R., Azzinnari, D., Spinelli, S., Seifritz, E., Tegethoff, M., Meinlschmidt, G., 2011. Helplessness: a systematic translational review of theory and evidence for its relevance to understanding and treating depression. Pharmacol. Ther. 132, 242–267.

Pulipparacharuvil, S., Renthal, W., Hale, C.F., Taniguchi, M., Xiao, G., Kumar, A., et al., 2008. Cocaine regulates MEF2 to control synaptic and behavioral plasticity. Neuron 59, 621–633.

Ramírez-Rodríguez, G., Ocaña-Fernández, M.A., Vega-Rivera, N.M., Torres-Pérez, O.M., Gómez-Sánchez, A., Estrada-Camarena, E., Ortiz-López, L., 2014. Environmental enrichment induces neuroplastic changes in middle age female BalbC mice and increases the hippocampal levels of BDNF, p-Akt and p-MAPK1/2. Neuroscience 260, 158–170.

Raval, A.P., Borges-Garcia, R., Javier Moreno, W., Perez-Pinzon, M.A., Bramlett, H., 2013. Periodic 17β-estradiol pretreatment protects rat brain from cerebral ischemic damage via estrogen receptor-β. PLoS One 8, e60716.

Recio-Pinto, E., Lang, F.F., Ishii, D.N., 1984. Insulin and insulin-like growth factor II permit nerve growth factor binding and the neurite formation response in cultured human neuroblastoma cells. Proc. Natl. Acad. Sci. U.S.A. 81, 2562–2566.

Reger, M., Watson, G., Frey, I., Baker, L., Cholerton, B., Keeling, M., et al., 2006. Effects of intranasal insulin on cognition in memory-impaired older adults: modulation by APOE genotype. Neurobiol. Aging 27, 451–458.

Reger, M.A., Watson, G.S., Green, P.S., Baker, L.D., Cholerton, B., Fishel, M.A., et al., 2008. Intranasal insulin administration dose-dependently modulates verbal memory and plasma amyloid-beta in memory-impaired older adults. J. Alzheimers Dis. 13, 323–331.

Rhee, J.S., Betz, A., Pyott, S., Reim, K., Varoqueaux, F., Augustin, I., et al., 2002. Beta phorbol ester- and diacylglycerol-induced augmentation of transmitter release is mediated by Munc13s and not by PKCs. Cell 108, 121–133.

Ridley, A.J., 2006. Rho GTPases and actin dynamics in membrane protrusions and vesicle trafficking. Trends Cell Biol. 16, 522–529.

Robleto, K., Poulos, A.M., Thompson, R.F., 2004. Brain mechanisms of extinction of the classically conditioned eyeblink response. Learn. Mem. 11, 517–524.

Romero, A.M., Renau-Piqueras, J., Pilar Marin, M., Timoneda, J., Berciano, M.T., Lafarga, M., Esteban-Pretel, G., 2013. Chronic alcohol alters dendritic spine development in neurons in primary culture. Neurotox. Res. 24, 532–548.

Rossman, K.L., Der, C.J., Sondek, J., 2005. GEF means go: turning on RHO GTPases with guanine nucleotide-exchange factors. Nat. Rev. Mol. Cell Biol. 6, 167–180.

Rozkalne, A., Hyman, B.T., Spires-Jones, T.L., 2011. Calcineurin inhibition with FK506 ameliorates dendritic spine density deficits in plaque-bearing Alzheimer model mice. Neurobiol. Dis. 41, 650–654.

Sandstrom, N.J., Williams, C.L., 2001. Memory retention is modulated by acute estradiol and progesterone replacement. Behav. Neurosci. 115, 384–393.

Schaffer, S., Asseburg, H., Kuntz, S., Muller, W.E., Eckert, G.P., 2012. Effects of polyphenols on brain ageing and Alzheimer's disease: focus on mitochondria. Mol. Neurobiol. 46, 161–178.

Schmechel, D.E., Saunders, A.M., Strittmatter, W.J., Crain, B.J., Hulette, C.M., Joo, S.H., et al., 1993. Increased amyloid beta-peptide deposition in cerebral cortex as a consequence of apolipoprotein E genotype in late-onset Alzheimer disease. Proc. Natl. Acad. Sci. U.S.A. 90, 9649–9653.

Schoenfeld, T.J., Gould, E., 2012. Stress, stress hormones, and adult neurogenesis. Exp. Neurol. 233, 12–21.

Schwabe, L., Joëls, M., Roozendaal, B., Wolf, O.T., Oitzl, M.S., 2012. Stress effects on memory: an update and integration. Neurosci. Biobehav. Rev. 36, 1740–1749.

Scott, R., Bourtchuladze, R., Gossweiler, S., Dubnau, J., Tully, T., 2002. CREB and the discovery of cognitive enhancers. J. Mol. Neurosci. 19, 171–177.

Sen, A., Alkon, D.L., Nelson, T.J., 2012. Apolipoprotein E3 (ApoE3) but not ApoE4 protects against synaptic loss through increased expression of protein kinase C epsilon. J. Biol. Chem. 287, 15947–15958.

Shipman, S.L., Nicoll, R.A., 2012. Dimerization of postsynaptic neuroligin drives synaptic assembly via transsynaptic clustering of neurexin. Proc. Natl. Acad. Sci. U.S.A. 109, 19432–19437.

Shirai, Y., Kouzuki, T., Kakefuda, K., Moriguchi, S., Oyagi, A., Horie, K., et al., 2010. Essential role of neuron-enriched diacylglycerol kinase (DGK), DGKβ in neurite spine formation, contributing to cognitive function. PLoS One 5, e11602.

Sivaprasad, U., Shankar, E., Basu, A., 2007. Downregulation of Bid is associated with PKCε-mediated TRAIL resistance. Cell Death Differ. 14, 851–857.

Smith, L., Chen, L., Reyland, M.E., DeVries, T.A., Talanian, R.V., Omura, S., Smith, J.B., 2000. Activation of atypical protein kinase C zeta by caspase processing and degradation by the ubiquitin-proteasome system. J. Biol. Chem. 275, 40620–40627.

Sometani, A., Nomoto, H., Nitta, A., Furukawa, Y., Furukawa, S., 2002. 4-Methylcatechol stimulates phosphorylation of Trk family neurotrophin receptors and MAP kinases in cultured rat cortical neurons. J. Neurosci. Res. 70, 335–339.

Sosa, M.S., Lewin, N.E., Choi, S.H., Blumberg, P.M., Kazanietz, M.G., 2009. Biochemical characterization of hyperactive β2-chimaerin mutants revealed an enhanced exposure of C1 and Rac-GAP domains. Biochemistry 48, 8171–8178.

Stafford, R.L., Ear, J., Knight, M.J., Bowie, J.U., 2011. The molecular basis of the Caskin1 and Mint1 interaction with CASK. J. Mol. Biol. 412, 3–13.

Steinberg, S.F., 2008. Structural basis of protein kinase C isoform function. Physiol. Rev. 88, 1341–1378.

Südhof, T.C., Rizo, J., 1996. Synaptotagmins: C2-domain proteins that regulate membrane traffic. Neuron 17, 379–388.

Sun, M.K., Alkon, D.L., 2005. Dual effects of bryostatin-1 on spatial memory and depression. Eur. J. Pharmacol. 512, 43–51.

Sun, M.K., Alkon, D.L., 2008. Effects of 4-methylcatechol on spatial memory and depression. Neuroreport 19, 355–359.

Sun, M.K., Hongpaisan, J., Nelson, T.J., Alkon, D.L., 2008. Poststroke neuronal rescue and synaptogenesis mediated in vivo by protein kinase C in adult brains. Proc. Natl. Acad. Sci. U.S.A. 105, 13620–13625.

Sun, M.K., Hongpaisan, J., Alkon, D.L., 2009. Postischemic PKC activation rescues retrograde and anterograde long-term memory. Proc. Natl. Acad. Sci. U.S.A. 106, 14676–14680.

Tabuchi, K., Biederer, T., Butz, S., Sudhof, T.C., 2002. CASK participates in alternative tripartite complexes in which Mint 1 competes for binding with caskin 1, a novel CASK-binding protein. J. Neurosci. 22, 4264–4273.

Tanaka, M., Sawada, M., Miura, M., Marunouchi, T., 1998. Insulin-like growth factor-I analogue prevents apoptosis mediated through an interleukin-1 beta converting enzyme (caspase-1)-like protease of cerebellar external granular layer neurons: developmental stage-specific mechanisms of neuronal cell death. Neuroscience 84, 89–100.

Teasdale, G.M., Nicoll, J.A.R., Murray, G., Fiddes, M., 1997. Association of apolipoprotein E polymorphism with outcome after head injury. Lancet 350, 1069–1071.

Terry, R.D., Masliah, E., Salmon, D.P., Butters, N., DeTeresa, R., Hill, R., et al., 1991. Physical basis of cognitive alterations in Alzheimer's disease: synapse loss is the major correlate of cognitive impairment. Ann. Neurol. 30, 572–580.

Timmermans, W., Xiong, H., Hoogenraad, C.C., Krugers, H.J., 2013. Stress and excitatory synapses: from health to disease. Neuroscience 248, 626–636.

Tolias, K.F., Bikoff, J.B., Burette, A., Paradis, S., Harrar, D., Tavazoie, S., et al., 2005. The Rac1-GEF Tiam1 couples the NMDA receptor to the activity-dependent development of dendritic arbors and spines. Neuron 45, 525–538.

Tolias, K.F., Bikoff, J.B., Kane, C.G., Tolias, C.S., Hu, L., Greenberg, M.E., 2007. The Rac1 guanine nucleotide exchange factor Tiam1 mediates EphB receptor-dependent dendritic spine development. Proc. Natl. Acad. Sci. U.S.A. 104, 7265–7270.

Tolias, K.F., Duman, J.G., Um, K., 2011. Control of synapse development and plasticity by Rho GTPase regulatory proteins. Prog. Neurobiol. 94, 133–148.

Valladolid-Acebes, I., Fole, A., Martín, M., Morales, L., Victoria Cano, M., Ruiz-Gayo, M., Olmo, N.D., 2013. Spatial memory impairment and changes in hippocampal morphology are triggered by high-fat diets in adolescent mice. Is there a role of leptin? Neurobiol. Learn. Mem. 106C, 18–25.

Van de Ven, T.J., VanDongen, H.M., VanDongen, A.M., 2005. The nonkinase phorbol ester receptor α1-chimerin binds the NMDA receptor NR2A subunit and regulates dendritic spine density. J. Neurosci. 25, 9488–9496.

Van Den Heuvel, C., Blumbergs, P.C., Finnie, J.W., Manavis, J., Jones, N.R., Reilly, P.L., Pereira, R.A., 1999. Upregulation of amyloid precursor protein messenger RNA in response to traumatic brain injury: an ovine head impact model. Exp. Neurol. 159, 441–450.

Wallace, M.J., Newton, P.M., McMahon, T., Connolly, J., Huibers, A., Whistler, J., Messing, R.O., 2009. PKCε regulates behavioral sensitivity, binding and tolerance to the CB1 receptor agonist WIN55,212-2. Neuropsychopharmacology 34, 1733–1742.

Walton, M.R., Dragunow, I., 2000. Is CREB a key to neuronal survival? Trends Neurosci. 23, 48–53.

Wang, T., Yang, Y.J., Wu, P.F., Wang, W., Hu, Z.L., Long, L.H., et al., 2011. Tetrahydroxystilbene glucoside, a plant-derived cognitive enhancer, promotes hippocampal synaptic plasticity. Eur. J. Pharmacol. 650, 206–214.

Wang, X.D., Su, Y.A., Wagner, K.V., Avrabos, C., Scharf, S.H., Hartmann, J., et al., 2013. Nectin-3 links CRHR1 signaling to stress-induced memory deficits and spine loss. Nat. Neurosci. 16, 706–713.

Wei, J., Yuen, E.Y., Liu, W., Li, X., Zhong, P., Karatsoreos, I.N., et al., 2013. Estrogen protects against the detrimental effects of repeated stress on glutamatergic transmission and cognition. Mol. Psychiatry 19, 588–598.

Wojcik, S.M., Brose, N., 2007. Regulation of membrane fusion in synaptic excitation secretion coupling: speed and accuracy matter. Neuron 55, 11–24.

Woolley, C.S., McEwen, B.S., 1992. Estradiol mediates fluctuation in hippocampal synapse density during the estrous cycle in the adult rat. J. Neurosci. 12, 2549–2554.

Wu, G., Malinow, R., Cline, H.T., 1996. Maturation of a central glutamatergic synapse. Science 274, 972–976.

Xia, Y., Wang, C.Z., Liu, J., Anastasio, N.C., Johnson, K.M., 2010. Brain-derived neurotrophic factor prevents phencyclidine-induced apoptosis in developing brain by parallel activation of both the ERK and PI-3K/Akt pathways. Neuropharmacology 58, 330–336.

Yamada, K., Nabeshima, T., 2003. Brain-derived neurotrophic factor/TrkB signaling in memory processes. J. Pharmacol. Sci. 91, 267–270.

Yan, J.Z., Xu, Z., Ren, S.Q., Hu, B., Yao, W., Wang, S.H., Liu, S.Y., Lu, W., 2011. Protein kinase C promotes N-methyl-D-aspartate (NMDA) receptor trafficking by indirectly triggering calcium/calmodulin-dependent protein kinase II (CaMKII) autophosphorylation. J. Biol. Chem. 286, 25187–25200.

Yang, C.P., Gilley, J.A., Zhang, G., Kernie, S.G., 2011. ApoE is required for maintenance of the dentate gyrus neural progenitor pool. Development 138, 4351–4362.

Zeng, Y., Liu, Y., Wu, M., Liu, J., Hu, Q., 2012. Activation of TrkB by 7,8-dihydroxyflavone prevents fear memory defects and facilitates amygdalar synaptic plasticity in aging. J. Alzheimers Dis. 31, 765–778.

Zhang, H., Etherington, L.A., Hafner, A.S., Belelli, D., Coussen, F., Delagrange, P., et al., 2013. Regulation of AMPA receptor surface trafficking and synaptic plasticity by a cognitive enhancer and antidepressant molecule. Mol. Psychiatry 18, 471–484.

Zhang, H., Webb, D.J., Asmussen, H., Niu, S., Horwitz, A.F., 2005. A GIT1/PIX/Rac/PAK signaling module regulates spine morphogenesis and synapse formation through MLC. J. Neurosci. 25, 3379–3388.

Zhang, Y., Luan, Z., Liu, A., Hu, G., 2001. The scaffolding protein CASK mediates the interaction between rabphilin3a and beta-neurexins. FEBS Lett. 497, 99–102.

Zhao, W., Chen, H., Xu, H., Moore, E., Meiri, N., Quon, M.J., Alkon, D.L., 1999. Brain insulin receptors and spatial memory. Correlated changes in gene expression, tyrosine phosphorylation, and signaling molecules in the hippocampus of water maze trained rats. J. Biol. Chem. 274, 34893–34902.

Zhao, W., Meiri, N., Xu, H., Cavallaro, S., Quattrone, A., Zhang, L., Alkon, D.L., 2000. Spatial learning induced changes in expression of the ryanodine type II receptor in the rat hippocampus. FASEB J. 14, 290–300.

Zhou, L., Jones, E.V., Murai, K.K., 2012. EphA signaling promotes actin-based dendritic spine remodeling through slingshot phosphatase. J. Biol. Chem. 287, 9346–9359.

Zlokovic, B.V., Deane, R., Sagare, A.P., Bell, R.D., Winkler, E.A., 2010. Low-density lipoprotein receptor-related protein-1: a serial clearance homeostatic mechanism for controlling Alzheimer's amyloid beta-peptide elimination from the brain. J. Neurochem. 115, 1077–1089.

Zohar, O., Lavy, R., Zi, X., Nelson, T.J., Hongpaisan, J., Pick, C.G., Alkon, D.L., 2011. PKC activator therapeutic for mild traumatic brain injury in mice. Neurobiol. Dis. 41, 329–337.

Chapter 3

Molecular Mechanisms of Drug-Induced Cognitive Enhancement

Shira Knafo[1] and Jose A. Esteban[2]

[1]*Unidad de Biofísica, CSIC, UPV/EHU, Universidad del País Vasco, Ikerbasque, The Basque Foundation for Science, Leioa, Spain;* [2]*Centro de Biología Molecular Severo Ochoa, Consejo Superior de Investigaciones Científicas/Universidad Autónoma de Madrid, Spain*

INTRODUCTION

It is becoming increasingly accepted that molecular and cellular processes in neurons may be modulated not only to treat mental illness but also to enhance cognitive function above physiological levels in healthy individuals. Obviously, these two aspects of cognitive enhancement are not unrelated. The growing knowledge of the molecular mechanisms underlying learning and memory is allowing us to propose specific manipulations that may improve information acquisition and/or retention. On the one hand, these manipulations help us to better understand the link between neuronal communication and cognitive behavior. On the other hand, if cognitive enhancement is indeed achieved, one can hope that these same manipulations may also be useful for the treatment of disorders where cognitive function is impaired, even if the pathogenic alteration is not fully understood. Therefore, investigations on mechanisms leading to cognitive enhancement will have both basic and translational interest.

Genetic studies on animal models have already offered a catalog of molecular alterations that result in enhanced cognition (Lee and Silva, 2009). Notably, most of these genetic changes can be related more or less directly with the process of synaptic plasticity, particularly long-term potentiation (LTP) and long-term depression (LTD). Indeed, this is one of the strongest arguments for these forms of synaptic plasticity as important underlying mechanisms for learning and memory (Bliss and Collingridge, 1993). Therefore, an emerging view is that cognitive enhancement may be achieved by facilitating or improving synaptic plasticity mechanisms. However, this is not a trivial task. Synaptic plasticity is an activity (experience)-dependent process, as learning is. Therefore, we cannot expect that simply enhancing synaptic strength (bypassing physiological stimuli) would be

Cognitive Enhancement. http://dx.doi.org/10.1016/B978-0-12-417042-1.00003-6

beneficial for cognition. In fact, it is more likely that such manipulations would be detrimental for cognitive function. Conversely, we would propose that successful cognitive enhancers would be those leaving intact basic synaptic plasticity mechanisms, while operating on modulatory aspects of these key mechanisms. Still, the number and nature of such potential agents would be too large to be covered in this chapter. Therefore, we have chosen to discuss a few examples that highlight some major mechanisms (or regulatory points) that we consider as suitable targets for cognitive enhancement. To this end, we have concentrated on synaptic plasticity mechanisms dependent on NMDA receptor activation, because this is a well-established process underlying learning and memory. Then, we have divided this process into three general stages, and we discuss a few agents (cognitive enhancers) that would act on each level (Figure 3.1):

- Induction: modulators of NMDA receptor function
  - Glycine/D-serine
- Signaling: neuromodulators acting on intracellular signaling pathways mediating synaptic plasticity
  - FGL
  - Ghrelin
- Expression: effectors of AMPA receptor function
  - Ampakines

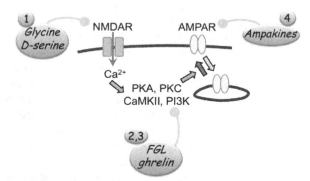

FIGURE 3.1 **Schematic representation of three potential sites for cognitive intervention based on the general process of NMDA receptor-dependent synaptic plasticity.** (1) Enhancement of NMDA receptor function, based on the availability of the coagonists glycine and/or d-serine. (2, 3) Modulation of the signaling pathways activated during synaptic plasticity downstream from NMDA receptor activation. Of the pathways represented in the figure, only CaMKII is directly sensitive to Ca^{2+} entry from NMDA receptors. Nevertheless, there is significant cross-talk between pathways, and all these kinases have been shown to participate at some level in the process of synaptic plasticity. The pharmacological agent FGL and the natural hormone ghrelin will be presented as modulators of these pathways with potential for cognitive enhancement. (4) To a major extent, these forms of synaptic plasticity are expressed by changes in the number or function of AMPA receptors at synapses. Enhancement of AMPA receptor function by ampakines will be discussed. (This figure is reproduced in color in the color plate section).

TARGETING THE INDUCTION OF PLASTICITY: GLYCINE, D-SERINE

NMDA receptors are the critical initiators of synaptic plasticity forms underlying learning and memory (Morris et al., 1986; Tsien et al., 1996). As such, they have been the target of multiple pharmacological and genetic manipulations to investigate cognitive performance and the potential for cognitive enhancement (Collingridge et al., 2013; Lee and Silva, 2009). In this chapter we will concentrate on two related molecules, glycine and D-serine, that together with glutamate, act as co-agonists for the activation of the NMDA receptor, and therefore, for the induction of synaptic plasticity.

Mechanisms of Action

The co-agonist role of glycine and D-serine at the NMDA receptor was discovered more than 25 years ago (Johnson and Ascher, 1987; Kleckner and Dingledine, 1988). These molecules bind to the GluN1 subunit of the receptor, whereas the "classic" agonist, glutamate, binds to the GluN2 subunits. Concomitant binding of these two sites is needed for full activation of the receptor (Laube et al., 1997). Given that glutamate is released from presynaptic terminals during excitatory synaptic transmission, it is expected that the extracellular availability of the coagonist will effectively modulate NMDA receptor function and affect synaptic plasticity. This is the case for both D-serine (Yang et al., 2003) and glycine (Martina et al., 2004). Interestingly, D-serine levels and serine racemase, the major catalytic activity for its synthesis, decline with aging in the hippocampus (Turpin et al., 2011). This limitation can be corrected pharmacologically by exogenous addition of D-serine, which restores synaptic plasticity in hippocampal slices from aged rats (Turpin et al., 2011) and from a mouse model with accelerated senescence (SAMP8) (Yang et al., 2005). In addition, D-serine administration increases neurogenesis in vivo and in vitro (Sultan et al., 2013).

The fact that glycine and D-serine appear to have similar effects on NMDA receptor function has complicated the identification of the endogenous ligand for the GluN1 site. Although this issue still remains controversial, experiments biochemically degrading endogenous D-serine (Mothet et al., 2000) or knocking-down serine racemase (Benneyworth et al., 2012) strongly suggest that most NMDA receptor–mediated synaptic currents and induction of synaptic plasticity are endogenously gated by D-serine. Nevertheless, recent results suggest that the location and subunit composition of the NMDA receptor may determine the identity of the coagonist. Thus, D-serine would be the major agonist for synaptic, GluN1-GluN2A–containing NMDA receptors, whereas glycine would mostly act on extrasynaptic, GluN1-GluN2B–containing receptors (Papouin et al., 2012). These details may have interesting implications for the therapeutic manipulation of NMDA receptor function, as mentioned below.

Effects on Cognition

The effects of the coagonists glycine and D-serine on synaptic plasticity are also translated into cognitive function. Thus, impairing D-serine synthesis by knocking-out serine racemase impairs fear-conditioning memory, and this deficiency is rescued by chronic D-serine treatment (Balu et al., 2013). In aged rats, which endogenously express reduced levels of serine racemase, administration of D-cycloserine, a partial agonist related to D-serine, or raising endogenous glycine levels with inhibitors of glycine transporters, improves spatial memory (Baxter et al., 1994; Harada et al., 2012). This cognitive enhancement may also be observed over physiological levels. For example, systemic administration of D-serine in adult wild-type mice has been shown to improve object recognition memory and working memory (Bado et al., 2011).

Clinical Implications and Future Prospects

The therapeutic potential of enhancing NMDA receptor function with glycine/D-serine has received a lot of attention relative to cognitive deficits in schizophrenia. This is because of the hypothesis of NMDA receptor hypofunction for schizophrenia (Laruelle, 2014). In agreement with this notion, administration of D-serine or inhibition of glycine uptake improves social recognition (Shimazaki et al., 2010). In fact, preliminary studies on schizophrenic patients indicate cognitive improvement (Tsai and Lin, 2010). Nevertheless, enhancing NMDA receptor function is inherently risky. It may lead to excessive calcium entry and neuronal death, a process that has been related to neurodegeneration in Alzheimer disease (Wenk, 2006). Indeed, current palliative therapies for Alzheimer patients involve inhibition (not enhancement) of NMDA receptor function (Lipton, 2007). However, increasing evidence points to extrasynaptic NMDA receptors as the major mediators for excitotoxicity-triggered neuronal death and Alzheimer-related neuronal dysfunctions (Li et al., 2009, 2011; Talantova et al., 2013). Therefore, it is tempting to speculate that selective enhancement of NMDA receptor function at synaptic sites may allow specific improvement of synaptic plasticity and cognitive abilities without detrimental excitotoxic effects. This may be achievable, given the proposed compartmentalization of D-serine and glycine as co-agonists for synaptic and extrasynaptic NMDA receptors (Papouin et al., 2012). According to this scenario, potentiating D-serine action would preferentially target synaptic NMDA receptors and may display the most beneficial effects. One potential approach to this purpose is the inhibition of the enzyme D-amino acid oxidase (DAAO), which catalyzes D-amino acid removal. In fact, knock-out mice lacking DAAO display increased spatial learning (Maekawa et al., 2005). However, it is unclear whether pharmacological inhibition of DAAO will result in a significant elevation of D-serine levels in brain regions relevant for learning and memory (Strick et al., 2011). Nevertheless, these are encouraging considerations for modulating NMDA receptor functions to specifically target cognitive performance.

INTERPLAY BETWEEN CELL ADHESION AND GROWTH FACTOR SIGNALING: FGL

The development of the cognitive enhancer FGL peptide had been possible due to the discovery of the exact region in the second F3 module of neural cell adhesion molecule (NCAM) that binds to and activates the fibroblast growth factor receptor 1 (FGFR1) (Kiselyov et al., 2003). FGL was therefore synthesized with a sequence identical to this region and, like NCAM, it binds to and activates FGFR1 in vitro and in vivo (Cambon et al., 2004; Kiselyov et al., 2003; Knafo et al., 2012). This binding results in activation of various downstream FGFR-dependent signaling cascades (Knafo et al., 2012), including the MAPK pathway, the PIP_3 pathway and the PKC pathway (Knafo et al., 2012). There are several versions of FGL varying in sequence and structure. FGL_L is a pentadecapeptide (EVYVVAENQQGKSKA) with dendrimeric structure in which four peptides are connected to a three-lysine backbone through their C termini (Hansen et al., 2010). Alternatively FGL_L can be synthesized in a dimeric form by linking two monomers through their N-terminal ends with iminodiacetic acid (*N*-carboxymethyl)-glycine (Secher et al., 2006). These complex structures enable the peptide to bind to two to four molecules of FGFR simultaneously and to bring them together, a crucial step for receptor phosphorylation and downstream signaling (Beenken and Mohammadi, 2009). The shorter version of FGL (FGL_S, decapeptide, AENQQGKSKA) also acts as a cognitive enhancer (Bisaz et al., 2011; Knafo et al., 2012), and due to better solubility it is more commonly used currently.

Mechanisms of Action

Facilitation of AMPAR Synaptic Delivery

We recently discovered that FGL increases the extent of synaptic potentiation in naive hippocampal slices, and similarly, it enhances the capacity for spatial learning in healthy, young adult rats (Knafo et al., 2012). Therefore, FGL can act as a synaptic and cognitive enhancer over physiological levels. Similar to ampakines, the results obtained with FGL support the notion that synaptic and cognitive mechanisms can be adjusted to run above normal physiological levels. FGL acts through a facilitation of AMPA receptor synaptic delivery, an effect that seems to be the link between the synaptic effect and the enhanced spatial learning (Knafo et al., 2012). Importantly, since FGL requires NMDAR and CaMKII activation, its effect on AMPA receptor delivery is defined as activity dependent. Therefore, FGL is not acting as a direct trigger but as a facilitator for AMPAR synaptic insertion. This mechanism differs considerably from other neurotrophin-related synaptic modulators, such as BDNF or tumor necrosis factor-α (TNFα), which trigger AMPAR synaptic delivery while bypassing standard LTP signaling (Kramár et al., 2012; Rex et al., 2006; Simmons et al., 2009; Stellwagen et al., 2005).

This is a significant distinction, since an effective cognitive enhancer may be expected to facilitate synaptic plasticity events, rather than provoke them in a manner unrelated to ongoing circuit activity.

Enhancement of Synaptic Transmission and LTP

Since FGL requires NMDAR and CaMKII activation, FGL is sensitizing the "classical" LTP pathway. Administration of FGL enhances LTP in young adult rats (Knafo et al., 2012) and attenuates impairment in LTP normally seen in aged rats (Downer et al., 2010). When FGL is injected locally to the dentate gyrus in vivo before applying high-frequency stimulation (HFS) to the medial perforant path, it facilitates both the induction and maintenance of LTP (Dallerac et al., 2011).

Increase of Neurotransmitter Release

FGL causes both a short-term facilitation of transmitter release (1 h) and a long-term (48 h) increase of synaptic efficacy in primary cultured neurons (Cambon et al., 2004). Nevertheless, no effect of FGL was observed on paired-pulse facilitation (a sort of presynaptic plasticity) in organotypic slice cultures, a preparation considered to be more physiological (Knafo et al., 2012). This finding suggests that FGL should be further tested in vivo, before getting to a final conclusion on its effect on presynaptic function.

Anti-inflammatory Function

Microglial cell activity increases in the rat hippocampus during normal brain aging. Administration of FGL to aged rats suppresses the activation of microglia, and the levels of proinflammatory interleukin-1β (IL-1β). FGL also has a stimulatory effect on neuronal CD200 that results from enhancement of interleukin-4 (IL-4) release from glial cells (Downer et al., 2010). Moreover, FGL corrects the age-related imbalance in hippocampal levels of insulin-like growth factor-1 (IGF-1) and proinflammatory interferon-γ and subsequently attenuates the glial reactivity associated with aging (Downer et al., 2009). Thus, by correcting the age-related imbalance in hippocampal inflammatory components, FGL attenuates hippocampal inflammation associated with aging.

Effects on Cognition

FGL improves hippocampus-dependent learning and memory. Specifically, FGL enhances memory for context (Cambon et al., 2004) and spatial navigation in the Morris water maze when administrated before (Knafo et al., 2012) or after (Cambon et al., 2004) training. FGL also has a positive effect on behavioral flexibility as measured with a reversal learning task (Cambon et al., 2004). FGL enhances social memory retention in rats (Secher et al., 2006) and has been shown to prevent cognitive impairment induced by stress (Bisaz et al., 2011; Borcel et al., 2008) and by oligomeric β-amyloid (Klementiev et al., 2007). Moreover, FGL has antidepressant-like effects in rats (Turner et al., 2008).

Side Effects

To date, no side effects were observed after treatment with FGL in rodents. FGL does not affect weight gain, and rodents treated with FGL do not present signs of illness or overt behavioral changes (Cambon et al., 2003, 2004). In addition, when tested in an open field, FGL treated rats do not present changes in locomotion, speed, percentage of freezing, percentage of time spent in either the inner or the outer zone, zone crossings, and in defecations (Cambon et al., 2004). It is important to note, though, that FGL has never been given for prolonged periods, so data on side effects after chronic or semi-chronic treatments are unavailable.

Clinical Trials

ENKAM Pharmaceuticals is currently (2014) conducting the first clinical trial with FGL_S in Alzheimer disease patients.

MODIFYING SYNAPSES WITH THE "HUNGER HORMONE" GHRELIN

Ghrelin is a well-known orexigenic hormone that is secreted into the blood stream by endocrine cells in the gastrointestinal mucosa, particularly in the stomach, in response to fasting (Inui et al., 2004). Ghrelin stimulates energy production and signals directly to the hypothalamic regulatory nuclei that control energy homeostasis (Inui, 2001). Nevertheless, the ghrelin receptor (growth-hormone secretagogue type 1a receptor, or GHS-R1a) is also abundantly expressed in the hippocampus, substantia nigra, and ventral tegmental area (Guan et al., 1997), brain regions undergoing intense synaptic plasticity processes related to learning, memory, and reward. Indeed, there is increasing evidence for a role of ghrelin in the modulation of neuronal function outside the hypothalamic system (Andrews, 2011), including enhancement of hippocampus-dependent memory (McNay, 2007).

Mechanism of Action

Ghrelin is a natural ligand for GSH-R1a, which is a G-protein–coupled receptor (GPCR). Ghrelin binding to GSH-R1a signals via $G_{q/11}$ to activate phospholipase C (PLC) leading to the mobilization of calcium from intracellular stores, production of diacyl glycerol (DAG) and activation of protein kinase C (PKC) (Camina, 2006). Activation of the ghrelin receptor has also been linked to PKA activation (Kohno et al., 2003), MAPK and PI3K pathways (Camina, 2006), although the mechanisms are still far from clear and may involve heterodimerization with other GPCRs (Schellekens et al., 2013). Despite the uncertainties in the underlying signaling pathways, ghrelin has been shown to have strong effects on neuronal and synaptic function in the hippocampus. Thus, it has been shown that circulating ghrelin can enter the hippocampus, where it has a synaptogenic effect in vivo

(Diano et al., 2006) and in cortical neuronal cultures (Stoyanova and le Feber, 2014). This effect may be mediated by remodeling of the actin cytoskeleton within dendritic spines (Berrout and Isokawa, 2012; Cuellar and Isokawa, 2011). This growth-promoting action of ghrelin appears to be mediated by the PI3K pathway and is correlated with potentiation of synaptic transmission in the dentate gyrus (Chen et al., 2011). Interestingly, this form of potentiation is independent from NMDA receptors and does not contribute to LTP induced by theta burst stimulation (Diano et al., 2006), although it extends the duration of LTP induced by high-frequency stimulation (Chen et al., 2011). According to the rationale discussed above, this form of synaptic strengthening is not necessarily conducive to the improvement of cognitive function. However, ghrelin has also been shown to enhance LTP, possibly mediated by separate signaling mechanisms (Ribeiro et al., 2014). Thus, in organotypic hippocampal slices, ghrelin potentiates synaptic transmission by inducing the delivery of AMPA receptors into synapses. This effect requires NMDA receptor activation and leads to LTP enhancement. The mobilization of AMPA receptors is accompanied by GluA1 and stargazin phosphorylation and is mediated by PKA and PKC activities (Ribeiro et al., 2014). In agreement, it has been shown that ghrelin induces CREB phosphorylation in hippocampal slices, in a process that requires NMDA receptor activation and is mediated by cAMP-PKA (Cuellar and Isokawa, 2011). Therefore, although the intracellular mechanisms are still far from clear, it appears that ghrelin-GSHR1a signaling may play modulatory roles that rely on intrinsic synaptic plasticity mechanisms, leading to a facilitation or enhancement of the actual synaptic plasticity process.

Effects on Cognition

As explained here, by facilitating synaptic plasticity mechanisms in memory-related brain areas, such as the hippocampus, ghrelin is a good candidate for cognitive enhancement. In fact, subcutaneous injection of ghrelin or a ghrelin receptor agonist has been shown to enhance working memory when administered before the behavioral task (Diano et al., 2006). Interestingly, ghrelin also enhanced memory retention when administered intracerebroventricularly immediately after training (Carlini et al., 2002; Diano et al., 2006). This effect on memory consolidation may be related to its activity on CREB-induced gene expression (Cuellar and Isokawa, 2011). Ghrelin also induces proliferation and differentiation of neuronal progenitors in the hippocampus of adult mice (Moon et al., 2009), a process that is thought to be important for learning and memory (Zhao et al., 2008) (although it may also facilitate memory erasure (Akers et al., 2014)).

Clinical Implications and Future Prospects

The broad metabolic actions of ghrelin signaling make it an interesting therapeutic candidate for diseases involving altered energy balance, cardiovascular defects, or systemic inflammation (DeBoer, 2012). However, this becomes a complication when considering cognitive applications. In addition, ghrelin is known to engage food reward circuits in the brain (Skibicka and Dickson, 2011), involving mesolimbic dopaminergic neurons (Malik et al., 2008; Naleid et al., 2005). These actions are probably related to the enhanced sensitization to drugs of abuse induced by ghrelin (Jerlhag et al., 2009). Nevertheless, it is becoming increasingly clear that some of the diverse actions of ghrelin on neuronal circuits and behavioral outputs are mediated by heterodimerization with other GPCRs, which result in extensive crosstalk with multiple signaling systems (Schellekens et al., 2013). These include dopamine receptors, chiefly involved in food reward and drug seeking behaviors (Jiang et al., 2006). These are still recent and controversial observations, and it is difficult to predict whether specific heterodimers will mediate ghrelin-GHSR1a signaling in the hippocampus. Nevertheless, this is an exciting possibility to eventually target individual receptor combinations to specifically intervene in cognitive processes with therapeutic purposes.

PROLONGING AMPA RECEPTOR EXCITATION: AMPAKINES

AMPA receptors are ionotropic channels that by converting chemical to electrical signals mediate most of the synaptic transmission in the brain. By controlling synaptic transmission, a process considered as the substance of information processing in the brain, AMPA receptors control cognitive function. Accordingly, alterations in AMPA receptor transmission are seen in conditions involving cognitive impairment, such as aging (Henley and Wilkinson, 2013) and Alzheimer disease (Liu et al., 2010). AMPA receptors are therefore regarded as potential therapeutic targets for clinical intervention for cognitive impairment (Chang et al., 2012). Here we will discuss the idea that improving AMPA receptor transmission might facilitate information processing and therefore cognition.

AMPA receptor desensitization regulates the decay of excitatory postsynaptic currents, a mechanism granting neuroprotection at central neurons (Stern-Bach et al., 1998). Ampakines are benzoylpiperidine drugs that slow the desensitization rate of AMPA receptors (Hampson et al., 1998), thereby enhancing AMPA-receptor-gated currents. Ampakines cross the blood–brain barrier and improve memory encoding in animals across a variety of experimental paradigms. Consequently, in the last two decades these drugs have been considered as strong candidates for use as cognitive enhancers in humans.

Mechanisms of Action

Ampakines act through several mechanisms, all of which can be easily association with cognitive function:

Enhancement of Synaptic Transmission

Ampakines increase the size of fast, AMPA receptor-mediated excitatory synaptic responses (Lynch and Gall, 2013). Therefore, the efficacy of ampakines has been tested in numerous animal models in which synaptic weakening in cortical networks seem to account for cognitive impairment.

Enhancement of LTP

As direct effectors of AMPA receptor ion channel function, ampakines do not appear to fulfill our initial criterion for cognitive enhancers as facilitators, rather than executioners of synaptic changes. However, through their effect on the size of AMPAR-mediated excitatory synaptic responses, ampakines produce greater net depolarizing in response to high-frequency stimulation and thus a greater likelihood of producing an NMDA receptor–mediated current (Hampson et al., 1998). The larger NMDA receptor currents reduce the amount of afferent activity needed to induce LTP (Lynch and Gall, 2006). Consequently, ampakines facilitate the induction of LTP and increase its magnitude. Ampakines also rescue LTP in conditions of LTP impairment, such as in a mouse model of Angelman syndrome where it was suggested to act through promotion of spine actin polymerization (Baudry et al., 2012). Given the clear links between stronger LTP and cognitive enhancement (Lee and Silva, 2009), LTP increase by ampakines is probably one of the mechanisms by which ampakines enhance cognitive function.

Recruitment of Additional Neurons to a Cognitive Task

Immediately after administration of ampakines the number of hippocampal neurons that fire in response to particular components of a test problem increases (Hampson et al., 1998). Thus, ampakines trigger an expansion of the cortical networks engaged by a difficult problem (Lynch and Gall, 2006). Given that the number of neurons forming a cortical network related to a specific memory encoding is correlated with performance in the cognitive task (Reijmers et al., 2007), this effect of ampakines is another mechanisms that can explain its influence over cognitive function.

Upregulation of Neurotrophic Factors

Ampakines significantly and reversibly increase the levels of brain-derived neurotrophic factor (BDNF) mRNA and protein, thereby enhancing the trophic effects of excitatory transmission (Lauterborn et al., 2000, 2003). Ampakines can therefore be employed to increase the availability of endogenous BDNF in the brain (Kramár et al., 2012). Probably through this effect, (Scharfman et al., 2005), ampakines also positively regulate neurogenesis (Schitine et al., 2012) that by itself can enhance cognitive function (Wezenberg et al., 2007).

Effects on Cognition

Ampakines improve performance in a number of behavioral tasks under either normal or pathological conditions. For example, in 1-day-old chicks, ampakines enhance passive avoidance learning task when injected after training

(Samartgis et al., 2012). In mice, acute treatment with ampakines reverses the deficit in sociability in a model of autism (Silverman et al., 2013). In a mouse model of Huntington disease, long-term ampakine treatment significantly slows the deterioration of striatal neuropathology and locomotor function (Simmons et al., 2011). In rats, ampakines improved performance in a spatial variant of the delayed-nonmatch-to-sample paradigm (Hampson et al., 1998). Moreover, ampakines improve retention scores in radial mazes (Staubli et al., 1994), facilitate the acquisition of a conditioned response (Shors et al., 1995), and reduce the number of trials needed to form stable olfactory memory (Larson et al., 1995). In rat models of schizophrenia ampakines reverse deficits in the novel object recognition task (Damgaard et al., 2010) and when combined with clozapine they improve measures of attention and memory (Goff et al., 2001). In rats with cognitive deficits caused by bilateral vestibular deafferentation, the ampakine CX717 improves the performance in a five choice serial reaction time but produced a detrimental effect in the object recognition memory task (Zheng et al., 2011). Altogether these findings imply that ampakines generally improve cognitive function in rodents but that their effect on cognition may be task dependent.

In monkeys, the ampakine CX717 administered in conditions of sleep deprivation prevents behavioral impairment and even return performance to above-normal levels (Porrino et al., 2005). This effect on cognition is accompanied by increased activity in prefrontal cortex, dorsal striatum, and medial temporal lobe, including hippocampus (Porrino et al., 2005).

In preliminary trials in human subjects, ampakines improved visual associations, recognition of odors, acquisition of a visuospatial maze, and location and identity of playing cards. Ampakines do not improve scores in a task requiring cued recall of verbal information (Ingvar et al., 1997). Evidence has also shown that ampakines have a positive effect on the delayed recall of nonsense syllables as well as on several commonplace forms of memory in humans (Lynch et al., 1996). Ampakines given to healthy individuals also counteract effects of sleep deprivation on attention-based tasks (Boyle et al., 2012).

Side Effects

Despite the enhancement of excitatory transmission in behaving animals, ampakines do not cause seizures or excitotoxic damage. In humans, CX516 is associated with fatigue, insomnia and epigastric discomfort but is generally well tolerated (Goff et al., 2008).

Clinical Trials

The ampakine CX516 was evaluated in a clinical trial for cognitive enhancement in schizophrenia patients. Stable schizophrenia patients treated with antipsychotic drugs were cotreated with CX516 or placebo for 4 weeks. Cognitive battery assessment revealed that CX516 was not effective for improving cognition or for alleviating symptoms of schizophrenia (Goff et al., 2008). Thus, after two decades of intensive investigation, it seems that treatment with ampakines in humans is not able to recapitulate the enhancing effects found in laboratory animals.

Future Prospect

Although the initial intention was to use ampakines as cognitive enhancers, currently they are suggested mainly for other purposes. For example, recent studies support the use of ampakines to reduce respiratory depression in humans treated with opioids (Lorier et al., 2010; Oertel et al., 2010) and to prevent and rescue propofol-induced severe apnea (Ren et al., 2013). Another study suggests ampakines as respiratory stimulants in postoperative patients (Golder et al., 2013).

REFERENCES

Akers, K.G., Martinez-Canabal, A., Restivo, L., Yiu, A.P., De Cristofaro, A., Hsiang, H.L., 2014. Hippocampal neurogenesis regulates forgetting during adulthood and infancy. Science 344 (6184), 598–602.

Andrews, Z.B., 2011. The extra-hypothalamic actions of ghrelin on neuronal function. Trends Neurosci. 34 (1), 31–40.

Bado, P., Madeira, C., Vargas-Lopes, C., Moulin, T.C., Wasilewska-Sampaio, A.P., Maretti, L., 2011. Effects of low-dose D-serine on recognition and working memory in mice. Psychopharmacology (Berl.) 218 (3), 461–470.

Balu, D.T., Li, Y., Puhl, M.D., Benneyworth, M.A., Basu, A.C., Takagi, S., 2013. Multiple risk pathways for schizophrenia converge in serine racemase knockout mice, a mouse model of NMDA receptor hypofunction. Proc. Natl. Acad. Sci. U.S.A. 110 (26), E2400–E2409.

Baudry, M., Kramar, E., Xu, X., Zadran, H., Moreno, S., Lynch, G., 2012. Ampakines promote spine actin polymerization, long-term potentiation, and learning in a mouse model of Angelman syndrome. Neurobiol. Dis. 47 (2), 210–215.

Baxter, M.G., Lanthorn, T.H., Frick, K.M., Golski, S., Wan, R.Q., Olton, D.S., 1994. D-cycloserine, a novel cognitive enhancer, improves spatial memory in aged rats. Neurobiol. Aging 15 (2), 207–213.

Beenken, A., Mohammadi, M., 2009. The FGF family: biology, pathophysiology and therapy. Nat. Rev. Drug Discov. 8 (3), 235–253.

Benneyworth, M.A., Li, Y., Basu, A.C., Bolshakov, V.Y., Coyle, J.T., 2012. Cell selective conditional null mutations of serine racemase demonstrate a predominate localization in cortical glutamatergic neurons. Cell. Mol. Neurobiol. 32 (4), 613–624.

Berrout, L., Isokawa, M., 2012. Ghrelin promotes reorganization of dendritic spines in cultured rat hippocampal slices. Neurosci. Lett. 516 (2), 280–284.

Bisaz, R., Schachner, M., Sandi, C., 2011. Causal evidence for the involvement of the neural cell adhesion molecule, NCAM, in chronic stress-induced cognitive impairments. Hippocampus 21 (1), 56–71.

Bliss, T.V., Collingridge, G.L., 1993. A synaptic model of memory: long-term potentiation in the hippocampus. Nature 361 (6407), 31–39.

Borcel, E., Perez-Alvarez, L., Herrero, A.I., Brionne, T., Varea, E., Berezin, V., 2008. Chronic stress in adulthood followed by intermittent stress impairs spatial memory and the survival of new-born hippocampal cells in aging animals: prevention by FGL, a peptide mimetic of neural cell adhesion molecule. Behav. Pharmacol. 19 (1), 41–49.

Boyle, J., Stanley, N., James, L.M., Wright, N., Johnsen, S., Arbon, E.L., 2012. Acute sleep deprivation: the effects of the AMPAKINE compound CX717 on human cognitive performance, alertness and recovery sleep. J. Psychopharmacol. 26 (8), 1047–1057.

Cambon, K., Hansen, S.M., Venero, C., Herrero, A.I., Skibo, G., Berezin, V., 2004. A synthetic neural cell adhesion molecule mimetic peptide promotes synaptogenesis, enhances presynaptic function, and facilitates memory consolidation. J. Neurosci. 24 (17), 4197–4204.

Cambon, K., Venero, C., Berezin, V., Bock, E., Sandi, C., 2003. Post-training administration of a synthetic peptide ligand of the neural cell adhesion molecule, C3d, attenuates long-term expression of contextual fear conditioning. Neuroscience 122 (1), 183–191.

Camina, J.P., 2006. Cell biology of the ghrelin receptor. J. Neuroendocrinol. 18 (1), 65–76.

Carlini, V.P., Monzon, M.E., Varas, M.M., Cragnolini, A.B., Schioth, H.B., Scimonelli, T.N., 2002. Ghrelin increases anxiety-like behavior and memory retention in rats. Biochem. Biophys. Res. Commun. 299 (5), 739–743.

Collingridge, G.L., Volianskis, A., Bannister, N., France, G., Hanna, L., Mercier, M., 2013. The NMDA receptor as a target for cognitive enhancement. Neuropharmacology 64, 13–26.

Cuellar, J.N., Isokawa, M., 2011. Ghrelin-induced activation of cAMP signal transduction and its negative regulation by endocannabinoids in the hippocampus. Neuropharmacology 60 (6), 842–851.

Chang, P.K., Verbich, D., McKinney, R.A., 2012. AMPA receptors as drug targets in neurological disease–advantages, caveats, and future outlook. Eur. J. Neurosci. 35 (12), 1908–1916.

Chen, L., Xing, T., Wang, M., Miao, Y., Tang, M., Chen, J., 2011. Local infusion of ghrelin enhanced hippocampal synaptic plasticity and spatial memory through activation of phosphoinositide 3-kinase in the dentate gyrus of adult rats. Eur. J. Neurosci. 33 (2), 266–275.

Dallerac, G., Zerwas, M., Novikova, T., Callu, D., Leblanc-Veyrac, P., Bock, E., 2011. The neural cell adhesion molecule-derived peptide FGL facilitates long-term plasticity in the dentate gyrus in vivo. Learn. Mem. 18 (5), 306–313.

Damgaard, T., Larsen, D.B., Hansen, S.L., Grayson, B., Neill, J.C., Plath, N., 2010. Positive modulation of alpha-amino-3-hydroxy-5-methyl-4-isoxazolepropionic acid (AMPA) receptors reverses sub-chronic PCP-induced deficits in the novel object recognition task in rats. Behav. Brain Res. 207 (1), 144–150.

De Boer, M.D., 2012. The use of ghrelin and ghrelin receptor agonists as a treatment for animal models of disease: efficacy and mechanism. Curr. Pharm. Des. 18 (31), 4779–4799.

Diano, S., Farr, S.A., Benoit, S.C., McNay, E.C., da Silva, I., Horvath, B., 2006. Ghrelin controls hippocampal spine synapse density and memory performance. Nat. Neurosci. 9 (3), 381–388.

Downer, E.J., Cowley, T.R., Cox, F., Maher, F.O., Berezin, V., Bock, E., 2009. A synthetic NCAM-derived mimetic peptide, FGL, exerts anti-inflammatory properties via IGF-1 and interferon-gamma modulation. J. Neurochem. 109 (5), 1516–1525.

Downer, E.J., Cowley, T.R., Lyons, A., Mills, K.H., Berezin, V., Bock, E., 2010. A novel anti-inflammatory role of NCAM-derived mimetic peptide, FGL. Neurobiol. Aging 31 (1), 118–128.

Goff, D.C., Lamberti, J.S., Leon, A.C., Green, M.F., Miller, A.L., Patel, J., 2008. A placebo-controlled add-on trial of the Ampakine, CX516, for cognitive deficits in schizophrenia. Neuropsychopharmacology 33 (3), 465–472.

Goff, D.C., Leahy, L., Berman, I., Posever, T., Herz, L., Leon, A.C., 2001. A placebo-controlled pilot study of the ampakine CX516 added to clozapine in schizophrenia. J. Clin. Psychopharmacol. 21 (5), 484–487.

Golder, F.J., Hewitt, M.M., McLeod, J.F., 2013. Respiratory stimulant drugs in the post-operative setting. Respir. Physiol. Neurobiol. 189 (2), 395–402.

Guan, X.M., Yu, H., Palyha, O.C., McKee, K.K., Feighner, S.D., Sirinathsinghji, D.J., 1997. Distribution of mRNA encoding the growth hormone secretagogue receptor in brain and peripheral tissues. Brain Res. Mol. Brain Res. 48 (1), 23–29.

Hampson, R.E., Rogers, G., Lynch, G., Deadwyler, S.A., 1998. Facilitative effects of the ampakine CX516 on short-term memory in rats: correlations with hippocampal neuronal activity. J. Neurosci. 18 (7), 2748–2763.

Hansen, S.M., Li, S., Bock, E., Berezin, V., 2010. Synthetic NCAM-derived ligands of the fibroblast growth factor receptor. Adv. Exp. Med. Biol. 663, 355–372.

Harada, K., Nakato, K., Yarimizu, J., Yamazaki, M., Morita, M., Takahashi, S., 2012. A novel glycine transporter-1 (GlyT1) inhibitor, ASP2535 (4-[3-isopropyl-5-(6-phenyl-3-pyridyl)-4H-1,2,4-triazol-4-yl]-2,1,3-benzoxadiazol e), improves cognition in animal models of cognitive impairment in schizophrenia and Alzheimer's disease. Eur. J. Pharmacol. 685 (1–3), 59–69.

Henley, J.M., Wilkinson, K.A., 2013. AMPA receptor trafficking and the mechanisms underlying synaptic plasticity and cognitive aging. Dialogues Clin. Neurosci. 15 (1), 11–27.

Ingvar, M., Ambros-Ingerson, J., Davis, M., Granger, R., Kessler, M., Rogers, G.A., 1997. Enhancement by an ampakine of memory encoding in humans. Exp. Neurol. 146 (2), 553–559.

Inui, A., 2001. Ghrelin: an orexigenic and somatotrophic signal from the stomach. Nat. Rev. Neurosci. 2 (8), 551–560.

Inui, A., Asakawa, A., Bowers, C.Y., Mantovani, G., Laviano, A., Meguid, M.M., 2004. Ghrelin, appetite, and gastric motility: the emerging role of the stomach as an endocrine organ. FASEB J. 18 (3), 439–456.

Jerlhag, E., Egecioglu, E., Landgren, S., Salome, N., Heilig, M., Moechars, D., 2009. Requirement of central ghrelin signaling for alcohol reward. Proc. Natl. Acad. Sci. U.S.A. 106 (27), 11318–11323.

Jiang, H., Betancourt, L., Smith, R.G., 2006. Ghrelin amplifies dopamine signaling by cross talk involving formation of growth hormone secretagogue receptor/dopamine receptor subtype 1 heterodimers. Mol. Endocrinol. 20 (8), 1772–1785.

Johnson, J.W., Ascher, P., 1987. Glycine potentiates the NMDA response in cultured mouse brain neurons. Nature 325 (6104), 529–531.

Kiselyov, V.V., Skladchikova, G., Hinsby, A.M., Jensen, P.H., Kulahin, N., Soroka, V., 2003. Structural basis for a direct interaction between FGFR1 and NCAM and evidence for a regulatory role of ATP. Structure 11 (6), 691–701.

Kleckner, N.W., Dingledine, R., 1988. Requirement for glycine in activation of NMDA-receptors expressed in *Xenopus* oocytes. Science 241 (4867), 835–837.

Klementiev, B., Novikova, T., Novitskaya, V., Walmod, P.S., Dmytriyeva, O., Pakkenberg, B., 2007. A neural cell adhesion molecule-derived peptide reduces neuropathological signs and cognitive impairment induced by Abeta25-35. Neuroscience 145 (1), 209–224.

Knafo, S., Venero, C., Sanchez-Puelles, C., Pereda-Perez, I., Franco, A., Sandi, C., 2012. Facilitation of AMPA receptor synaptic delivery as a molecular mechanism for cognitive enhancement. PLoS Biol. 10 (2), e1001262.

Kohno, D., Gao, H.Z., Muroya, S., Kikuyama, S., Yada, T., 2003. Ghrelin directly interacts with neuropeptide-Y-containing neurons in the rat arcuate nucleus: Ca^{2+} signaling via protein kinase A and N-type channel-dependent mechanisms and cross-talk with leptin and orexin. Diabetes 52 (4), 948–956.

Kramár, E.A., Chen, L.Y., Lauterborn, J.C., Simmons, D.A., Gall, C.M., Lynch, G., 2012. BDNF upregulation rescues synaptic plasticity in middle-aged ovariectomized rats. Neurobiol. Aging 33 (4), 708–719.

Larson, J., Lieu, T., Petchpradub, V., LeDuc, B., Ngo, H., Rogers, G.A., 1995. Facilitation of olfactory learning by a modulator of AMPA receptors. J. Neurosci. 15 (12), 8023–8030.

Laruelle, M., 2014. Schizophrenia: from dopaminergic to glutamatergic interventions. Curr. Opin. Pharmacol. 14, 97–102.

Laube, B., Hirai, H., Sturgess, M., Betz, H., Kuhse, J., 1997. Molecular determinants of agonist discrimination by NMDA receptor subunits: analysis of the glutamate binding site on the NR2B subunit. Neuron 18 (3), 493–503. pii:S0896-6273(00)81249-0.

Lauterborn, J.C., Lynch, G., Vanderklish, P., Arai, A., Gall, C.M., 2000. Positive modulation of AMPA receptors increases neurotrophin expression by hippocampal and cortical neurons. J. Neurosci. 20 (1), 8–21.

Lauterborn, J.C., Truong, G.S., Baudry, M., Bi, X., Lynch, G., Gall, C.M., 2003. Chronic elevation of brain-derived neurotrophic factor by ampakines. J. Pharmacol. Exp. Ther. 307 (1), 297–305.

Lee, Y.S., Silva, A.J., 2009. The molecular and cellular biology of enhanced cognition. Nat. Rev. Neurosci. 10 (2), 126–140.

Li, S., Hong, S., Shepardson, N.E., Walsh, D.M., Shankar, G.M., Selkoe, D., 2009. Soluble oligomers of amyloid Beta protein facilitate hippocampal long-term depression by disrupting neuronal glutamate uptake. Neuron 62 (6), 788–801.

Li, S., Jin, M., Koeglsperger, T., Shepardson, N.E., Shankar, G.M., Selkoe, D.J., 2011. Soluble Abeta oligomers inhibit long-term potentiation through a mechanism involving excessive activation of extrasynaptic NR2B-containing NMDA receptors. J. Neurosci. 31 (18), 6627–6638.

Lipton, S.A., 2007. Pathologically-activated therapeutics for neuroprotection: mechanism of NMDA receptor block by memantine and S-nitrosylation. Curr. Drug Targets 8 (5), 621–632.

Liu, S.J., Gasperini, R., Foa, L., Small, D.H., 2010. Amyloid-beta decreases cell-surface AMPA receptors by increasing intracellular calcium and phosphorylation of GluR2. J. Alzheimers Dis. 21 (2), 655–666.

Lorier, A.R., Funk, G.D., Greer, J.J., 2010. Opiate-induced suppression of rat hypoglossal motoneuron activity and its reversal by ampakine therapy. PLoS One 5 (1), e8766.

Lynch, G., Gall, C.M., 2006. Ampakines and the threefold path to cognitive enhancement. Trends Neurosci. 29 (10), 554–562.

Lynch, G., Gall, C.M., 2013. Mechanism based approaches for rescuing and enhancing cognition. Front. Neurosci. 7, 143.

Lynch, G., Kessler, M., Rogers, G., Ambros-Ingerson, J., Granger, R., Schehr, R.S., 1996. Psychological effects of a drug that facilitates brain AMPA receptors. Int. Clin. Psychopharmacol. 11 (1), 13–19.

Maekawa, M., Watanabe, M., Yamaguchi, S., Konno, R., Hori, Y., 2005. Spatial learning and long-term potentiation of mutant mice lacking D-amino-acid oxidase. Neurosci. Res. 53 (1), 34–38.

Malik, S., McGlone, F., Bedrossian, D., Dagher, A., 2008. Ghrelin modulates brain activity in areas that control appetitive behavior. Cell Metab. 7 (5), 400–409.

Martina, M., Gorfinkel, Y., Halman, S., Lowe, J.A., Periyalwar, P., Schmidt, C.J., 2004. Glycine transporter type 1 blockade changes NMDA receptor-mediated responses and LTP in hippocampal CA1 pyramidal cells by altering extracellular glycine levels. J. Physiol. 557 (Pt 2), 489–500.

McNay, E.C., 2007. Insulin and ghrelin: peripheral hormones modulating memory and hippocampal function. Curr. Opin. Pharmacol. 7 (6), 628–632.

Moon, M., Kim, S., Hwang, L., Park, S., 2009. Ghrelin regulates hippocampal neurogenesis in adult mice. Endocr. J. 56 (3), 525–531.

Morris, R.G., Anderson, E., Lynch, G.S., Baudry, M., 1986. Selective impairment of learning and blockade of long-term potentiation by an N-methyl-D-aspartate receptor antagonist, AP5. Nature 319 (6056), 774–776.

Mothet, J.P., Parent, A.T., Wolosker, H., Brady Jr, R.O., Linden, D.J., Ferris, C.D., 2000. D-serine is an endogenous ligand for the glycine site of the N-methyl-D-aspartate receptor. Proc. Natl. Acad. Sci. U.S.A. 97 (9), 4926–4931.

Naleid, A.M., Grace, M.K., Cummings, D.E., Levine, A.S., 2005. Ghrelin induces feeding in the mesolimbic reward pathway between the ventral tegmental area and the nucleus accumbens. Peptides 26 (11), 2274–2279.

Oertel, B.G., Felden, L., Tran, P.V., Bradshaw, M.H., Angst, M.S., Schmidt, H., 2010. Selective antagonism of opioid-induced ventilatory depression by an ampakine molecule in humans without loss of opioid analgesia. Clin. Pharmacol. Ther. 87 (2), 204–211.

Papouin, T., Ladepeche, L., Ruel, J., Sacchi, S., Labasque, M., Hanini, M., 2012. Synaptic and extrasynaptic NMDA receptors are gated by different endogenous coagonists. Cell 150 (3), 633–646.

Porrino, L.J., Daunais, J.B., Rogers, G.A., Hampson, R.E., Deadwyler, S.A., 2005. Facilitation of task performance and removal of the effects of sleep deprivation by an ampakine (CX717) in nonhuman primates. PLoS Biol. 3 (9), e299.

Reijmers, L.G., Perkins, B.L., Matsuo, N., Mayford, M., 2007. Localization of a stable neural correlate of associative memory. Science 317 (5842), 1230–1233.

Ren, J., Lenal, F., Yang, M., Ding, X., Greer, J.J., 2013. Coadministration of the AMPAKINE CX717 with propofol reduces respiratory depression and fatal apneas. Anesthesiology 118 (6), 1437–1445.

Rex, C.S., Lauterborn, J.C., Lin, C.Y., Kramar, E.A., Rogers, G.A., Gall, C.M., 2006. Restoration of long-term potentiation in middle-aged hippocampus after induction of brain-derived neurotrophic factor. J. Neurophysiol. 96 (2), 677–685.

Ribeiro, L.F., Catarino, T., Santos, S.D., Benoist, M., van Leeuwen, J.F., Esteban, J.A., 2014. Ghrelin triggers the synaptic incorporation of AMPA receptors in the hippocampus. Proc. Natl. Acad. Sci. U.S.A. 111 (1), E149–E158.

Samartgis, J.R., Schachte, L., Hazi, A., Crowe, S.F., 2012. Piracetam, an AMPAkine drug, facilitates memory consolidation in the day-old chick. Pharmacol. Biochem. Behav. 103 (2), 353–358.

Scharfman, H., Goodman, J., Macleod, A., Phani, S., Antonelli, C., Croll, S., 2005. Increased neurogenesis and the ectopic granule cells after intrahippocampal BDNF infusion in adult rats. Exp. Neurol. 192 (2), 348–356.

Schellekens, H., Dinan, T.G., Cryan, J.F., 2013. Taking two to tango: a role for ghrelin receptor heterodimerization in stress and reward. Front. Neurosci. 7, 148.

Schitine, C., Xapelli, S., Agasse, F., Sarda-Arroyo, L., Silva, A.P., De Melo Reis, R.A., 2012. Ampakine CX546 increases proliferation and neuronal differentiation in subventricular zone stem/progenitor cell cultures. Eur. J. Neurosci. 35 (11), 1672–1683.

Secher, T., Novitskaia, V., Berezin, V., Bock, E., Glenthoj, B., Klementiev, B., 2006. A neural cell adhesion molecule-derived fibroblast growth factor receptor agonist, the FGL-peptide, promotes early postnatal sensorimotor development and enhances social memory retention. Neuroscience 141 (3), 1289–1299.

Shimazaki, T., Kaku, A., Chaki, S., 2010. D-Serine and a glycine transporter-1 inhibitor enhance social memory in rats. Psychopharmacology (Berl.) 209 (3), 263–270.

Shors, T.J., Servatius, R.J., Thompson, R.F., Rogers, G., Lynch, G., 1995. Enhanced glutamatergic neurotransmission facilitates classical conditioning in the freely moving rat. Neurosci. Lett. 186 (2–3), 153–156.

Silverman, J.L., Oliver, C.F., Karras, M.N., Gastrell, P.T., Crawley, J.N., 2013. AMPAKINE enhancement of social interaction in the BTBR mouse model of autism. Neuropharmacology 64, 268–282.

Simmons, D.A., Mehta, R.A., Lauterborn, J.C., Gall, C.M., Lynch, G., 2011. Brief ampakine treatments slow the progression of Huntington's disease phenotypes in R6/2 mice. Neurobiol. Dis. 41 (2), 436–444.

Simmons, D.A., Rex, C.S., Palmer, L., Pandyarajan, V., Fedulov, V., Gall, C.M., 2009. Up-regulating BDNF with an ampakine rescues synaptic plasticity and memory in Huntington's disease knockin mice. Proc. Natl. Acad. Sci. U.S.A. 106 (12), 4906–4911.

Skibicka, K.P., Dickson, S.L., 2011. Ghrelin and food reward: the story of potential underlying substrates. Peptides 32 (11), 2265–2273.

Staubli, U., Rogers, G., Lynch, G., 1994. Facilitation of glutamate receptors enhances memory. Proc. Natl. Acad. Sci. U.S.A. 91 (2), 777–781.

Stellwagen, D., Beattie, E.C., Seo, J.Y., Malenka, R.C., 2005. Differential regulation of AMPA receptor and GABA receptor trafficking by tumor necrosis factor-α. J. Neurosci. 25 (12), 3219–3228.

Stern-Bach, Y., Russo, S., Neuman, M., Rosenmund, C., 1998. A point mutation in the glutamate binding site blocks desensitization of AMPA receptors. Neuron 21 (4), 907–918.

Stoyanova II, le Feber, J., 2014. Ghrelin accelerates synapse formation and activity development in cultured cortical networks. BMC Neurosci. 15, 49.

Strick, C.A., Li, C., Scott, L., Harvey, B., Hajos, M., Steyn, S.J., 2011. Modulation of NMDA receptor function by inhibition of D-amino acid oxidase in rodent brain. Neuropharmacology 61 (5–6), 1001–1015.

Sultan, S., Gebara, E.G., Moullec, K., Toni, N., 2013. D-serine increases adult hippocampal neurogenesis. Front. Neurosci. 7, 155.

Talantova, M., Sanz-Blasco, S., Zhang, X., Xia, P., Akhtar, M.W., Okamoto, S., 2013. Abeta induces astrocytic glutamate release, extrasynaptic NMDA receptor activation, and synaptic loss. Proc. Natl. Acad. Sci. U.S.A. 110 (27), E2518–E2527.

Tsai, G.E., Lin, P.Y., 2010. Strategies to enhance N-methyl-D-aspartate receptor-mediated neurotransmission in schizophrenia, a critical review and meta-analysis. Curr. Pharm. Des. 16 (5), 522–537.

Tsien, J.Z., Huerta, P.T., Tonegawa, S., 1996. The essential role of hippocampal CA1 NMDA receptor-dependent synaptic plasticity in spatial memory. Cell 87 (7), 1327–1338.

Turner, C.A., Gula, E.L., Taylor, L.P., Watson, S.J., Akil, H., 2008. Antidepressant-like effects of intracerebroventricular FGF2 in rats. Brain Res. 1224, 63–68.

Turpin, F.R., Potier, B., Dulong, J.R., Sinet, P.M., Alliot, J., Oliet, S.H., 2011. Reduced serine racemase expression contributes to age-related deficits in hippocampal cognitive function. Neurobiol. Aging 32 (8), 1495–1504.

Wenk, G.L., 2006. Neuropathologic changes in Alzheimer's disease: potential targets for treatment. J. Clin. Psychiatry 67 (Suppl. 3), 3–7. quiz 23.

Wezenberg, E., Verkes, R.J., Ruigt, G.S., Hulstijn, W., Sabbe, B.G., 2007. Acute effects of the ampakine farampator on memory and information processing in healthy elderly volunteers. Neuropsychopharmacology 32 (6), 1272–1283.

Yang, S., Qiao, H., Wen, L., Zhou, W., Zhang, Y., 2005. D-serine enhances impaired long-term potentiation in CA1 subfield of hippocampal slices from aged senescence-accelerated mouse prone/8. Neurosci. Lett. 379 (1), 7–12.

Yang, Y., Ge, W., Chen, Y., Zhang, Z., Shen, W., Wu, C., 2003. Contribution of astrocytes to hippocampal long-term potentiation through release of D-serine. Proc. Natl. Acad. Sci. U.S.A. 100 (25), 15194–15199.

Zhao, C., Deng, W., Gage, F.H., 2008. Mechanisms and functional implications of adult neurogenesis. Cell 132 (4), 645–660.

Zheng, Y., Balabhadrapatruni, S., Masumura, C., Darlington, C.L., Smith, P.F., 2011. Effects of the putative cognitive-enhancing ampakine, CX717, on attention and object recognition memory. Curr. Alzheimer Res. 8 (8), 876–882.

Chapter 4

Role of Environment, Epigenetics, and Synapses in Cognitive Enhancement

Ciaran M. Regan[1]

[1]*School of Biomolecular and Biomedical Science, UCD Conway Institute, University College Dublin, Belfield, Dublin, Ireland*

SETTING THE SCENE

Thomas Aquinas (1225–1274), Dominican friar, priest, and philosopher, defined sensible experience to be both cognitive in our perception of the world and affective by the feelings and emotions that allow us to understand the world. In his view, this "external sense-cognition is achieved solely by the modification of the sense by the sensible" (as cited in Haldane, 1983). Yet, how an optimal course of action might be achieved by an organism comparing incoming sensory information with stored representation of world structure remains largely unknown. Moreover, how current knowledge might predict behavioral actions, and how the brain provides the necessary functional capabilities, lack any significant degree of biological certainty.

The patterns of behavior that evolve from signals that emerge from complex and ever-changing environments seem to be specific to each organism, and these changes, which can be enduring, underscore the remarkable plasticity of the brain. Songbirds, for example, have an innate vocalization pattern, yet they require hearing the song of conspecifics before they can acquire the mature song necessary for successful mating (Nottebohm and Liu, 2010). These modifications to song quality appear to require subtle structural change to occur in the song-generating motor neurons. The remarkable array of song repertoires, thus generated, is unlikely to be subject to mechanisms of genetic variation and natural selection. These processes are far too slow, given that genes and traits propagate or are lost by differential mortality and reproductive success. Genes encode for protein, not function and, in truth, genes cannot alter behavior. Genes must, therefore, employ other mechanisms to alter the fundamental nature of brain and body that, in turn, alter behavior. A constant interaction between the

Cognitive Enhancement. http://dx.doi.org/10.1016/B978-0-12-417042-1.00004-8

genome and the environment is required, one by which the environment regulates the cellular signals and functions that control the operation of the genome. Epigenetic mechanisms may be the ideal device for regulating cellular adaptation to environmental signals as many of these regulatory events involve genes that alter neuronal structure and function, often in a lasting way. This concept of epigenetics, the word being derived from the Greek *epi* meaning "upon" and genetics, is an aspect of Darwinian evolution that remains to be more fully explored. The idea was proposed originally by Conrad Waddington in 1957.

EPIGENETIC REGULATION OF THE GENOME

The activation or repression of gene activity is regulated by a class of proteins called transcription factors. These proteins bind to regions of DNA and regulate the extent to which gene transcription is permitted. One major epigenetic mechanism that dictates the degree to which transcription factors can access and dock to their DNA binding sites is the post-translational modification of histone proteins. These proteins form the core of the nucleosome that wraps around a DNA unit containing approximately 150 base pairs, which together are termed chromatin. Partly due to the electrostatic interactions between the positively charged histone proteins and the negatively charged DNA, the histone proteins and DNA exist as a tight complex that significantly reduces gene transcription. Post-translational modification of the histone protein tails, as occurs through the binding of histone acetyltransferase (HAT) and the covalent attachment of acetyl groups to lysine amino acids, can profoundly relax the histone-DNA interactions and improve transcription factor binding and gene transcription (Grunstein, 1997). Histone deacetylases (HDACs) have the opposite action of removing the acetyl groups from the histone proteins thereby generating a closed chromatin structure and decreased transcription factor binding and gene transcription (see Figure 4.1). Many other post-translational modifications to

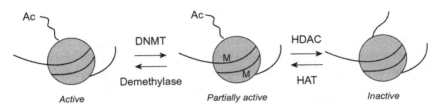

FIGURE 4.1   Epigenetic regulation of transcriptional state. The filled spheres represent the histone proteins, around which is wrapped the DNA chain (thin black line) to form units of chromatin. Regulation operates at the level of DNA by DNA methylation, or by the post-translational modification of the chromatin histone proteins. The thicker black lines represent the covalent attachment of acetyl groups to the histone proteins, which can also undergo numerous other post-translational modifications. DNMT, DNA methyltransferase; HAT, histone acetyltransferase; HDAC, histone deacetylase; Ac, acetyl group; M, methyl group.

histone protein tails also regulate gene transcription and these include methylation, phosphorylation, and ubiquitination.

The second most commonly reported epigenetic mechanism involves the addition of methyl groups to DNA cytosine bases by DNA methyltransferase (DNMT) or their removal by a demethylase (Razin and Riggs, 1980). These methylations result in gene silencing by swathes of methylated DNA preventing transcription factor binding or their interaction with methylated-DNA binding proteins and HDACs to form repressor protein complexes (see Figure 4.1). This latter mechanism occurs largely in the brain regions with dynamic variations in gene transcription, such as the hypothalamus (Semaco and Neul, 2011).

The regulated binding of transcription factors has been most commonly associated with environmental programming of gene expression. Environmental impact on developmental ontogeny, such as stress-related change in hormone signaling, have been associated with structural and functional alteration of DNA and persisting complex effects on the adult phenotype (Weaver et al., 2004; Champagne et al., 2008). Further, epigenetic modifications can often exhibit stochastic variations that have no apparent biological function but are believed to be mediated by both extrinsic and intrinsic factors (Bjornsson et al., 2008; Fraga et al., 2005; Wong et al., 2010). While clear mechanistic insights remain to be established, it would appear that substantial epigenetic change contributes to environment-induced phenotypes, that the biological primacy of these interactions is dependent on context, and that the most pertinent question relates to how these contextual influences are stored as long-term memory.

EPIGENETIC SIGNALING AND BEHAVIORAL PLASTICITY

Recent studies have demonstrated a role for epigenetic mechanisms, such as DNA methylation and chromatin modification, in experience-dependent behavioral modification (Day and Sweatt, 2011). Some intracellular signals involved in learning and memory are enzymes capable of modifying histone proteins. The CREB-binding protein (CBP) is a histone acetyltransferase essential for normal cognition (Alarcón et al., 2004). CBP is particularly involved in the consolidation of learning paradigms, such as contextual fear conditioning, and modulations in histone protein acetylation are observed in the brain regions processing the relevant information, such as the hippocampus, amygdala, and prefrontal cortex (Korzus et al., 2004; Yeh et al., 2004; Wood et al., 2006). The role of CBP in these histone modifications is further highlighted by the long-term memory impairments observed in mice harboring dysfunctional forms of this protein and in the ability of HDAC inhibitors, such as trichostatin A, to act through CBP and ameliorate these deficits (Bourtchouladze et al., 2003; Vecsey et al., 2007).

The role of post-translational acetylation of histone proteins in memory formation has also been demonstrated by transgenic studies in mice. Neuron-specific overexpression of HDAC2, for example, impairs memory formation and this is associated with an attenuation of neural plasticity, including suppression of dendritic spine density and synapse number (Guan et al., 2009). Conversely, genetic deletion of HDAC2 results in enhanced memory formation and synaptic plasticity. This latter effect is similar to that obtained with HDAC inhibitors. MS-275, a benzamide inhibitor specific to the HDAC1-3 class I isoforms, has been demonstrated to enhance task acquisition and consolidation and cell adhesion molecule-mediated neural plasticity (Foley et al., 2012). These effects of HDAC2 inhibition are most likely to arise from altered gene transcription as this isoform localizes predominantly to the nucleus where it can mediate its actions through the formation of stable transcriptional complexes with SIN3A, NuRD, and CoReST (Kazantsev and Thompson, 2008). Similar results have been found for other post-translational modifications of histone proteins. Protein phosphatase 1, for example, which removes histone phosphorylation marks, has been shown to enhance long-term memory formation (Koshibu et al., 2009) and the genetic deletion of histone-specific methyltransferase has been found to impair memory consolidation of a contextual fear conditioning paradigm (Gupta et al., 2010).

The covalent attachment of methyl groups to the cytosines of DNA may also constitute an epigenetic code, one that acts in tandem with the histone epigenetic code and provides a critical molecular mechanism to regulate synaptic plasticity in the formation and maintenance of long-term memory (Miller et al., 2008). Of particular interest is the role of the methyl CpG binding protein 2 (MeCP2) in memory formation (Samaco and Neul, 2011). MeCP2, which is mutated in Rett syndrome, regulates transcriptional repression through its interaction with methylated DNA and HDAC1 and HDAC2, and this interaction results in the dramatic alteration of hippocampal synaptic plasticity and memory formation. MeCP2 becomes phosphorylated in response to neuronal activity, a modification necessary for modulating expression of the gene encoding brain-derived neurotrophic factor (BDNF), which is associated with dendritic growth and spine maturation (Zhou et al., 2006) (see Figure 4.2).

Mouse models of altered *Mecp2* gene dosage exist and, remarkably, loss of MeCP2 function has been found to lead to neurological syndromes that overlap with those caused by gain of MeCP2 function, suggesting that these disorders arise from a failure of synaptic homeostasis (Ramocki and Zoghbi, 2008). Homeostatic responses are necessary to re-establish an appropriate balance between excitation and inhibition in order to return an affected system to a set point following a given neurodevelopmental or environmental perturbation. The loss or gain in protein or RNA dose that results in altered synaptic output and leads to overlapping phenotypes suggests that the molecules involved tightly control homeostatic mechanisms. Thus, any lack of homeostatic compensation leads to neural networks with weakened synaptic flexibility and loss of phenotypic resolution. At a molecular level, this homeostatic plasticity appears to require chromatin remodeling that changes gene expression and repression, the profile of protein production and turnover, and cytoskeletal rearrangements that are essential to synapse remodeling. In the adult animal, this plasticity has the

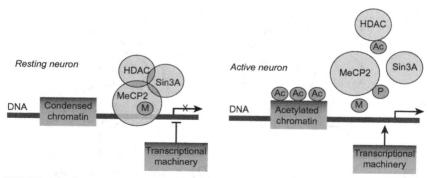

FIGURE 4.2 Potential mechanism for the regulation of gene expression through DNA methylation. Within inactive neurons, the linking of a methyl group binding protein, in this case MeCP2, to methylated DNA results in the recruitment of the Sin3A-HDAC corepressor complex, which leads to chromatin condensation and the inaccessibility of promoters required for gene transcription. Enhanced neuronal activity leads to calcium influx, the activation of CaMKII, MeCP2 phosphorylation, and release of the repressor complex. Membrane depolarization also results in cAMP-mediated phosphorylation of transcription factor CREB by protein kinase A, its association with CBP, the acetylation of nearby histones, and further promotion of transcriptional activity. Details of these mechanisms are further elaborated in Tsankova et al. (2007) and Chahrour and Zoghbi (2007). Ac, acetyl group; CaMKII, Ca^{2+}/calmodulin-dependent protein kinase II; CBP, histone acetyltransferase CREB-binding protein; CREB, cAMP-response element binding protein; HDAC, histone deacetylase; MeCP2, methyl CpG binding protein two; M, methyl group; P, phosphate group; Sin3A, corepressor protein.

potential to lead to modifications of the nervous system in response to environmental events and culminate in altered behaviors which are broadly termed learning and memory.

LEARNING AND MEMORY AND SYNAPSE PLASTICITY

The most dominant idea underpinning the role of synapse plasticity in learning and memory undoubtedly is based on Hebb's formulation in which memory networks are established by retuning the strength of existing synapses (Hebb, 1949). Sometimes referred to as the cell assembly hypothesis, these proposed networks are distinguished by the composition of cell synapses that are co-activated in accordance with local neural activity (see Figure 4.3). This idea of biophysical change in synapse strength was first confirmed by Bliss and Lømo (1973) when they directly demonstrated that increased synapse strength was generated as pre- and post-synaptic activities co-occurred, an event they termed long-term potentiation (LTP). Later, the modulatory action of neurotransmitter dopamine was found to play a role in the strengthening of coactivated synapses and in the absence of this transmitter the strength of these coactivated synapses was weakened, a consequence termed long-term depression (LTD) (Chen et al., 1996). Finally, the observation that spatial novelty could enhance LTP (Li et al., 2003) linked change in synaptic strength in accordance with local activity to be

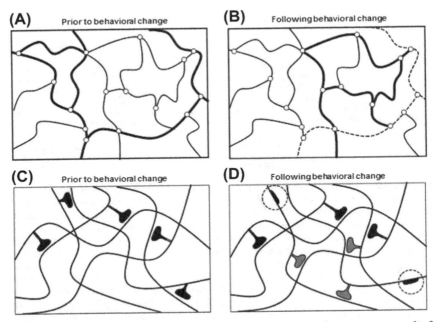

FIGURE 4.3 **Selective strengthening or weakening of populations of synapses as a result of behavioral modification.** In the cell assembly mechanism behavioral change is suggested to result in the network of cell synapses that are strengthened in various circuits (bold) and weakened in others (dashed) due to the degree of coactivation dictated by local neural activity (Panels (A) and (B)). In the synapse assembly hypothesis, new synapses are suggested to be created by experience and incorporated into the network (light-colored synapses) and the redundant supernumerary synapses (dashed circle) to be eliminated by a pruning mechanism (Panels (C) and (D)).

the empirical rule of learning and the enduring association of separate events (Bliss and Collingridge, 1993).

Memory, particularly declarative forms, however, is both instantaneous and permanent and, therefore, requires structural change to ensure its permanence. Indeed, as stated by Hebb (1949):

> *The conception of a transient, unstable reverberatory trace is therefore useful, if it is possible to suppose also that some more permanent structural change reinforces it.*

Structural change has been associated with the functional alterations induced by long-lasting LTP. These changes have been related to the synthesis and directed delivery of plasticity-related proteins to synapses "tagged" by LTP. Synapses, thus, are strengthened, or "captured," within the newly activated neural circuit (Redondo and Morris, 2011). Conversely, synapses weakened through the induction of LTD do not have delivery of plasticity-related proteins, shrink, and possibly become eliminated from the neural circuit. These dendritic spines, highly dynamic structures that emerge as tiny protrusions and form the postsynaptic sites for excitatory synapses, emerge within minutes in response to change in neural activity, and have been postulated to be a possible mechanism to explain the enduring nature of LTP.

Electron microscopy has been employed to analyze the morphology of synapses following the induction of LTP, and this has identified transient remodeling of the postsynaptic membrane followed by an increase in the number of postsynaptic sites contacting several dendritic spines (Toni et al., 1999). Spine proliferation in the hippocampal dentate gyrus becomes detectable at 30 min following the induction of LTP and returns to baseline values at 60 min post-stimulation (Wosiski-Kuhn and Stranahan, 2012). Surprisingly, LTP-induced spine proliferation is unaffected by inhibitors of transcription or protein synthesis and the relevance of these spine proliferation changes to the induction and maintenance of LTP has been challenged. For example, mice with functionally impaired L-alpha-amino-3-hydroxy-5-methylisoxazole-4-propionate (AMPA) receptors, which otherwise exhibit normal development and synaptic complement, do not express LTP in CA3 to CA1 synapses but retain hippocampal spatial reference memory learning ability in the water maze, whereas hippocampal-independent spatial working memory is impaired (Zamanillo et al., 1999; Schmitt et al., 2005). This dichotomy between the inability to induce hippocampal LTP and yet retain the ability for spatial learning ability suggests that AMPA receptor subunit composition controls LTP expression in the hippocampus, but not all types of cognitive function.

Dendritic spines are, however, the basic functional units of neuronal integration and, in addition to being rapidly formed, they can be selectively stabilized over time as synapses form in response to learning. One of the earliest demonstrations of morphological change in response to an environmental stimulus was demonstrated in the sea slug *Aplysia californica* (Bailey and Chen, 1983). Here, the formation of the associative reflexes of habituation and sensitization were found to result in the number, size, and vesicle complement of sensory neuron active zones, being larger in animals showing long-term sensitization and smaller in animals showing long-term habituation. These changes were proposed to represent an anatomical substrate for the consolidation of these forms of memory. Many other empirical studies now support a role for dendritic spines in the structural plasticity linked to memory-associated reorganization of neural circuits. Nevertheless, the search for cellular correlates of learning remains a major challenge in neurobiology.

The hippocampal formation is important for learning spatial relations, and the long-lasting consequence of this form of learning is alteration of the size, shape, and number of excitatory synapses in the basal dendrites of the hippocampal CA1 region (Moser et al., 1994). Trace eye-blink conditioning, an associative form of memory, has also been shown to induce significant and persisting increases in hippocampal CA1 spine density, along with multiple synapse boutons that form on more than one dendritic spine (Geinisman et al., 2001; Leuner et al., 2003). Indeed, in a meta-analysis study published in 2007, the available literature on morphological change following hippocampal-dependent learning showed significant and long-lived increases in persistent hippocampal dendritic complexity, spine density, and the size of perforated postsynaptic densities

(Marrone, 2007). It is also important to note that spine density changes within the hippocampal circuitry has been related to natural neuronal activity that is active during the associative learning of experience (Kitanishi et al., 2009).

The use of in vivo imaging of spines has further contributed to our understanding of learning-associated change in morphological parameters within the cortex. Repeated imaging of dendritic spines in the mouse barrel cortex for 1 month after trimming alternate whiskers has been found to result in the stabilization of new spines and destabilization of previously persistent spines, changes suggested to underlie experience-dependent remodeling of specific neocortical circuits (Holtmaat et al., 2006). Novel motor skills that persist following repetitive practice also result in the selective elimination of spines that existed before training (Xu et al., 2009). These eliminated spines were rapidly replaced by the formation of post-synaptic dendritic spines within the primary motor cortex. These spines stabilized with subsequent training, and their synapses persisted long after training had ceased. Similarly, novel sensory experience can also induce a cycle of cortical spine elimination, and de novo synapse formation over a protracted period of time (Yang et al., 2009). Only a small fraction of these new spines correlate with behavioral improvement, but these endure over a prolonged period of time as a stable connected synaptic network.

Behavioral learning, therefore, would appear to occur when the instructive experience stabilizes and strengthens synapse formation on neurons important for the control of the learned behavior. Structural plasticity at the axo–dendritic interface may therefore provide a mechanism for information processing, one that transcends the classical Hebbian learning scheme. In this discernment, which has been termed the synapse assembly hypothesis, new synapses are created by experience and incorporated into the learning network following the selective pruning of redundant synapses (Doyle et al., 1992a; Lichtman and Colman, 2000; Ziv and Ahissar, 2009) (see Figure 4.3). Moreover, this mechanism of synapse gain and/or elimination allows the elaboration of a network of specific groups of novel synapses in a connectivity scheme that provides a long-lasting memory trace optimized for each experience. Identifying the mechanisms underpinning this type of synapse plasticity poses a unique challenge, which is partly due to our limited understanding of how structure relates to function in the nervous system.

NEURODEVELOPMENTAL PRINCIPLES AND MEMORY-RELATED SYNAPSE REMODELING

The idea that synapse growth and change are associated with learning has conceptual parallels relating to neurodevelopmental principles (Marcus et al., 1994). There are analogies between cell phenotypes and properties that are triggered by developmental and environmental milieus and cognitive-behavioral memory, given that the information is acquired through experience and remains available for recall over a lifetime.

The developmental specification of neuronal networks throughout the nervous system would appear to be generated through the selective stabilization of synapses from a population that is transiently overproduced (Changeux and Danchin, 1976; Huttenlocher, 1979; Schuster et al., 1996). Similarly, within the molecular layer of adult hippocampal granule cells, transient increases in both spine and synapse numbers have been shown to occur in response to the acquisition and consolidation of several behavioral paradigms (O'Malley et al., 1998, 2000; Eyre et al., 2003). This learning-associated increase in spine density, which is instantiated by the acquisition of experience and necessary for its storage, occurs in a strictly time-dependent manner. Spine and synapse formation manifest specifically at the 6–9 h post-training time and returns to basal levels by the 72 h post-training time. Spine formation is strictly experience-dependent, as it is not observed in animals exposed to context alone. Furthermore, synapse remodeling is more dominant in the dorsal region of the hippocampus following spatial learning, whereas that associated with an avoidance task extends over the entire dorso-ventral aspect of the hippocampal formation, regions known to be essential for processing either spatial or emotional information (Scully et al., 2012). These transient populations of synapses associated with memory consolidation appear to be formed de novo as there is no evidence that they arise from synapse perforation and splitting. In addition, these synapses appear to be fully functional, as all express a significant complement of presynaptic vesicles and fully formed post-synaptic densities (Scully et al., 2012). Finally, although the numerical magnitude of synapse formation is the same as that observed following the induction of LTP, it is important to note that the temporal appearance and nature of the transient experience-dependent synapse population is distinctly different. Following the induction of LTP, mature synapses are observed within 30 min of change in neural activity, and the synapse population formed includes a heterogeneous mix of simple, perforated, and multiple synapse boutons (Toni et al., 2001; Mezey et al., 2004).

There is yet another conundrum associated with the simple idea of neural activity rapidly inducing synapse remodeling, and this is particularly relevant to the phenomenon of LTP. Synapses are recognized by characteristic ultrastructural features such as the apposition of pre- and post-synaptic plasma membranes, a synaptic cleft, and presynaptic vesicles, particularly at the level of the electron microscope. It is not unreasonable to assume, therefore, that these structural specializations evolve slowly during the elaboration of new synapses. Secondly, there is the implicit requirement that synapses relevant to the transiently produced populations, as described above, form and mature synchronously over time. Providing a molecular basis for this requirement is a formidable problem. One possibility is that the molecules involved in activity-dependent events of neuronal development are later called upon again to orchestrate synaptic stabilization, growth, and elimination during long-term plasticity.

Unlike the peripheral nervous system, where motor axon presynaptic compartments are located at their termini, the vertebrate central nervous system can form many presynaptic sites (varicosities) along the length of the axonal segments as the evolving neuropil is continually remodeled. Dynamically, axons vigorously extend and retract lateral protrusions containing preassembled precursors of presynaptic boutons, or prototerminals, to sites of contact on nearby axons. (Vaughn, 1989; Roos and Kelly, 2000; Ziv and Garner, 2004). An important assumption is that prototerminal recruitment into mature synapses requires cell adhesion molecules to stabilize these short-lived axodendritic contacts for a period long enough to allow more specialized membrane proteins to interact with their counterparts and activate specific intracellular cascades to induce pre- and postsynaptic differentiation. An example of the importance of cell adhesion molecules in activity-dependent synapse elaboration has been provided by live-imaging studies (Sytnyk et al., 2002). In these studies, intracellular organelles of trans-golgi network origin have been found to link to clusters of extracellular-facing cell adhesion molecules, and that these complexes travel together along axons until they are trapped at axodendritic contacts sites. Such observations suggest a major role for adhesion molecules in activity-dependent neural remodeling and the stabilization of axodendritic contacts for a period sufficient to allow the interaction of more specialized membrane proteins and the activation of specific intracellular cascades.

ROLE OF CELL ADHESION MOLECULES IN EXPERIENCE-DEPENDENT SYNAPSE REMODELING

Activity-dependent transduction of signals from the extracellular environment to the nucleus of the neuron is crucial to understanding how synapse remodeling modifies brain structure and function during the encoding of recent perceptions. This process of memory consolidation seems to be regulated, in part, by transmembrane cell adhesion molecules (CAMs) located in the synapse, such as integrins, and those characterized by immunoglobulin-like domains. These cell-surface macromolecules appear to be capable of regulating the extent of synapse signaling by modulating the degree of cell–cell interaction in a manner that allows rapid change in synapse efficacy, connectivity pattern, or both.

A compelling case for the role of CAMs in synapse remodeling initially came from studies on long-term sensitization in the sea slug *Aplysia california* and using an avoidance conditioning paradigm in adult Wistar rats (Doyle et al., 1992b; Mayford et al., 1992). These observations centered on the role that the neural cell adhesion molecule (NCAM) and apCAM, its *Aplysia* homolog. NCAM, originally described as a synaptic membrane protein (Jorgenson and Bock, 1974), was the first CAM to be isolated and characterized (Thiery et al., 1977) and was demonstrated to be uniquely modified by the post-translational addition of α2-8-linked sialic acid residues (polysialic acid, PSA) (Finne et al., 1983). A member of the immunoglobulin superfamily of CAMs, NCAM is characterized by a number of splice variants. There are three main isoforms of NCAM, which arise from alternative splicing of a single gene. NCAM-140 and NCAM-180 are type I transmembrane proteins that differ in the length of their cytosolic tail, whereas

NCAM-120 is linked to the membrane via a glycosylphosphatidylinositol anchor (Cunningham et al., 1987). The three isoforms share a common extracellular structure consisting of five immunoglobulin (Ig) domains and two fibronectin type III repeats (FN1 and FN2). NCAM 180, in particular, is distinguished by its localization to post-synaptic membranes, notably in the hippocampus (Pollerberg et al., 1986; Persohn et al., 1989), and ability to mediate signal transduction and regulation of intracellular Ca^{2+} concentrations (Schuch et al., 1989).

In the studies on *Aplysia*, long-term sensitization, as evidenced by gill withdrawal in response to a noxious stimulus, had been associated with the formation of new synapses between the sensory neurons and their motorneuron targets. These long-term functional changes were demonstrated to be dependent on the synthesis of macromolecules during the period between the accompanying enhancement of neural activity and structural change (Bailey and Chen, 1983; Bailey et al., 1992). In vitro, the synaptic structural change could be mimicked by application of serotonin (5-HT), and this was found to be preceded by a rapid increase in the regulation of newly synthesized apCAM and the internalization and degradation of existing apCAM from the surface of the sensory neurons. Thus, application of 5-HT to cultures of sensory and motor neurons linked change in presynaptic sprouting and synapse formation to modulations of cell adhesion molecule function.

At the same time, interventive studies involving the infusion of antibodies to NCAM demonstrated a functional requirement for this cell adhesion molecule, specifically at the 6 h post-training period following acquisition of an avoidance conditioning paradigm (Doyle et al., 1992b). Later studies, using a peptide antagonist of NCAM–NCAM homophilic binding, revealed an additional requirement for NCAM function just following task acquisition (0 h) that, when blocked, resulted in impaired NCAM internalization and degradation and memory consolidation (Foley et al., 2000). Thus, this activity-dependent downregulation of adhesion molecule function suggests a common mechanism linking transient patterns of neural activity to adhesive changes in synapses and that their destabilization and/or elimination may serve as a clearing event before subsequent synaptic growth and memory consolidation.

The learning-associated synaptic growth, described in the preceding section, immediately follows NCAM internalization and appears to be dependent on enhanced NCAM synthesis as NCAM–NCAM homophilic binding, and signaling is also required at the 6 h post-training period (Doyle et al., 1992b; Foley et al., 2000). This NCAM–NCAM homophilic binding requirement is consistent with in vitro observations demonstrating neurite outgrowth necessitates homophilic binding at a specific NCAM protein threshold and with in vivo studies that have confirmed an increase in hippocampal NCAM to accompany the consolidation of a spatial learning paradigm (Doherty et al., 1990; Venero et al., 2006). It is also worth noting that the temporal action of anti-NCAM is specific to the 6 h post-training time, as it is not observed with other antibodies that induce amnesia when administered at earlier time points (Nolan et al., 1987; Doyle et al., 1990). Secondly, infusions of anti-NCAM in the 6 h post-training were found to require task re-exposure to elicit their amnesic action as the amnesia becomes apparent only following subsequent recall trials (Doyle et al., 1992b; Alexinsky et al., 1997). These observations suggest that NCAM may in some way be involved in an activity-dependent strengthening of de novo synapse formation, as might be required for enhancing the salience of information being processed for long-term memory formation.

Although synapse remodeling obviously plays an important in establishing novel circuit-connectivity pattern, the process of eliminating the supernumerary synapses may be of greater interest. Synapse elimination has the potential to remove competition from redundant inputs thereby ensuring that those synapses relevant to establishing a more indelible memory trace are selectively strengthened. Synapse elimination also provides a mechanism by which large numbers of circuits may be specifically created from an initial set of more diffuse and redundant connections. There are reasons to believe that polysialylated NCAM may play a specific role in the elimination of supernumerary synapses in an evolving memory trace.

REGULATION OF NCAM POLYSIALYLATION STATE

A unique post-translational modification of NCAM is the attachment of linear polymers of PSA. The negative charge of these basal units of PSA forms a hydration shell that increases the hydrodynamic radius of the NCAM carrier, enlarges the space between adjacent cells, and inhibits cell–cell interactions as well as intracellular signaling (Yang et al., 1992; Krushel et al., 1999; Burgess and Aubert, 2006). Polysialylation of NCAM is mediated by two polysialyltransferases. That termed ST8SiaII is also known as STX and is mainly expressed in the developing brain (Livingston and Paulson, 1993). The second form is referred to as ST8SiaIV, or PST, and this is predominantly expressed in the mature brain (Eckhardt et al., 1995).

The regulation of polysialyltransferase expression is poorly defined but appears to involve both transcriptional and nontranscriptional mechanisms. Nontranscriptional control has been argued to involve a calcium-dependent regulatory mechanism (Brusés and Rutishauser, 1998) and polysialyltransferase phosphorylation that directly influences the degree of enzyme activity (Gallagher et al., 2001; Conboy et al., 2009). A calcium-dependent mechanism has also been proposed to regulate a rapid, activity-dependent delivery of presynthesized NCAM PSA to the cell surface (Kiss et al., 1994).

REGULATION OF NCAM PSA EXPRESSION DURING ACTIVITY-DEPENDENT NEURAL REMODELING

There is now extensive evidence to suggest that NCAM PSA expression is intimately involved in the neural remodeling associated with novel sensory experience in the adult central nervous system. NCAM PSA expression in the suprachiasmatic nucleus, for example, is responsible for light-induced phase shifts in circadian rhythm (Prosser et al., 2003), and this activity-dependent remodeling of hypothalamic neurons occurs in response to the intrinsic stimuli that govern parturition and lactation (Hoyk et al., 2001). Secondly, studies on animals reared in complex environments have been central in correlating modulation of activity-related brain plasticity to behavioral responses that arise from signals emanating from the external milieu. For example, the increases in hippocampal polysialylated cell frequency associated with rearing in a complex environment have been directly correlated with improved performance in the water maze learning paradigm (Murphy et al., 2006). Although these correlations do not demonstrate causation, it is encouraging to note that chronic administration of acetylcholinesterase inhibitors, such as tacrine, results in a significant correlation between increased hippocampal polysialylated cell number and the associated procognitive action in water-maze learning to precisely the same extent as that obtained by environmental enrichment (Murphy et al., 2006). The potential role of NCAM PSA in extrinsic, experience-dependent neural remodeling is further reinforced by the consistent observation of upregulated expression of NCAM PSA during the consolidation of a diverse range of learning paradigms, including spatial learning, avoidance and contextual fear conditioning, odor discrimination, and LTP (Fox et al., 1995; Murphy et al., 1996; Foley et al., 2003; Sandi et al., 2004). Moreover, these increases in NCAM PSA expression are necessary for memory consolidation, as cleavage of PSA from NCAM by infusions of endoneuraminidase-N results in task amnesia (Becker et al., 1996; Venero et al., 2006).

Importantly, many studies have demonstrated these learning-associated increases in NCAM PSA to be associated with hippocampal granule cells located in the infragranular zone, and to a discrete population of neurons in layer II of the entorhinal cortex and extending to the piriform cortex (Doyle et al., 1992c; Fox et al., 1995, 2000; Murphy et al., 1996; O'Connell et al., 1997). In addition to their spatial resolution, these polysialylated cells exhibit a strict temporal resolution, increasing the number of cells expressing NCAM PSA only in the 12 h post-training period, and returning to basal values within a 24-h period. Secondly, these polysialylated cells repeatedly modulate their numbers in response to sequential exposure to alternative tasks, providing the tasks are separated by an interparadigm period of 2 h (Murphy and Regan, 1999), and these increases are more dominant in the dorsal region of the hippocampus following spatial learning, but extended over the entire dorso-ventral aspect of the hippocampal formation after avoidance conditioning (Lopez-Fernandez et al., 2007; Scully et al., 2012). Thirdly, these polysialylated granule cells appear to be involved in strengthening the evolving memory trace, as a significant correlation exists between the strength of learning and the number of cells glycosylated at the 12 h post-training time (Sandi et al., 2004). Finally, as was observed using antibodies directed to NCAM, infusions of anti-PSA in the 10 h post-training time were found to be amnesic, but only following task re-exposure, which suggests that NCAM PSA is involved in an activity-dependent mechanism involved in task consolidation (Seymour et al., 2008).

Not all studies have supported the contention of NCAM PSA playing a functional role in memory consolidation. The injection of NCAM PSA-Fc chimeras or free PSA, but not NCAM, into the dorsal hippocampus of wild-type mice before fear conditioning, has been found to impair the formation of hippocampus-dependent contextual memory (Senkov et al., 2006). The possibility exists, however, that the NCAM PSA-Fc employed in these studies may function as a competitive antagonist capable of abolishing NCAM PSA-mediated synaptogenesis, as a cyclic oligopeptide PSA mimetic that acts as a noncompetitive agonist enhances acquisition and consolidation of a spatial learning paradigm in a manner that is consistent with the requirement of post-training increases in NCAM polysialylation state necessary for successful spatial learning (Torregrossa et al., 2004; Florian et al., 2006).

As neurogenesis occurs at the infragranular zone of the adult dentate gyrus, it is not surprising that some of the NCAM PSA-immunopositive cells have been recently generated and might be available for incorporation into the existing neural structure (Seki, 2002; Toni et al., 2007; Dupret et al., 2007). This phenomenon has been proposed to be a mechanism that allows the development of a relational network suggested to be necessary for pattern separation during the prolonged period of memory consolidation (Rolls and Kesner, 2006; Deng et al., 2010). This population of newly-generated cells has to be small, as many studies have failed to associate increased NCAM PSA-mediated plasticity with neurogenesis (Fox et al., 1995; Pham et al., 2005; Knafo et al., 2005; van der Borght et al., 2005). Moreover, learning-associated increases in NCAM-polysialylated cell frequency occur in brain regions that do not support adult neurogenesis, such as layer II of the medial temporal lobe (O'Connell et al., 1997; Fox et al., 2000).

The mechanisms by which neural remodeling is mediated by the temporal and spatial resolution of NCAM PSA expression remains to be precisely established. Polysialic acid can only be a general modulator, a permissive signal that allows the appropriate degree of cell–cell interaction at relevant times and locations. NCAM PSA, however, has the potential to facilitate the elimination of redundant supernumerary synapses, as polysialylation is known to restrain synapse signaling through NMDA receptors, particularly those containing GluN2B subunits (Kochlamazashvili et al., 2010), most likely by steric hindrance of receptor–ligand interactions (Burgess and Aubert, 2006). Secondly, removal of PSA can also induce differentiation and growth in synapses selected for retention by increasing BDNF-binding capacity and that of other growth factors, such as glial cell line-derived neurotrophic factor (Muller et al., 2000; Paratcha et al., 2003; Tyler and Pozzo-Miller, 2003). These two mechanisms may operate in tandem during the synaptic remodeling associated with memory consolidation as inhibition of PKCδ, and the concomitant activation of PSA expression would allow selection of synapses marked for elimination whereas those not polysialylated would be amenable to growth factor–induced growth and selection. Moreover, these separate mechanisms exhibit a temporal and spatial resolution that allows them operate in tandem in the hippocampus, specifically at the 12 h post-training period when both are necessary for memory consolidation (Gallagher et al., 2001; Rossato et al., 2009; Conboy et al., 2009).

It is important to also note that other PKC-dependent mechanisms have been implicated in learning-associated neural plasticity and the associated enhancement of hippocampal polysialylated cell frequency. For example, the synaptic remodeling and improved spatial learning induced by a mimetic peptide that encompasses an interactive domain of NCAM for the fibroblast growth factor receptor has been demonstrated to be specifically mediated by an initial activation of PKC, followed by a long-lasting enhancement of synaptic transmission and a persistent activation of calcium/calmodulin-dependent protein kinase II (Knafo et al., 2012). Secondly, the ability of PKCα or β to activate sphingosine-1-phosphate and its acetylation of H3 histone proteins by HDAC1 and HDAC2 in promotor repressor complexes may play an indirect role in the regulation of NCAM polysialylation state, as valproate, and its analogs, are known to inhibit HDAC and significantly enhance H3 histone protein acetylation, ST8SiaIV transcription, and NCAM PSA expression (Beecken et al., 2005; Lampen et al., 2005; Hait et al., 2009; Morquecho-León et al., 2014; Foley et al., 2014) Other than these PKC-mediated mechanisms, no other second-messenger system has been reported to regulate the activity of NCAM-dependent polysialyltransferases. The overarching implication of these observations is that regulation of PKC activity provides a potential mechanism to allow a constant interaction between the environment and the regulation of cellular signals involved in synapse remodeling and the operational control of the genome.

SYNAPSE REMODELING AND MEMORY CONSOLIDATION

The evolutionary necessity of ensuring the gradual betterment of adaptive behaviors capable of informing future value decisions also requires that sensory data be incorporated into stored knowledge. A neural system is therefore required to allow subjective values be appended to decisions and how these values are learned, stored, and represented. The associative learning of rewarding events, for example, can be observed in the phasic firing of midbrain dopaminergic neurons, and their potentiation or depression of connection strengths permits the implementation of a prediction error rule (Sutton and Barto, 1998; for a recent overview see Regan, 2014). This rule relates rational expectation of future rewards with current stored knowledge and the learned revision of such expectations. Thus, the modulation of midbrain dopaminergic neuron phasic activity modulates output from the *substantia nigra* to regions of the frontal cortex that control motor movements, and those from the ventral tegmental area (VTA) that increase the motivational drive required for the reward response (Montague et al., 1996; Schultz et al., 1997).

The prediction error rule may provide a rationale for understanding how the greatest number of rewards may be obtained, but it does not explain how sustained behavior is necessary for achieving more distant rewards. This requires more prolonged tonic dopamine signaling within the striatum, as has been observed in rats navigating mazes to obtain rewards (Howe et al., 2013). Furthermore, these signals ramp as the animal approaches the reward and appear to be influenced by the location of the reward, as if they are responding to a spatial cognitive map formed by place-cell assemblies in the hippocampus.

Functional interactions that regulate motivation and place-reward associations are known to exist between the hippocampus and ventral striatum (Ito et al., 2008). This means that the ramping of dopaminergic neuronal firing in the striatum as an animal navigates toward a reward may be correlated to hippocampal theta rhythms that, in turn, provide a mechanism for the consolidation and recall of reward-based spatial experience in a given environment (Skaggs et al., 1996; O'Keefe and Recce, 1993). It is not necessarily the case that these dopaminergic signals influence reward-based decisions; they could equally represent reward estimations that influence goal-directed behavior over time. In this regard, unexpected rewards allow novelty-dependent dopaminergic activity in the VTA to be looped to the hippocampus CA1 region, where it is compared to previously stored memory delivered via the CA3 and dentate gyrus (Rolls and Kesner, 2006; Luo et al., 2011). In turn, the estimated extent of novelty is returned to the VTA, where it further modulates dopaminergic firing and enhances the value of previously positive but unrewarded associative memories, provided that they are explicitly remembered. Simultaneously, the new information delivered by the hippocampus–VTA loop is interleaved into that already consolidated as long-term memory in cortical neuronal ensembles.

The idea that the hippocampus encodes all episodic memory in distributed neuronal assemblies comes from studies showing that patients with damage to the medial temporal lobe had difficulty in recalling recent events, but not those of the more distant past (Ribot, 1882). This temporally graded amnesia on declarative memory tasks led to the concept of memory consolidation. This suggests that the hippocampal formation rapidly encodes episodic information in distributed neuronal assemblies that act to index information for neuronal transfer to cortical ensembles, and that over time the binding of this information results in coherent cortical representations of memory (Alvarez and Squire, 1994). The cortical ensembles that constitute a given memory trace may also be reactivated to bind with additional and emerging traces that share information about the initial experience (Nadel and Moscovitch, 1997). The integration of additional information into an existing cognitive framework requires matching it to details of previous learning events, as these provide the set of expectations associated with the prior event and permit the selective strengthening of shared elements. Common features of memory, sometimes termed schemas, allow rapid incorporation of new information, in part, due to a greater functional coupling between the hippocampus and the medial prefrontal cortex (Tse et al., 2007, 2011; van Kesteren et al., 2010). In contrast, the need to form a new schema necessitates a much longer period of information processing within the hippocampus and within the loops between the hippocampal and cortical ensembles.

The mechanisms associated with the consolidation of new schemas and the reactivation and reconsolidation of previously formed schemas appear to be distinctly different. For example, both consolidation and reconsolidation require protein synthesis; however, the synthesis of brain-derived neurotrophic factor (BDNF) is necessary for consolidation but not reconsolidation, whereas that of transcription factor Zif268 is necessary for reconsolidation but not consolidation (Lee et al., 2004; Morris et al., 2006; Rodriguez-Ortiz et al., 2008). Furthermore, reconsolidation recruits only a subset of the immediate-early genes that are induced during consolidation (von Hertzen and Giese, 2005; Hoeffer et al., 2011). Although these findings point to separate encoding mechanisms being involved in the consolidation and reconsolidation of memory, they also reinforce the idea that the system initially encoding memory content may be different to that which later stores the information (McClelland et al., 1995). For example, the formation of schemas for noncongruent information may be a feature of memory consolidation prior and during their migration to point of storage, and those schemas for congruent information might be formed in migrated traces by processes of reconsolidation.

The synaptic consolidation processes considered in this review involve the generation of a transient learning-associated population of supernumerary synapses, from which synapse selection and elimination form the memory trace at the cellular level. This is believed to provide the foundation for systems consolidation by a continuing interplay between hippocampal and neocortical assemblies to allow the newly acquired information be slowly incorporated into cortical representations. This reinforcement loop would therefore permit repeated activation of memory to progressively build new schematic representations of relationships between environmental stimuli and add and strengthen relevant features of this information into existing schemas. Selection, not instruction, is therefore viewed as providing the mechanism for learning and involves increasing the strength of one set of synaptic connections while weakening or eliminating others. Further, the information to be encoded occurs within the same circuit and at the same time as the information redistributes among other circuits.

Many features of this learning-associated model of synapse plasticity are consistent with a role in memory consolidation. These include spatial restriction to the medial temporal lobe (Fox et al., 1995, 2000), repetitive reactivations of synapse remodeling in response to alternate environmental stimuli (Murphy et al., 1996), the requirement of BDNF and synapse growth (O'Malley et al., 1998, 2000; Rossato et al., 2009), the need to strengthen the synaptic trace by context re-exposure (Foley et al., 2000), and a temporal resolution of 24–48 h (Murphy and Regan, 1999). The role of synapse remodeling in the reconsolidation of existing schemas is much less certain. Previous studies have suggested that transcription factor Zif268 to be necessary for reconsolidation but not consolidation (Lee et al., 2004). However, mutant mice homozygous for Zif268 function show deficits for both consolidation and reconsolidation of a contextual fear-conditioning paradigm, whereas the heterozygous mutants display a selective deficit Zof reconsolidation, and only if the memory was recently encoded (Besnard et al., 2013). Although these results point to a close relationship between Zif268 expression and memory processing, they blur the distinction between mechanisms of consolidation and reconsolidation and, moreover, the associated role of the hippocampus. Evidence associating neural plasticity with the formation of congruent schemas within the migrated trace remains to be acquired.

FINAL COMMENT

The brain is generally accepted to be a highly dynamic organ that exists in permanent relationship between the environment and the actions of the individual. The elementary feature of this relationship is that of declarative memory by which encoding of internal and external representations form explicit relationships between specific items and events. This information is flexibly generalized and integrated for use in the continual updating of our response to novel situations. This general concept has been variously reformulated as the phenomenon of plasticity in which experience impacts on the neuronal structure in a manner that modifies the efficiency of information transfer beyond that which is innate. The concept also implies that the synapse may be altered by experience, and that such morphological changes alter the geometry of neuronal interactions and their synaptic connectivity pattern to result in behavioral change. These changes in our neural structure require *gene × environment* interactions mediated primarily by transcription factors controlled by external signals that facilitate the genome in operating in a context-dependent manner in order to exert persisting effects on phenotype.

The idea that our behavioral phenotype involves growth and functional change in the existing neural structure has been restated many times since Tanzi (1893) first wrote:

Perhaps every representation immediately determines a functional hypertrophy of the protoplasmic processes and axons concerned; molecular vibrations become more intense and diffuse themselves, momentarily altering the form of dendrites; and thus, if the conditions are favorable, new expansions and collaterals originate and become permanent. Each fresh occurrence of the same conscious phenomenon in the form of recollection strengthens the mnemonic capacity, because it determines the formation of new impressions that are substituted for or added to those that were there.

REFERENCES

Alarcón, J.M., Malleret, G., Touzani, K., Vronskaya, S., Ishii, S., Kandel, E.R., Barco, A., 2004. Chromatin acetylation, memory, and LTP are impaired in CBP[+/-] mice: a model for the cognitive deficit in Rubinstein-Taybi syndrome and its amelioration. Neuron 42, 947–959.

Alexinsky, T., Przybyslawski, J., Mileusnic, R., Rose, S.P., Sara, S.J., 1997. Antibody to day-old chick brain glycoprotein produces amnesia in adult rats. Neurobiol. Learn Mem. 67, 14–20.

Alvarez, P., Squire, L.R., 1994. Memory consolidation and the medial temporal lobe: a simple network model. Proc. Natl. Acad. Sci. U.S.A. 91, 7041–7045.

Bailey, C.H., Chen, M., 1983. Morphological basis of long-term habituation and sensitization in Aplysia. Science 220, 91–93.

Bailey, C.H., Montarolo, P., Chen, M., Kandel, E.R., Schacher, S., 1992. Inhibitors of protein and RNA synthesis block structural changes that accompany long-term heterosynaptic plasticity in Aplysia. Neuron 9, 749–758.

Becker, C.G., Artola, A., Gerardy-Schahn, R., Becker, T., Welzl, H., Schachner, M., 1996. The polysialic acid modification of the neural cell adhesion molecule is involved in spatial learning and hippocampal long-term potentiation. J. Neurosci. Res. 45, 143–152.

Beecken, W.D., Engl, T., Ogbomo, H., Relja, B., Cinatl, J., Bereiter-Hahn, J., Oppermann, E., Jonas, D., Blaheta, R.A., 2005. Valproic acid modulates NCAM polysialylation and polysialyltransferase mRNA expression in human tumor cells. Int. Immunopharmacol. 5, 757–769.

van der Borght, K., Wallinga, A.E., Luiten, P.G., Eggen, B.J., Van der Zee, E.A., 2005. Morris water maze learning in two rat strains increases the expression of the polysialylated form of the neural cell adhesion molecule in the dentate gyrus but has no effect on hippocampal neurogenesis. Behav. Neurosci. 119, 926–932.

Besnard, A., Caboche, J., Laroche, S., 2013. Recall and reconsolidation of contextual fear memory: differential control by ERK and Zif268 expression dosage. PLoS One 8, e72006.

Bliss, T.V., Collingridge, G.L., 1993. A synaptic model of memory: long-term potentiation in the hippocampus. Nature 361, 31–39.

Bliss, T.V., Lømo, T., 1973. Long-lasting potentiation of synaptic transmission in the dentate area of the anaesthetized rabbit following stimulation of the perforant path. J. Physiol. 232, 331–356.

Bourtchouladze, R., Lidge, R., Catapano, R., Stanley, J., Gossweiler, S., Romashko, D., Scott, R., Tully, T., 2003. A mouse model of Rubinstein-Taybi syndrome: defective long-term memory is ameliorated by inhibitors of phosphodiesterase 4. Proc. Natl. Acad. Sci. U.S.A. 100, 10518–10522.

Bjornsson, H.T., Sigurdsson, M.I., Fallin, M.D., Irizarry, R.A., Aspelund, T., Cui, H., Yu, W., Rongione, M.A., Ekström, T.J., Harris, T.B., Launer, L.J., Eiriksdottir, G., Leppert, M.F., Sapienza, C., Gudnason, V., Feinberg, A.P., 2008. Intra-individual change over time in DNA methylation with familial clustering. JAMA 299, 2877–2883.

Brusés, J.L., Rutishauser, U., 1998. Regulation of neural cell adhesion molecule polysialylation: evidence for nontranscriptional control and sensitivity to an intracellular pool of calcium. J. Cell Biol. 140, 1177–1186.

Burgess, A., Aubert, I., 2006. Polysialic acid limits choline acetyltransferase activity induced by brain-derived neurotrophic factor. J. Neurochem. 99, 797–806.

Chahrour, M., Zoghbi, H.Y., 2007. The story of Rett syndrome: from clinic to neurobiology. Neuron 56, 422–437.

Champagne, D.L., Bagot, R.C., van Hasselt, F., Ramakers, G., Meaney, M.J., de Kloet, E.R., Joëls, M., Krugers, H., 2008. Maternal care and hippocampal plasticity: evidence for experience-dependent structural plasticity, altered synaptic functioning, and differential responsiveness to glucocorticoids and stress. J. Neurosci. 28, 6037–6045.

Changeux, J.P., Danchin, A., 1976. Selective stabilisation of developing synapses as a mechanism for the specification of neuronal networks. Nature 264, 705–712.

Chen, Z., Ito, K., Fujii, S., Miura, M., Furuse, H., Sasaki, H., Kaneko, K., Kato, H., Miyakawa, H., 1996. Roles of dopamine receptors in long-term depression: enhancement via D1 receptors and inhibition via D2 receptors. Receptors Channels 4, 1–8.

Conboy, L., Foley, A.G., O'Boyle, N.M., Lawlor, M., Gallagher, H.C., Murphy, K.J., Regan, C.M., 2009. Curcumin-induced degradation of PKCδ is associated with enhanced dentate NCAM PSA expression and spatial learning in adult and aged Wistar rats. Biochem. Pharmacol. 77, 1254–1265.

Cunningham, B.A., Hemperly, J.J., Murray, B.A., Prediger, E.A., Brackenbury, R., Edelman, G.M., 1987. Neural cell adhesion molecule: structure, immunoglobulin-like domains, cell surface modulation, and alternative RNA splicing. Science 236, 799–806.

Day, J.J., Sweatt, J.D., 2011. Epigenetic mechanisms in cognition. Neuron 70, 813–829.

Deng, W., Aimone, J.B., Gage, F.H., 2010. New neurons and new memories: how does adult hippocampal neurogenesis affect learning and memory? Nat. Rev. Neurosci. 11, 339–350.

Doherty, P., Fruns, M., Seaton, P., Dickson, G., Barton, C.H., Sears, T.A., Walsh, F.S., 1990. A threshold effect of the major isoforms of NCAM on neurite outgrowth. Nature 343, 464–466.

Doyle, E., Bruce, M.T., Breen, K.C., Smith, D.C., Anderton, B., Regan, C.M., 1990. Intraventricular infusion of antibodies to amyloid-β-protein precursor impair the acquisition of a passive avoidance response in the rat. Neurosci. Lett. 115, 97–102.

Doyle, E., Nolan, P.M., Bell, R., Regan, C.M., 1992a. Neurodevelopmental events underlying information acquisition and storage. Network 3, 89–94.

Doyle, E., Nolan, P., Bell, R., Regan, C.M., 1992b. Intraventricular infusions of anti-neural cell adhesion molecules in a discrete post-training period impair consolidation of a passive avoidance response in the rat. J. Neurochem. 59, 1570–1573.

Doyle, E., Bell, R., Regan, C.M., 1992c. Hippocampal NCAM180 transiently increases sialylation during the acquisition and consolidation of a passive avoidance response in the adult rat. J. Neurosci. Res. 31, 513–523.

Dupret, D., Fabre, A., Döbrössy, M.D., Panatier, A., Rodríguez, J.J., Lamarque, S., Lemaire, V., Oliet, S.H., Piazza, P.V., Abrous, D.N., 2007. Spatial learning depends on both the addition and removal of new hippocampal neurons. PLoS Biol. 5, e214.

Eckhardt, M., Mühlenhoff, M., Bethe, A., Koopman, J., Frosch, M., Gerardy-Schahn, R., 1995. Molecular characterization of eukaryotic polysialyltransferase-1. Nature 373, 715–718.

Eyre, M.D., Richter-Levin, G., Avital, A., Stewart, M.G., 2003. Morphological changes in hippocampal dentate gyrus synapses following spatial learning in rats are transient. Eur. J. Neurosci. 17, 1973–1980.

Finne, J., Finne, U., Deagostini-Bazin, H., Goridis, C., 1983. Occurrence of alpha 2-8 linked polysialosyl units in a neural cell adhesion molecule. Biochem. Biophys. Res. Commun. 112, 482–487.

Florian, C., Foltz, J., Norreel, J.-C., Rougon, G., Roullet, P., 2006. Post-training intrahippocampal injection of synthetic poly-α-2,8-sialic acid-neural cell adhesion molecule mimetic peptide improves spatial long-term performance in mice. Learn Mem. 13, 335–341.

Foley, A.G., Hartz, B.P., Gallagher, H.C., Rønn, L.C.B., Berezin, V., Bock, E., Regan, C.M., 2000. A synthetic peptide ligand of NCAM Ig1 domain prevents NCAM internalization and disrupts passive avoidance learning. J. Neurochem. 74, 2607–2613.

Foley, A.G., Rønn, L.C.B., Murphy, K.J., Regan, C.M., 2003. Distribution of polysialylated neural cell adhesion molecule in the rat septal nuclei and septohippocampal pathway: transient increase of polysialylated cells in sub-triangular septal zone during memory consolidation. J. Neurosci. Res. 74, 807–817.

Foley, A.F., Gannon, S., Rombach-Mullan, N., Prendergast, A., Barry, C., Cassidy, A.W., Regan, C.M., 2012. Class I histone deacetylase inhibition ameliorates social cognition and cell adhesion molecule plasticity deficits in a rodent model of autism spectrum disorders. Neuropharmacology 63, 750–760.

Foley, A.G., Cassidy, A.W., & Regan, C.M., 2014. Pentyl-4-yn-VPA, a histone deacetylase inhibitor, ameliorates deficits in social behavior and cognition in a rodent model of autism spectrum disorders. Eur. J. Pharmacol. 727, 80–86.

Fox, G.B., O'Connell, A.W., Murphy, K.J., Regan, C.M., 1995. Memory consolidation induces a transient and time-dependent increase in the frequency of neural cell adhesion molecule polysialylated cells in the adult rat hippocampus. J. Neurochem. 65, 2796–2799.

Fox, G.B., Fichera, G., Barry, T., O'Connell, A.W., Gallagher, H.C., Murphy, K.J., Regan, C.M., 2000. Consolidation of passive avoidance learning is associated with transient increases of polysialylated neurons in layer II of the rat medial temporal cortex. J. Neurobiol. 45, 135–141.

Fraga, M.F., Ballestar, E., Paz, M.F., Ropero, S., Setien, F., Ballestar, M.L., Heine-Suñer, D., Cigudosa, J.C., Urioste, M., Benitez, J., Boix-Chornet, M., Sanchez-Aguilera, A., Ling, C., Carlsson, E., Poulsen, P., Vaag, A., Stephan, Z., Spector, T.D., Wu, Y.Z., Plass, C., Esteller, M., 2005. Epigenetic differences arise during the lifetime of monozygotic twins. Proc. Natl. Acad. Sci. U.S.A. 102, 10604–10609.

Gallagher, H.C., Murphy, K.J., Foley, A.G., Regan, C.M., 2001. Protein kinase C delta regulates neural cell adhesion molecule polysialylation state in the rat brain. J. Neurochem. 77, 425–434.

Geinisman, Y., Berry, R.W., Disterhoft, J.F., Power, J.M., Van der Zee, E.A., 2001. Associative learning elicits the formation of multiple-synapse boutons. J. Neurosci. 21, 5568–5573.

Grunstein, M., 1997. Histone acetylation in chromatin structure and transcription. Nature 389, 349–352.

Guan, J.S., Haggarty, S.J., Giacometti, E., Dannenberg, J.H., Joseph, N., Gao, J., Nieland, T.J., Zhou, Y., Wang, X., Mazitschek, R., Bradner, J.E., DePinho, R.A., Jaenisch, R., Tsai, L.H., 2009. HDAC2 negatively regulates memory formation and synaptic plasticity. Nature 459, 55–60.

Gupta, S., Kim, S.Y., Artis, S., Molfese, D.L., Schumacher, A., Sweatt, J.D., Paylor, R.E., Lubin, F.D., 2010. Histone methylation regulates memory formation. J. Neurosci. 30, 3589–3599.

Hait, N.C., Allegood, J., Maceyka, M., Strub, G.M., Harikumar, K.B., Singh, S.K., Luo, C., Marmorstein, R., Kordula, T., Milstien, S., Spiegel, S., 2009. Regulation of histone acetylation in the nucleus by sphingosine-1-phosphate. Science 325, 1254–1257.

Haldane, J.J., 1983. Aquinas on sense-perception. Phil. Rev. XCII, 233–239.

Hebb, D.O., 1949. The Organization of Behaviour: A Neuropsychological Theory. Wiley.

Hoeffer, C.A., Cowansage, K.K., Arnold, E.C., Banko, J.L., Moerke, N.J., Rodriguez, R., Schmidt, E.K., Klosi, E., Chorev, M., Lloyd, R.E., Pierre, P., Wagner, G., LeDoux, J.E., Klann, E., 2011. Inhibition of the interactions between eukaryotic initiation factor 4E and 4G impairs long-term associative memory consolidation but not reconsolidation. Proc. Natl. Acad. Sci. U.S.A. 108, 3383–3388.

Holtmaat, A., Wilbrecht, L., Knott, G.W., Welker, E., Svoboda, K., 2006. Experience-dependent and cell-type-specific spine growth in the neocortex. Nature 441, 979–983.

Howe, M.W., Tierney, P.L., Sandberg, S.G., Phillips, P.E., Graybiel, A.M., 2013. Prolonged dopamine signalling in striatum signals proximity and value of distant rewards. Nature 500, 575–579.

von Hertzen, L.S.I., Giese, K.P., 2005. Memory reconsolidation engages only a subset of immediate-early genes induced during consolidation. J. Neurosci. 25, 1935–1942.

Hoyk, Zs., Parducz, A., Theodosis, D.T., 2001. The highly sialylated isoform of the neural cell adhesion molecule is required for estradiol-induced morphological plasticity in the adult arcuate nucleus. Eur. J. Neurosci. 13, 649–656.

Huttenlocher, P.R., 1979. Synaptic density in human frontal cortex - developmental changes and effects of aging. Brain Res. 163, 195–205.

Ito, R., Robbins, T.W., Pennartz, C.M., Everitt, B.J., 2008. Functional interaction between the hippocampus and nucleus accumbens shell is necessary for the acquisition of appetitive spatial context conditioning. J. Neurosci. 28, 6950–6959.

Jørgensen, O.S., Bock, E., 1974. Brain specific synaptosomal membrane proteins demonstrated by crossed immunoelectrophoresis. J. Neurochem. 23, 879–880.

Kazantsev, A.G., Thompson, L.M., 2008. Therapeutic application of histone deacetylase inhibitors for central nervous system disorders. Nat. Rev. Drug Discov. 7, 854–868.

Kiss, J.Z., Wang, C., Olive, S., Rougon, G., Lang, J., Baetens, D., Harry, D., Pralong, W.F., 1994. Activity-dependent mobilization of the adhesion molecule polysialic NCAM to the cell surface of neurons and endocrine cells. EMBO J. 13, 5284–5292.

Kitanishi, T., Ikegaya, Y., Matsuki, N., 2009. Behaviorally evoked transient reorganization of hippocampal spines. Eur. J. Neurosci. 30, 560–566.

van Kesteren, M.T., Rijpkema, M., Ruiter, D.J., Fernández, G., 2010. Retrieval of associative information congruent with prior knowledge is related to increased medial prefrontal activity and connectivity. J. Neurosci. 30, 15888–15894.

Knafo, S., Venero, C., Sánchez-Puelles, C., Pereda-Peréz, I., Franco, A., Sandi, C., Suárez, L.M., Solís, J.M., Alonso-Nanclares, L., Martín, E.D., Merino-Serrais, P., Borcel, E., Li, S., Chen, Y., Gonzalez-Soriano, J., Berezin, V., Bock, E., Defelipe, J., Esteban, J.A., 2012. Facilitation of AMPA receptor synaptic delivery as a molecular mechanism for cognitive enhancement. PLoS Biol. 10 (2), e1001262.

Knafo, S., Barkai, E., Herrero, A.I., Libersat, F., Sandi, C., Venero, C., 2005. Olfactory learning-related NCAM expression is state, time, and location specific and is correlated with individual learning capabilities. Hippocampus 15, 316–325.

Kochlamazashvili, G., Senkov, O., Grebenyuk, S., Robinson, C., Xiao, M.-F., Stummeyer, K., Gerardy-Schahn, R., Engel, A.K., Feig, L., Semynaov, A., Suppiramaniam, V., Schachner, M., Dityatev, A., 2010. Neural cell adhesion molecule-associated polysialic acid regulates synaptic plasticity and learning by restraining the signaling through gluN2B-containing NMDA receptors. J. Neurosci. 30, 4171–4183.

Korzus, E., Rosenfeld, M.G., Mayford, M., 2004. CBP histone acetyltransferase activity is a critical component of memory consolidation. Neuron 42, 961–972.

Koshibu, K., Gräff, J., Beullens, M., Heitz, F.D., Berchtold, D., Russig, H., Farinelli, M., Bollen, M., Mansuy, I.M., 2009. Protein phosphatase 1 regulates the histone code for long-term memory. J. Neurosci. 29, 13079–13089.

Krushel, L.A., Cunningham, B.A., Edelman, G.M., Crossin, K.L., 1999. NF-κB activity is induced by neural cell adhesion molecule binding to neurons and astrocytes. J. Biol. Chem. 274, 2432–2439.

Lampen, A., Grimaldi, P.A., Nau, H., 2005. Modulation of peroxisome proliferator-activated receptor delta activity affects neural cell adhesion molecule and polysialyltransferase ST8SiaIV induction by teratogenic valproic acid analogs in F9 cell differentiation. Mol. Pharmacol. 68, 193–203.

Lee, J.L., Everitt, B.J., Thomas, K.L., 2004. Independent cellular processes for hippocampal memory consolidation and reconsolidation. Science 304, 839–843.

Leuner, B., Falduto, J., Shors, T.J., 2003. Associative memory formation increases the observation of dendritic spines in the hippocampus. J. Neurosci. 23, 659–665.

Li, S., Cullen, W.K., Anwyl, R., Rowan, M.J., 2003. Dopamine-dependent facilitation of LTP induction in hippocampal CA1 by exposure to spatial novelty. Nat. Neurosci. 6, 526–531.

Lichtman, J.W., Colman, H., 2000. Synapse elimination and indelible memory. Neuron 25, 269–278.

Livingston, B.D., Paulson, J.C., 1993. Polymerase chain reaction cloning of a developmentally regulated member of the sialyltransferase gene family. J. Biol. Chem. 268, 11504–11507.

Lopez-Fernandez, M.A., Montaron, M.-F., Varea, E., Rougon, G., Venero, C., Abrous, D.N., Sandi, C., 2007. Upregulation of polysialylated neural cell adhesion molecule in the dorsal hippocampus after ontextual fear conditioning is involved in long-term memory formation. J. Neurosci. 27, 4552–4561.

Luo, A.H., Tahsili-Fahadan, P., Wise, R.A., Lupica, C.R., Aston-Jones, G., 2011. Linking context with reward: a functional circuit from hippocampal CA3 to ventral tegmental area. Science 333, 353–357.

Mayford, M., Barzilai, A., Keller, F., Schacher, S., Kandel, E.R., 1992. Modulation of an NCAM-related adhesion molecule with long-term synaptic plasticity in Aplysia. Science 256, 638–644.

Marcus, E.A., Emptage, N.J., Marois, R., Carew, T.J., 1994. A comparison of the mechanistic relationships between development and learning in Aplysia. Prog. Brain Res. 100, 179–188.

Marrone, D.F., 2007. Ultrastructural plasticity associated with hippocampal-dependent learning: a meta-analysis. Neurobiol. Learn Mem. 87, 361–371.

McClelland, J.L., McNaughton, B.L., O'Reilly, R.C., 1995. Why there are complementary learning systems in the hippocampus and neocortex: insights from the successes and failures of connectionist models of learning and memory. Psychol. Rev. 102, 419–457.

Mezey, S., Doyère, V., De Souza, I., Harrison, E., Cambon, K., Kendal, C.E., Davies, H., Laroche, S., Stewart, M.G., 2004. Long-term synaptic morphometry changes after induction of long-term potentiation and long-term depression in the dentate gyrus of awake rats are not simply mirror phenomena. Eur. J. Neurosci. 19, 2310–2318.

Miller, C.A., Campbell, S.L., Sweatt, J.D., 2008. DNA methylation and histone acetylation work in concert to regulate memory formation and synaptic plasticity. Neurobiol. Learn Mem. 89, 599–603.

Montague, P.R., Dayan, P., Sejnowski, T.J., 1996. A framework for mesencephalic dopamine systems based on predictive Hebbian learning. J. Neurosci. 16, 1936–1947.

Morquecho-León, M.A., Bazúa-Valenti, S., Romero-Ávila, M.T., García-Sáinz, J.A., 2014. Isoforms of protein kinase C involved in phorbol ester-induced sphingosine 1-phosphate receptor 1 phosphorylation and desensitization. Biochim. Biophys. Acta 1843, 327–334.

Morris, R.G.M., Inglis, J., Ainge, J.A., Olverman, H.J., Tulloch, J., Dudai, Y., Kelly, P.A., 2006. Memory reconsolidation: sensitivity of spatial memory to inhibition of protein synthesis in dorsal hippocampus during encoding and retrieval. Neuron 50, 479–489.

Moser, M.B., Trommald, M., Andersen, P., 1994. An increase in dendritic spine density on hippocampal CA1 pyramidal cells following spatial learning in adult rats suggests the formation of new synapses. Proc. Natl. Acad. Sci. U.S.A. 91, 12673–12675.

Muller, D., Djebbara-Hannas, Z., Jourdain, P., Vutskits, L., Durbec, P., Rougon, G., Kiss, J.Z., 2000. Brain-derived neurotrophic factor restores long-term potentiation in polysialic acid-neural cell adhesion molecule-deficient hippocampus. Proc. Natl. Acad. Sci. U.S.A. 97, 4315–4320.

Murphy, K.J., Foley, A.G., O'Connell, A., Regan, C.M., 2006. Chronic exposure of rats to cognition enhancing drugs produces a neuroplastic response identical to that obtained by complex environment rearing. Neuropsychopharmacology 31, 93–100.

Murphy, K.J., O'Connell, A.W., Regan, C.M., 1996. Repetitive and transient increases in hippocampal neural cell adhesion molecule polysialylation state following multi-trial spatial training. J. Neurochem. 67, 1268–1274.

Murphy, K.J., Regan, C.M., 1999. Sequential training in separate paradigms impairs second task consolidation and learning-associated modulations of hippocampal NCAM polysialylation. Neurobiol. Learn. Mem. 72, 28–38.

Nadel, L., Moscovitch, M., 1997. Memory consolidation, retrograde amnesia and the hippocampal complex. Curr. Opin. Neurobiol. 7, 217–227.

Nolan, P.M., Bell, R., Regan, C.M., 1987. Acquisition of a brief behavioural experience in the rat is inhibited by a brain-specific monoclonal antibody, F3-87-8. Neurosci. Lett. 79, 346–350.

Nottebohm, F., Liu, W.-C., 2010. The origins of vocal learning: new sounds, new circuits, new cells. Brain Lang. 115, 3–17.

O'Connell, A.W., Fox, G.B., Murphy, K.J., Fichera, G., Kelly, J., Regan, C.M., 1997. Spatial learning activates neural cell adhesion molecule polysialylation in a cortico-hippocampal pathway within the medial temporal lobe. J. Neurochem. 68, 2538–2546.

O'Keefe, J., Recce, M.L., 1993. Phase relationship between hippocampal place units and the EEG theta rhythm. Hippocampus 3, 317–330.

O'Malley, A., O'Connell, C., Regan, C.M., 1998. Ultrastructural analysis reveals avoidance conditioning to induce a transient increase in hippocampal dentate spine density in the 6h post-training period of consolidation. Neuroscience 87, 607–613.

O'Malley, A., O'Connell, C., Murphy, K.J., Regan, C.M., 2000. Transient spine density increases in the mid-molecular layer of hippocampal dentate gyrus accompany consolidation of a spatial learning task in the rodent. Neuroscience 99, 229–232.

Paratcha, G., Ledda, F., Ibáñez, C.F., 2003. The neural cell adhesion molecule NCAM is an alternative signaling receptor for GDNF family ligands. Cell 113, 867–879.

Persohn, E., Pollerberg, G.E., Schachner, M., 1989. Immunoelectron-microscopic localization of the 180 kD component of the neural cell adhesion molecule N-CAM in postsynaptic membranes. J. Comp. Neurol. 288, 92–100.

Pham, K., McEwen, B.S., LeDoux, J.E., Nader, K., 2005. Fear learning transiently impairs hippocampal cell proliferation. Neuroscience 130, 17–24.

Pollerberg, G.E., Schachner, M., Davoust, J., 1986. Differentiation state-dependent surface mobilities of two forms of the neural cell adhesion molecule. Nature 324, 462–465.

Prosser, R.A., Rutishauser, U., Ungers, G., Fedorkova, L., Glass, J.D., 2003. Intrinsic role of polysialylated neural cell adhesion molecule in photic phase resetting of the mammalian circadian clock. J. Neurosci. 23, 652–658.

Ramocki, M.B., Zoghbi, H.Y., 2008. Failure of neuronal homeostasis results in common neuropsychiatric phenotypes. Nature 455, 912–918.

Razin, A., Riggs, A.D., 1980. DNA methylation and gene function. Science 210, 604–610.

Redondo, R.L., Morris, R.G.M., 2011. Making memories last: the synaptic tagging and capture hypothesis. Nat. Rev. Neurosci. 12, 17–30.

Regan, C.M., 2014. Decisions, dopamine, and degeneracy in complex biological systems. Neurosci. Neuroeconomics 3, 11–18.

Ribot, T.A., 1882. Diseases of Memory. Appleton-Century-Crofts, New York.

Rodriguez-Ortiz, C.J., Garcia De La Torre, P., Benavidez, E., Ballesteros, M.A., Bermudez-Rattoni, F., 2008. Intrahippocampal anisomycin infusions disrupt previously consolidated spatial memory only when memory is updated. Neurobiol. Learn. Mem. 89, 352–359.

Rolls, E.T., Kesner, R.P., 2006. A computational theory of hippocampal function, and empirical tests of the theory. Prog. Neurobiol. 79, 1–48.

Roos, J., Kelly, R.B., 2000. Preassembly and transport of nerve terminals: a new concept of axonal transport. Nat. Neurosci. 3, 415–417.

Rossato, J.I., Bevilaqua, L.R., Izquierdo, I., Medina, J.H., Cammarota, M., 2009. Dopamine controls persistence of long-term memory storage. Science 325, 1017–1020.

Samaco, R.C., Neul, J.L., 2011. Complexities of Rett syndrome and MeCP2. J. Neurosci. 31, 7951–7959.

Sandi, C., Cordero, M.I., Merino, J.J., Kruyt, N.D., Regan, C.M., Murphy, K.J., 2004. Neurobiological and endocrine correlates of individual differences in spatial learning ability. Learn. Mem. 11, 244–252.

Schmitt, W.B., Sprengel, R., Mack, V., Draft, R.W., Seeburg, P.H., Deacon, R.M., Rawlins, J.N., Bannerman, D.M., 2005. Restoration of spatial working memory by genetic rescue of GluR-A-deficient mice. Nat. Neurosci. 11, 270–272.

Schuch, U., Lohse, M.J., Schachner, M., 1989. Neural cell adhesion molecules influence second messenger systems. Neuron 3, 13–20.

Schultz, W., Dayan, P., Montague, P.R., 1997. A neural substrate of prediction and reward. Science 275, 1593–1599.

Schuster, C.M., Davis, G.W., Fetter, R.D., Goodman, C.S., 1996. Genetic dissection of structural and functional components of synaptic plasticity. I. Fasciclin II controls synaptic stabilization and growth. Neuron 17, 641–654.

Scully, D., Fedriani, R., DeSouza, I.E.J., Murphy, K.J., Regan, C.M., 2012. Regional dissociation of paradigm-specific synapse remodelling during memory consolidation in the adult rat dentate gyrus. Neuroscience 209, 74–83.

Seki, T., 2002. Hippocampal neurogenesis occurs in a microenvironment provided by PSA-NCAM-expressing immature neurons. J. Neurosci. Res. 69, 772–783.

Senkov, O., Sun, M., Weinhold, B., Gerardy-Schahn, R., Schachner, M., Dityatev, A., 2006. Polysialylated neural cell adhesion molecule is involved in induction of long-term potentiation and memory acquisition and consolidation in a fear-conditioning paradigm. J. Neurosci. 26, 10888–109898.

Seymour, C.M., Foley, A.G., Murphy, K.J., Regan, C.M., 2008. Intraventricular infusions of anti-NCAM PSA impair the process of consolidation of both avoidance conditioning and spatial learning paradigms in Wistar rats. Neuroscience 157, 813–820.

Skaggs, W.E., McNaughton, B.L., Wilson, M.A., Barnes, C.A., 1996. Theta phase precession in hippocampal neuronal populations and the compression of temporal sequences. Hippocampus 6, 149–172.

Sutton, R., Barto, A., 1998. Reinforcement Learning. MIT Press, Cambridge (MA).

Sytnyk, V., Leshchyns'ka, I., Delling, M., Dityateva, G., Dityatev, A., Schachner, M., 2002. Neural cell adhesion molecule promotes accumulation of TGN organelles at sites of neuron-to-neuron contacts. J. Cell Biol. 159, 649–661.

Tanzi, E., 1893. I fatti i le induzione nell'odierna istologia del sistema nervoso. Riv Sper Freniatr Med. Leg Alienazioni Ment. 19, 419–472.

Thiery, J.-P., Brackenbury, T., Rutishauser, U., Edelman, G.M., 1977. Adhesion among neural cells of the chick embryo: II Purfication and characterisation of a cell adhesion molecule from neural retina. J. Biol. Chem. 252, 6841–6845.

Toni, N., Buchs, P.A., Nikonenko, I., Bron, C.R., Muller, D., 1999. LTP promotes formation of multiple spine synapses between a single axon terminal and a dendrite. Nature 402, 421–425.

Toni, N., Buchs, P.A., Nikonenko, I., Povilaitite, P., Parisi, L., Muller, D., 2001. Remodeling of synaptic membranes after induction of long-term potentiation. J. Neurosci. 21, 6245–6251.

Toni, N., Teng, E.M., Bushong, E.A., Aimone, J.B., Zhao, C., Consiglio, A., et al., 2007. Synapse formation on neurons born in the adult hippocampus. Nat. Neurosci. 10, 727–734.

Torregrossa, P., Buhl, L., Bancila, M., Durbec, P., Schafer, C., Schachner, M., Rougon, G., 2004. Selection of poly-α-2,8-sialic acid mimotopes from a random phage peptide library and analysis of their bioactivity. J. Biol. Chem. 279, 30707–30714.

Tsankova, N., Renthal, W., Kumar, A., Nestler, E.J., 2007. Epigenetic regulation in psychiatric disorders. Nat. Rev. Neurosci. 8, 355–367.

Tse, D., Langston, R.F., Kakeyama, M., Bethus, I., Spooner, P.A., Wood, E.R., et al., 2007. Schemas and memory consolidation. Science 316, 76–82.

Tse, D., Takeuchi, T., Kakeyama, M., Kajii, Y., Okuno, H., Tohyama, C., et al., 2011. Schema-dependent gene activation and memory encoding in neocortex. Science 333, 891–895.

Tyler, W.J., Pozzo-Miller, L., 2003. Miniature synaptic transmission and BDNF modulate dendritic spine growth and form in rat CA1 neurones. J. Physiol. 553, 497–509.

Vaughn, J.E., 1989. Fine structure of synaptogenesis in the vertebrate central nervous system. Synapse 3, 255–285.

Vecsey, C.G., Hawk, J.D., Lattal, K.M., Stein, J.M., Fabian, S.A., Attner, M.A., et al., 2007. Histone deacetylase inhibitors enhance memory and synaptic plasticity via CREB: CBP-dependent transcriptional activation. J. Neurosci. 27, 6128–6140.

Venero, C., Herrero, A.I., Touyarot, K., Cambon, K., López-Fernández, M.A., Berezin, V., et al., 2006. Hippocampal up-regulation of NCAM expression and polysialylation plays a key role on spatial memory. Eur. J. Neurosci. 23, 1585–1595.

Waddington, C.H., 1957. The Strategy of the Genes: A Discussion of Some Aspects of Theoretical Biology. Allen & Unwin, London.

Weaver, I.C., Cervoni, N., Champagne, F.A., D'Alessio, A.C., Sharma, S., Seckl, J.R., et al., 2004. Epigenetic programming by maternal behavior. Nat. Neurosci. 7, 847–854.

Wong, C.C., Caspi, A., Williams, B., Craig, I.W., Houts, R., Ambler, A., et al., 2010. A longitudinal study of epigenetic variation in twins. Epigenetics 5, 516–526.

Wood, M.A., Attner, M.A., Oliveira, A.M., Brindle, P.K., Abel, T., 2006. A transcription factor-binding domain of the coactivator CBP is essential for long-term memory and the expression of specific target genes. Learn. Mem. 13, 609–617.

Wosiski-Kuhn, M., Stranahan, A.M., 2012. Transient increases in dendritic spine density contribute to dentate gyrus long-term potentiation. Synapse 66, 661–664.

Xu, T., Yu, X., Perlik, A.J., Tobin, W.F., Zweig, J.A., Tennant, K., et al., 2009. Rapid formation and selective stabilization of synapses for enduring motor memories. Nature 462, 915–919.

Yang, P., Yin, X., Rutishauser, U., 1992. Intercellular space is affected by the polysialic acid content of NCAM. J. Cell Biol. 116, 1487–1496.

Yang, G., Pan, F., Gan, W.-B., 2009. Stably maintained dendritic spines are associated with lifelong memories. Nature 462, 920–924.

Yeh, S.H., Lin, C.H., Gean, P.W., 2004. Acetylation of nuclear factor-kappaB in rat amygdala improves long-term but not short-term retention of fear memory. Mol. Pharmacol. 65, 1286–1292.

Zamanillo, D., Sprengel, R., Hvalby, O., Jensen, V., Burnashev, N., Rozov, A., et al., 1999. Importance of AMPA receptors for hippocampal synaptic plasticity but not for spatial learning. Science 284, 1805–1811.

Zhou, Z., Hong, E.J., Cohen, S., Zhao, W.N., Ho, H.Y., Schmidt, L., et al., 2006. Brain-specific phosphorylation of MeCP2 regulates activity-dependent *Bdnf* transcription, dendritic growth, and spine maturation. Neuron 52, 255–269.

Ziv, N.E., Garner, C.C., 2004. Cellular and molecular mechanisms of presynaptic assembly. Nat. Rev. Neurosci. 5, 385–399.

Ziv, N.E., Ahissar, E., 2009. New tricks and old spines. Nature 462, 859–861.

Chapter 5

Transgenic Mice with Enhanced Cognition

Yong-Seok Lee
Department of Life Science, College of Natural Science, Chung-Ang University, Seoul, Republic of Korea

Genetic engineering technology along with the classical pharmacological approaches allows scientists to study the role of specific molecules implicated in cognitive functions such as learning and memory at multiple levels. Since the introduction of knock-out technique to neuroscience field in the early 1990s (Grant et al., 1992; Silva et al., 1992a,b), a number of genetically engineered mice have been generated and their cognitive functions have been tested (Anagnostopoulos et al., 2001; Bolivar et al., 2000; Matynia et al., 2002). Now, a PubMed search with the keywords "mutant mice and learning" yields more than 1500 publications. Most of those mutations result in deficits in cognitive functions. However, it is fascinating to find that there are many transgenic/knock-out mice with enhanced cognition (Lee and Silva, 2009). In this chapter, mutant mice that show better performance in several well-characterized learning and memory-related behavioral tasks were classified into several groups according to the affected signal transduction pathways (Table 5.1). I also briefly summarize how each genetic manipulation affects synaptic plasticity.

GENERATING MUTANT MICE

Simple forms of mutant mice can be generated with the targeted disruption (knock-out) or overexpression (transgenenic) of gene of interests. To derive transgenic mice, the pronucleus of fertilized eggs is injected with the gene of interest expressed under the regulation of an appropriate promoter. The injected eggs are implanted into the oviduct of a surrogate mother. Some of the resulting progeny exhibit germline transformation and their offspring also contain the transgene. In this simple transgenic method, the injected DNA integrates at a random position in the genome. In contrast, knock-out mice are generated by introducing the targeted mutation into embryonic stem (ES) cells by site-specific recombination mechanisms. Then, the ES cells with successful recombination are selected and introduced into the normal blastocysts to derive mice lines with the targeted mutation. The knock-out

Cognitive Enhancement. http://dx.doi.org/10.1016/B978-0-12-417042-1.00005-X
87

TABLE 5.1 List of Mutant Mice with Enhanced Memory

Signaling Pathway	Mutant Mice[a]	References
NMDA receptors	NR2B *Tg*, KIF17 *Tg*, Cdk5 KO, p25 *Tg* (transient), ORL1 KO	Fischer et al. (2005), Hawasli et al. (2007), Manabe et al. (1998), Tang et al. (1999), Wong et al. (2002)
CREB and its related molecules	CREB-y134F *Tg*, CREB-DIEDML *Tg*, GCN2 KO, EGFP-AZIP *Tg*, eIF2α$^{+/S51A}$ KI, CaMKIV *Tg*, AC1 *Tg*, PDE4D KO, PDE8B KO, calcineurin CI, PP1 CI	Chen et al. (2003), Costa-Mattioli et al. (2005), Costa-Mattioli et al. (2007), Fukushima et al. (2008), Genoux et al. (2002), Li et al. (2011), Malleret et al. (2001), Suzuki et al. (2011), Tsai et al. (2012)
Translational regulations	PAIP2A KO, FKBP12 KO	Hoeffer et al. (2008), Khoutorsky et al. (2013)
Epigenetic regulations	HDAC2 KO	Guan et al. (2009)
Excitation and inhibition	GABAAR α4 KO, MAGL KO, PKR KO, GABAAR α5 KO, GRPR KO, BEC1 KO, Kvβ1.1 KO	Collinson et al. (2002), Miyake et al. (2009), Moore et al. (2010), Murphy et al. (2004), Pan et al. (2011), Shumyatsky et al. (2002), Zhu et al. (2011)
MicroRNA	Dicer1 KO	Konopka et al. (2010)
Extracellular factors	MMP-9 *Tg*, tPA *Tg*, HB-GAM *Tg*	(Fragkouli et al. (2012), Madani et al. (1999), Pavlov et al. (2002)

Tg, transgenic; KO, knock-out; KI, knock-in; CI, conditional inhibition.
[a]*Not all the mice in this table are mentioned in the text.*

method can be modified to target specific gene domains or even specific base pairs (knock-in). Early studies with the α-calcium-calmodulin–dependent protein kinase II (αCaMKII) knock-out (Silva et al., 1992a,b) and the tyrosine kinase Fyn knock-out mice (Grant et al., 1992) demonstrated that the knock-out techniques combined with behavioral and electrophysiological assays provide a unique opportunity to study the cellular and molecular mechanism of cognition.

In addition to these simple methods, advanced techniques were developed to temporally and spatially regulate the expression of transgenes or the deletion of target genes (Matynia et al., 2002; Mayford and Kandel, 1999). Using cell-type specific promoters in the transgenic vector allows the expression of transgenes in desired cell types such as excitatory neurons or inhibitory neurons. Also, the Cre-loxP system was used to gain spatial-specificity in knock-out mice (Tsien et al., 1996a). For example, a transgenic mouse expressing Cre recombinase of which expression is driven by αCaMKII promoter can be crossed with another mouse line harboring a loxP-flanked target gene to delete this target gene only in principal neurons of the postnatal forebrain.

Temporal control of transgene expression was achieved by employing the tetracycline system (Mayford et al., 1996). Tetracycline-controlled transactivator (tTA) can be expressed under control of the αCaMKII promoter to gain a spatial control and doxycycline is used to temporally turn on or off the transgene expression (Matynia et al., 2002; Mayford et al., 1996; Mayford and Kandel, 1999). More recently, chemical-regulated transgene expression was demonstrated as another useful tool to investigate the role of specific genes in animal models. For example, a target protein fused with the ligand-binding domain (LBDm) of a modified estrogen receptor can be activated by tamoxifen treatment at specific times (Kida et al., 2002). Furthermore, combined with these genetic tools, using various viral vectors provides more options for manipulating gene expression with higher spatial and temporal resolution in specific cell types in specific brain areas.

SYNAPTIC PLASTICITY AND MEMORY

Investigating the mechanisms of synaptic plasticity largely relies on the belief that our experiences from daily life including learning are encoded into persisting memories by long-lasting changes in synaptic strength in the brain. This idea has been initially proposed by Donald Hebb, who proposed that synaptic connections between neurons that are repeatedly coactivated during learning are strengthened, and that these changes in synapses serves as a cellular basis of learning and memory. Indeed, Bliss and Lomo found the activity-dependent long-lasting synaptic change in the dentate gyrus of the hippocampus in 1973 (Bliss and Gardner-Medwin, 1973; Bliss and Lomo, 1973). The idea that long-term synaptic plasticity is the cellular mechanism of learning and memory has been supported and also challenged by numerous studies (Bliss and Collingridge, 1993; Eichenbaum, 1996; Malenka and Nicoll, 1999; Matynia et al., 2002; Silva, 2003). However, recent studies strongly suggest that such a long-lasting change, long-term potentiation (LTP), is induced by learning in the hippocampus and amygdala (McKernan and Shinnick-Gallagher, 1997; Rogan et al., 1997; Whitlock et al., 2006).

It has been shown that both positive and negative regulators play critical roles in synaptic plasticity (Abel et al., 1998; Kandel, 2001). For example, the activations of several protein kinases such as of αCaMKII, protein kinase A (PKA), and mitogen-activated protein kinase (MAPK) promote the induction of LTP, whereas a set of phosphatases including protein phosphatase-1 (PP-1) repress the LTP (Malenka and Nicoll, 1999). Turning off the positive regulators of LTP,

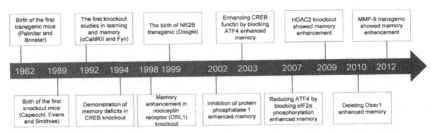

FIGURE 5.1 Timeline for the critical discoveries in the studies of smart mutants.

for example by genetic deletion of αCaMKII, impaired spatial learning and hippocampal LTP (Silva et al., 1992a,b). On the other hand, the overexpression of components of synaptic plasticity such as *N*-methyl-D-aspartate (NMDA) receptor subtype NR2B enhanced learning and memory (Tang et al., 1999). Accordingly, there have been many attempts to enhance memory by shifting the balance in favor of the induction of LTP either by augmenting the positive signaling or by removing the inhibitory constraints as reviewed next (Figure 5.1).

ENHANCING COGNITION BY AUGMENTING NMDA RECEPTOR FUNCTION

Activation of NMDA receptors (NMDARs) and subsequent Ca^{2+} influx activates a variety of signaling molecules including αCaMKII (Figure 5.2) (Lisman et al., 2002; Malenka and Nicoll, 1999; Sanes and Lichtman, 1999; Silva, 2003). The critical roles of NMDA receptors in memory and synaptic plasticity have been extensively addressed through genetic and pharmacological manipulations (Bliss and Collingridge, 1993; Matynia et al., 2002). In the 1980s, a classical study performed by Morris and his colleagues showed that intraventricular infusion of NMDAR blocker AP5 impaired spatial learning and LTP (Morris et al., 1986). A decade later, this finding was reinvestigated by using elegant gene knock-out technology. Hippocampal CA1-specific deletion of NR1, an obligatory subunit for channel function, impaired LTP and spatial memory without confounding nonspatial learning ability (Tsien et al., 1996b). More recently, hippocampal subregion-specific deletion of NR1 in CA3 and dentate gyrus also impaired different aspects of memory (McHugh et al., 2007; Nakazawa et al., 2002, 2003). In addition to NR1, NMDARs require other subunits including NR2 (A, B, C, and D) and NR3 (A and B) with their compositions change during development (Monyer et al., 1992, 1994; Sheng et al., 1994). Deleting NR2A, which is the dominantly expressed NR2 subunit in the adult brain, also resulted in deficits in hippocampal LTP and hippocampus-dependent learning tasks (Kiyama et al., 1998; Sakimura et al., 1995). While its expression is decreased during the development, the duration of NR2B-mediated current is longer than that of NR2A, which can allow more Ca^{2+} influx through NMDA receptor (Monyer et al., 1994). However, the learning and memory could not be examined in NR2B-deficient mice since they died shortly after birth (Kutsuwada et al., 1996).

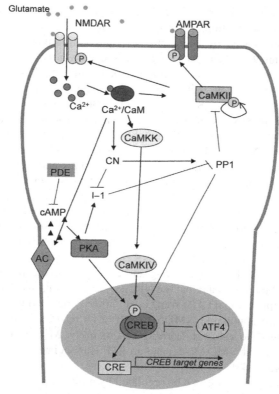

FIGURE 5.2   NMDA receptor–dependent signaling pathways in the postsynaptic neuron.
Ca^{2+} influx through the N-methyl-D-aspartate (NMDA) receptors (NMDARs) activates a variety of
signaling molecules including α-calcium-calmodulin–dependent protein kinase II (αCaMKII) and
protein kinase A (PKA). Activations of these signaling cascades eventually turn on the transcription factor, cAMP responsive element binding protein (CREB), in the nucleus. The detailed roles
of these molecules in LTP and learning are described in the text. AMPAR, α-amino-3-hydroxy-
5-methyl-4-isoxazolepropionic acid receptor; CaM, calmodulin; CaMKK, calcium-calmodulin–
dependent protein kinase kinase; CN, calcineurin; I-1, inhibitor-1; PP1, protein phosphatase 1;
PDE, phosphodiesterase; AC, adenylyl cyclase; CaMKIV, calcium-calmodulin–dependent protein
kinase IV; ATF4, Activating transcription factor 4; CRE, cAMP-responsive element. (This figure is
reproduced in color in the color plate section.)

To investigate the role of NR2B in memory and synaptic plasticity, Tsien
and his collaborators overexpressed NR2B in the mouse forebrain, which
resulted in the birth of the "smart" mice, *doogie* (Tang et al., 1999). The prolonged NMDAR activation led to the enhancement of LTP in the transgenic
mice hippocampus, which is consistent with the finding from juvenile brain
in which NR2B expression is higher than the adult (Harris and Teyler, 1984).
Moreover, *doogie* were superior in several learning and memory tasks. First, the
transgenic mice showed better performance than their wild-type littermates in

the hidden-platform version of water maze which is a spatial task that requires intact hippocampal functions (Morris et al., 1982). Second, associative forms of memory were tested by using classic fear conditioning. As described in detail in Chapter 9, in this task, animals associate a nonaversive conditioned stimulus such as tone or context with an aversive unconditioned stimulus like an electric shock on their feet to develop a range of conditioned responses (Kim and Fanselow, 1992; Kim et al., 1992). Both contextual and cued fear memory were found to be enhanced in *doogie* mice. In addition, fear extinction, which is NMDAR dependent and thought to be another form of active learning (Walker and Davis, 2002), was also facilitated in NR2B mutant. A recent follow-up study showed that this superiority of learning and memory is retained in aged transgenic mice, too (Cao et al., 2007). The memory enhancing effect of NR2B overexpresion was not limited to the hippocampus-dependent tasks. NR2B transgenic mice also showed enhanced working memory function in delay non-match-to-place T-maze task (Cui et al., 2011). Similar to the findings in the hippocampus, cortical LTP was also enhanced in NR2B mutant mice (Cui et al., 2011). To demonstrate that the NR2B serves as a rate-limiting molecule in memory in multiple species, Wang and colleagues overexpressed NR2B in the forebrain of rat and found that the NR2B transgenic rats also show enhanced memory and hippocampal LTP (Wang et al., 2009). These studies demonstrated that either NR2B containing NMDAR itself or its related signaling molecules can be the targets to enhance learning and memory. Moreover, these studies support the idea that NMDAR-dependent LTP is associated with memory in a set of behavioral tasks.

The function of proteins can be regulated by multiple post-translational regulations such as covalent modifications, subcellular localization, and degradation. The trafficking of glutamate receptors from the cytoplasm to synaptic sites play important roles in LTP and learning and memory (Malinow and Malenka, 2002; Rumpel et al., 2005). NR2B was shown to be transported along microtubules by a neuron-specific motor protein KIF17 (Setou et al., 2000). To investigate the role of the motor protein of NR2B, Wong and colleagues generated transgenic mice overexpressing KIF17 and found that the transgenic showed better performance in water maze and working memory tasks (Wong et al., 2002). Interestingly, both the mRNA and protein level of NR2B were found to be increased although the amount of NR2B in synaptic sites were not directly examined in the transgenic mice. Moreover, the phosphorylation of cAMP-responsive element binding protein (CREB) was also increased. Evidence from cultured neuron transfected with a dominant negative form of KIF17 supports that KIF17 is involved in delivering NR2B to synapses, suggesting enhanced transport of NR2B could be attributed, at least to some degree, to the enhanced learning ability (Guillaud et al., 2003).

The degradation of NMDA receptors can be regulated by Ca^{2+}-dependent protease calpain (Dong et al., 2006; Simpkins et al., 2003; Wu et al., 2005). Calpain is activated by Ca^{2+} entering through NMDARs and rapidly cleaves

NMDAR subunits, which are clustered with the scaffolding protein complex containing PSD-95, and this cleavage results in the decrease of functional NMDAR (Husi et al., 2000; Simpkins et al., 2003). Recently, conditional knock-out mice of cyclin-dependent kinase 5 (Cdk5) were generated to address the role of Cdk5 in learning and memory (Hawasli et al., 2007). Deletion of Cdk5 in adult mouse forebrain improved contextual fear conditioning, fear extinction, reversal water maze learning, and LTP. Interestingly, loss of Cdk5 reduced NR2B degradation, which results in the augmentation of NMDAR-mediated currents. It was suggested that, in addition to its kinase activity, physical interactions of Cdk5 with NR2B and calpain play an important role in regulating proteolysis of NR2B, which can control synaptic plasticity and learning.

Since Cdk5 has a variety of substrates and also binds to many different cofactors, the role of Cdk5 in learning and memory was not clear (Angelo et al., 2006; Hawasli and Bibb, 2007). Chronic activation of p25, a strong activator of Cdk5 caused neuronal loss in the cortex and hippocampus and severely impaired learning and synaptic plasticity (Cruz et al., 2003; Fischer et al., 2005). However, transient expression of p25 in mice forebrain enhanced synaptic plasticity and hippocampus-dependent memory including contextual fear conditioning and water maze (Fischer et al., 2005). Interestingly, the number of dendritic spines and synapses were also increased by transient activation of p25 (Fischer et al., 2005). To investigate the mechanism of LTP enhancement in transient activation of p25, Fischer and colleagues analyzed NR2A phosphorylation and NMDA-mediated current and found that both are increased after transient overexpression of p25 (Fischer et al., 2005). It would be interesting to investigate whether calpain-mediated NR2B cleavage and/or the NR2B-mediated current are also changed in transient p25-overexpressing mice.

There are other manipulations that indirectly enhance NMDAR function and subsequently enhance memory. Mice lacking a nociception receptor opioid receptor-like 1 (ORL1) showed enhanced learning and memory in the Morris water maze, passive avoidance task, and contextual fear conditioning (Mamiya et al., 2003; Manabe et al., 1998). Moreover, LTP was significantly enhanced in this mutant. Since ORL1 was initially reported to inhibit adenylyl cyclase via G protein (Henderson and McKnight, 1997), increased cAMP level was postulated to be an underlying mechanism of enhanced plasticity and learning in ORL1 knock-out mice. However, a recent study showed that the deletion of ORL1 increased CaMKII activity and enhanced NMDAR function, suggesting that enhanced NMDAR function might be responsible for the enhanced cognition in ORL1 knock-out mice (Mamiya et al., 2003).

Transgenic mice overexpressing hepatocyte growth factor (HGF) also showed enhanced learning and memory performance in the Morris water maze (Kato et al., 2012). Biochemical analysis revealed that NR2A and NR2B expressions were significantly increased in the hippocampus of HGF transgenic mice.

Taken together, these studies demonstrate that upregulation of NMDAR function is one of the most common molecular mechanisms of genetic enhancement of learning and memory.

cAMP-CREB SIGNALING

The crucial roles of cAMP signaling in synaptic plasticity and memory are evolutionary well conserved and the molecules in this pathway have been considered as key targets to develop memory enhancing drugs (Kandel, 2001; Tully et al., 2003). Adenylyl cyclases (ACs) play important roles in synaptic plasticity and memory by coupling Ca^{2+} signaling through NMDAR to cAMP signaling in mammalian brain (Figure 5.2) (Wong et al., 1999). Of ACs, AC1 and AC8 are neuron-specific (Wong et al., 1999). To examine whether upregulation of AC1 can enhance memory, Wang and colleagues overexpressed AC1 in mouse forebrain (Wang et al., 2004). AC1 overexpression enhanced LTP and AC1 transgenic mice showed enhanced memory in object recognition task. After training in the object recognition task, activation of MAPK and CREB was significantly higher in mutants than control mice. Although contextual and cued fear conditioning was not improved, the rate of contextual memory extinction was slower in transgenic mice.

Phosphodiesterases (PDEs) compose a family of 11 enzymes that hydrolyze cAMP in mammals. A PDE4 inhibitor rolipram enhances LTP induction and contextual fear memory in wild type mice (Barad et al., 1998) and it also rescues memory deficits in a mouse model of Rubinstein-Taybi syndrome (Bourtchouladze et al., 2003), suggesting that PDEs can be promising targets for memory enhancing drug development. Among four subtypes of PDE4 (A, B, C, and D), PDE4D knock-out mice showed memory enhancement in radial arm maze, Morris water maze, and object recognition test (Li et al., 2011). Activation of CREB (phosphorylated CREB or p-CREB) was increased in PDE4D knock-out. More recently, deletion of another PDE family, PDE8B was also shown to enhance memory (Tsai et al., 2012). PDE8B knock-out showed memory enhancement in contextual fear conditioning, Morris water maze and appetitive instrumental conditioning task (Tsai et al., 2012). These studies show that learning and memory function can be enhanced by shifting balance between synthesis and degradation of cAMP.

In addition to gating plasticity and memory as discussed, cAMP signaling activates transcription in the nucleus via regulating CREB. CREB, a basic leucine zipper transcription factor, is involved in long-term plasticity and memory in the nervous systems of both invertebrates and vertebrates (Bartsch et al., 1998; Bourtchuladze et al., 1994; Kandel, 2001; Kida et al., 2002; Lee et al., 2008; Matynia et al., 2002; Silva et al., 1998; Yin et al., 1994). In the mammal, CREB-deficient mice displayed impaired LTP and long-term memory (Bourtchuladze et al., 1994). In contrast, the threshold for late phase LTP (L-LTP) was lowered in the hippocampus of mice expressing the constitutively active form of CREB (VP16-CREB) (Barco et al., 2002). However, due to the excessively high level of CREB activation, it was not easy to draw a consistent conclusion about the role of active CREB in memory (Gruart et al., 2012; Viosca et al., 2009a,b). To address the effects of moderate upregulation of CREB on cognition, Kida and colleagues generated two transgenic mice expressing dominant active CREB mutant in the forebrain: CREB-Y134F that displays a higher affinity to PKA; and CREB-DIEDML that constitutively interacts with CBP (Suzuki et al., 2011). CREB-Y134F mutant mice showed enhanced memory in social recognition, contextual fear conditioning, context discrimination, and Morris water maze task. Similarly, CREB-DIEDML mutant also showed enhanced memory in social recognition and contextual fear conditioning, which are hippocampus-dependent tasks (Suzuki et al., 2011). LTP was also enhanced in CREB-Y134F mutant mice, demonstrating that CREB positively regulates synaptic plasticity and memory.

CREB activity can be modulated by other regulatory proteins such as cAMP-responsive element modulator (CREM) and activating transcription factor-1 (ATF-1) (Shaywitz and Greenberg, 1999). In invertebrates, repressor forms of CREB have been characterized (Yin et al., 1994). Transgenic *Drosophila* expressing the dominant negative member of CREB family, dCREB-2b, showed deficits in long-term memory (Yin et al., 1994). Overexpression of CREB2 in *Aplysia* also blocked long-term synaptic plasticity, while inhibiting CREB-2 lowered the threshold for the long-term synaptic plasticity induced by serotonin treatments (Bartsch et al., 1995; Lee et al., 2003), suggesting that the balance between positive and negative regulation of CREB can determine the polarity and/or strength of synaptic plasticity and memory.

Activating transcription factor 4 (ATF4), a mammalian homolog of *Aplysia* CREB-2, which interacts with the CCAAT/enhancer binding protein (C/EBP) family of transcription factors has been cloned as a negative regulator of CREB in vertebrates (Karpinski et al., 1992). Since the deletion of ATF4 resulted in impaired lens development or severe fetal anemia, learning and memory could not be tested in ATF knock-out mice (Masuoka and Townes, 2002; Tanaka et al., 1998). Chen and colleagues expressed a broad dominant negative inhibitor of C/EBP family (EGFP-AZIP) in the mouse forebrain (Chen et al., 2003). They found that EGFP-AZIP preferentially suppresses the repressor isoforms of the C/EBP family proteins and that the expression of ATF4 was reduced in the transgenic mice expressing EGFP-AZIP. This manipulation shifts the transcriptional balance in favor of activation of CREB-downstream genes. Attenuating transcriptional suppression resulted in lowering the threshold for LTP and memory formation. Mutant mice showed enhanced learning when they were trained with weak protocol in Morris water maze (Chen et al., 2003). In parallel, one pulse of tetanus which induces only E-LTP can induce transcription-dependent L-LTP, whereas LTD induction was reduced in hippocampal slices from mutant mice. These data suggest that relief of transcriptional repression can be an evolutionarily conserved strategy to enhance learning and memory. However, it is still possible that expression of EGFP-AZIP can interfere with the function of nonspecific target proteins. Enhanced paired-pulse facilitation (a form of presynaptic plasticity) in this mutant might be caused by such a nonspecific effect of AZIP on unspecified presynaptic proteins.

Phosphorylation of an α subunit of eukaryotic initiation factor 2 (eIF2) can stimulate the mRNA translation of ATF4, while it inhibits general translation (Harding et al., 2000; Sonenberg and Dever, 2003). Deletion of general control nonderepressible 2 (GCN2), a conserved eIF2α kinase, reduced phosphorylation of eIF2α and subsequently suppressed the translation of ATF4 mRNA (Costa-Mattioli et al., 2005). With enhanced CREB-mediated gene expression, threshold for L-LTP was lowered and spatial learning was enhanced when the mutants were trained with weak training protocol. Interestingly, deletion of GCN2 was shown to prevent deficits in synaptic plasticity and spatial memory in an Alzheimer's disease model mice (Ma et al., 2013).

To more directly investigate the role of eIF2α phosphorylation in synaptic plasticity and learning and memory, eIF2α heterozygous mice (eIF2α$^{+/S51A}$) in which the phosphorylation of eIF2α is blocked were generated (Costa-Mattioli et al., 2007). Only the protein level of ATF4, but not its mRNA was significantly reduced in this mutant mouse. Consistently with the previous findings, threshold for L-LTP was lowered. The memory-enhancing phenotype was more striking in eIF2α$^{+/S51A}$ than GCN2$^{-/-}$ or EGFP-AZIP mice. Specifically, spatial learning was enhanced with both weak and strong training protocol. This mutant showed improved learning and memory in a variety of behavioral tasks including contextual and cued fear conditioning, conditioned taste aversion, and latent inhibition (Costa-Mattioli et al., 2007). Recently, it has been shown that the deletion of protein kinase RNA (PKR)-like ER kinase (PERK), another eIF2α kinase, rescues the deficits in synaptic plasticity and spatial memory in mice that express familial Alzheimer's disease-causing mutations in amyloid precursor protein (APP) and presenilin 1 (PSEN1) (Ma et al., 2013), suggesting that eIF2α may be an potential target to enhance synaptic plasticity and memory in both normal and diseased brain. In addition, these studies on eIF2α not only highlight the importance of CREB in memory function but also suggest that the regulation of protein translation can be another tipping point for memory enhancement.

TRANSLATIONAL REGULATION AND ENHANCED COGNITION

The formation of long-term memory requires synthesis of new mRNA and proteins. Synaptic stimulation or learning activates multiple signaling pathways to orchestrate gene transcription and translation. Translation initiation is facilitated by poly(A)-binding protein (PABP), whose activity is negatively regulated by PABP-interacting protein 2 (PAIP2). PAIP2A is degraded in response to in vitro neural activation and in vivo learning in contextual fear conditioning

(Khoutorsky et al., 2013). To examine whether PAIP2A is involved in memory formation by regulating protein translation, Khoutorsky and colleagues generated *Paip2a* knock-out mice (Khoutorsky et al., 2013). *Paip2a* null mutant showed memory enhancements in multiple behavioral tasks including Morris water maze, contextual fear conditioning, and object-location memory tasks, all of which depend on the hippocampus. Accordingly, *Paip2a* knock-out mice showed a lowered threshold for the induction of L-LTP. Furthermore, biochemical analysis showed that the translation of αCaMKII mRNA is increased in the hippocampus of the knock-out mice following training in contextual fear conditioning (Khoutorsky et al., 2013).

Mammalian target of rapamycin (mTOR) signaling regulates the translation initiation and plays important roles in memory formation and synaptic plasticity (Bekinschtein et al., 2007; Tang et al., 2002). Dysregulation of mTOR signaling is also associated with cognitive disorders such as seen in tuberous sclerosis (Ehninger et al., 2008; Krab et al., 2008). Activity of mTOR can be regulated by several interacting proteins. Among those, FK506-binding protein 12 (FKBP12) binds rapamycin and inhibits mTOR. Activation of mTOR signaling is enhanced in the brain-specific FKBP12 knock-out mice (Hoeffer et al., 2008). L-LTP was enhanced in FKBP12 knock-out mice and the LTP enhancement was sensitive to anisomycin but not to rapamycin. Contextual fear memory was also enhanced in the knock-out mice. However, interestingly, the FKBP12 mutant mice also showed autistic preservative behaviors in the water maze, Y-maze reversal task and novel object recognition task, suggesting that memory enhancement might have unexpected behavioral costs (Hoeffer et al., 2008).

EPIGENETIC REGULATION AND ENHANCED COGNITION

Epigenetic regulations such as histone modifications and DNA methylation are also involved in regulating learning and synaptic plasticity. Pharmacological manipulations of histone acetylations by treating histone deacetylase (HDAC) inhibitors have been shown to enhance memory and synaptic plasticity in both mammals and invertebrates (Levenson and Sweatt, 2005; Si et al., 2004). Also, mice with reduced histone acetyltransferase activity showed deficits in both long-lasting forms of memory and LTP (Bourtchouladze et al., 2003; Korzus et al., 2004). Guan and colleagues generated both transgenics and knock-outs of HDACs (Guan et al., 2009). HDAC2, but not HDAC1-overexpressing mice show deficits in memory and LTP, suggesting that HDAC2 might be a major target of HDAC inhibitors associated with memory enhancement (Guan et al., 2009). Consistently, HDAC2 knock-out mice showed enhanced memory in contextual fear conditioning and increased LTP. Chromatin immunoprecipitation experiment revealed that HDAC2 is associated with genes that are previously known to be involved in synaptic plasticity and synaptic remodeling such as *Bdnf, Egr1, Fos, Camk2a, Creb1, Crebbp, NRXN3,* and the NMDAR subunits (Guan et al., 2009).

REDUCING INHIBITION AND ENHANCED COGNITION

Maintaining a normal balance between excitatory and inhibitory synaptic transmission is critical for intact brain functions. Interestingly, there are multiple lines of evidence suggesting that modulating inhibition may enhance memory, for example, pharmacological reduction of inhibition enhanced memory consolidation (Izquierdo and Medina, 1991; McGaugh and Roozendaal, 2009). Also, reduction of inhibitory synaptic transmission lowered the threshold for LTP induction (Abraham et al., 1986). To examine the effect of genetic reduction of tonic inhibition, $GABA_AR$ $\alpha 4$ subunit knock-out mice were tested in fear conditioning (Moore et al., 2010). $GABA_AR$ $\alpha 4$ mutant mice showed enhanced trace and contextual fear conditioning, suggesting that reducing tonic inhibition enhances hippocampus-dependent memory (Moore et al., 2010). In addition to the direct manipulation of GABA receptors, there are other smart mutants showing decreased inhibition through indirect mechanisms.

Monoacelglycerol lipase (MAGL) is an enzyme that hydrolyzes an endocannabinoid 2-arachidonoylglycerol (2-AG). Cannabinoid receptor CB1 is dominantly expressed in the inhibitory neurons and thus endocannabinoids can regulate the inhibitory synaptic transmissions. Deletion of MAGL increases the level of 2-AG and suppressed the $GABA_AR$-mediated inhibition in the hippocampus (Pan et al., 2011). Contrary to the exogenous cannabinoid that impairs learning and memory, increasing the level of endocannabinoid 2-AG in the MAGL knock-out mice enhanced learning and memory in the Morris water maze and object recognition task (Pan et al., 2011). The cognitive enhancement is also accompanied by the enhanced LTP in the hippocampus (Pan et al., 2011).

GABA release can be also inhibited by interferon-γ, whose translation is negatively regulated by a double-stranded RNA-activated protein kinase (PKR) and eIF2α. Either deletion of PKR or eIF2α^{S51A} mutation increases the translation of PKR and subsequently reduces GABAergic inhibition (Zhu et al., 2011). PKR knock-out mice showed memory enhancement in the Morris water maze and contextual and auditory fear conditioning. Memory extinction in contextual fear conditioning was also enhanced in PKR mutants. Due to the reduced GABAergic inhibition, network excitability is increased in the hippocampal slices of PKR knock-out mice, suggesting that modulating the network excitability causes memory enhancement (Zhu et al., 2011).

One of the key factors for determining neuronal excitability is the potassium channel. BEC1 (KCNH3) is a member of the *ether-a-go-go* (KCNH) family voltage-gated K^+ channels that is preferentially expressed in the forebrain. Deletion of BEC1 increased the excitability of the hippocampal pyramidal neurons and also enhanced working memory, spatial memory, and attention (Miyake et al., 2009). Consistently, overexpression of BEC1 in the forebrain impaired memory and LTP (Miyake et al., 2009). Taken together, manipulating excitation/inhibition (E/I) balance either by reducing inhibition or by increasing network excitability within an adequate range might be a promising candidate for developing cognitive enhancing strategy. However, manipulating E/I balance may cause unexpected complications, since disruptions in excitation/inhibition balance have been proposed as underlying mechanisms for psychiatric disorders such as schizophrenia, autism, and learning disabilities (Cui et al., 2008; Lee and Silva, 2011; Shilyansky et al., 2010).

MicroRNA AND ENHANCED COGNITION

MicroRNAs (miRNAs) are small noncoding RNA molecules that can block the translation of specific mRNAs by binding to their untranslated regions. miRNAs regulate various cellular functions including cellular differentiation and survival, neuronal development, synaptic plasticity, and learning and memory (Kosik, 2006). The expression of miRNA has been shown to be dynamically altered by NMDA-dependent neuronal activation or behavioral learning (Kye et al., 2011). Dicer is an RNase III that is responsible for producing the mature form of miRNAs. Konopka and colleagues investigated the effect of miRNA loss in the adult mouse brain by using conditioning knock-out mice expressing Cre recombinase under the control of tamoxifen (Konopka et al., 2010). Deletion of *Dicer1* in the adult brain reduced the abundance of the mature miRNAs but did not cause neuronal death or abnormalities in motor function, in anxiety, or in circadian rhythm up to 14 weeks after the induction of *Dicer1* mutation. Interestingly, *Dicer1* conditional knock-out mice showed enhanced learning and memory in the Morris water maze and fear conditioning (Konopka et al., 2010). *Dicer1* deletion also alters morphology of dendritic spines and increased the levels of synaptic plasticity-related proteins such as BDNF, AMPAR, PSD-95, and MMP-9 (Konopka et al., 2010).

EXTRACELLULAR FACTORS AND ENHANCED COGNITION

Long-term plasticity accompanies synaptic structural remodeling and, therefore, the molecules that modify synaptic structures are interesting candidates to modulate synaptic and memory efficacy. Matrix metalloproteinases (MMPs) are zinc-dependent proteases that are activated by proteolytic cleavage. MMPs are involved in remodeling of pericellular environment by degrading extracellular matrix. Including the discussion in the previous section, multiple lines of evidence suggest that MMP-9 plays a role in synaptic plasticity and learning and memory (Konopka et al., 2010; Wang et al., 2008). Indeed, transgenic mice overexpressing MMP-9 in the forebrain displayed enhanced performance in the Morris water maze and object recognition task and accordingly, LTP was also enhanced in the MMP-9 transgenic mice (Fragkouli et al., 2012).

Tissue-type plasminogen activator (tPA) is an extracellular serine protease which was identified as an activity-induced gene in the hippocampus (Qian et al., 1993). Genetic deletion of tPA resulted in deficits in L-LTP and several forms of memory and supported the idea that tPA plays an important role in LTP and memory (Calabresi et al., 2000; Carmeliet et al., 1994; Huang et al., 1996). Neuronal overexpression of tPA enhanced both LTP and hippocampus-dependent spatial memory (Madani et al., 1999). PPF was also enhanced but LTD was not altered in transgenic mice. Nevertheless, the mechanism underlying enhanced memory and LTP had remained unclear. Recently, it was reported that tPA converts the brain-derived neurotrophic factor (BDNF) precursor, pro-BDNF, to mature BDNF (mBDNF) by activating plasmin, and this conversion of BDNF is critical for L-LTP in the mouse hippocampus (Pang et al., 2004). BDNF is currently thought to be one of the key molecules involved in L-LTP and long-term memory (for the details of BDNF, please see comprehensive reviews: Nagappan and Lu, 2005; Pang and Lu, 2004). It is possible to speculate that the enhanced LTP and memory in tTA transgenic mice might be achieved through upregulating BDNF function.

CONCLUSION

The human brain is the most complex organ, consisting of more than 100 billion neurons, which form countless numbers of synapses. Furthermore, numerous signal transduction pathways interact with each other in every single neuron. Considering this complexity, it might be too naive to believe that manipulating single molecules or signaling pathways in limited areas of the brain can enhance cognitive functions such as learning and memory. In this chapter, nevertheless, we show that the genetic manipulations of single genes result in memory enhancement in many mutant mice. Although the number of mutants can be changed depending on the stringency of criteria for memory enhancement in mice, it still should be more than a negligible number which can be considered as fortunate mistakes. Then, are there any rules or common mechanisms which can be found from those smart mutants? Despite some controversy on the connections between memory and LTP, the studies of these smart mice present a strong evidence for critical roles of LTP in memory. As shown in LTP studies, the positive modulations of a signaling axis composed of NMDAR-ACs-CREB are shown to enhance memory. However, this does not guarantee that any manipulation that enhances LTP can modulate memory to the same direction. For example, genetic deletion of PSD-95 enhanced LTP, but spatial learning was severely impaired in this mutant (Migaud et al., 1998). This suggests that the increase of LTP alone is not sufficient for memory enhancement. In addition, genetic manipulation can affect other forms of synaptic plasticity such as LTD, which also plays crucial roles in memory (Bear, 1996; Zeng et al., 2001). Since most of the mutant mice have been generated by targeting a set of known molecules from LTP studies, we cannot exclude the possibility that the positive correlation between LTP and memory shown in those mice might be biased or exaggerated. As an alternative for the target molecule-driven studies, a phenotype-driven top-down approach using the smart mutants may help to unravel other hidden core mechanisms of memory enhancement (Lee and Silva, 2009). Also, there has been a big effort in the field of pharmacology to develop memory-enhancing drugs (Mehlman, 2004). Some drugs are based on specific targets like AMPA receptors (Lynch, 1998), but targets still needs to be characterized for many other drugs. Investigating the signaling pathways modulated by those drugs can be one of the complementary approaches.

It is worthwhile to address several practical issues to be overcome in the search for the memory enhancing mechanism using mutant mice. First, most of the mutants discussed in this chapter are from a different genetic background. It is well recognized that different lines of inbred mice show different performance in learning and memory-related behavioral tasks (Nguyen et al., 2000). Moreover, changing genetic background can reduce or remove the behavioral phenotypes of transgenic animal (Murphy et al., 2004). Thus, enhanced memory in some mutants can be simply claimed as a genetic compensation in certain genetic backgrounds, rather than as a genuine memory enhancing effect of transgenes. Second, some mutant mice were challenged with only a limited number of behavioral tasks and it is unclear if they are normal or worse in other tasks. It is possible that a mutant showing better performance in one task can show normal or worse phenotypes in another task and there can be many explanations for the discrepancy. Deletion or expression of any specific gene can have different effects in different brain regions. For example, the deletion of HCN1, a subunit of HCN (hyperpolarization-activated, cyclic nucleotide–gated, cation-nonselective), channel from the entire mouse results in the alteration in the integrative properties of cerebellar Purkinje cells and causes deficits in motor learning (Nolan et al., 2003). However, forebrain-specific deletion of HCN1 enhances hippocampal-dependent learning and memory (Nolan et al., 2004). Moreover, it is becoming clear that hippocampal subregions play a distinct role in memory processing, for example, in pattern separation and completion (McHugh et al., 2007; Nakazawa et al., 2002) (also please see in Chapter 9 a comprehensive review on the role of the different hippocampal subregions). Thus, it is necessary to recruit more carefully designed behavioral analyses. In addition, not only hippocampus-dependent learning tasks, but other behavioral tasks requiring cortical functions need to be examined. Third, other factors in combination with genes can affect the cognitive functions in mutant animals. Several lines of mutants such as mice lacking voltage-gated potassium channel subunit Kvβ1.1 and mice overexpressing extracellular superoxide dismutase showed enhanced learning only in old ages (Hu et al., 2006; Murphy et al., 2004). Even within a single mutant line, there seems to be some degree of individual differences in their behavioral phenotype depending on the level of transgene expression (Holahan et al., 2007; Routtenberg et al., 2000).

Another important issue is that genetic enhancement of memory can be accompanied by changes in other physiological or cognitive functions, and even by unexpected adverse behavioral costs. For example, NR2B transgenic mice, *doogie*, exhibited enhanced chronic pain (Wei et al., 2001). NR2B was also overexpressed in the pain-related forebrain areas of the transgenic mice (Wei et al., 2001). NR2B transgenic mice and wild type mice showed similar responses in acute pain test, but the transgenic mice displayed enhanced responsiveness to peripheral injection of inflammatory stimuli that induce chronic pain, suggesting that the overexpression of NR2B in the forebrain can affect pain perception in mice (Wei et al., 2001). Moreover, enhancing memory strength is sometimes accompanied by the loss of memory flexibility. While AC1 transgenic mice showed better performance in the object recognition test, this mutant showed slower extinction in contextual fear memory (Wang et al., 2004). Considering that the fear extinction is suggested as a new learning for the animal to learn that the context is not dangerous any more (Phelps et al., 2004), slower extinction suggests that the mutants are impaired in this type of new learning. Similarly, FKBP12 knock-out mice that showed enhanced memory in contextual fear conditioning also lost behavioral flexibilities (Hoeffer et al., 2008). The mutant mice showed deficits in the repeated acquisition paradigm water maze and the Y-maze reversal task that measure behavioral flexibility (Hoeffer et al., 2008). Also, FKBP12 mutant showed preference for the familiar object over the novel object in the object recognition test (Hoeffer et al., 2008). Although it is not highlighted in this review, it should be also carefully estimated whether the enhancement of memory is a secondary effect of alterations of other cognitive functions such as changes in anxiety or attention status.

We may be just beginning our journey from the early stage of cognitive studies using genetic and molecular tools to a more sophisticated approach to understand how to achieve memory enhancement. However, it is without any doubt that all these findings will help to develop treatments for improving cognitive functions of patients suffering from cognitive deficits including memory loss.

ACKNOWLEDGMENT

I would like to give special thanks to Dr. Alcino J. Silva for his enthusiasm for this project.

REFERENCES

Abel, T., Martin, K.C., Bartsch, D., Kandel, E.R., 1998. Memory suppressor genes: inhibitory constraints on the storage of long-term memory. Science 279 (5349), 338–341.

Abraham, W.C., Gustafsson, B., Wigstrom, H., 1986. Single high strength afferent volleys can produce long-term potentiation in the hippocampus in vitro. Neurosci. Lett. 70 (2), 217–222.

Anagnostopoulos, A.V., Mobraaten, L.E., Sharp, J.J., Davisson, M.T., 2001. Transgenic and knock-out databases: behavioral profiles of mouse mutants. Physiol. Behav. 73 (5), 675–689.

Angelo, M., Plattner, F., Giese, K.P., 2006. Cyclin-dependent kinase 5 in synaptic plasticity, learning and memory. J. Neurochem. 99 (2), 353–370.

Barad, M., Bourtchouladze, R., Winder, D.G., Golan, H., Kandel, E., 1998. Rolipram, a type IV-specific phosphodiesterase inhibitor, facilitates the establishment of long-lasting long-term potentiation and improves memory. Proc. Natl. Acad. Sci. U.S.A. 95 (25), 15020–15025.

Barco, A., Alarcon, J.M., Kandel, E.R., 2002. Expression of constitutively active CREB protein facilitates the late phase of long-term potentiation by enhancing synaptic capture. Cell 108 (5), 689–703.

Bartsch, D., Casadio, A., Karl, K.A., Serodio, P., Kandel, E.R., 1998. CREB1 encodes a nuclear activator, a repressor, and a cytoplasmic modulator that form a regulatory unit critical for long-term facilitation. Cell 95 (2), 211–223.

Bartsch, D., Ghirardi, M., Skehel, P.A., Karl, K.A., Herder, S.P., Chen, M., Kandel, E.R., 1995. Aplysia CREB2 represses long-term facilitation: relief of repression converts transient facilitation into long-term functional and structural change. Cell 83 (6), 979–992.

Bear, M.F., 1996. A synaptic basis for memory storage in the cerebral cortex. Proc. Natl. Acad. Sci. U.S.A. 93 (24), 13453–13459.

Bekinschtein, P., Katche, C., Slipczuk, L.N., Igaz, L.M., Cammarota, M., Izquierdo, I., Medina, J.H., 2007. mTOR signaling in the hippocampus is necessary for memory formation. Neurobiol. Learn Mem. 87 (2), 303–307.

Bliss, T.V., Collingridge, G.L., 1993. A synaptic model of memory: long-term potentiation in the hippocampus. Nature 361 (6407), 31–39.

Bliss, T.V., Gardner-Medwin, A.R., 1973. Long-lasting potentiation of synaptic transmission in the dentate area of the unanaestetized rabbit following stimulation of the perforant path. J. Physiol. 232 (2), 357–374.

Bliss, T.V., Lomo, T., 1973. Long-lasting potentiation of synaptic transmission in the dentate area of the anaesthetized rabbit following stimulation of the perforant path. J. Physiol. 232 (2), 331–356.

Bolivar, V., Cook, M., Flaherty, L., 2000. List of transgenic and knockout mice: behavioral profiles. Mamm. Genome 11 (4), 260–274.

Bourtchouladze, R., Lidge, R., Catapano, R., Stanley, J., Gossweiler, S., Romashko, D., Tully, T., 2003. A mouse model of Rubinstein-Taybi syndrome: defective long-term memory is ameliorated by inhibitors of phosphodiesterase 4. Proc. Natl. Acad. Sci. U.S.A. 100 (18), 10518–10522.

Bourtchuladze, R., Frenguelli, B., Blendy, J., Cioffi, D., Schutz, G., Silva, A.J., 1994. Deficient long-term memory in mice with a targeted mutation of the cAMP-responsive element-binding protein. Cell 79 (1), 59–68.

Calabresi, P., Napolitano, M., Centonze, D., Marfia, G.A., Gubellini, P., Teule, M.A., Gulino, A., 2000. Tissue plasminogen activator controls multiple forms of synaptic plasticity and memory. Eur. J. Neurosci. 12 (3), 1002–1012.

Cao, X., Cui, Z., Feng, R., Tang, Y.P., Qin, Z., Mei, B., Tsien, J.Z., 2007. Maintenance of superior learning and memory function in NR2B transgenic mice during ageing. Eur. J. Neurosci. 25 (6), 1815–1822.

Carmeliet, P., Schoonjans, L., Kieckens, L., Ream, B., Degen, J., Bronson, R., Mulligan, R.C., 1994. Physiological consequences of loss of plasminogen activator gene function in mice. Nature 368 (6470), 419–424.

Chen, A., Muzzio, I.A., Malleret, G., Bartsch, D., Verbitsky, M., Pavlidis, P., Kandel, E.R., 2003. Inducible enhancement of memory storage and synaptic plasticity in transgenic mice expressing an inhibitor of ATF4 (CREB-2) and C/EBP proteins. Neuron 39 (4), 655–669.

Collinson, N., Kuenzi, F.M., Jarolimek, W., Maubach, K.A., Cothliff, R., Sur, C., Rosahl, T.W., 2002. Enhanced learning and memory and altered GABAergic synaptic transmission in mice lacking the alpha 5 subunit of the GABA(A) receptor. J. Neurosci. 22 (13), 5572–5580.

Costa-Mattioli, M., Gobert, D., Harding, H., Herdy, B., Azzi, M., Bruno, M., Sonenberg, N., 2005. Translational control of hippocampal synaptic plasticity and memory by the eIF2alpha kinase GCN2. Nature 436 (7054), 1166–1173.

Costa-Mattioli, M., Gobert, D., Stern, E., Gamache, K., Colina, R., Cuello, C., Sonenberg, N., 2007. eIF2alpha phosphorylation bidirectionally regulates the switch from short- to long-term synaptic plasticity and memory. Cell 129 (1), 195–206.

Cruz, J.C., Tseng, H.C., Goldman, J.A., Shih, H., Tsai, L.H., 2003. Aberrant Cdk5 activation by p25 triggers pathological events leading to neurodegeneration and neurofibrillary tangles. Neuron 40 (3), 471–483.

Cui, Y., Costa, R.M., Murphy, G.G., Elgersma, Y., Zhu, Y., Gutmann, D.H., Silva, A.J., 2008. Neurofibromin regulation of ERK signaling modulates GABA release and learning. Cell 135 (3), 549–560.

Cui, Y., Jin, J., Zhang, X., Xu, H., Yang, L., Du, D., Cao, X., 2011. Forebrain NR2B overexpression facilitating the prefrontal cortex long-term potentiation and enhancing working memory function in mice. PLoS One 6 (5), e20312.

Dong, Y.N., Wu, H.Y., Hsu, F.C., Coulter, D.A., Lynch, D.R., 2006. Developmental and cell-selective variations in N-methyl-D-aspartate receptor degradation by calpain. J. Neurochem. 99 (1), 206–217.

Ehninger, D., Han, S., Shilyansky, C., Zhou, Y., Li, W., Kwiatkowski, D.J., Silva, A.J., 2008. Reversal of learning deficits in a Tsc2$^{+/-}$ mouse model of tuberous sclerosis. Nat. Med.

Eichenbaum, H., 1996. Learning from LTP: a comment on recent attempts to identify cellular and molecular mechanisms of memory. Learn Mem. 3 (2–3), 61–73.

Fischer, A., Sananbenesi, F., Pang, P.T., Lu, B., Tsai, L.H., 2005. Opposing roles of transient and prolonged expression of p25 in synaptic plasticity and hippocampus-dependent memory. Neuron 48 (5), 825–838.

Fragkouli, A., Papatheodoropoulos, C., Georgopoulos, S., Stamatakis, A., Stylianopoulou, F., Tsilibary, E.C., Tzinia, A.K., 2012. Enhanced neuronal plasticity and elevated endogenous sAPPalpha levels in mice over-expressing MMP9. J. Neurochem. 121 (2), 239–251.

Fukushima, H., Maeda, R., Suzuki, R., Suzuki, A., Nomoto, M., Toyoda, H., Kida, S., 2008. Upregulation of calcium/calmodulin-dependent protein kinase IV improves memory formation and rescues memory loss with aging. J. Neurosci. 28 (40), 9910–9919.

Genoux, D., Haditsch, U., Knobloch, M., Michalon, A., Storm, D., Mansuy, I.M., 2002. Protein phosphatase 1 is a molecular constraint on learning and memory. Nature 418 (6901), 970–975.

Grant, S.G., O'Dell, T.J., Karl, K.A., Stein, P.L., Soriano, P., Kandel, E.R., 1992. Impaired long-term potentiation, spatial learning, and hippocampal development in fyn mutant mice. Science 258 (5090), 1903–1910.

Gruart, A., Benito, E., Delgado-Garcia, J.M., Barco, A., 2012. Enhanced cAMP response element-binding protein activity increases neuronal excitability, hippocampal long-term potentiation, and classical eyeblink conditioning in alert behaving mice. J. Neurosci. 32 (48), 17431–17441.

Guan, J.S., Haggarty, S.J., Giacometti, E., Dannenberg, J.H., Joseph, N., Gao, J., Tsai, L.H., 2009. HDAC2 negatively regulates memory formation and synaptic plasticity. Nature 459 (7243), 55–60.

Guillaud, L., Setou, M., Hirokawa, N., 2003. KIF17 dynamics and regulation of NR2B trafficking in hippocampal neurons. J. Neurosci. 23 (1), 131–140.

Harding, H.P., Novoa, I., Zhang, Y., Zeng, H., Wek, R., Schapira, M., Ron, D., 2000. Regulated translation initiation controls stress-induced gene expression in mammalian cells. Mol. Cell 6 (5), 1099–1108.

Harris, K.M., Teyler, T.J., 1984. Developmental onset of long-term potentiation in area CA1 of the rat hippocampus. J. Physiol. 346, 27–48.

Hawasli, A.H., Benavides, D.R., Nguyen, C., Kansy, J.W., Hayashi, K., Chambon, P., Bibb, J.A., 2007. Cyclin-dependent kinase 5 governs learning and synaptic plasticity via control of NMDAR degradation. Nat. Neurosci. 10 (7), 880–886.

Hawasli, A.H., Bibb, J.A., 2007. Alternative roles for Cdk5 in learning and synaptic plasticity. Biotechnol. J. 2 (8), 941–948.

Henderson, G., McKnight, A.T., 1997. The orphan opioid receptor and its endogenous ligand–nociceptin/orphanin FQ. Trends Pharmacol. Sci. 18 (8), 293–300.

Hoeffer, C.A., Tang, W., Wong, H., Santillan, A., Patterson, R.J., Martinez, L.A., Klann, E., 2008. Removal of FKBP12 enhances mTOR-Raptor interactions, LTP, memory, and perseverative/repetitive behavior. Neuron 60 (5), 832–845.

Holahan, M.R., Honegger, K.S., Tabatadze, N., Routtenberg, A., 2007. GAP-43 gene expression regulates information storage. Learn Mem. 14 (6), 407–415.

Hu, D., Serrano, F., Oury, T.D., Klann, E., 2006. Aging-dependent alterations in synaptic plasticity and memory in mice that overexpress extracellular superoxide dismutase. J. Neurosci. 26 (15), 3933–3941.

Huang, Y.Y., Bach, M.E., Lipp, H.P., Zhuo, M., Wolfer, D.P., Hawkins, R.D., Carmeliet, P., 1996. Mice lacking the gene encoding tissue-type plasminogen activator show a selective interference with late-phase long-term potentiation in both Schaffer collateral and mossy fiber pathways. Proc. Natl. Acad. Sci. U.S.A. 93 (16), 8699–8704.

Husi, H., Ward, M.A., Choudhary, J.S., Blackstock, W.P., Grant, S.G., 2000. Proteomic analysis of NMDA receptor-adhesion protein signaling complexes. Nat. Neurosci. 3 (7), 661–669.

Izquierdo, I., Medina, J.H., 1991. GABAA receptor modulation of memory: the role of endogenous benzodiazepines. Trends Pharmacol. Sci. 12 (7), 260–265.

Kandel, E.R., 2001. The molecular biology of memory storage: a dialogue between genes and synapses. Science 294 (5544), 1030–1038.

Karpinski, B.A., Morle, G.D., Huggenvik, J., Uhler, M.D., Leiden, J.M., 1992. Molecular cloning of human CREB-2: an ATF/CREB transcription factor that can negatively regulate transcription from the cAMP response element. Proc. Natl. Acad. Sci. U.S.A. 89 (11), 4820–4824.

Kato, T., Funakoshi, H., Kadoyama, K., Noma, S., Kanai, M., Ohya-Shimada, W., Nakamura, T., 2012. Hepatocyte growth factor overexpression in the nervous system enhances learning and memory performance in mice. J. Neurosci. Res. 90 (9), 1743–1755.

Khoutorsky, A., Yanagiya, A., Gkogkas, C.G., Fabian, M.R., Prager-Khoutorsky, M., Cao, R., Sonenberg, N., 2013. Control of synaptic plasticity and memory via suppression of poly(A)-binding protein. Neuron 78 (2), 298–311.

Kida, S., Josselyn, S.A., de Ortiz, S.P., Kogan, J.H., Chevere, I., Masushige, S., Silva, A.J., 2002. CREB required for the stability of new and reactivated fear memories. Nat. Neurosci. 5 (4), 348–355.

Kim, J.J., Fanselow, M.S., 1992. Modality-specific retrograde amnesia of fear. Science 256 (5057), 675–677.

Kim, J.J., Fanselow, M.S., DeCola, J.P., Landeira-Fernandez, J., 1992. Selective impairment of long-term but not short-term conditional fear by the N-methyl-D-aspartate antagonist APV. Behav. Neurosci. 106 (4), 591–596.

Kiyama, Y., Manabe, T., Sakimura, K., Kawakami, F., Mori, H., Mishina, M., 1998. Increased thresholds for long-term potentiation and contextual learning in mice lacking the NMDA-type glutamate receptor epsilon1 subunit. J. Neurosci. 18 (17), 6704–6712.

Konopka, W., Kiryk, A., Novak, M., Herwerth, M., Parkitna, J.R., Wawrzyniak, M., Schutz, G., 2010. MicroRNA loss enhances learning and memory in mice. J. Neurosci. 30 (44), 14835–14842.

Korzus, E., Rosenfeld, M.G., Mayford, M., 2004. CBP histone acetyltransferase activity is a critical component of memory consolidation. Neuron 42 (6), 961–972.

Kosik, K.S., 2006. The neuronal microRNA system. Nat. Rev. Neurosci. 7 (12), 911–920.

Krab, L.C., Goorden, S.M., Elgersma, Y., 2008. Oncogenes on my mind: ERK and MTOR signaling in cognitive diseases. Trends Genet. 24 (10), 498–510.

Kutsuwada, T., Sakimura, K., Manabe, T., Takayama, C., Katakura, N., Kushiya, E., Mishina, M., 1996. Impairment of suckling response, trigeminal neuronal pattern formation, and hippocampal LTD in NMDA receptor epsilon 2 subunit mutant mice. Neuron 16 (2), 333–344.

Kye, M.J., Neveu, P., Lee, Y.S., Zhou, M., Steen, J.A., Sahin, M., Silva, A.J., 2011. NMDA mediated contextual conditioning changes miRNA expression. PLoS One 6 (9), e24682.

Lee, J.A., Kim, H., Lee, Y.S., Kaang, B.K., 2003. Overexpression and RNA interference of Ap-cyclic AMP-response element binding protein-2, a repressor of long-term facilitation, in Aplysia kurodai sensory-to-motor synapses. Neurosci. Lett. 337 (1), 9–12.

Lee, Y.S., Bailey, C.H., Kandel, E.R., Kaang, B.K., 2008. Transcriptional regulation of long-term memory in the marine snail Aplysia. Mol. Brain 1, 3.

Lee, Y.S., Silva, A.J., 2009. The molecular and cellular biology of enhanced cognition. Nat. Rev. Neurosci. 10 (2), 126–140.

Lee, Y.S., Silva, A.J., 2011. Modeling hyperactivity: of mice and men. Nat. Med. 17 (5), 541–542.

Levenson, J.M., Sweatt, J.D., 2005. Epigenetic mechanisms in memory formation. Nat. Rev. Neurosci. 6 (2), 108–118.

Li, Y.F., Cheng, Y.F., Huang, Y., Conti, M., Wilson, S.P., O'Donnell, J.M., Zhang, H.T., 2011. Phosphodiesterase-4D knock-out and RNA interference-mediated knock-down enhance memory and increase hippocampal neurogenesis via increased cAMP signaling. J. Neurosci. 31 (1), 172–183.

Lisman, J., Schulman, H., Cline, H., 2002. The molecular basis of CaMKII function in synaptic and behavioural memory. Nat. Rev. Neurosci. 3 (3), 175–190.

Lynch, G., 1998. Memory and the brain: unexpected chemistries and a new pharmacology. Neurobiol. Learn Mem. 70 (1–2), 82–100.

Ma, T., Trinh, M.A., Wexler, A.J., Bourbon, C., Gatti, E., Pierre, P., Klann, E., 2013. Suppression of eIF2alpha kinases alleviates Alzheimer's disease-related plasticity and memory deficits. Nat. Neurosci. 16 (9), 1299–1305.

Madani, R., Hulo, S., Toni, N., Madani, H., Steimer, T., Muller, D., Vassalli, J.D., 1999. Enhanced hippocampal long-term potentiation and learning by increased neuronal expression of tissue-type plasminogen activator in transgenic mice. Embo J. 18 (11), 3007–3012.

Malenka, R.C., Nicoll, R.A., 1999. Long-term potentiation–a decade of progress? Science 285 (5435), 1870–1874.

Malinow, R., Malenka, R.C., 2002. AMPA receptor trafficking and synaptic plasticity. Annu. Rev. Neurosci. 25, 103–126.

Malleret, G., Haditsch, U., Genoux, D., Jones, M.W., Bliss, T.V., Vanhoose, A.M., Mansuy, I.M., 2001. Inducible and reversible enhancement of learning, memory, and long-term potentiation by genetic inhibition of calcineurin. Cell 104 (5), 675–686.

Mamiya, T., Yamada, K., Miyamoto, Y., Konig, N., Watanabe, Y., Noda, Y., Nabeshima, T., 2003. Neuronal mechanism of nociceptin-induced modulation of learning and memory: involvement of N-methyl-D-aspartate receptors. Mol. Psychiatry 8 (8), 752–765.

Manabe, T., Noda, Y., Mamiya, T., Katagiri, H., Houtani, T., Nishi, M., Takeshima, H., 1998. Facilitation of long-term potentiation and memory in mice lacking nociceptin receptors. Nature 394 (6693), 577–581.

Masuoka, H.C., Townes, T.M., 2002. Targeted disruption of the activating transcription factor 4 gene results in severe fetal anemia in mice. Blood 99 (3), 736–745.

Matynia, A., Kushner, S.A., Silva, A.J., 2002. Genetic approaches to molecular and cellular cognition: a focus on LTP and learning and memory. Annu. Rev. Genet. 36, 687–720.

Mayford, M., Bach, M.E., Huang, Y.Y., Wang, L., Hawkins, R.D., Kandel, E.R., 1996. Control of memory formation through regulated expression of a CaMKII transgene. Science 274 (5293), 1678–1683.

Mayford, M., Kandel, E.R., 1999. Genetic approaches to memory storage. Trends Genet. 15 (11), 463–470.

McGaugh, J.L., Roozendaal, B., 2009. Drug enhancement of memory consolidation: historical perspective and neurobiological implications. Psychopharmacology (Berl) 202 (1–3), 3–14.

McHugh, T.J., Jones, M.W., Quinn, J.J., Balthasar, N., Coppari, R., Elmquist, J.K., Tonegawa, S., 2007. Dentate gyrus NMDA receptors mediate rapid pattern separation in the hippocampal network. Science 317 (5834), 94–99.

McKernan, M.G., Shinnick-Gallagher, P., 1997. Fear conditioning induces a lasting potentiation of synaptic currents in vitro. Nature 390 (6660), 607–611.

Mehlman, M.J., 2004. Cognition-enhancing drugs. Milbank Q. 82 (3), 483–506 (table of contents).

Migaud, M., Charlesworth, P., Dempster, M., Webster, L.C., Watabe, A.M., Makhinson, M., Grant, S.G., 1998. Enhanced long-term potentiation and impaired learning in mice with mutant post-synaptic density-95 protein. Nature 396 (6710), 433–439.

Miyake, A., Takahashi, S., Nakamura, Y., Inamura, K., Matsumoto, S., Mochizuki, S., Katou, M., 2009. Disruption of the ether-a-go-go K+ channel gene BEC1/KCNH3 enhances cognitive function. J. Neurosci. 29 (46), 14637–14645.

Monyer, H., Burnashev, N., Laurie, D.J., Sakmann, B., Seeburg, P.H., 1994. Developmental and regional expression in the rat brain and functional properties of four NMDA receptors. Neuron 12 (3), 529–540.

Monyer, H., Sprengel, R., Schoepfer, R., Herb, A., Higuchi, M., Lomeli, H., Seeburg, P.H., 1992. Heteromeric NMDA receptors: molecular and functional distinction of subtypes. Science 256 (5060), 1217–1221.

Moore, M.D., Cushman, J., Chandra, D., Homanics, G.E., Olsen, R.W., Fanselow, M.S., 2010. Trace and contextual fear conditioning is enhanced in mice lacking the alpha4 subunit of the GABA(A) receptor. Neurobiol. Learn Mem. 93 (3), 383–387.

Morris, R.G., Anderson, E., Lynch, G.S., Baudry, M., 1986. Selective impairment of learning and blockade of long-term potentiation by an N-methyl-D-aspartate receptor antagonist, AP5. Nature 319 (6056), 774–776.

Morris, R.G., Garrud, P., Rawlins, J.N., O'Keefe, J., 1982. Place navigation impaired in rats with hippocampal lesions. Nature 297 (5868), 681–683.

Murphy, G.G., Fedorov, N.B., Giese, K.P., Ohno, M., Friedman, E., Chen, R., Silva, A.J., 2004. Increased neuronal excitability, synaptic plasticity, and learning in aged Kvbeta1.1 knockout mice. Curr. Biol. 14 (21), 1907–1915.

Nagappan, G., Lu, B., 2005. Activity-dependent modulation of the BDNF receptor TrkB: mechanisms and implications. Trends Neurosci. 28 (9), 464–471.

Nakazawa, K., Quirk, M.C., Chitwood, R.A., Watanabe, M., Yeckel, M.F., Sun, L.D., Tonegawa, S., 2002. Requirement for hippocampal CA3 NMDA receptors in associative memory recall. Science 297 (5579), 211–218.

Nakazawa, K., Sun, L.D., Quirk, M.C., Rondi-Reig, L., Wilson, M.A., Tonegawa, S., 2003. Hippocampal CA3 NMDA receptors are crucial for memory acquisition of one-time experience. Neuron 38 (2), 305–315.

Nguyen, P.V., Abel, T., Kandel, E.R., Bourtchouladze, R., 2000. Strain-dependent differences in LTP and hippocampus-dependent memory in inbred mice. Learn Mem. 7 (3), 170–179.

Nolan, M.F., Malleret, G., Dudman, J.T., Buhl, D.L., Santoro, B., Gibbs, E., Morozov, A., 2004. A behavioral role for dendritic integration: HCN1 channels constrain spatial memory and plasticity at inputs to distal dendrites of CA1 pyramidal neurons. Cell 119 (5), 719–732.

Nolan, M.F., Malleret, G., Lee, K.H., Gibbs, E., Dudman, J.T., Santoro, B., Morozov, A., 2003. The hyperpolarization-activated HCN1 channel is important for motor learning and neuronal integration by cerebellar Purkinje cells. Cell 115 (5), 551–564.

Pan, B., Wang, W., Zhong, P., Blankman, J.L., Cravatt, B.F., Liu, Q.S., 2011. Alterations of endocannabinoid signaling, synaptic plasticity, learning, and memory in monoacylglycerol lipase knock-out mice. J. Neurosci. 31 (38), 13420–13430.

Pang, P.T., Lu, B., 2004. Regulation of late-phase LTP and long-term memory in normal and aging hippocampus: role of secreted proteins tPA and BDNF. Ageing Res. Rev. 3 (4), 407–430.

Pang, P.T., Teng, H.K., Zaitsev, E., Woo, N.T., Sakata, K., Zhen, S., Lu, B., 2004. Cleavage of proBDNF by tPA/plasmin is essential for long-term hippocampal plasticity. Science 306 (5695), 487–491.

Pavlov, I., Voikar, V., Kaksonen, M., Lauri, S.E., Hienola, A., Taira, T., Rauvala, H., 2002. Role of heparin-binding growth-associated molecule (HB-GAM) in hippocampal LTP and spatial learning revealed by studies on overexpressing and knockout mice. Mol. Cell Neurosci. 20 (2), 330–342.

Phelps, E.A., Delgado, M.R., Nearing, K.I., LeDoux, J.E., 2004. Extinction learning in humans: role of the amygdala and vmPFC. Neuron 43 (6), 897–905.

Qian, Z., Gilbert, M.E., Colicos, M.A., Kandel, E.R., Kuhl, D., 1993. Tissue-plasminogen activator is induced as an immediate-early gene during seizure, kindling and long-term potentiation. Nature 361 (6411), 453–457.

Rogan, M.T., Staubli, U.V., LeDoux, J.E., 1997. Fear conditioning induces associative long-term potentiation in the amygdala. Nature 390 (6660), 604–607.

Routtenberg, A., Cantallops, I., Zaffuto, S., Serrano, P., Namgung, U., 2000. Enhanced learning after genetic overexpression of a brain growth protein. Proc. Natl. Acad. Sci. U.S.A. 97 (13), 7657–7662.

Rumpel, S., LeDoux, J., Zador, A., Malinow, R., 2005. Postsynaptic receptor trafficking underlying a form of associative learning. Science 308 (5718), 83–88.

Sakimura, K., Kutsuwada, T., Ito, I., Manabe, T., Takayama, C., Kushiya, E., et al., 1995. Reduced hippocampal LTP and spatial learning in mice lacking NMDA receptor epsilon 1 subunit. Nature 373 (6510), 151–155.

Sanes, J.R., Lichtman, J.W., 1999. Can molecules explain long-term potentiation? Nat. Neurosci. 2 (7), 597–604.

Setou, M., Nakagawa, T., Seog, D.H., Hirokawa, N., 2000. Kinesin superfamily motor protein KIF17 and mLin-10 in NMDA receptor-containing vesicle transport. Science 288 (5472), 1796–1802.

Shaywitz, A.J., Greenberg, M.E., 1999. CREB: a stimulus-induced transcription factor activated by a diverse array of extracellular signals. Annu. Rev. Biochem. 68, 821–861.

Sheng, M., Cummings, J., Roldan, L.A., Jan, Y.N., Jan, L.Y., 1994. Changing subunit composition of heteromeric NMDA receptors during development of rat cortex. Nature 368 (6467), 144–147.

Shilyansky, C., Lee, Y.S., Silva, A.J., 2010. Molecular and cellular mechanisms of learning disabilities: a focus on NF1. Annu. Rev. Neurosci. 33, 221–243.

Shumyatsky, G.P., Tsvetkov, E., Malleret, G., Vronskaya, S., Hatton, M., Hampton, L., Bolshakov, V.Y., 2002. Identification of a signaling network in lateral nucleus of amygdala important for inhibiting memory specifically related to learned fear. Cell 111 (6), 905–918.

Si, K., Lindquist, S., Kandel, E., 2004. A possible epigenetic mechanism for the persistence of memory. Cold Spring Harb. Symp. Quant. Biol. 69, 497–498.

Silva, A.J., 2003. Molecular and cellular cognitive studies of the role of synaptic plasticity in memory. J. Neurobiol. 54 (1), 224–237.

Silva, A.J., Kogan, J.H., Frankland, P.W., Kida, S., 1998. CREB and memory. Annu. Rev. Neurosci. 21, 127–148.

Silva, A.J., Paylor, R., Wehner, J.M., Tonegawa, S., 1992a. Impaired spatial learning in alpha-calcium-calmodulin kinase II mutant mice. Science 257 (5067), 206–211.

Silva, A.J., Stevens, C.F., Tonegawa, S., Wang, Y., 1992b. Deficient hippocampal long-term potentiation in alpha-calcium-calmodulin kinase II mutant mice. Science 257 (5067), 201–206.

Simpkins, K.L., Guttmann, R.P., Dong, Y., Chen, Z., Sokol, S., Neumar, R.W., Lynch, D.R., 2003. Selective activation induced cleavage of the NR2B subunit by calpain. J. Neurosci. 23 (36), 11322–11331.

Sonenberg, N., Dever, T.E., 2003. Eukaryotic translation initiation factors and regulators. Curr. Opin. Struct. Biol. 13 (1), 56–63.

Suzuki, A., Fukushima, H., Mukawa, T., Toyoda, H., Wu, L.J., Zhao, M.G., Kida, S., 2011. Upregulation of CREB-mediated transcription enhances both short- and long-term memory. J. Neurosci. 31 (24), 8786–8802.

Tanaka, T., Tsujimura, T., Takeda, K., Sugihara, A., Maekawa, A., Terada, N., Akira, S., 1998. Targeted disruption of ATF4 discloses its essential role in the formation of eye lens fibres. Genes Cells 3 (12), 801–810.

Tang, S.J., Reis, G., Kang, H., Gingras, A.C., Sonenberg, N., Schuman, E.M., 2002. A rapamycin-sensitive signaling pathway contributes to long-term synaptic plasticity in the hippocampus. Proc. Natl. Acad. Sci. U.S.A. 99 (1), 467–472.

Tang, Y.P., Shimizu, E., Dube, G.R., Rampon, C., Kerchner, G.A., Zhuo, M., Tsien, J.Z., 1999. Genetic enhancement of learning and memory in mice. Nature 401 (6748), 63–69.

Tsai, L.C., Chan, G.C., Nangle, S.N., Shimizu-Albergine, M., Jones, G.L., Storm, D.R., Zweifel, L.S., 2012. Inactivation of Pde8b enhances memory, motor performance, and protects against age-induced motor coordination decay. Genes Brain Behav. 11 (7), 837–847.

Tsien, J.Z., Chen, D.F., Gerber, D., Tom, C., Mercer, E.H., Anderson, D.J., Tonegawa, S., 1996a. Subregion- and cell type-restricted gene knockout in mouse brain. Cell 87 (7), 1317–1326.

Tsien, J.Z., Huerta, P.T., Tonegawa, S., 1996b. The essential role of hippocampal CA1 NMDA receptor-dependent synaptic plasticity in spatial memory. Cell 87 (7), 1327–1338.

Tully, T., Bourtchouladze, R., Scott, R., Tallman, J., 2003. Targeting the CREB pathway for memory enhancers. Nat. Rev. Drug Discov. 2 (4), 267–277.

Viosca, J., Lopez de Armentia, M., Jancic, D., Barco, A., 2009a. Enhanced CREB-dependent gene expression increases the excitability of neurons in the basal amygdala and primes the consolidation of contextual and cued fear memory. Learn Mem. 16 (3), 193–197.

Viosca, J., Malleret, G., Bourtchouladze, R., Benito, E., Vronskava, S., Kandel, E.R., Barco, A., 2009b. Chronic enhancement of CREB activity in the hippocampus interferes with the retrieval of spatial information. Learn Mem. 16 (3), 198–209.

Walker, D.L., Davis, M., 2002. The role of amygdala glutamate receptors in fear learning, fear-potentiated startle, and extinction. Pharmacol. Biochem. Behav. 71 (3), 379–392.

Wang, D., Cui, Z., Zeng, Q., Kuang, H., Wang, L.P., Tsien, J.Z., Cao, X., 2009. Genetic enhancement of memory and long-term potentiation but not CA1 long-term depression in NR2B transgenic rats. PLoS One 4 (10), e7486.

Wang, H., Ferguson, G.D., Pineda, V.V., Cundiff, P.E., Storm, D.R., 2004. Overexpression of type-1 adenylyl cyclase in mouse forebrain enhances recognition memory and LTP. Nat. Neurosci. 7 (6), 635–642.

Wang, X.B., Bozdagi, O., Nikitczuk, J.S., Zhai, Z.W., Zhou, Q., Huntley, G.W., 2008. Extracellular proteolysis by matrix metalloproteinase-9 drives dendritic spine enlargement and long-term potentiation coordinately. Proc. Natl. Acad. Sci. U.S.A. 105 (49), 19520–19525.

Wei, F., Wang, G.D., Kerchner, G.A., Kim, S.J., Xu, H.M., Chen, Z.F., Zhuo, M., 2001. Genetic enhancement of inflammatory pain by forebrain NR2B overexpression. Nat. Neurosci. 4 (2), 164–169.

Whitlock, J.R., Heynen, A.J., Shuler, M.G., Bear, M.F., 2006. Learning induces long-term potentiation in the hippocampus. Science 313 (5790), 1093–1097.

Wong, R.W., Setou, M., Teng, J., Takei, Y., Hirokawa, N., 2002. Overexpression of motor protein KIF17 enhances spatial and working memory in transgenic mice. Proc. Natl. Acad. Sci. U.S.A. 99 (22), 14500–14505.

Wong, S.T., Athos, J., Figueroa, X.A., Pineda, V.V., Schaefer, M.L., Chavkin, C.C., Storm, D.R., 1999. Calcium-stimulated adenylyl cyclase activity is critical for hippocampus-dependent long-term memory and late phase LTP. Neuron 23 (4), 787–798.

Wu, H.Y., Yuen, E.Y., Lu, Y.F., Matsushita, M., Matsui, H., Yan, Z., Tomizawa, K., 2005. Regulation of N-methyl-D-aspartate receptors by calpain in cortical neurons. J. Biol. Chem. 280 (22), 21588–21593.

Yin, J.C., Wallach, J.S., Del Vecchio, M., Wilder, E.L., Zhou, H., Quinn, W.G., Tully, T., 1994. Induction of a dominant negative CREB transgene specifically blocks long-term memory in Drosophila. Cell 79 (1), 49–58.

Zeng, H., Chattarji, S., Barbarosie, M., Rondi-Reig, L., Philpot, B.D., Miyakawa, T., Tonegawa, S., 2001. Forebrain-specific calcineurin knockout selectively impairs bidirectional synaptic plasticity and working/episodic-like memory. Cell 107 (5), 617–629.

Zhu, P.J., Huang, W., Kalikulov, D., Yoo, J.W., Placzek, A.N., Stoica, L., Costa-Mattioli, M., 2011. Suppression of PKR promotes network excitability and enhanced cognition by interferon-gamma-mediated disinhibition. Cell 147 (6), 1384–1396.

Chapter 6

The Use of Viral Vectors to Enhance Cognition

Tsuneya Ikezu

Laboratory of Molecular NeuroTherapeutics, Departments of Pharmacology & Experimental Therapeutics and Neurology, Boston University School of Medicine, Boston, MA, USA

INTRODUCTION

Recovering cognitive function of human by viral gene therapy sounds futuristic, and regarded as a subject matter of Hollywood blockbuster movies rather than real health care. Indeed, the recent science fiction movie *Rise of the Planet of the Apes (2011)* depicts humanization of primate cognitive function by viral delivery of neuroregenerative genes. This was intended to cure Alzheimer's disease (AD); instead the virus killed human and triggered the evolution of primates. Gene therapy is conceptually simple: researchers deliver the gene of interest into the specific region of brains to protect neurons, enhance neural regeneration, and promote cognitive function. There are many promising results from animal studies that this chapter will cover. However, for their clinical application, the viral gene therapy itself had several stumbles at the pioneering phase of clinical trials: the most notable case is the adenovirus-mediated gene delivery of ornithine transcarbamylase into a young volunteer who had a moderate deficiency of the enzyme, who died of a massive immune response after hepatic injection of the purified viral particles (Teichler Zallen, 2000). Another inflammatory arthritis patient on a clinical trial of adeno-associated virus (AAV)-mediated gene delivery of tumor necrosis factor-α (TNF-α) inhibitors later died from different complications (Evans et al., 2008). As a natural consequence, the US Food and Drug Administration and the European Medicines Agency have not approved any viral human gene therapy products for sale. However, increasing number of clinical trials use viral vectors for specific disease applications, such as AD, Canavan disease, cystic fibrosis, hemophilia B, Leber congenital amaurosis, lipoprotein lipase deficiency, muscular dystrophy Parkinson disease, and rheumatoid arthritis (Aalbers et al., 2011). The commonly approved viral vectors for clinical trials are exclusively AAV vectors (Aalbers et al., 2011), which are extensively covered in this chapter.

Cognitive Enhancement. http://dx.doi.org/10.1016/B978-0-12-417042-1.00006-1

111

ADENO-ASSOCIATED VIRUS

AAV is currently the most common viral vector for gene therapy clinical trials focused on neurodegeneration (Lim et al., 2010). Discovered in 1965 as a contaminant of adenovirus preparations (Atchison et al., 1965; Hoggan et al., 1966), AAV is a small-sized (20 nm in diameter), nonenveloped, replication-defective virus and a member of the Parvoviridae family. This is about 1/100th of the size of adenoviruses, which are 90–100 nm in diameter. It is classified in the *Dependovirus* genus because a productive lytic cycle of DNA replication, amplification, and its packaging into progeny virions requires coinfection with a helper virus, such as adenovirus (Ad) or herpes simplex virus (HSV) (Atchison et al., 1965; Casto et al., 1967; Berns et al., 1988; Yakobson et al., 1989; Russell et al., 1995).

The structure of AAV is extremely simple (Figure 6.1). AAV has a linear single-stranded DNA (ssDNA) genome of approximately 4.7-kilobases (kb), with two 145-nucleotide-long inverted terminal repeats (ITRs). Its genome does not encode a DNA/RNA polymerase; thus, it relies on cellular polymerases for genomic replication. The ITRs flank the two viral genes: *rep* (replication), which encodes four nonstructural proteins involved in genome replication and packing into the nuclear capsid (King et al., 2001), and *cap* (capsid), which encodes three structural proteins (virion protein VP1, VP2, and VP3) for the capsid formation. The ITRs are the only *cis* elements required for genome replication, packaging, and integration into the viral capsid (McLaughlin et al., 1988; Samulski et al., 1989). Recombinant AAVs (rAAVs) are commonly produced by replacing the *rep* and *cap* genes with a promoter and gene of interest and by supplying *rep* and *cap* genes in *trans* from a separate plasmid lacking ITRs.

AAV has been highly promising as a vector for gene therapy in the central nervous system (CNS) for several reasons. (1) Unlike the larger retroviruses, it can infect both dividing and nondividing cells after a single delivery. (2) Unlike

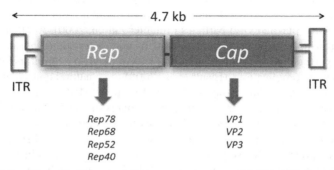

FIGURE 6.1 Schematic diagram of the genomic structure of AAV2. ITR, inverted terminal repeat (145 nucleotides); *Rep*, replication gene encoding four different Rep proteins; *Cap*, capsid gene encoding three different viral particle (VP) proteins.

adenovirus herpes virus, or lentivirus, AAV infection show minimal pathogenicity, immune reactions, or toxicity. (3) ITR-flanked genomic sequence integrates into infected host genome, leading to long-term transgene expression (Berns et al., 1975). Moreover, AAV serotype 8 (AAV8) and AAV1 shows a stronger transduction efficiency than AAV2 (Weinberg et al., 2013). Modern rAAV vectors have 96% of the viral genome removed from the vector; because only the two 145-bp ITRs are remaining viral DNA, no de novo viral protein synthesis can occur after transduction. AAV is also favorable because it has no association with any known human etiologies and very low incidence of antigen-specific immunity, which is a major problem of the adenovirus system (Chirmule et al., 1999).

AAV's unique site-specific genomic integration could reduce the risk of insertional mutagenesis, which randomly occurs after retrovirus or adenovirus infection and is a major cause of tumorigenesis. Through nonhomologous recombination, AAV2 specifically integrates into the human genome at chromosome 19q13.4 via AAV2 Rep proteins (Kotin et al., 1990; Samulski et al., 1991; Weitzman et al., 1994; Balague et al., 1997). After AAV infection, the AAV genome enters a nonproductive, latent, non–progeny-producing state in which it exists as a provirus integrated into the chromosomal genome of the host cell (Cheung et al., 1980). The potential for unwanted viral spread is limited by the requirement of helper virus functions for a productive AAV lytic cycle.

So far AAV serotypes 1–12 are documented (Table 6.1). Transduced AAV genomes confer long-term expression in a variety of cell types and tissues dependent on the viral serotype, including retina (Flannery et al., 1997), muscle (Xiao et al., 1996; Fisher et al., 1997), liver (Ponnazhagan et al., 1997), and the CNS (Kaplitt et al., 1994; McCown et al., 1996; Xiao et al., 1997). Long-term expression (greater than 1.5 years) has also been demonstrated in a number of AAV-infected animals, including murine, hamster, and canine (Xiao et al., 1996; Monahan et al., 1998; Li et al., 2003).

STRATEGIES TO INCREASE EFFICIENCY AND SPECIFICITY OF GENE TRANSFER

Many innovations have been made in rAAV vector development to allow increased specificity, efficiency and spread of gene transfer, including hybrid serotypes, rationally designed capsids, split vectors, and specific promoter/enhancer additions. rAAV transduction efficiency can be 20 to thousands of vector particles per transducing unit, although this varies depending on cell type and differences in infectivity assays (Grieger and Samulski, 2012).

One fundamental aspect of AAV specificity for targeting of relevant cell types and brain areas is AAV serology. AAV serotypes, of which there are currently 12 known naturally occurring and laboratory-defined, are classified based on their cell surface antigens in the capsid protein motifs (Table 6.1). A "new" serotype is defined as one that does not crossreact with neutralizing sera that

TABLE 6.1 AAV Serotypes

Serotype	Natural Host/Origin	Tissue/Cell Type Transduced	CNS Area Transduced	Viral Receptor	Viral Coreceptor	Disease Targets
AAV1	Monkey	Muscle, liver, CNS	SNpc, SNpr, midbrain, hippocampus, medial septum, striatum, spinal cord, motor cortex	2,3N/2,6N-sialic acid	Unknown	Lipoprotein lipase deficiency
AAV2	Human	Kidney, muscle, lung, eye, liver, CNS	SNpc, dentate gyrus, midbrain	HSPG	LamR, FGFR1, integrins, HGFR, c-met	Leber congenital amaurosis, Parkinson disease, rheumatoid arthritis, AD
AAV3	Human	Liver cancer cells		HSPG	LamR, FGFR1, HGF	
AAV4	Monkey	CNS, lung, ependymal cells	Retina, midbrain	2,3-O-linked sialic acid	Unknown	
AAV5	Human	Muscle, liver, CNS	SNpc, SNpr, hippocampus, medial septum, striatum, spinal cord, motor cortex, cerebellum, retina	2,3N-sialic acid	PDGFR	Rheumatoid arthritis
AAV6	Human	Muscle, liver, spinal cord	Spinal cord	2,3N/2,6N-sialic acid	EGFR	
AAV7	Monkey	Muscle, liver		N-sialic acid	PDGFR	

AAV8	Monkey	Liver, heart, pancreas, muscle, CNS, eye	Hippocampus, retina	Unknown	LamR	Hemophilia B
AAV9	Monkey	Heart, lung, muscle, liver, CNS, blood–brain barrier	Hippocampus, striatum, cortex, dorsal root ganglia, spinal cord	N-galactose	LamR	
AAV10	Monkey	CNS, muscle, liver, spleen, lymph node	Striatum, nucleus accumbens	Unknown	Unknown	
AAV11	Monkey	Spleen, lymph node		Unknown	Unknown	
AAV12	Monkey	Nasal epithelia		Unknown	Unknown	
AAV2.5	Recombinant	Muscle				Duchenne muscular dystrophy

Abbreviations: SNpc, substantia nigra pars compacta; SNpr, substantia nigra pars reticulata; HSPG, heparan sulfate proteoglycan; HCFR, hepatic growth factor receptor; EGFR, epidermal growth factor receptor; FGFR1, fibroblast growth factor receptor 1; PDCFR, platelet-derived growth factor receptor; LamR, 37/67-kDa Laminin receptor. *References:* AAV1 (Burger et al., 2004; Gao et al., 2004; Wu et al., 2006a; Stroes et al., 2008; Dodiya et al., 2010; Miyake et al., 2012; AAV2 (Summerford and Samulski, 1998; Qing et al., 1999; Summerford et al., 1999; Davidson et al., 2000; Burger et al., 2004; Takeda et al., 2004; Kashiwakura et al., 2005; Akache et al., 2006; Asokan et al., 2006; Arvanitakis Z, 2007; Bishop et al., 2008; Glushakova et al., 2009; Maguire et al., 2009; Mease et al., 2009; Hadaczek et al., 2010; Mandel, 2010; Miyake et al., 2012), AAV3 (Rabinowitz et al., 2002; Akache et al., 2006; Ling et al., 2010; Miyake et al., 2012), AAV4 (Davidson et al., 2000; Kaludov et al., 2001; Weber et al., 2003; Klein et al., 2008; Miyake et al., 2012), AAV5 (Davidson et al., 2000; Walters et al., 2001; Di Pasquale et al., 2003; Weber et al., 2003; Burger et al., 2004; Adriaansen et al., 2007; Dodiya et al., 2010; Miyake et al., 2012), AAV6 (Wu et al., 2006a; Weller et al., 2010; Miyake et al., 2012), AAV7 (Gao et al., 2004; Miyake et al., 2012), AAV8 (Gao et al., 2002; Akache et al., 2006; Cearley and Wolfe, 2006; Klein et al., 2006; Dodiya et al., 2010; Allay et al., 2011; Miyake et al., 2012), AAV9 (Xiao et al., 1999; Blankinship et al., 2004; Gao et al., 2004; Akache et al., 2006; Cearley and Wolfe, 2006; Klein et al., 2008; Foust et al., 2008; Bevan et al., 2011; Gray et al., 2011a; Shen et al., 2011; Fang et al., 2012), AAV10 (Anderson et al., 2008; Klein et al., 2008; Mori et al., 2008; Miyake et al., 2012), AAV11(Mori et al., 2008), AAV12 (Quinn et al., 2011), AAV2.5 (Bowles et al., 2012).

are specific for existing serotypes. Based on this definition, AAV6 is not a true serotype because the serology of AAV6 is nearly identical to that of AAV1 (Wu et al., 2006b). AAV2 was the first serotype to be cloned into bacterial plasmids (Samulski et al., 1982) and has since been widely used. The following discovery and study of other serotypes has highlighted not only their ability to evade naturally occurring human AAV2-neutralizing antibodies but also their ability for increased CNS gene transfer compared with AAV2, both in terms of total transduced brain volume and total number of transduced cells (Burger et al., 2004; Cearley and Wolfe, 2006; Klein et al., 2008). Because the capsid motif governs the way AAV enters the host cell, each serotype has a unique transduction efficacy, and this can be taken advantage of by researchers for infection of particular cell types or tissues using naturally occurring serotypes as well as for design of hybrid serotypes for tissue or cell-specific targeting.

AAV hybrid serotypes have capsid protein modifications that increase the specificity and efficiency of viral, which are essential for targeting the tissue and cell type of interest and minimizing dose infection (Choi et al., 2005). One variety of hybrid serotype is obtained through trans-capsidation, or packaging the genome containing ITRs (*cis*-acting) from one serotype into the capsid of a different serotype (*trans*-acting virion shell). The tropism or host-cell specificity is determined by the *cap* gene-encoded VP1, VP2, and VP3 proteins; tropism of an AAV vector during transduction can thus be changed by exchanging the *rep/cap* gene serotypes. Most vectors that were developed prior to the development of hybrid vectors have been AAV2, and these are most used as ITRs for crosspackaging in capsids of another serotype. This is because the integration sites of AAV2 ITRs in human genome are defined and are known to be safe. Transcapsidation of the AAV2 genome allows the genome from this well-characterized serotype to target cell types that do not express receptors utilized by AAV2. In addition, AAV2 genomic integration is present in ~80–90% of the population; AAV2-neutralizing antibodies were found in humans in early AAV studies (Parks et al., 1970) and are now known to be more prevalent than AAV1-neutralizing antibodies in humans (Xiao et al., 1999). Thus, since tropism is determined by the *cap* genes, rAAV has been developed with AAV2 ITRs and *rep* and *cap* genes of alternative serotypes, thereby avoiding actions of AAV2-neutralizing antibodies.

By packaging the capsids of different serotypes with AAV2 ITRs, the transduction efficiencies of naturally occurring AAV serotype vectors in different tissues and cell types have been compared, providing a vast amount of information on specific serotypes in the literature.

Keeping in mind inter-study variation in AAV promoters, transgenes, titers and doses, comparative efficiency of transduction in major tissues has been established (see Table 6.1 for summary) (Wu et al., 2006b; Zincarelli et al., 2008). AAV2 transduces a wide range of cell types and tissues with moderate efficiency (liver, muscle, lung, CNS). AAV9 has a similar profile to AAV2 but shows more efficient transduction (Gao et al., 2004). In skeletal muscle, AAV1 and AAV7 show rapid onset and high transduction levels (Gao et al., 2004). AAV6, because it differs from AAV1 by only six amino acids, also transduces skeletal muscle.

In the CNS, AAV 1, 2, 5, 8, and 9 have been the most widely studied serotypes, with AAV 1 and 5 conferring a superior transduction efficiency than AAV2, and AAV8 and 9 conferring further superior transduction over AAV1 and 5 in the rodent CNS (Burger et al., 2004; Klein et al., 2006; Wu et al., 2006b; Klein et al., 2008; Gray et al., 2011a). In comparison to AAV2, most serotypes show greater CNS transduction in terms of total transduced brain volume and total number of transduced cells but also in some cases, higher level of gene expression per cell (Burger et al., 2004; Klein et al., 2006). Burger et al. assessed CNS transduction of AAV1, 2, and 5 capsids flanked with AAV2 ITRs injected into different regions of the rat brain (Burger et al., 2004). While all constructs primarily transduced neurons, AAV1 and AAV5 capsids showed higher transduction efficiency than AAV2 in all CNS regions injected, including the hippocampus, striatum, globus pallidus, substantia nigra, and spinal cord. In the hippocampus, AAV1 and 5 capsids mostly transduced pyramidal neurons in CA1-CA3 regions, while AAV2 mostly transduced neurons in the granular and hilar region of the dentate gyrus. AAV8 showed superior transduction to AAV1, 2, and 5 in the hippocampus of the rat brain, although in one study this efficient gene transfer by AAV8 might have caused neurotoxic level of green fluorescent protein expression (Klein et al., 2006). In contrast to findings in rodents, a study in adult cynomolgus monkeys showed superior transduction by AAV1 and AAV5 compared with AAV8 in the striatum (Dodiya et al., 2010). Klein et al. showed that AAV9 conferred more efficient gene transfer in the brain than AAV2 or AAV8 in rat tauopathy models (Klein et al., 2008). A recent study demonstrated serotype-specificity in transduction of recombinant AAV in different neuronal cell types in different brain regions (Table 6.2) (Aschauer et al., 2013). For AD studies, researchers may be interested in injecting into many regions but perhaps specifically the hippocampal region, where early neurodegeneration occurs. Thus, for targeting the hippocampus in rodent studies, AAV8 (Klein et al., 2006) and AAV9 (Klein et al., 2008) may be superior.

AAV9 has been studied for its unique ability to cross the blood–brain barrier (BBB) when injected into neonate rodents, allowing the CNS administration from the periphery (Foust et al., 2009; Bevan et al., 2011; Gray et al., 2011a; Dayton et al., 2012). However, in adult mice, AAV9 administered peripherally showed transduction of mainly neurons in the hippocampus and striatum, but mainly astrocytes in the cortex (Gray et al., 2011a); an opposing study reported robust transduction of astrocytes throughout the CNS with limited neuronal transduction (Foust et al., 2009). To highlight the need for caution in extrapolating transduction efficiencies between species, AAV9 showed reduced transduction efficiency and a switch from primarily neuronal to primarily glial expression in nonhuman primates, which could be attributed to differential AAV receptor expression, promoter regulation, or differential levels of preexisting

TABLE 6.2 AAV Serotype Specificity of CNS Transduction

	Serotype	AAV1	AAV2	AAV5	AAV6	AAV8	AAV9
	Cortex	+	±	+	+	+	++
	Hippocampus	+	±	++	±	+	++
	Striatum	+	±	++	+	+	+
Cortex	Oligodendrocytes	+	±	+	±	+	+
	Microglia	+	±	+	±	+	+
	Astrocytes	+	±	+	±	+++	+
	Neurons	±	±	±	±	±	+
	Inhibitory neurons	+	+	±	±	+	++
Hippocampus	Oligodendrocytes	+	+	±	+	+	+
	Microglia	+	±	+	+	++	±
	Astrocytes	+	±	±	+	+	+
	Neurons	+	±	±	±	++	+
	Inhibitory neurons	+	±	+	+	++	+
Striatum	Oligodendrocytes	+	±	+	+	±	+
	Microglia	++	±	±	±	+	±
	Astrocytes	+	±	+	±	+	±
	Neurons	++	±	+	+	+	+
	Inhibitory neurons	+	±	+	+	+	+

AAV-neutralizing antibodies in the primates (Allay et al., 2011). However, another study reported neuron-specific infection in the macaque and marmoset brain by AAV8-EGFP and AAV9-EGFP (Masamizu et al., 2011). Although AAV9 is the only naturally occurring serotype known to show BBB permeability, numerous chimeric and directed evolution vectors have been constructed to cross the BBB, allowing peripheral administration of a CNS-targeted therapeutic gene (e.g., Gray et al., 2010). Due to their increased specificity and transduction efficacy, pseudotyped vectors are now the primary choice for rAAV clinical trials (2012). However, despite the focus on comparing serotypes, some researchers posit that serotype differences have a minimal overall effect on transduction efficacy (e.g., Klein et al., 2008).

In addition to hybrid serotypes involving trans-capsidation, rationally designed AAV capsids have driven the customization of AAV vectors to improve efficacy for clinical use, which include chimeric and mosaic capsids and its mutants. For example, a capsid termed AAV2.5 was developed using AAV2 with five amino acid mutations from AAV1, in order to harness the muscle-transducing abilities of AAV1 with the receptor binding properties of AAV2 and to decrease antigenic crossreactivity against both parental serotypes. AAV2.5 was subsequently used in a Phase I clinical trial for Duchenne muscular dystrophy (Bowles et al., 2012). Additional AAV capsids have been designed to achieve unique tropisms and to improve transduction efficiency (for review, see Grieger and Samulski, 2012).

Promoters and enhancers are frequent components of rAAV vectors that can be used to boost specificity of gene expression. Recombinant AAV constructed for use in neurological disease accordingly contain CNS cell type-specific promoters, including platelet-derived growth factor (PDGF) promoter (Peel and Klein, 2000), neuron-specific enolase (NSE) promoter, and less specific chicken β-actin (CBA) or cytomegalovirus (CMV) promoter. The CMV promoter confers high neuron-selective transgene expression in rodents (Kaplitt et al., 1994; Gray et al., 2011b), but some studies observed different durations of expression of vectors with this promoter depending on the brain region, implying region-specific CMV promoter suppression mechanism (McCown et al., 1996; Gray et al., 2011b). CMV hybrid promoters, such as a CMV/CBA promoter, can prevent this attenuation of CMV promoter activity (Niwa et al., 1991). CMV/CBA hybrid vectors were additionally found to transduce more cells than NSE vectors in rat hippocampus (Klein et al., 2002). Alternatively, CMV promoters may be used for the long-term expression of recombinant genes. Gray et al. reported that CBA promoters show ubiquitous and high neural expression but low expression in motor neurons (Gray et al., 2011b). This was bypassed by development of an 800-bp hybrid CBA promoter that shows high expression in motor neurons and all cell types transduced by native CBA and CMV promoters (Gray et al., 2011b).

Some studies may aim for glial expression of transgene, in which case glial-specific promoters can be used. This may be useful for studying the involvement of glial cells in AD, as well as for many autoimmune neurodegenerative disorders involving demyelination and axonal degeneration such as multiple sclerosis, Charcot-Marie-Tooth disease and various leukodystrophies. The glial fibrillary acidic protein (GFAP) promoter has successfully been used for astrocyte-specific gene expression, while the myelin basic protein (MBP) promoter can be used for oligodendrocyte-specific gene expression (Chen et al., 1999; Feng et al., 2004; Lawlor et al., 2009).

The recent AAV expression vectors also contain the woodchuck hepatitis virus (WHV) post-transcriptional regulatory element (WPRE), a commonly used 3'-UTR enhancer used to increase viral titer and transgene expression (Loeb et al., 1999). Klein et al. reported an 11-fold increase in transgene expression levels with incorporation of the WPRE into a CBA promoter vector in rat hippocampus (Klein et al., 2002).

TRANS-SPLICING AAV

Due to the small size of the AAV genome, other viral vectors typically have a greater capacity with which to insert transgenes, but this has mostly been overcome by vector constructs specially engineered to carry large transgenes. For instance, split vectors have been made in which the transgene cassette is split into two constructs, which have a slight sequence overlap with each other so that recombination after vector nuclear entry leads to the intact transgene product being expressed (Yan et al., 2000). Using this *trans*-splicing method, therapeutic genes up to 9 kb have been delivered in the retina, lung and muscle, although these vectors are less efficient than normal rAAV vectors (Daya and Berns, 2008). Alternatively, Gray et al. developed a short neuronal promoter that can package larger transgenes into AAV vectors because of the relatively reduced size of the promoter—a 229-bp fragment of the mouse methyl-CpG-binding protein-2 (MeCP2) (Gray et al., 2011b).

ADVANCEMENTS IN rAAV PACKAGING AND PURIFICATION

As a complement to innovations in vector design, improvements in methods for rAAV manufacturing have advanced AAV gene therapy for human use. These include the engineering of plasmids carrying adenovirus helper functions without the complete AD genome, stable "producer" cell lines providing helper functions, and purification methods resulting in large rAAV yields appropriate for clinical use.

Recombinant AAV was historically produced after gene construction by using wild-type adenovirus as a helper virus. This method involves transfecting cell lines that stably harbor AAV *rep/cap* genes with wild-type adenovirus and the AAV vector DNA. Although this can be scaled up to produce vectors with high titers, it is difficult to avoid adenovirus contamination in this method even with the use of repeated cesium chloride gradients. This has been overcome by the development of the "mini-Ad genome," plasmids carrying only the adenovirus helper genes (which include the E1a, E1b, E2a, E4, and VA RNA genes). This adenovirus-free method involves transient transfection of all elements required for AAV production into host cells (such as human embryonic kidney 293 cells (HEK293)): an rAAV ITR-containing plasmid carrying the gene of interest, a plasmid that carries AAV *rep* and *cap* genes, and a helper plasmid with only the adenovirus helper genes. This triple transfection "helper-free" method was first used with the mini-Ad genome plasmid PXX6 (Xiao et al., 1998) and since then similar plasmids have been developed, such as pFD13, which has an 8-kb deletion in the adenovirus E2B region and most of the late genes (Xiao et al., 1999). The mini-adenovirus genome preceded the development of pDG, a plasmid with AAV2 packaging functions and adenovirus helper functions (AAV2 *rep* and *cap* genes and VA, E2A, and E4 genes of adenovirus 5), allowing for transfection of only two plasmids (Grimm et al., 1998). Additional helper viruses based on pDG, with its original AAV2 *cap* genes replaced by *cap* genes from AAV1 and AAV3-6 were engineered by the same group, in order to achieve increased efficacy in varied cell types (Table 6.1) (Grimm et al., 2003) (Box 6.1).

Box 6.1 *cis* and *trans* Genes

cis genes: genes that regulate the transcription of their own region.
trans genes: genes that regulate the transcription of other regions.

Other innovations have been developed for maximized AAV growth and scalability of production. "Producer" stable cell lines, such as the AAV293 cell line, provide adenovirus genes to support AAV growth and produce higher viral titers (Agilent Technologies, Santa Clara, CA). AAV293 cells are human embryonic kidney cells derived from the commonly used HEK293 cells that have been transformed by sheared adenovirus type 5 DNA. AAV293 cells produce the adenovirus E1 gene in *trans*, allowing the production of infectious AAV particles when cells are cotransfected with three AAV helper-free system plasmids (an ITR-containing plasmid, pAAV-RC which supplies *rep* and *cap* genes in *trans*, and an E1-deleted helper plasmid). Another producer cell line, 84-31 cells (Human Applications Laboratory, University of Pennsylvania), are a subclone of HEK293 cells that stably express E4 of the adenovirus genome and are used in the same manner as AAV293 (Xiao et al., 1999). Production technologies have recently been improved to allow production methods that are more scalable than using adherent HEK293 cells for rAAV production. These include HEK293 cell lines that can grow in serum-free suspension, the dual rHSV infection system of suspension baby hamster kidney cells, and the baculovirus expression vector system (BEVS) using *Spodoptera frugiperda* 9 (Sf9) insect cells (see Grieger and Samulski, 2012). These systems are especially appropriate for clinical applications, where scalability of rAAV production is essential.

In addition to the preparation of rAAV in large quantities, it must also be purified in large quantities for clinical use. Purification rids the preparation of contaminants such as "empty shells" (AAV particles lacking viral nucleic acid), or Ad particles if Ad is used as a helper virus. The traditionally used method of sedimentation through cesium chloride gradients is not scalable, and has been replaced by nonionic iodixanol gradient purification or ammonium sulfate precipitation, followed by ion exchange or heparin/agarose column chromatography (Zolotukhin et al., 1999). This method is based on the finding that AAV2 binds to the heparin sulfate proteoglycan surface molecule (Summerford and Samulski, 1998). AAV6 is also known to bind heparin with moderate affinity, but despite its high sequence homology with AAV1 (~99.2%), AAV1 does not exhibit this quality (Halbert et al., 2001) and must therefore be purified using other methods such as ion exchange chromatography (Zolotukhin et al., 1999). Wu et al. identified a single amino acid (K531) that is essential for conferring the heparin binding characteristics of AAV6, and that introduction of an E531K change in AAV1 yields a heparin binding ability similar to that of AAV6 (Wu et al., 2006b).

GENE DELIVERY TO THE CNS

There are many potential risks associated with viral gene delivery in humans, and therefore certain considerations must be made for studies involving the CNS gene delivery. Unless AAV9 is used in neonates, therapeutic vectors must be administered directly into the CNS. This requires bilateral stereotaxic surgery on anesthetized subjects, which could lead to significant side effects (Tuszynski et al., 2005; Mandel, 2010). In this case, gene transfer must be locally restricted to minimize the risks of serious adverse effects that can result from broad distribution. Thus, intracranial injections must be optimized, and vectors must be designed in order to maximize efficiency and specificity of transduction to minimize required dose. Though the first rAAV clinical trials used AAV2, most recent clinical trials use AAV2 ITRs pseudotyped with capsids of other serotypes such as AAV5 or 8 (e.g., Wu et al., 2005; Bowles et al., 2012), allowing increased transduction efficiency of targeted cell types, as well as avoidance of AAV2-neutralizing antibodies, which is important for minimizing the viral dose.

Although simple injection methods using a constant flow rate have proven to work well for rAAV delivery, some researchers have developed methods that may improve brain delivery of rAAV. For example, convection-enhanced delivery (CED) is a method developed specifically for CNS delivery of large compounds that are normally BBB impermeable, in which a constant pressure gradient is applied to the infusate to cause bulk flow, rather than diffusion, through the interstitium (Bobo et al., 1994; Bankiewicz et al., 2000). Step cannulae may also be used for injection, which prevent reflux into the track of injection (Krauze et al., 2005). If a study is designed for systemic delivery to the CNS, therapeutic genes may be delivered via intracerebroventricular, intrathecal, or peripheral methods. AAV9, as it is BBB permeable, may be delivered intravenously in the periphery, avoiding the potential hazards and difficulties of intracranial injection. However, adult animals may show a low neuronal versus glial transduction efficiency with AAV9, and significant amounts of peripheral tissue may likely be transduced when vector is delivered peripherally (Gray et al., 2011a). Other delivery methods include targeting brain areas via retrograde transport from muscle to spinal neurons (Towne et al., 2010). In certain diseases or disease states, such as stroke, timing of therapy may be crucial for outcome. In AD or other slow-progressing neurodegenerative diseases, therapy may be effective at the earliest disease stage.

COGNITIVE ENHANCEMENT AND NEUROGENESIS

Adult neurogenesis is the process of neuronal proliferation and maturation in specific brain regions, and it is not only involved in CNS maintenance but also in the formation of new memories that new evidence suggests may be linked to synaptic plasticity affected by environmental or behavioral factors (Bruel-Jungerman et al., 2007; Deng et al., 2009, 2010; Tronel et al., 2012). Neural stem cells (NSCs) are always present in the adult CNS by self-renewal where they have the ability to differentiate into neurons, astrocytes, and oligodendrocytes. However, the process appears to be strictly controlled by local cues that keep the production of new neurons to a certain level (Dayer et al., 2005; Tamura et al., 2007). The production of new neurons in adulthood is mainly seen in the subventricular zone (SVZ), where neuroblasts migrate to the olfactory bulb, and in the subgranular zone (SGZ) of the dentate gyrus of hippocampal formation, where the neurons are involved in hippocampal regeneration, the process of contextual and long-term memory formation and learning, and the regulation of mood (Ming and Song, 2005; Franklin and Ffrench-Constant, 2008). These areas have a network with high demand for the production of new neurons because they are constantly exposed to novel stimuli (Carpentier and Palmer, 2009). Only a small subset of NSCs created in the SGZ reach maturity after integration into the neural network, meaning a majority of the newborn cells undergo apoptosis within the first 4 days after creation (Sierra et al., 2010). It was shown by a number of researchers that exposure to novel smells in the olfactory bulb stimulated the production and retention of new neurons (Magavi et al., 2005; So et al., 2008), and it was likewise shown in the hippocampus that environmental enrichment, physical activity, and the act of learning promoted the production of new neurons (Emsley et al., 2005; Duan et al., 2008). Oddly enough, both depression and olfactory deficits are early indications of neurodegeneration in both AD and Parkinson's disease (Bruck et al., 2004; Hawkes, 2006; Gabryelewicz et al., 2007; Matsuda, 2007; Poewe, 2008).

NEUROGENESIS IN AGING AND AD

One study demonstrated that an age-dependent increase in specific blood-borne factors associated with proinflammatory (M1) microglia, as shown by the presence of the M1 marker, CCL11, may contribute to the inhibition of neurogenesis in healthy aging humans, as was seen when young mice were joined to the systemic environments of old mice by heterochronic parabiosis. This also resulted in decreased synaptic plasticity and impaired contextual fear conditioning, spatial memory, and learning (Villeda et al., 2011). There have been several contradictory reports that show how neurogenesis is particularly altered in the AD brain as well (for review, see Waldau and Shetty, 2008). Investigators have demonstrated that, while there is some reduction in neuronal maturation in the presenile post-mortem AD hippocampus, there is an increase in cellular proliferation in the hippocampus (Jin et al., 2004; Boekhoorn et al., 2006). Therefore, despite the supposed increase in neurogenesis due to increased proliferation, there is an overall reduction in neurogenesis because these newly proliferated cells do not become mature neurons. The chronic neuroinflammation seen in AD has been shown to be the major contributor to overall suppression of neurogenesis in the SVZ and SGZ (Monje et al., 2003; Hoehn et al., 2005; Deng et al., 2010).

ANIMAL MODELS OF AD

The development of transgenic mouse models that partly recapitulate behavioral and pathological aspects of AD has proved to be an invaluable tool for studying the disease etiology and effectiveness of therapeutics. The first report of a transgenic mouse displaying AD pathology was that of the PDAPP mouse in 1995, which overexpresses mutant β-amyloid precursor protein (APP) leading to Aβ plaque deposition in relevant brain areas (Games et al., 1995). Tg2576, another line expressing mutant APP developed soon after, shows similar pathology as well as age-related cognitive decline (Hsiao et al., 1996). Transgenic mice expressing familial AD-linked mutants of APP and presenilin-1 (PS1) (APP/PS1 mice) have also proved to be valuable tools in AD investigations, as transgene expression leads to Alzheimer-like pathology and phenotype including hippocampal and cortical Aβ deposits and deficits in spatial memory. This spatial memory deficit makes these mice especially useful for spatial memory testing, such as in the radial arm water maze (RAWM) test.

One of the most notable therapeutic developments from the AD mouse models was Aβ immunotherapies, which have shown improvements in amyloid clearance and spatial learning in mouse models expressing mutant APP and have been the main focus of therapeutic development (Schenk et al., 1999; Morgan et al., 2000). Recently, an independent academic group reported that their analysis of results of a Phase 3 trial of Solanezumab, Eli Lilly and Company's humanized monoclonal Aβ antibody, revealed small but significant improvements in cognition in mild-stage AD (Callaway, 2012). However, these changes were only very small and require further analyses. Despite the lack of translation of amyloid-β antibody therapies from mice to humans, animal models remain useful for easily exploring many features of the disease and the extent to which genetic insults affect disease.

ASSESSING OUTCOMES OF AD GENE THERAPY: BEHAVIORAL TESTING AND NEUROPHYSIOLOGY

For the treatment AD by viral gene delivery, optimization of transduction efficiency and specificity is important for targeting affected brain areas. AD is characterized by accumulation of intracellular microtubule-binding protein tau (τ) and extracellular β-amyloid (Aβ) plaques, which are thought to lead to synaptic degeneration and progressive cognitive impairment. This pathology in the AD brain starts in the entorhinal cortex and spreads to hippocampal subregions and cortical areas (Harris et al., 2010).

AD leads to cognitive deficits including learning and memory dysfunction, which correlate with synapse loss and widespread neuron degeneration particularly in the hippocampus (West and Gundersen, 1990; Sze et al., 1997). Relevant measures of outcome of therapeutic interventions in experimental animals thus include spatial memory behavioral testing, electrophysiological assessment of neuron function, and histological analysis of neuron and synapse morphology.

To measure changes in behavior after AD gene therapy, spatial memory tests are often used, one of which is the RAWM test. The RAWM measures the ability of a mouse or rat to remember the location of a hidden underwater platform in repeated trials. Double transgenic APP/PS1 mice show spatial memory deficit as measured by this test (Arendash et al., 2001; Kiyota et al., 2009, 2012). Changes in function at the synaptic level can also be measured by electrophysiology. Young PDAPP(J20) and PDAPP(J9) mice, which contain human APP carrying familial AD Swedish (K670N/M671L) and Indiana (V717F) mutations, show a deficit in hippocampal basal synaptic transmission prior to the formation of Aβ plaques, as measured by change in field excitatory post-synaptic potential (fEPSP) slope (Hsia et al., 1999). Similarly, Chapman et al. showed that aged Tg2576 mice display normal fast synaptic transmission and short-term plasticity but are impaired in long-term potentiation (LTP) in CA1 and the dentate gyrus (Chapman et al., 1999). Prominent hippocampal synaptic loss is seen in AD patients, especially in CA1 (West and Gundersen, 1990); thus, measures of synaptic transmission in this region may reveal the efficacy of a certain treatment for AD. Basal synaptic transmission, LTP, and long-term depression are common electrophysiological measures of synaptic function and plasticity that can easily be applied to AD studies using AAV gene therapy.

Despite the widespread neuronal loss is seen in AD, it is believed to be a disease of synaptic failure. This synaptic failure, thought to be caused by the toxicity of amyloid plaques and neurofibrillary tangles, correlates with cognitive decline and is believed to be the initial cause of memory impairment prior to neuron loss (Selkoe, 2002). This is supported by electrophysiological studies as outlined previously (Chapman et al., 1999; Hsia et al., 1999), as well as by studies of synapse density and expression of synaptic markers. Whereas amyloid plaque load and neuron death do not correlate with cognitive decline (Terry et al., 1991), loss of the presynaptic vesicle protein synaptophysin seen in AD patients in the hippocampus (Sze et al., 1997) and prefrontal cortex (Terry et al., 1991) correlates with cognitive decline. Histological examination of the brain readily reveals changes in synapse morphology and density that correlate with cognitive decline in AD. Synapse density can be measured immunohisto-chemically using antibodies against synaptophysin or other synaptic proteins. Hsia et al. used this method to show that PDAPP (J9) mice show significantly decreased synaptophysin-positive terminals in the CA1 region of the hippocampus at as early as 2–3 months of age (Hsia et al., 1999). Neuronal loss can also be measured with neuronal markers such as microtubule-associated protein 2 (MAP2, dendritic marker) or β3-tubulin (axonal marker).

Increasing evidence shows that adult neurogenesis in the neurogenic regions (subventricular zone and subgranular zone of the dentate gyrus) may be dys-regulated in AD, which may be linked to age-dependent memory loss (Galvan and Bredesen, 2007; Abdipranoto et al., 2008). APP/PS1 mice also show a significant inhibition of neurogenesis (Biscaro et al., 2009; Kiyota et al., 2010, 2012). Neurogenesis may be assessed using markers such as doublecortin (Dcx, a marker of newly generated neurons), nestin (a marker of neuronal precursor cells), and bromodeoxyuridine, which is incorporated into newly born cells. Thus, with behavioral, electrophysiological and histological examination, outcomes of AAV gene therapy for AD can be thoroughly assessed.

CURRENT AAV THERAPIES IN AD ANIMAL STUDIES AND CLINICAL TRIALS

Neurotrophic Factor Genes

To date, 80 clinical trials using AAV gene therapy strategies in humans have been completed, are open, or have been reviewed, 17% of which are for neurological disease, and two of which are trials for AD therapies (Grieger and Samulski, 2012; Gene Therapy Clinical Trials Worldwide Database http://www.wiley.com/legacy/wileychi/genmed/clinical/).

Most preclinical and clinical studies for Alzheimer gene therapy so far have used neurotrophic growth factors, including nerve growth factor (NGF), fibroblast growth factor 2 (FGF2), and brain-derived neurotrophic growth factor (BDNF) to counteract inhibition of neurogenesis (Nagahara et al., 2009). The first gene therapy used in AD patients tested ex vivo gene delivery of human β-NGF, which has been shown to prevent cholinergic neuron degeneration (Hefti, 1986), with primary fibroblasts transduced using retroviral vectors. This phase I trial, completed in 2003, involved forebrain implantation of autologous fibroblasts in eight patients with mild-stage AD (Tuszynski et al., 2005). Although two patients were excluded from the trial due to movement during stereotaxic injection, a 22-month follow-up in the six remaining subjects revealed no long-term adverse effects of NGF, an decrease in the rate of cognitive decline, while serial positron emission tomography (PET) scans showed significant increases in cortical glucose uptake function (as measured by the glucose analog 18-fluorodeoxyglucose) after treatment.

The two gene therapy clinical trials using AAV also tested intracranial delivery of NGF using AAV2 (AAV2-NGF a.k.a. CERE-110; Ceregene, Inc.) (Mandel, 2010). Initial animal studies showed that AAV-mediated NGF expression in the rat basal forebrain (AAV2-NGF) (Bishop et al., 2008) or medial septum (AAV2/5-NGF) (Wu et al., 2005) leads to neuroprotection from cholinergic neuron axotomy. A phase I trial involving delivery of AAV2-NGF (CERE-110) to 10 patients with mild to moderate AD was completed in 2010 (ClinicalTrials.gov identifier: NCT00087789) (Arvanitakis, 2007), and 50 patients are now being recruited for a CERE-110 phase II trial (ClinicalTrials.gov identifier: NCT00876863), although results from the first trial have not been published.

FGF2, an established neurogenic factor of proliferation and differentiation for multipotent neural progenitors (Kuhn et al., 1997; Tao et al., 1997; Mudo et al., 2009), is additionally under investigation for AD gene therapy. FGF2 is expressed in neurogenic regions in the CNS, and has been implicated in the control of adult neurogenesis because of its effect on proliferation and fate choice of adult neural progenitor cells (Jin et al., 2003; Baldauf and Reymann, 2005). Our lab has recently shown that bilateral delivery of FGF2 to the hippocampi of APP/PS-1 bigenic mice using an AAV serotype 2/1 hybrid (AAV2/1-FGF2) results in significantly improved spatial learning in the radial arm water maze test, enhanced neurogenesis as measured by number of doublecortin, BrdU/NeuN, and c-fos–positive cells in the dentate gyrus, and enhanced clearance of fibrillar amyloid-β peptide (Aβ) in the hippocampus. AAV2/1-FGF2 injection was also shown to enhance long-term potentiation in another APP mouse model (J20) compared with control AAV2/1-GFP–injected littermates (Kiyota et al., 2011).

Anti-Inflammatory Genes

The suppression of proinflammatory activation by nonsteroidal anti-inflammatory drugs (NSAIDs), glatiramer acetate, or interleukin (IL)-4 gene delivery in the APP, PS1, or APP+PS1 mouse brain restored the suppression of neurogenesis seen in the SGZ (Wen et al., 2004; Chevallier et al., 2005; Butovsky et al., 2006a,b; Kiyota et al., 2010). The anti-inflammatory cytokines mediate the neuroprotective responses of microglia: IL-4 stimulation of microglia reduced the production of TNF-α and upregulated production of insulin-like growth factor-1, an important neuroprotective factor for neural maturation (Butovsky et al., 2005, 2006b).

While growth factors have shown beneficial effects as AD gene therapies, our lab has also shown that AAV-mediated delivery of certain anti-inflammatory chemokine and cytokine genes may counteract the variety of inflammatory processes involved in AD progression. AAV2 ITRs/AAV1 rep/cap hybrid vector (AAV2/1)-mediated delivery of the anti-inflammatory cytokine IL-4 into the hippocampus resulted in sustained expression of IL-4, reduced astro/microgliosis, Aβ oligomerization and deposition, enhanced neurogenesis, and improved spatial learning (Kiyota et al., 2010).

Similarly, AAV2/1-mediated hippocampal neuronal expression of the mouse anti-inflammatory cytokine IL-10 gene ameliorated cognitive dysfunction and was associated with reduced astro/microgliosis, enhanced plasma Aβ levels, enhanced neurogenesis, and improved spatial learning in APP/PS-1 mice (Kiyota et al., 2012).

Along the same lines, suppressing expression of the proinflammatory chemokine CCL2 via AAV2/1-mediated delivery of 7ND, a dominant-negative CCL2 mutant, in APP/PS-1 mice reduced astro/microgliosis, β-amyloidosis, and improved spatial learning (Kiyota et al., 2009). Whether delivering growth factors to reverse neurodegeneration and promote neurogenesis, or cytokines and chemokines to counteract harmful neuroinflammation in AD, these studies highlight the AAV2/1 system as a useful tool for the CNS gene delivery.

FUTURE DIRECTIONS

There is still no successful therapy available to halt and reverse the devastating neurodegeneration seen in AD, but the evidence leads one to conclude that the best treatment for AD may be a combined therapeutic with anti-inflammatory and proneurogenic components. While none have been thoroughly tested, BDNF, FGF2, IL-4, and IL-10 signaling proteins have proven to be promising targets for further research. Regardless of the various potentials of these therapeutic targets, it is clear that there is still a lack of understanding of the complicated relationship between neurotropism, inflammation, and cognitive enhancements in AD that warrants further investigation.

REFERENCES

Aalbers, C.J., Tak, P.P., Vervoordeldonk, M.J., 2011. Advancements in adeno-associated viral gene therapy approaches: exploring a new horizon. F1000 Med. Rep. 3, 17.

Abdipranoto, A., Wu, S., Stayte, S., Vissel, B., 2008. The role of neurogenesis in neurodegenerative diseases and its implications for therapeutic development. CNS Neurol. Disord. Drug Targets 7, 187–210.

Adriaansen, J., Khoury, M., de Cortie, C.J., Fallaux, F.J., Bigey, P., Scherman, D., et al., 2007. Reduction of arthritis following intra-articular administration of an adeno-associated virus serotype 5 expressing a disease-inducible TNF-blocking agent. Ann. Rheum. Dis. 66, 1143–1150.

Akache, B., Grimm, D., Pandey, K., Yant, S.R., Xu, H., Kay, M.A., 2006. The 37/67-kilodalton laminin receptor is a receptor for adeno-associated virus serotypes 8, 2, 3, and 9. J. Virol. 80, 9831–9836.

Allay, J.A., Sleep, S., Long, S., Tillman, D.M., Clark, R., Carney, G., et al., 2011. Good manufacturing practice production of self-complementary serotype 8 adeno-associated viral vector for a hemophilia B clinical trial. Hum. Gene Ther. 22, 595–604.

Anderson, S.M., Famous, K.R., Sadri-Vakili, G., Kumaresan, V., Schmidt, H.D., Bass, C.E., et al., 2008. CaMKII: a biochemical bridge linking accumbens dopamine and glutamate systems in cocaine seeking. Nat. Neurosci. 11, 344–353.

Arendash, G.W., King, D.L., Gordon, M.N., Morgan, D., Hatcher, J.M., Hope, C.E., et al., 2001. Progressive, age-related behavioral impairments in transgenic mice carrying both mutant amyloid precursor protein and presenilin-1 transgenes. Brain Res. 891, 42–53.

Arvanitakis Z, P.S., Bartus, R.T., Bennett, D., 2007. A phase I clinical trial of CERE-110 (AAV-NGF) gene delivery in Alzheimer's disease. In: American Academy of Neurology Annual Meeting. Boston, MA.

Aschauer, D.F., Kreuz, S., Rumpel, S., 2013. Analysis of transduction efficiency, tropism and axonal transport of AAV serotypes 1, 2, 5, 6, 8 and 9 in the mouse brain. PLoS ONE 8, e76310.

Asokan, A., Hamra, J.B., Govindasamy, L., Agbandje-McKenna, M., Samulski, R.J., 2006. Adeno-associated virus type 2 contains an integrin alpha5beta1 binding domain essential for viral cell entry. J. Virol. 80, 8961–8969.

Atchison, R.W., Casto, B.C., Hammon, W.M., 1965. Adenovirus-associated defective virus particles. Science 149, 754–756.

Balague, C., Kalla, M., Zhang, W.W., 1997. Adeno-associated virus Rep78 protein and terminal repeats enhance integration of DNA sequences into the cellular genome. J. Virol. 71, 3299–3306.

Baldauf, K., Reymann, K.G., 2005. Influence of EGF/bFGF treatment on proliferation, early neurogenesis and infarct volume after transient focal ischemia. Brain Res. 1056, 158–167.

Bankiewicz, K.S., Eberling, J.L., Kohutnicka, M., Jagust, W., Pivirotto, P., Bringas, J., et al., 2000. Convection-enhanced delivery of AAV vector in parkinsonian monkeys; in vivo detection of gene expression and restoration of dopaminergic function using pro-drug approach. Exp. Neurol. 164, 2–14.

Berns, K.I., Kotin, R.M., Labow, M.A., 1988. Regulation of adeno-associated virus DNA replication. Biochim. Biophys. Acta 951, 425–429.

Berns, K.I., Pinkerton, T.C., Thomas, G.F., Hoggan, M.D., 1975. Detection of adeno-associated virus (AAV)-specific nucleotide sequences in DNA isolated from latently infected Detroit 6 cells. Virology 68, 556–560.

Bevan, A.K., Duque, S., Foust, K.D., Morales, P.R., Braun, L., Schmelzer, L., et al., 2011. Systemic gene delivery in large species for targeting spinal cord, brain, and peripheral tissues for pediatric disorders. Mol. Ther. 19, 1971–1980.

Biscaro, B., Lindvall, O., Hock, C., Ekdahl, C.T., Nitsch, R.M., 2009. Abeta immunotherapy protects morphology and survival of adult-born neurons in doubly transgenic APP/PS1 mice. J. Neurosci. 29, 14108–14119.

Bishop, K.M., Hofer, E.K., Mehta, A., Ramirez, A., Sun, L., Tuszynski, M., et al., 2008. Therapeutic potential of CERE-110 (AAV2-NGF): targeted, stable, and sustained NGF delivery and trophic activity on rodent basal forebrain cholinergic neurons. Exp. Neurol. 211, 574–584.

Blankinship, M.J., Gregorevic, P., Allen, J.M., Harper, S.Q., Harper, H., Halbert, C.L., et al., 2004. Efficient transduction of skeletal muscle using vectors based on adeno-associated virus serotype 6. Mol. Ther. 10, 671–678.

Bobo, R.H., Laske, D.W., Akbasak, A., Morrison, P.F., Dedrick, R.L., Oldfield, E.H., 1994. Convection-enhanced delivery of macromolecules in the brain. Proc. Natl. Acad. Sci. U.S.A. 91, 2076–2080.

Boekhoorn, K., Joels, M., Lucassen, P.J., 2006. Increased proliferation reflects glial and vascular-associated changes, but not neurogenesis in the presenile Alzheimer hippocampus. Neurobiol. Dis. 24, 1–14.

Bowles, D.E., McPhee, S.W., Li, C., Gray, S.J., Samulski, J.J., Camp, A.S., et al., 2012. Phase 1 gene therapy for Duchenne muscular dystrophy using a translational optimized AAV vector. Mol. Ther. 20, 443–455.

Bruck, A., Kurki, T., Kaasinen, V., Vahlberg, T., Rinne, J.O., 2004. Hippocampal and prefrontal atrophy in patients with early non-demented Parkinson's disease is related to cognitive impairment. J. Neurol. Neurosurg. Psychiatry 75, 1467–1469.

Bruel-Jungerman, E., Rampon, C., Laroche, S., 2007. Adult hippocampal neurogenesis, synaptic plasticity and memory: facts and hypotheses. Rev. Neurosci. 18, 93–114.

Burger, C., Gorbatyuk, O.S., Velardo, M.J., Peden, C.S., Williams, P., Zolotukhin, S., et al., 2004. Recombinant AAV viral vectors pseudotyped with viral capsids from serotypes 1, 2, and 5 display differential efficiency and cell tropism after delivery to different regions of the central nervous system. Mol. Ther. 10, 302–317.

Butovsky, O., Talpalar, A.E., Ben-Yaakov, K., Schwartz, M., 2005. Activation of microglia by aggregated beta-amyloid or lipopolysaccharide impairs MHC-II expression and renders them cytotoxic whereas IFN-gamma and IL-4 render them protective. Mol. Cell Neurosci. 29, 381–393.

Butovsky, O., Koronyo-Hamaoui, M., Kunis, G., Ophir, E., Landa, G., Cohen, H., et al., 2006a. Glatiramer acetate fights against Alzheimer's disease by inducing dendritic-like microglia expressing insulin-like growth factor 1. Proc. Natl. Acad. Sci. U.S.A. 103, 11784–11789.

Butovsky, O., Ziv, Y., Schwartz, A., Landa, G., Talpalar, A.E., Pluchino, S., et al., 2006b. Microglia activated by IL-4 or IFN-gamma differentially induce neurogenesis and oligodendrogenesis from adult stem/progenitor cells. Mol. Cell Neurosci. 31, 149–160.

Callaway, E., 2012. Alzheimer's drugs take a new tack. Nature 489, 13–14.

Carpentier, P.A., Palmer, T.D., 2009. Immune influence on adult neural stem cell regulation and function. Neuron 64, 79–92.

Casto, B.C., Atchison, R.W., Hammon, W.M., 1967. Studies on the relationship between adeno-associated virus type I (AAV-1) and adenoviruses. I. Replication of AAV-1 in certain cell cultures and its effect on helper adenovirus. Virology 32, 52–59.

Cearley, C.N., Wolfe, J.H., 2006. Transduction characteristics of adeno-associated virus vectors expressing cap serotypes 7, 8, 9, and Rh10 in the mouse brain. Mol. Ther. 13, 528–537.

Chapman, P.F., White, G.L., Jones, M.W., Cooper-Blacketer, D., Marshall, V.J., Irizarry, M., et al., 1999. Impaired synaptic plasticity and learning in aged amyloid precursor protein transgenic mice. Nat. Neurosci. 2, 271–276.

Chen, H., McCarty, D.M., Bruce, A.T., Suzuki, K., 1999. Oligodendrocyte-specific gene expression in mouse brain: use of a myelin-forming cell type-specific promoter in an adeno-associated virus. J. Neurosci. Res. 55, 504–513.

Cheung, A.K., Hoggan, M.D., Hauswirth, W.W., Berns, K.I., 1980. Integration of the adeno-associated virus genome into cellular DNA in latently infected human Detroit 6 cells. J. Virol. 33, 739–748.

Chevallier, N.L., Soriano, S., Kang, D.E., Masliah, E., Hu, G., Koo, E.H., 2005. Perturbed neurogenesis in the adult hippocampus associated with presenilin-1 A246E mutation. Am. J. Pathol. 167, 151–159.

Chirmule, N., Propert, K., Magosin, S., Qian, Y., Qian, R., Wilson, J., 1999. Immune responses to adenovirus and adeno-associated virus in humans. Gene Ther. 6, 1574–1583.

Choi, V.W., McCarty, D.M., Samulski, R.J., 2005. AAV hybrid serotypes: improved vectors for gene delivery. Curr. Gene Ther. 5, 299–310.

Davidson, B.L., Stein, C.S., Heth, J.A., Martins, I., Kotin, R.M., Derksen, T.A., et al., 2000. Recombinant adeno-associated virus type 2, 4, and 5 vectors: transduction of variant cell types and regions in the mammalian central nervous system. Proc. Natl. Acad. Sci. U.S.A. 97, 3428–3432.

Daya, S., Berns, K.I., 2008. Gene therapy using adeno-associated virus vectors. Clin. Microbiol. Rev. 21, 583–593.

Dayer, A.G., Cleaver, K.M., Abouantoun, T., Cameron, H.A., 2005. New GABAergic interneurons in the adult neocortex and striatum are generated from different precursors. J. Cell Biol. 168, 415–427.

Dayton, R.D., Wang, D.B., Klein, R.L., 2012. The advent of AAV9 expands applications for brain and spinal cord gene delivery. Expert Opin. on Biol. Ther. 12, 757–766.

Deng, W., Aimone, J.B., Gage, F.H., 2010. New neurons and new memories: how does adult hippocampal neurogenesis affect learning and memory? Nat. Rev. Neurosci. 11, 339–350.

Deng, W., Saxe, M.D., Gallina, I.S., Gage, F.H., 2009. Adult-born hippocampal dentate granule cells undergoing maturation modulate learning and memory in the brain. J. Neurosci. 29, 13532–13542.

Di Pasquale, G., Davidson, B.L., Stein, C.S., Martins, I., Scudiero, D., Monks, A., et al., 2003. Identification of PDGFR as a receptor for AAV-5 transduction. Nat. Med. 9, 1306–1312.

Dodiya, H.B., Bjorklund, T., Stansell III, J., Mandel, R.J., Kirik, D., Kordower, J.H., 2010. Differential transduction following basal ganglia administration of distinct pseudotyped AAV capsid serotypes in nonhuman primates. Mol. Ther. 18, 579–587.

Duan, X., Kang, E., Liu, C.Y., Ming, G.L., Song, H., 2008. Development of neural stem cell in the adult brain. Curr. Opin. Neurobiol. 18, 108–115.

Emsley, J.G., Mitchell, B.D., Kempermann, G., Macklis, J.D., 2005. Adult neurogenesis and repair of the adult CNS with neural progenitors, precursors, and stem cells. Prog. Neurobiol. 75, 321–341.

Evans, C.H., Ghivizzani, S.C., Robbins, P.D., 2008. Arthritis gene therapy's first death. Arthritis Res. Ther. 10, 110.

Fang, H., Lai, N.C., Gao, M.H., Miyanohara, A., Roth, D.M., Tang, T., et al., 2012. Comparison of adeno-associated virus serotypes and delivery methods for Cardiac gene Transfer. Hum. Gene Ther. Methods 23 (4), 234–41.

Feng, X., Eide, F.F., Jiang, H., Reder, A.T., 2004. Adeno-associated viral vector-mediated ApoE expression in Alzheimer's disease mice: low CNS immune response, long-term expression, and astrocyte specificity. Front. Biosci. 9, 1540–1546.

Fisher, K.J., Jooss, K., Alston, J., Yang, Y., Haecker, S.E., High, K., et al., 1997. Recombinant adeno-associated virus for muscle directed gene therapy. Nat. Med. 3, 306–312.

Flannery, J.G., Zolotukhin, S., Vaquero, M.I., LaVail, M.M., Muzyczka, N., Hauswirth, W.W., 1997. Efficient photoreceptor-targeted gene expression in vivo by recombinant adeno-associated virus. Proc. Natl. Acad. Sci. U.S.A. 94, 6916–6921.

Foust, K.D., Nurre, E., Montgomery, C.L., Hernandez, A., Chan, C.M., Kaspar, B.K., 2009. Intravascular AAV9 preferentially targets neonatal neurons and adult astrocytes. Nat. Biotechnol. 27, 59–65.

Franklin, R.J., Ffrench-Constant, C., 2008. Remyelination in the CNS: from biology to therapy. Nat. Rev. Neurosci. 9, 839–855.

Gabryelewicz, T., Styczynska, M., Luczywek, E., Barczak, A., Pfeffer, A., Androsiuk, W., et al., 2007. The rate of conversion of mild cognitive impairment to dementia: predictive role of depression. Int. J. Geriatr. Psychiatry 22, 563–567.

Galvan, V., Bredesen, D.E., 2007. Neurogenesis in the adult brain: implications for Alzheimer's disease. CNS Neurol. Disord. Drug Targets 6, 303–310.

Games, D., Adams, D., Alessandrini, R., Barbour, R., Berthelette, P., Blackwell, C., et al., 1995. Alzheimer-type neuropathology in transgenic mice overexpressing V717F beta-amyloid precursor protein. Nature 373, 523–527.

Gao, G., Vandenberghe, L.H., Alvira, M.R., Lu, Y., Calcedo, R., Zhou, X., et al., 2004. Clades of Adeno-associated viruses are widely disseminated in human tissues. J. Virol. 78, 6381–6388.

Gao, G.P., Alvira, M.R., Wang, L., Calcedo, R., Johnston, J., Wilson, J.M., 2002. Novel adeno-associated viruses from rhesus monkeys as vectors for human gene therapy. Proc. Natl. Acad. Sci. U.S.A. 99, 11854–11859.

Glushakova, L.G., Lisankie, M.J., Eruslanov, E.B., Ojano-Dirain, C., Zolotukhin, I., Liu, C., et al., 2009. AAV3-mediated transfer and expression of the pyruvate dehydrogenase E1 alpha subunit gene causes metabolic remodeling and apoptosis of human liver cancer cells. Mol. Genet. Metab. 98, 289–299.

Gray, S.J., Matagne, V., Bachaboina, L., Yadav, S., Ojeda, S.R., Samulski, R.J., 2011a. Preclinical differences of intravascular AAV9 delivery to neurons and glia: a comparative study of adult mice and nonhuman primates. Mol. Ther. 19, 1058–1069.

Gray, S.J., Blake, B.L., Criswell, H.E., Nicolson, S.C., Samulski, R.J., McCown, T.J., et al., 2010. Directed evolution of a novel adeno-associated virus (AAV) vector that crosses the seizure-compromised blood-brain barrier (BBB). Mol. Ther. 18, 570–578.

Gray, S.J., Foti, S.B., Schwartz, J.W., Bachaboina, L., Taylor-Blake, B., Coleman, J., et al., 2011b. Optimizing promoters for recombinant adeno-associated virus-mediated gene expression in the peripheral and central nervous system using self-complementary vectors. Hum. Gene Ther. 22, 1143–1153.

Grieger, J.C., Samulski, R.J., 2012. Adeno-associated virus vectorology, manufacturing, and clinical applications. Methods Enzymol. 507, 229–254.

Grimm, D., Kay, M.A., Kleinschmidt, J.A., 2003. Helper virus-free, optically controllable, and two-plasmid-based production of adeno-associated virus vectors of serotypes 1 to 6. Mol. Ther. 7, 839–850.

Grimm, D., Kern, A., Rittner, K., Kleinschmidt, J.A., 1998. Novel tools for production and purification of recombinant adenoassociated virus vectors. Hum. Gene Ther. 9, 2745–2760.

Hadaczek, P., Eberling, J.L., Pivirotto, P., Bringas, J., Forsayeth, J., Bankiewicz, K.S., 2010. Eight years of clinical improvement in MPTP-lesioned primates after gene therapy with AAV2-hAADC. Mol. Ther. 18, 1458–1461.

Halbert, C.L., Allen, J.M., Miller, A.D., 2001. Adeno-associated virus type 6 (AAV6) vectors mediate efficient transduction of airway epithelial cells in mouse lungs compared with that of AAV2 vectors. J. Virol. 75, 6615–6624.

Harris, J.A., Devidze, N., Verret, L., Ho, K., Halabisky, B., Thwin, M.T., et al., 2010. Transsynaptic progression of amyloid-beta-induced neuronal dysfunction within the entorhinal-hippocampal network. Neuron 68, 428–441.

Hawkes, C., 2006. Olfaction in neurodegenerative disorder. Adv. Otorhinolaryngol. 63, 133–151.

Hefti, F., 1986. Nerve growth factor promotes survival of septal cholinergic neurons after fimbrial transections. J. Neurosci. 6, 2155–2162.

Hoehn, B.D., Palmer, T.D., Steinberg, G.K., 2005. Neurogenesis in rats after focal cerebral ischemia is enhanced by indomethacin. Stroke 36, 2718–2724.

Hoggan, M.D., Blacklow, N.R., Rowe, W.P., 1966. Studies of small DNA viruses found in various adenovirus preparations: physical, biological, and immunological characteristics. Proc. Natl. Acad. Sci. U.S.A. 55, 1467–1474.

Hsia, A.Y., Masliah, E., McConlogue, L., Yu, G.Q., Tatsuno, G., Hu, K., et al., 1999. Plaque-independent disruption of neural circuits in Alzheimer's disease mouse models. Proc. Natl. Acad. Sci. U.S.A. 96, 3228–3233.

Hsiao, K., Chapman, P., Nilsen, S., Eckman, C., Harigaya, Y., Younkin, S., et al., 1996. Correlative memory deficits, Abeta elevation, and amyloid plaques in transgenic mice. Science 274, 99–102.

Jin, K., Peel, A.L., Mao, X.O., Xie, L., Cottrell, B.A., Henshall, D.C., et al., 2004. Increased hippocampal neurogenesis in Alzheimer's disease. Proc. Natl. Acad. Sci. U.S.A. 101, 343–347.

Jin, K., Sun, Y., Xie, L., Batteur, S., Mao, X.O., Smelick, C., et al., 2003. Neurogenesis and aging: FGF-2 and HB-EGF restore neurogenesis in hippocampus and subventricular zone of aged mice. Aging Cell 2, 175–183.

Kaludov, N., Brown, K.E., Walters, R.W., Zabner, J., Chiorini, J.A., 2001. Adeno-associated virus serotype 4 (AAV4) and AAV5 both require sialic acid binding for hemagglutination and efficient transduction but differ in sialic acid linkage specificity. J. Virol. 75, 6884–6893.

Kaplitt, M.G., Leone, P., Samulski, R.J., Xiao, X., Pfaff, D.W., O'Malley, K.L., et al., 1994. Long-term gene expression and phenotypic correction using adeno-associated virus vectors in the mammalian brain. Nat. Genet. 8, 148–154.

Kashiwakura, Y., Tamayose, K., Iwabuchi, K., Hirai, Y., Shimada, T., Matsumoto, K., et al., 2005. Hepatocyte growth factor receptor is a coreceptor for adeno-associated virus type 2 infection. J. Virol. 79, 609–614.

King, J.A., Dubielzig, R., Grimm, D., Kleinschmidt, J.A., 2001. DNA helicase-mediated packaging of adeno-associated virus type 2 genomes into preformed capsids. EMBO J. 20, 3282–3291.

Kiyota, T., Ingraham, K.L., Jacobsen, M.T., Xiong, H., Ikezu, T., 2011. FGF2 gene transfer restores hippocampal functions in mouse models of Alzheimer's disease and has therapeutic implications for neurocognitive disorders. Proc. Natl. Acad. Sci. U.S.A. 108, E1339–E1348.

Kiyota, T., Okuyama, S., Swan, R.J., Jacobsen, M.T., Gendelman, H.E., Ikezu, T., 2010. CNS expression of anti-inflammatory cytokine interleukin-4 attenuates Alzheimer's disease-like pathogenesis in APP+PS1 bigenic mice. FASEB J. 24, 3093–3102.

Kiyota, T., Ingraham, K.L., Swan, R.J., Jacobsen, M.T., Andrews, S.J., Ikezu, T., 2012. AAV serotype 2/1-mediated gene delivery of anti-inflammatory interleukin-10 enhances neurogenesis and cognitive function in APP+PS1 mice. Gene Ther. 19, 724–733.

Kiyota, T., Yamamoto, M., Schroder, B., Jacobsen, M.T., Swan, R.J., Lambert, M.P., et al., 2009. AAV1/2-mediated CNS gene delivery of dominant-negative CCL2 mutant suppresses gliosis, beta-amyloidosis, and learning impairment of APP/PS1 mice. Mol Ther. 17, 803–809.

Klein, R.L., Dayton, R.D., Tatom, J.B., Diaczynsky, C.G., Salvatore, M.F., 2008. Tau expression levels from various adeno-associated virus vector serotypes produce graded neurodegenerative disease states. Eur. J. Neurosci. 27, 1615–1625.

Klein, R.L., Dayton, R.D., Leidenheimer, N.J., Jansen, K., Golde, T.E., Zweig, R.M., 2006. Efficient neuronal gene transfer with AAV8 leads to neurotoxic levels of tau or green fluorescent proteins. Mol. Ther. 13, 517–527.

Klein, R.L., Hamby, M.E., Gong, Y., Hirko, A.C., Wang, S., Hughes, J.A., et al., 2002. Dose and promoter effects of adeno-associated viral vector for green fluorescent protein expression in the rat brain. Exp. Neurol. 176, 66–74.

Kotin, R.M., Siniscalco, M., Samulski, R.J., Zhu, X.D., Hunter, L., Laughlin, C.A., et al., 1990. Site-specific integration by adeno-associated virus. Proc. Natl. Acad. Sci. U.S.A. 87, 2211–2215.

Krauze, M.T., Saito, R., Noble, C., Tamas, M., Bringas, J., Park, J.W., et al., 2005. Reflux-free cannula for convection-enhanced high-speed delivery of therapeutic agents. J. Neurosurg. 103, 923–929.

Kuhn, H.G., Winkler, J., Kempermann, G., Thal, L.J., Gage, F.H., 1997. Epidermal growth factor and fibroblast growth factor-2 have different effects on neural progenitors in the adult rat brain. J. Neurosci. 17, 5820–5829.

Lawlor, P.A., Bland, R.J., Mouravlev, A., Young, D., During, M.J., 2009. Efficient gene delivery and selective transduction of glial cells in the mammalian brain by AAV serotypes isolated from nonhuman primates. Mol. Ther. 17, 1692–1702.

Li, J., Wang, D., Qian, S., Chen, Z., Zhu, T., Xiao, X., 2003. Efficient and long-term intracardiac gene transfer in delta-sarcoglycan-deficiency hamster by adeno-associated virus-2 vectors. Gene Ther. 10, 1807–1813.

Lim, S.T., Airavaara, M., Harvey, B.K., 2010. Viral vectors for neurotrophic factor delivery: a gene therapy approach for neurodegenerative diseases of the CNS. Pharmacol. Res. 61, 14–26.

Ling, C., Lu, Y., Kalsi, J.K., Jayandharan, G.R., Li, B., Ma, W., et al., 2010. Human hepatocyte growth factor receptor is a cellular coreceptor for adeno-associated virus serotype 3. Hum. Gene Ther. 21, 1741–1747.

Loeb, J.E., Cordier, W.S., Harris, M.E., Weitzman, M.D., Hope, T.J., 1999. Enhanced expression of transgenes from adeno-associated virus vectors with the woodchuck hepatitis virus posttranscriptional regulatory element: implications for gene therapy. Hum. Gene Ther. 10, 2295–2305.

Magavi, S.S., Mitchell, B.D., Szentirmai, O., Carter, B.S., Macklis, J.D., 2005. Adult-born and preexisting olfactory granule neurons undergo distinct experience-dependent modifications of their olfactory responses in vivo. J. Neurosci. 25, 10729–10739.

Maguire, A.M., et al., 2009. Age-dependent effects of RPE65 gene therapy for Leber's congenital amaurosis: a phase 1 dose-escalation trial. Lancet 374, 1597–1605.

Mandel, R.J., 2010. CERE-110, an adeno-associated virus-based gene delivery vector expressing human nerve growth factor for the treatment of Alzheimer's disease. Curr. Opin. Mol. Ther. 12, 240–247.

Masamizu, Y., Okada, T., Kawasaki, K., Ishibashi, H., Yuasa, S., Takeda, S., et al., 2011. Local and retrograde gene transfer into primate neuronal pathways via adeno-associated virus serotype 8 and 9. Neuroscience 193, 249–258.

Matsuda, H., 2007. The role of neuroimaging in mild cognitive impairment. Neuropathology 27, 570–577.

McCown, T.J., Xiao, X., Li, J., Breese, G.R., Samulski, R.J., 1996. Differential and persistent expression patterns of CNS gene transfer by an adeno-associated virus (AAV) vector. Brain Res. 713, 99–107.

McLaughlin, S.K., Collis, P., Hermonat, P.L., Muzyczka, N., 1988. Adeno-associated virus general transduction vectors: analysis of proviral structures. J. Virol. 62, 1963–1973.

Mease, P.J., Hobbs, K., Chalmers, A., El-Gabalawy, H., Bookman, A., Keystone, E., et al., 2009. Local delivery of a recombinant adenoassociated vector containing a tumour necrosis factor alpha antagonist gene in inflammatory arthritis: a phase 1 dose-escalation safety and tolerability study. Ann. Rheum. Dis. 68, 1247–1254.

Ming, G.L., Song, H., 2005. Adult neurogenesis in the mammalian central nervous system. Annu. Rev. Neurosci. 28, 223–250.

Miyake, K., Miyake, N., Yamazaki, Y., Shimada, T., Hirai, Y., 2012. Serotype-independent method of recombinant adeno-associated virus (AAV) vector production and purification. J. Nippon Med. Sch. 79, 394–402.

Monahan, P.E., Samulski, R.J., Tazelaar, J., Xiao, X., Nichols, T.C., Bellinger, D.A., et al., 1998. Direct intramuscular injection with recombinant AAV vectors results in sustained expression in a dog model of hemophilia. Gene Ther. 5, 40–49.

Monje, M.L., Toda, H., Palmer, T.D., 2003. Inflammatory blockade restores adult hippocampal neurogenesis. Science 302, 1760–1765.

Morgan, D., Diamond, D.M., Gottschall, P.E., Ugen, K.E., Dickey, C., Hardy, J., et al., 2000. A beta peptide vaccination prevents memory loss in an animal model of Alzheimer's disease. Nature 408, 982–985.

Mori, S., Takeuchi, T., Enomoto, Y., Kondo, K., Sato, K., Ono, F., et al., 2008. Tissue distribution of cynomolgus adeno-associated viruses AAV10, AAV11, and AAVcy.7 in naturally infected monkeys. Arch. Virol. 153, 375–380.

Mudo, G., Bonomo, A., Di Liberto, V., Frinchi, M., Fuxe, K., Belluardo, N., 2009. The FGF-2/FGFRs neurotrophic system promotes neurogenesis in the adult brain. J. Neural. Transm. 116, 995–1005.

Nagahara, A.H., Merrill, D.A., Coppola, G., Tsukada, S., Schroeder, B.E., Shaked, G.M., et al., 2009. Neuroprotective effects of brain-derived neurotrophic factor in rodent and primate models of Alzheimer's disease. Nature Medicine 15, 331–337.

Niwa, H., Yamamura, K., Miyazaki, J., 1991. Efficient selection for high-expression transfectants with a novel eukaryotic vector. Gene 108, 193–199.

Parks, W.P., Boucher, D.W., Melnick, J.L., Taber, L.H., Yow, M.D., 1970. Seroepidemiological and ecological studies of the adenovirus-associated satellite viruses. Infect. Immun. 2, 716–722.

Peel, A.L., Klein, R.L., 2000. Adeno-associated virus vectors: activity and applications in the CNS. J. Neurosci. Methods 98, 95–104.

Poewe, W., 2008. Non-motor symptoms in Parkinson's disease. Eur. J. Neurol. 15 (Suppl. 1), 14–20.

Ponnazhagan, S., Mukherjee, P., Yoder, M.C., Wang, X.S., Zhou, S.Z., Kaplan, J., et al., 1997. Adeno-associated virus 2-mediated gene transfer in vivo: organ-tropism and expression of transduced sequences in mice. Gene 190, 203–210.

Qing, K., Mah, C., Hansen, J., Zhou, S., Dwarki, V., Srivastava, A., 1999. Human fibroblast growth factor receptor 1 is a co-receptor for infection by adeno-associated virus 2. Nat. Med. 5, 71–77.

Quinn, K., Quirion, M.R., Lo, C.Y., Misplon, J.A., Epstein, S.L., Chiorini, J.A., 2011. Intranasal administration of adeno-associated virus type 12 (AAV12) leads to transduction of the nasal epithelia and can initiate transgene-specific immune response. Mol. Ther. 19, 1990–1998.

Rabinowitz, J.E., Rolling, F., Li, C., Conrath, H., Xiao, W., Xiao, X., et al., 2002. Cross-packaging of a single adeno-associated virus (AAV) type 2 vector genome into multiple AAV serotypes enables transduction with broad specificity. J. Virol. 76, 791–801.

Russell, D.W., Alexander, I.E., Miller, A.D., 1995. DNA synthesis and topoisomerase inhibitors increase transduction by adeno-associated virus vectors. Proc. Natl. Acad. Sci. U.S.A. 92, 5719–5723.

Samulski, R.J., Chang, L.S., Shenk, T., 1989. Helper-free stocks of recombinant adeno-associated viruses: normal integration does not require viral gene expression. J. Virol. 63, 3822–3828.

Samulski, R.J., Berns, K.I., Tan, M., Muzyczka, N., 1982. Cloning of adeno-associated virus into pBR322: rescue of intact virus from the recombinant plasmid in human cells. Proc. Natl. Acad. Sci. U.S.A. 79, 2077–2081.

Samulski, R.J., Zhu, X., Xiao, X., Brook, J.D., Housman, D.E., Epstein, N., et al., 1991. Targeted integration of adeno-associated virus (AAV) into human chromosome 19. EMBO J. 10, 3941–3950.

Schenk, D., et al., 1999. Immunization with amyloid-beta attenuates Alzheimer-disease-like pathology in the PDAPP mouse. Nature 400, 173–177.

Selkoe, D.J., 2002. Alzheimer's disease is a synaptic failure. Science 298, 789–791.

Shen, S., Bryant, K.D., Brown, S.M., Randell, S.H., Asokan, A., 2011. Terminal N-linked galactose is the primary receptor for adeno-associated virus 9. J. Biol. Chem. 286, 13532–13540.

Sierra, A., Encinas, J.M., Deudero, J.J., Chancey, J.H., Enikolopov, G., Overstreet-Wadiche, L.S., et al., 2010. Microglia shape adult hippocampal neurogenesis through apoptosis-coupled phagocytosis. Cell Stem Cell 7, 483–495.

So, K., Moriya, T., Nishitani, S., Takahashi, H., Shinohara, K., 2008. The olfactory conditioning in the early postnatal period stimulated neural stem/progenitor cells in the subventricular zone and increased neurogenesis in the olfactory bulb of rats. Neuroscience 151, 120–128.

Stroes, E.S., Nierman, M.C., Meulenberg, J.J., Franssen, R., Twisk, J., Henny, C.P., et al., 2008. Intramuscular administration of AAV1-lipoprotein lipase S447X lowers triglycerides in lipoprotein lipase-deficient patients. Arterioscler. Thromb. Vasc. Biol. 28, 2303–2304.

Summerford, C., Samulski, R.J., 1998. Membrane-associated heparan sulfate proteoglycan is a receptor for adeno-associated virus type 2 virions. J. Virol. 72, 1438–1445.

Summerford, C., Bartlett, J.S., Samulski, R.J., 1999. AlphaVbeta5 integrin: a co-receptor for adeno-associated virus type 2 infection. Nat. Med. 5, 78–82.

Sze, C.I., Troncoso, J.C., Kawas, C., Mouton, P., Price, D.L., Martin, L.J., 1997. Loss of the presynaptic vesicle protein synaptophysin in hippocampus correlates with cognitive decline in Alzheimer disease. J. Neuropathol. Exp. Neurol. 56, 933–944.

Takeda, S., Takahashi, M., Mizukami, H., Kobayashi, E., Takeuchi, K., Hakamata, Y., et al., 2004. Successful gene transfer using adeno-associated virus vectors into the kidney: comparison among adeno-associated virus serotype 1-5 vectors in vitro and in vivo. Nephron Exp. Nephrol. 96, e119–126.

Tamura, Y., Kataoka, Y., Cui, Y., Takamori, Y., Watanabe, Y., Yamada, H., 2007. Multi-directional differentiation of doublecortin- and NG2-immunopositive progenitor cells in the adult rat neocortex in vivo. Eur. J. Neurosci. 25, 3489–3498.

Tao, Y., Black, I.B., DiCicco-Bloom, E., 1997. In vivo neurogenesis is inhibited by neutralizing antibodies to basic fibroblast growth factor. J. Neurobiol. 33, 289–296.

Teichler Zallen, D., 2000. US gene therapy in crisis. Trends Genet. 16, 272–275.

Terry, R.D., Masliah, E., Salmon, D.P., Butters, N., DeTeresa, R., Hill, R., et al., 1991. Physical basis of cognitive alterations in Alzheimer's disease: synapse loss is the major correlate of cognitive impairment. Ann. Neurol. 30, 572–580.

Towne, C., Schneider, B.L., Kieran, D., Redmond Jr., D.E., Aebischer, P., 2010. Efficient transduction of non-human primate motor neurons after intramuscular delivery of recombinant AAV serotype 6. Gene Ther. 17, 141–146.

Tronel, S., Belnoue, L., Grosjean, N., Revest, J.M., Piazza, P.V., Koehl, M., et al., 2012. Adult-born neurons are necessary for extended contextual discrimination. Hippocampus. 22(2) 292–298.

Tuszynski, M.H., Thal, L., Pay, M., Salmon, D.P., U, H.S., Bakay, R., Patel, P., et al., 2005. A phase 1 clinical trial of nerve growth factor gene therapy for Alzheimer disease. Nat. Med. 11, 551–555.

Villeda, S.A., et al., 2011. The ageing systemic milieu negatively regulates neurogenesis and cognitive function. Nature 477, 90–94.

Waldau, B., Shetty, A.K., 2008. Behavior of neural stem cells in the Alzheimer brain. Cell Mol. Life Sci. 65, 2372–2384.

Walters, R.W., Yi, S.M., Keshavjee, S., Brown, K.E., Welsh, M.J., Chiorini, J.A., Zabner, J., 2001. Binding of adeno-associated virus type 5 to 2,3-linked sialic acid is required for gene transfer. J. Biol. Chem. 276, 20610–20616.

Weber, M., Rabinowitz, J., Provost, N., Conrath, H., Folliot, S., Briot, D., et al., 2003. Recombinant adeno-associated virus serotype 4 mediates unique and exclusive long-term transduction of retinal pigmented epithelium in rat, dog, and nonhuman primate after subretinal delivery. Mol. Ther. 7, 774–781.

Weinberg, M.S., Samulski, R.J., McCown, T.J., 2013. Adeno-associated virus (AAV) gene therapy for neurological disease. Neuropharmacology 69, 82–88.

Weitzman, M.D., Kyostio, S.R., Kotin, R.M., Owens, R.A., 1994. Adeno-associated virus (AAV) Rep proteins mediate complex formation between AAV DNA and its integration site in human DNA. Proc. Natl. Acad. Sci. U.S.A. 91, 5808–5812.

Weller, M.L., Amornphimoltham, P., Schmidt, M., Wilson, P.A., Gutkind, J.S., Chiorini, J.A., 2010. Epidermal growth factor receptor is a co-receptor for adeno-associated virus serotype 6. Nat. Med. 16, 662–664.

Wen, P.H., Hof, P.R., Chen, X., Gluck, K., Austin, G., Younkin, S.G., et al., 2004. The presenilin-1 familial Alzheimer disease mutant P117L impairs neurogenesis in the hippocampus of adult mice. Exp. Neurol. 188, 224–237.

West, M.J., Gundersen, H.J., 1990. Unbiased stereological estimation of the number of neurons in the human hippocampus. J. Comp. Neurol. 296, 1–22.

Wu, K., Meyer, E.M., Bennett, J.A., Meyers, C.A., Hughes, J.A., King, M.A., 2005. AAV2/5-mediated NGF gene delivery protects septal cholinergic neurons following axotomy. Brain Res. 1061, 107–113.

Wu, Z., Miller, E., Agbandje-McKenna, M., Samulski, R.J., 2006a. $\alpha2,3$ and $\alpha2,6$ N-linked sialic acids facilitate efficient binding and transduction by adeno-associated virus types 1 and 6. J. Virol. 80, 9093–9103.

Wu, Z., Asokan, A., Grieger, J.C., Govindasamy, L., Agbandje-McKenna, M., Samulski, R.J., 2006b. Single amino acid changes can influence titer, heparin binding, and tissue tropism in different adeno-associated virus serotypes. J. Virol. 80, 11393–11397.

Xiao, W., Chirmule, N., Berta, S.C., McCullough, B., Gao, G., Wilson, J.M., 1999. Gene therapy vectors based on adeno-associated virus type 1. J. Virol. 73, 3994–4003.

Xiao, X., Li, J., Samulski, R.J., 1996. Efficient long-term gene transfer into muscle tissue of immunocompetent mice by adeno-associated virus vector. J. Virol. 70, 8098–8108.

Xiao, X., Li, J., Samulski, R.J., 1998. Production of high-titer recombinant adeno-associated virus vectors in the absence of helper adenovirus. J. Virol. 72, 2224–2232.

Xiao, X., Li, J., McCown, T.J., Samulski, R.J., 1997. Gene transfer by adeno-associated virus vectors into the central nervous system. Exp. Neurol. 144, 113–124.

Yakobson, B., Hrynko, T.A., Peak, M.J., Winocour, E., 1989. Replication of adeno-associated virus in cells irradiated with UV light at 254 nm. J. Virol. 63, 1023–1030.

Yan, Z., Zhang, Y., Duan, D., Engelhardt, J.F., 2000. Trans-splicing vectors expand the utility of adeno-associated virus for gene therapy. Proc. Natl. Acad. Sci. U.S.A. 97, 6716–6721.

Zincarelli, C., Soltys, S., Rengo, G., Rabinowitz, J.E., 2008. Analysis of AAV serotypes 1-9 mediated gene expression and tropism in mice after systemic injection. Mol. Ther. 16, 1073–1080.

Zolotukhin, S., Byrne, B.J., Mason, E., Zolotukhin, I., Potter, M., Chesnut, K., et al., 1999. Recombinant adeno-associated virus purification using novel methods improves infectious titer and yield. Gene Ther. 6, 973–985.

Chapter 7

Advancing Fear Memory Research with Optogenetics

Inbal Goshen, Anat Shapir and Yanir Mor
Edmond and Lily Safra Center for Brain Sciences, The Hebrew University, Jerusalem, Israel

INTRODUCTION

One of the biggest mysteries in neuroscience, which attracts a great volume of research, is the way in which memories are formed, saved and extracted. In decades of using techniques such as physical, pharmacological, and genetic lesions of specific brain areas, together with electrical or pharmacological stimulation of these areas, pioneering studies had identified the major brain areas that are involved in the different stages of various memory tasks. However, the precise anatomical and functional connections between these different regions (as well as the contribution of other areas, hitherto considered irrelevant) remained only partially understood. The main obstacle was the inability to specifically control genetically defined neuronal populations in real-time, in behaving animals performing cognitive tasks. As Francis Crick envisioned 35 years ago (Crick, 1979), "a method by which all neurons of just one type could be inactivated, leaving the others more or less unaltered" was required to truly understand complex brain function as cognition and emotion.

The realization of this seemingly impossible vision came with the development of optogenetics—a method that allows real-time control of genetically defined neuronal populations with a millisecond precision. This accurate control is gained by expressing microbial light-sensitive proteins in neuronal cells and then manipulating the activity of the expressing cells with light (Deisseroth, 2010, 2011; Deisseroth and Schnitzer, 2013). Since the first successful use of opsins in neurons in 2005, the technique was enthusiastically embraced by the neuroscientific community, and led to a dramatic renaissance in this field (Reiner and Isacoff, 2013).

The major focus of this chapter will be recent optogenetics-driven breakthroughs in fear memory research, as this specific paradigm attracted a large enough mass of optogenetic studies to provide a comprehensive new picture of its underlying mechanisms. Finally, the use of optogenetics for memory generation and memory enhancement will be discussed.

CONTEMPORARY AND TRADITIONAL METHODS IN MEMORY RESEARCH

This section will provide a concise description of the major behavioral and optogenetic techniques that were used by the studies described in the following sections.

Fear Memory Induction and Testing

Classical fear conditioning (FC) is one of the most powerful experimental models for studying the neural basis of associative learning and memory formation in mammals (LeDoux, 2000; Maren, 2001; Maren et al., 2013; Maren and Quirk, 2004). The simultaneous presentation of a neutral (conditioned) stimulus (CS) and an aversive (unconditioned) stimulus (US) renders the formerly neutral stimulus a frightful quality, so that even when it appears by itself, without the aversive stimulus, it will elicit a fearful conditioned response (Maren, 2001) (see Figure 7.1). FC can be rapidly formed in humans and animals, even following a single conditioning trial, and is usually maintained for long periods

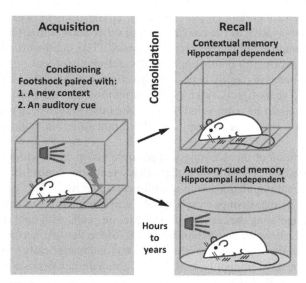

FIGURE 7.1 **The basic principles of fear conditioning.** The conditioning apparatus consists of a mouse chamber set up in a sound attenuated box (the context). Mice receive conditioning trials tone (CS) and a foot shock (US) delivered through the grid floor. For the context test, mice are located into the conditioning chamber and freezing to the context is assessed. For the tone test, mice are placed in a different chamber and then presented with the tones.

(Maren, 2001). In rodents, the dominant behavioral fear response is freezing (complete immobility), and the most commonly used aversive stimulus is the delivery of a weak short electrical shock (Fanselow, 2000). The conditioning process itself (i.e., the association between the neutral and aversive stimuli) is mediated primarily by the amygdala (LeDoux, 2000; Maren, 2001; Maren and Quirk, 2004), and by using different types of conditioned stimuli, the fear-conditioning paradigm enables differentiation between hippocampal dependent and independent functions (see Figure 7.1): When a simple perceptual conditioned stimulus (such as a light or an auditory cue) is used, the hippocampus is not required. However, when the conditioned stimulus is a new environment, a mental representation of this new context has to be created, so that the amygdala can associate this representation with the aversive stimulus; this function depends on hippocampal functioning (Fanselow, 2000; Maren and Holt, 2000; Maren et al., 2013). In the most commonly used version of the FC paradigm, animals are placed in a novel conditioning cage, in which they hear an auditory tone, followed by a short foot-shock. Thus, the animal can associate the aversive stimulus with the new context as well as with the tone. To test contextual FC, animals are placed again in the original conditioning cage, and freezing is measured. This task is hippocampus dependent, as it cannot be performed following hippocampal lesions (Fanselow, 2000). To test the hippocampus-independent auditory-cued FC, freezing is measured when the tone is sounded in a differently shaped context. In this case, hippocampal lesions have no detrimental effect on performance level (Fanselow, 2000; Maren and Holt, 2000; Maren and Quirk, 2004). In the trace variation of the FC paradigm (trace fear conditioning (TFC)), the neutral CS and the aversive US are separated by a stimulus-free time gap of several seconds, called the trace interval. After conditioning, similarly to regular FC, subjects express fear of the CS, but that response diminishes in intensity as the interval grows (Raybuck and Lattal, 2013). TFC seems to be at least partially different from regular FC in its underlying brain structure (Raybuck and Lattal, 2013): The hippocampus and amygdala are involved (Bangasser et al., 2006; Fanselow and LeDoux, 1999), but many high cortical brain areas like the prefrontal, anterior cingulated, and entorhinal cortices were also heavily implicated in forming the association between the temporally separated stimuli (Raybuck and Lattal, 2013). To sum up, the major strengths of the FC model are the defined anatomy of the basic neuronal circuit, and the well-defined temporal separation between different stages of memory; acquisition, consolidation, and recall.

Despite the vast repertoire of pioneering works examining the FC circuitry, many unsolved mysteries remained, especially concerning the real-time involvement of specific populations in normal hippocampal functioning. Physical, pharmacological, and genetic lesion studies have greatly enhanced our understanding of neural systems underlying FC, but despite their effectiveness, these methods typically involve tradeoffs between cellular and temporal precision. Optogenetics combine the advantages of all these methods while avoiding their drawbacks, as described in the next section.

Optogenetics

This revolutionary versatile approach allows genetically defined subpopulations of cells to be precisely controlled with millisecond precision using microbial opsins (Bernstein and Boyden, 2011; Deisseroth, 2010, 2011; Fenno et al., 2011; Yizhar et al., 2011a). Briefly, optogenetic control is achieved by first targeting microbe-derived light-sensitive proteins (opsins) to be expressed in specific cell populations and then illuminating these cells in order to activate the opsins and manipulate cellular activity.

Microbial Opsins

In recent years, opsins were engineered to offer a diverse toolbox for neuronal excitation or inhibition (Mattis et al., 2012), as well as control of intracellular signaling (Airan et al., 2009) (Table 7.1). These major groups are described below:

Excitatory Opsins

The microbial opsins used for neuronal excitation are light-sensitive cation channels that allow positively charged ions to flow into the cell upon illumination. These opsins require retinal, a vitamin A-related organic cofactor, for light

TABLE 7.1 Opsin Glossary: Main Properties of the Opsins Used in the Works Reviewed Here, Out of Many Available Opsins

	Opsin Name	Effect on Neurons	Mechanism of Action
Excitation	ChR2 Channelrhodopsin 2	Depolarization	Nonselective inward cation channel
	ChIEF A modified ChR2, faster and more stable	Depolarization	Nonselective inward cation channel
	SSFO Stable step function opsin	Prolonged depolarization	Nonselective inward cation channel
Inhibition	NpHR Natronomonas pharaonis Halorhodopsin	Hyperpolarization	Inward Cl⁻ pump
	Arch Halorubrum sodomense archaerhodopsin-3	Hyperpolarization	Outward H⁺ pump

sensing. Luckily, retinal is present in vertebrate tissues in sufficient amounts, thus the expression of the opsin in neurons is by itself functional, without requiring any added chemical (Deisseroth et al., 2006; Zhang et al., 2006). The first opsin to be used in neurons was channelrhodopsin 2 (ChR2) (Boyden et al., 2005), and since then a variety of excitatory opsins were designed in an attempt to allow a better imitation of the physiological activity of different populations (Lin et al., 2009; Mattis et al., 2012). For example, step function opsins (SFOs) have prolonged activity after the termination of the light stimulus; orders-of-magnitude higher than ChRs—from tens of seconds to longer than 30 min (Berndt et al., 2009; Yizhar et al., 2011b). Furthermore, SFOs can be deactivated by yellow light, allowing control over the termination of the stimulus. On the other hand, ChETA (Gunaydin et al., 2010) is an ultrafast ChR2 mutant, allowing high-frequency spike induction at 200 Hz or more over sustained trains, allowing a precise activation of inhibitory fast-spiking cells. Other engineering efforts were invested in developing red-shifted excitatory opsins like C1V1 and VChR1 (Yizhar et al., 2011b; Zhang et al., 2007) that are activated by higher wavelength than the regular ChR2, allowing for combinatorial activation of different cellular populations (e.g., one population with ChR2 or SFO, and one with C1V1 or VChR1). Finally, there are attempts to control the ionic permeability of the channel. For example, the Ca^{2+} translocating channelrhodopsin (CatCh) evokes more reliable Ca^{2+} elevations than ChR2 (Kleinlogel et al., 2011).

Inhibitory Opsins

Inhibition is mediated by light-activated ion pumps that hyperpolarize the expressing illuminated neurons. These proteins are sensitive to yellow/green light, thus allowing combinatorial manipulation together with ChR (Zhang et al., 2007). For example, NpHR (*Natronomonas pharaonis* Halorhodopsin) is a bacterial inward chloride pump hyperpolarizing cells in response to yellow light (Gradinaru et al., 2007, 2010; Zhang et al., 2007), and Arch (archaerhodopsin-3 from *Halorubrum sodomense*) is a light-driven outward proton pump (Chow et al., 2010), efficiently blocking neuronal activity in response to yellow light. Modifications done on NpHR and Arch in recent years have resulted in increased currents, higher expression, and precise intracellular targeting (Gradinaru et al., 2010; Mattis et al., 2012), which allowed for a successful use in behaving animals (Goshen et al., 2011; Tye et al., 2011; Witten et al., 2010).

Intracellular Signaling Manipulation

Engineering of chimeric proteins with the extracellular and membranous segments of bacterial rhodopsin, and the intracellular part of G protein-coupled receptor now allows light-control of intracellular signaling (Airan et al., 2009; Masseck et al., 2014). Two of these chimeras were initially cloned from the α1 (Gq-coupled) and β2 (Gs-coupled) adrenergic receptors but can now be used in any cellular population (Airan et al., 2009). A third group (Gi/o-coupled) was generated using vertebrate cone opsins (Masseck et al., 2014). All OptoGPCRs (Gq, Gs, and Gi/o) were successfully used in vivo (Airan et al., 2009; Masseck et al., 2014). An optically controlled metabotropic glutamate receptor (LiGluR) (Levitz et al., 2013) was also generated but has not been used in vivo yet.

Optogenetics in Behaving Animals

To use the great strengths of optogenetics in memory research, opsins are introduced into a specific neuronal population and subsequently activated with light in vivo. This section will describe the technical procedures allowing such experiments.

Targeting Opsins to Specific Cell Populations

To induce opsin expression in discrete brain cell populations, a foreign DNA sequence, encoding for the opsin has to be delivered into the brain. In most cases, this DNA is delivered using viral vectors. These vectors, generated from lentiviruses or adeno-associated viruses (AAVs), are injected into the brain area of interest, and infect the cell bodies (for an overview on AAVs, please refer to Chapter 6). Within days to weeks, the opsins are expressed throughout the cell membrane—including distant projections sent by the infected cell bodies to distant brain regions. Cell-type specific gene expression is determined by the regulatory DNA sequences called promoters. If the known unique promoter of a specific cellular population is strong and small enough it can be packed into the viral vector together with the foreign opsin DNA, and directly drive expression in the relevant cells. The viruses will infect all cells, and the promoters will determine which cells will produce the protein. This procedure was successfully used to express opsins specifically in hypocretin neurons (Adamantidis et al., 2007) and excitatory pyramidal neurons (Goshen et al., 2011; Lee et al., 2010; Sohal et al., 2009; Zhang et al., 2007), for example.

If the relevant promoter is too weak to drive sufficient expression or too large to be packed into a virus, transgenic animals can be used. Several mouse lines expressing opsins in the brain were developed (Arenkiel et al., 2007; Hagglund et al., 2010). While this tool does not require virus injection, it is costly and inflexible—when new opsins are developed, new mouse lines have to be generated. A more versatile strategy is to use transgenic mice that express Cre recombinase in a specific cellular population. These mice can then be injected with a virus containing any opsin DNA in an inverted orientation, flanked by two sets of incompatible Cre recombinase recognition sequences (double-floxed inverted open-reading-frame (DIO)) (Zhang et al., 2010). The virus will infect all the cells in the injected region, but only in the cells that transgenically express Cre the DNA sequence will be flipped into the correct orientation, allowing transcription of the coding region, under a strong ubiquitous promoter (Atasoy et al., 2008; Sohal et al., 2009; Tsai et al., 2009). This technique was widely used to manipulate dopaminergic (Kravitz et al., 2010; Tsai et al., 2009;

Tye et al., 2013), cholinergic (Witten et al., 2010), GABAergic (Brown et al., 2012; Tan et al., 2012), parvalbumin GABAergic neurons (Letzkus et al., 2011; Sohal et al., 2009; Yizhar et al., 2011b), and granular glutamatergic neurons in the dentate gyrus (DG) (Kheirbek et al., 2013), to name just a few. Furthermore, Cre-driver rat lines were recently developed, to allow targeting of opsins into dopaminergic and cholinergic neurons (Witten et al., 2011). This adaptable strategy allows the use of any new developed opsin in the population of interest.

New genetic tools now allow opsin expression based on cellular activity, providing an opportunity to specifically activate or inhibit a population of neurons that participated in a certain behavioral task, using optogenetic tools (Liu et al., 2012; Ramirez et al., 2013), as will be described in detail later in this chapter.

In vivo Illumination

To modulate the activity of opsin-expressing neurons, light has to be delivered to the brain region of interest. For deep brain structures, this is done by implanting an optical fiber (or a guide tube through which a fiber can be inserted) right above the region of interest. In experiments requiring projection targeting, cell bodies are infected in one brain region and their axonal projections are illuminated in another. The fiber is then connected into a light source, most commonly a laser diode (Aravanis et al., 2007; Yizhar et al., 2011a).

The use of optogenetics in behavioral studies offers a combination of advantages (cell-type specificity, high temporal and spatial resolution) without the tradeoffs between them that are inherent in other methods. The optogenetic toolbox is rapidly expanding, offering a range of possible modulations.

NOVEL FINDINGS IN MEMORY RESEARCH FROM OPTOGENETIC STUDIES

Since the introduction of optogenetics and its adaptation to studies in behaving animals, a major scientific effort was invested in the perturbation of the neural basis of memory. The following sections will show how the incorporation of optogenetic methods into memory research had revolutionized this field. This chapter will not cover the impressive works using other learning and memory paradigms (Gu et al., 2012; Narayanan et al., 2012; Steinberg et al., 2013) and will focus specifically on fear memory. We will present the major studies that were published in this field, and show the significant new insights we have gained, within such a short period of time, thanks to the integration of optogenetics. These novel studies address core issues in fear memory like the differential roles of the hippocampal subregions (DG, CA1-3) the significance of its axial components (dorsal vs ventral), the contribution of extrahippocampal regions to fear memory, and the transition from recent to remote memory.

As described above, the major brain areas involved in fear memory were recognized decades ago. However, it was impossible to pinpoint the roles of specific neuronal populations within these structures, or the functional connections between them. The introduction of optogenetics provided an opportunity to delve into the fine mechanisms underlying fear, and indeed, major breakthroughs in this field were evident in recent years. This section will describe the new knowledge gained regarding the different areas contributing to fear memory, the neurotransmitters involved, and the functional connections between the different regions. As the main focus of investigation was pointed toward the hippocampus, several aspects of this area's involvement will be discussed: the role of different hippocampal subregions in fear acquisition and retrieval, the functional differences along the hippocampal dorsoventral axis, the temporal involvement of this region in recent and remote memories, and the transition between the two.

The new findings in memory research using optogenetics tools are summarized in Figure 7.2.

The Brain Areas Mediating the Acquisition and Recall of Fear Memory

This section will concentrate on nonhippocampal regions involved in fear memory, mainly the amygdala, cortical, and striatal areas. Hippocampal involvement will be discussed at length in the following sections.

The Amygdala

As the amygdala is a core player in FC (LeDoux, 2000; Maren and Quirk, 2004), a major effort was invested in a fine examination of its role in FC using optogenetics. The amygdala is composed of several nuclei, different in their major neuronal populations, afferent and efferent connections, and functional significance. For example, the lateral nucleus (LA) is considered to be generating and storing the association between the CS and US (LeDoux, 2000; Maren and Quirk, 2004), whereas the central nucleus (CEA) is thought to underlie the autonomic and motor conditioned fear expression (Krettek and Price, 1978; LeDoux et al., 1988). However, it seems that this distinction is not clear, and that some functional overlap exists. For example, CEA was shown to be involved not only in fear expression, but also in memory acquisition (Goosens and Maren, 2003; Wilensky et al., 2006). The CEA has several substructures: its output neurons (projecting to the brain stem and the hypothalamus) reside mostly in its medial subdivision (CEm) and are inhibited by neurons in the lateral and capsular subdivisions of the CEA, together referred to as CEl (Huber et al., 2005; Sun et al., 1994).

Johansen et al. (2010) expressed ChR2 in excitatory neurons in the LA and showed that pairing a pure tone with LA optogenetic stimulation resulted in fear memory. Optogenetic activation induces a fear response during illumination, but can also serve as an US and paired with a tone can induce fear memory of the tone at a later time point, when illumination is absent (Johansen et al., 2010). This fear memory is weak (less than 20% freezing) compared to fear

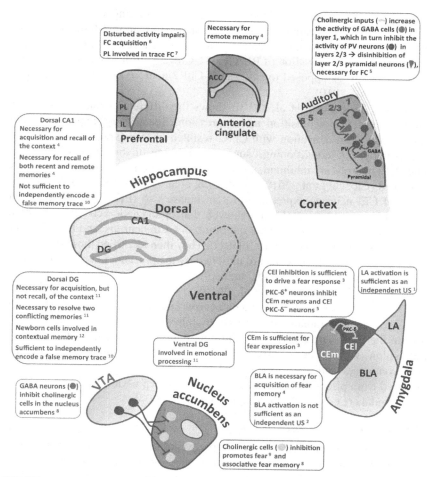

FIGURE 7.2 **Optogenetics-based findings in fear memory research.** This figure presents the different areas involved in fear memory that were implicated by optogenetics: amygdalar nuclei, primary and high cortical areas, striatum, and hippocampus. Each finding is marked by a number, signifying the corresponding published work, in the order they appear here: (1) Johansen et al. (2010); (2) Jasnow et al. (2013); (3) Ciocchi et al. (2010); (4) Goshen et al. (2011); (5) Letzkus et al. (2011); (6) Yizhar et al. (2011b); (7) Gilmartin et al. (2013); (8) Brown et al. (2012); (9) Witten et al. (2010); (10) Ramirez et al. (2013); (11) Kheirbek et al. (2013); (12) Gu et al. (2012). (This figure is reproduced in color in the plate section.)

induced by foot shock delivery, which could be explained by the fact that the general neuronal population of LA neurons was targeted, rather than the specific ensemble encoding for the paired tone (Han et al., 2007, 2009). This theory is partially supported by a study (Jasnow et al., 2013) showing that activation of basolateral amygdala (BLA) neurons in transgenic mice expressing ChR2 under the Thy-1 promoter did not affect freezing during training with a foot shock US, but decreased freezing during testing, suggesting an interference with the more precise ensemble representation of the amygdala cells that pair to the CS. Interestingly, light activation of BLA Thy-1-ChR2 neurons could not, by itself, serve as an US, as opposed to LA CamK-ChR2 neurons (Jasnow et al., 2013; Johansen et al., 2010).

A study by Ciocchi et al. (2010) shows the differential roles of the CEA sub-nuclei in fear acquisition and expression. Specifically, they report that optogenetic CEm activation with ChR2 resulted in fear expression (freezing). Interestingly, fear-conditioning causes disinhibition of the CEm by CEl, and when CEl neurons are inhibited, a nonconditioned, spontaneous fear response is generated (Ciocchi et al., 2010). Haubensak et al. (2010) identified a subpopulation of CEl neurons expressing protein kinase C-δ (PKC-δ), targeted them genetically to express ChR2 and showed that optogenetic activation of these CEl neurons results in a complete inhibition of CEm neurons, and in local inhibition of PKC-δ$^-$ neurons in the CEl itself. They then identified these PKC-δ$^+$ as CEl$_{off}$ units; that is, these cells are inhibited by the presentation of the CS, thus disinhibiting both CEm and CEl$_{on}$ units (the PKC-δ$^-$ neurons) and allowing the expression of fear (Haubensak et al., 2010).

These studies show that amygdala neurons are sufficient for the generation of FC. We demonstrated their necessity by bilaterally targeting excitatory neurons in the BLA with NpHR and inhibiting their activity with light during FC acquisition (Goshen et al., 2011). We found that this manipulation impaired both contextual and auditory-cued FC acquisition (Goshen et al., 2011), as expected from prior findings that acquisition and expression of fear depend on the amygdala (LeDoux, 2000; Maren and Quirk, 2004).

Primary and High Cortical Areas

A role for high cortical areas like the prefrontal cortex (PFCx) and the anterior cingulate cortex (ACC) was previously suggested mainly for fear memory extinction and remote memory consolidation and retrieval (Maren et al., 2013).

An impressive comprehensive study described a surprising role for the primary auditory cortex, beyond the mere perception of the tone, in auditory-cued fear-conditioning. Letzkus et al. (2011) defined the circuit, in which cholinergic inputs increase the activity of GABAergic cells in cortical layer 1, which in turn inhibit the activity of parvalbumin neurons in layers 2/3, resulting in increased firing of layer 2/3 pyramidal neurons (Letzkus et al., 2011). When parvalbumin neurons are optogenetically activated by ChR2 following foot shock (at the time when their activity is naturally suppressed by layer 1 neurons), auditory-cued FC is dramatically impaired (Letzkus et al., 2011).

Yizhar et al. (2011b) developed the stable step function opsin (SSFO), a ChR2 variant that can depolarize neurons for over 30 min in response to a brief light stimulation. They reported that hyper-activation of the PFCx during FC acquisition using SSFO in pyramidal neurons severely impaired both contextual and auditory-cued fear memory tested 1 day later. On the other hand, PFCx inhibition, achieved by SSFO activation of parvalbumin inhibitory neurons, had no effect on fear memory acquisition (Yizhar et al., 2011b). The observed over-excitation-induced acquisition failure is probably due to masking of the informative PFCx trace with a noisier opsin-induced signaling. The lack of effect of PFCx inhibition may be due to the low penetrance of the parvalbumin-Cre line. It is possible that a direct inhibition of pyramidal neurons with an inhibitory opsin would have resulted in a behavioral effect.

The PFCx, and especially its prelimbic (PL) area, was also implicated in TFC. For example, increased firing is observed in this region during the delay period between the CS and US (Baeg et al., 2001). Gilmartin et al. (2013) provided causal demonstration of the involvement of PL in trace conditioning by optogenetically inhibiting this area using ArchT during the 20-s interval between the CS (auditory cue) and US (electric shock). They showed that PL inhibition at that specific time significantly impaired the cued conditioning when tested 1 day later (Gilmartin et al., 2013). This is a striking demonstration of the temporal precision power of optogenetics.

Striatum

Another area that was implicated in associative fear memory is the dorsal striatum, including the nucleus accumbens (NAcc), but lesion studies provided inconsistent data (Everitt et al., 1999). One recurring finding was the development of a brief pause in cholinergic activity in the striatum as animals learn that a certain stimulus predicts an outcome (aversive or appetitive) (Apicella, 2007). This conditioned pause occurs upon presentation of the conditioned stimulus, and develops over several conditioning pairings (Apicella et al., 2011). Several optogenetic studies focused on the NAcc, mostly in the context of reward and addiction (Bock et al., 2013; Brown et al., 2012; Stuber et al., 2011; van Zessen et al., 2012; Witten et al., 2010), and some investigated memory as well:

Witten et al. (2010) showed that optogenetic inhibition of cholinergic neurons in the NAcc increased the activity of medium spiny neurons in this nucleus, and decreased cocaine-induced conditioned place preference. Interestingly, NAcc cholinergic inhibition with NpHR also increased freezing in the fear-conditioning context both immediately after shock delivery, as well as a day later during testing (Witten et al., 2010). This effect seems to be not on the memory itself, but on the general valence of the context. Interestingly, no effect on auditory-cued fear was observed (Witten et al., 2010).

Brown et al. (2012) then described a physiological circuit of NAcc cholinergic inhibition by GABAergic VTA neurons, and its involvement in fear memory: By injecting floxed ChR2-EYFP to the VTA of GAD-Cre mice they expressed ChR2 only in GABAergic neurons in this area. They then showed that projections of these neurons are in contact with cholinergic cells in the NAcc, and that these connections are functional, as when VTA GABAergic neurons were activated by ChR2 they, in turn, decreased the activity of NAcc cholinergic neurons (Brown et al., 2012). The causal proof of the involvement of VTA GABA neurons in associative fear memory was then achieved by activating these cells for 300 ms at the beginning of the CS$^+$ (followed by a shock), but not a different CS$^-$ (a different sound, not followed by a shock) during the 2 days of training. GAD-Cre$^-$ mice showed generalized fear from both stimuli (because of the intense training), but GAD-Cre$^+$ mice, in which the cholinergic neurons in NAcc were briefly inhibited at the beginning of the CS$^+$, showed a clear discrimination between this stimulus and the CS$^-$; they froze more in response to the CS$^+$ (Brown et al., 2012).

Nucleus Reuniens

A recent work identified a specific thalamic nucleus (the nucleus reuniens (NR)) as a major contributor to the specificity of contextual memory (Xu and Sudhof, 2013). The researchers stimulated NR neurons using ChIEF, a faster and more stable form of ChR2 (Lin et al., 2009), and found different effects on memory specificity, depending on the stimulation patters. Tonic stimulation induced higher precision, whereas phasic stimulation resulted in more generalization (Xu and Sudhof, 2013).

The Role of Different Hippocampal Subregions in Fear Memory

The hippocampus is composed of several subregions, with known connections between them: The DG, with over 1 million granule neurons (Rapp and Gallagher, 1996), is the primary target of the entorhinal cortex, and receives information from this region via the perforant path. Processed information from the DG region is then transferred via the mossy fibers to CA3, containing 80% less neurons (only about 220,000 pyramidal cells). CA3 projections in the Shaffer collaterals then innervate the 400,000 CA1 pyramidal neurons. Numerous theoretical models sought to explain the computational function of this sharp decrease (followed by a smaller expansion) in the number of cells, concentrating mainly on CA3, as the bottleneck of information. However, optogenetic memory experiments so far mainly shed light on the differences between the roles of DG and CA1 in fear memory.

To test the role of CA1 in memory acquisition and recall, we targeted pyramidal neurons in this region with NpHR, under control of the calcium/calmodulin-dependent protein kinase IIα (CaMKIIα) promoter, selective for excitatory glutamatergic neurons, and showed that continuous illumination of CA1 neurons inhibited spiking in vivo in a temporally precise, stable, and reversible manner (Goshen et al., 2011). We found that CA1 optogenetic inhibition by continuous green light during training prevented the acquisition of contextual fear memory. Furthermore, this effect is completely reversible, as when these mice were re-trained on the next day without light and then tested without light a day later they showed flawless memory (Goshen et al., 2011). We next retested the same mice with light delivery during recall, to examine whether dorsal CA1 optogenetic inhibition could also interfere with recall, and found that the memory that had been present on the previous day became unavailable for recall under illumination (Goshen et al., 2011). CA1 light-inhibition had no effect on auditory-cued fear memory acquisition when light was administered during training or on auditory-cued fear recall when illumination was administered during testing (Goshen et al., 2011). These experiments suggest a real-time involvement of CA1 excitatory cells in *both* acquisition and recall of contextual fear memory.

The role of dorsal DG in fear memory acquisition and recall was examined in a recent study (Kheirbek et al., 2013) by expressing opsins specifically in DG granular neurons using the pro-opiomelanocortin (POMC)-Cre mouse line. When double-floxed NpHR or ChR2 are expressed specifically in DG neurons, they induce inhibition or excitation of this region, respectively (Kheirbek et al., 2013). When the activity of dorsal DG neurons is inhibited during fear memory acquisition by illuminating NpHR throughout the conditioning trial, memory of the context on the next day is impaired, but auditory-cued fear memory acquisition is unaffected (Kheirbek et al., 2013). Interestingly, when DG functions normally during acquisition, but is inhibited during memory recall, no effect on memory is observed (Kheirbek et al., 2013).

What could be the reason for the necessity of CA1 signaling during recall while DG activity is not necessary at this stage? Several explanations may be offered: First, the DG participates in acquisition (and possibly consolidation) of the contextual memory trace, but then becomes unnecessary, while CA1 still plays a crucial role at this stage. An alternative explanation would be that since CA1 is the main output region of the hippocampus, any disruption of its activity will have a behavioral effect, even if the actual computation required for recall is performed elsewhere (in CA3, for example). Future experiments may clarify this issue. Other functional differences between DG and CA1, especially in the ways in which neuronal ensembles in these structures encode specific information, will be discussed later.

Interestingly, Kheirbek et al. (2013) further report that DG neurons inhibition had no effect on either the acquisition or the retrieval of a spatial task—active place avoidance, where mice were trained to avoid a stationary shock zone base on spatial cues in a circular arena. However, when the position of the shock zone was switched to the opposite side, requiring a rapid encoding of a new contingency and resolving two conflicting memories, POMC-NpHR mice were markedly impaired. These data suggest that the DG is necessary for rapid memory acquisition (single trial FC, or zone reversal) and cognitive flexibility (in the resolution of conflicting memories) but not in the recall of established memories.

As mentioned, DG inhibition impairs contextual memory acquisition but not recall. However, different results were obtained when DG cells were activated rather than inhibited: When ChR2 was expressed in DG granule cells and light was delivered during acquisition, encoding was impaired—as demonstrated by reduced fear expression during testing on the next day (Kheirbek et al., 2013). As opposed to DG inhibition, DG granule cells activation impaired memory recall even when light was delivered during testing. DG activation had no effect on auditory-cued memory when delivered either during training or during recall (Kheirbek et al., 2013). These hyperactivation-induced memory impairments are probably due to the fact that the information conveyed by the DG to the following hippocampal station are now meaningless, as not only the neuronal ensemble encoding the specific context is activated—but many other neurons, too. Indeed, the DG is characterized by sparse coding (Chawla et al., 2005; Leutgeb et al., 2007); that is, only a small fraction of the neurons in this area are activated by any specific behavioral experience. Thus, when a large population of DG cells is activated, less information (or competing information) is actually conveyed.

Another unique characteristic of the DG compared to other hippocampal areas is neurogenesis; the continuous differentiation and integration of newly formed neurons into this structure (Kempermann et al., 2002, 2004). General ablation of these new neurons can result in memory impairments, and it seems that their contribution changes as they integrate into the existing network (Aimone et al., 2011). To examine the time-dependent contribution of newly formed DG neurons to memory, Gu et al. (2012) targeted the inhibitory opsin Arch into newly formed neurons in the subgranular zone using retroviruses (targeting dividing cells). Four weeks later, mice were trained in an FC paradigm, and the 4-week-old new neurons (already integrated into the DG, forming synapses with CA3, and showing enhanced plasticity) were optically inhibited during fear memory recall (Gu et al., 2012). This manipulation impaired contextual, but not auditory-cued, fear recall. Interestingly, when 2-week- or 8-week-old neurons were silenced no behavioral effect was observed, providing a precise time window of functionally relevant hyperactive in newly formed cells. This is another elegant demonstration of the power of optogenetics—allowing the first opportunity for real-time control of a specific cellular population, in this case based on the age of the cells.

Axial Variations in Hippocampal Activity

Afferent and efferent connectivity varies greatly along the dorsoventral axis of the hippocampus, which led to the theory of differential roles for the dorsal and ventral hippocampus in cognitive and emotional functions (Bannerman et al., 2004; Fanselow and Dong, 2010): Specifically, the dorsal hippocampus projects extensively to associative cortical regions, suggesting a role for this area in spatial and contextual memory, whereas the ventral hippocampus projects to the PFCx, amygdala, and hypothalamus suggesting a role in emotional processing (Fanselow and Dong, 2010; Moser and Moser, 1998; Swanson and Cowan, 1977). Indeed, studies had shown that dorsal hippocampus lesions disrupted spatial memory, whereas ventral lesions spared spatial learning but had an anxiolytic effect (Bannerman et al., 2002, 1999; Kjelstrup et al., 2002; Moser et al., 1995; Richmond et al., 1999).

However, the real-time involvement of the dorsal and ventral hippocampus is still unclear, and it is also unknown if this axial distribution applies to each specific subregion (DG, CA1-3) independently. A recent study addressed these questions using optogenetics in either dorsal or ventral DG, and comparing the behavioral outcome of similar manipulations: Kheirbek et al. (2013) expressed either NpHR or ChR2 specifically in DG granular neurons using the POMC-Cre mouse line. The effect of either dorsal or ventral illumination on cognitive and emotional behaviors was then examined. They have reported that suppressing dorsal DG activity (using NpHR) during training significantly reduced freezing behavior when the animals were tested in the chamber without light stimulation 24 h later. This encoding deficit was specific to contextual FC because DG inhibition (either dorsal or ventral) did not severely affect auditory-cued FC (Kheirbek et al., 2013). Ventral-DG stimulation with ChR2, on the other hand, had no effect on memory acquisition and recall (Kheirbek et al., 2013). It did, however, have a striking effect on emotional behavior—exerting an anxiolytic effect in both the open field and the elevated plus maze (Kheirbek et al., 2013). This study is an elegant demonstration for the changing roles performed differentially by the hippocampus along its dorsoventral axis, at least in the DG sub-field.

Retrieval Strategies for Recent and Remote Fear Memories

The recall of contextual fear memory is based on different consolidation processes, depending on the time that had passed since the memory was acquired. The consolidation of remote memories relies on both synaptic processes on the timescale of minutes to hours, and circuit consolidation over weeks to years (Frankland and Bontempi, 2005; Squire and Bayley, 2007). Many findings from both human studies and animal research suggest that process of long-term contextual fear memory consolidation requires early involvement of the hippocampus, followed by the neocortex. Specifically, these studies showed that hippocampal lesions impair recent memory 1 day after training, but the same lesions have no effect on remote memory, several weeks after training (Anagnostaras et al., 1999; Bontempi et al., 1999; Debiec et al., 2002; Frankland et al., 2004; Kim and Fanselow, 1992; Kitamura et al., 2009; Maren et al., 1997; Maviel et al., 2004; Shimizu et al., 2000; Wang et al., 2003). Such graded retrograde amnesia is also observed in human patients with medial temporal lobe injuries (Kitamura et al., 2009; Squire and Bayley, 2007). Studies causing extensive hippocampal damage have reported nongraded retrograde amnesia for FC (Sutherland et al., 2008; Wang et al., 2009; Winocur et al., 2010). This and other work had led to the "multiple trace theory," suggesting that the hippocampal memory trace is not replaced by the cortical one but rather that both memories are in continuous interplay and the effect of hippocampal lesions may depend on both the nature of the task and the nature of the lesion (Cipolotti and Bird, 2006; Moscovitch et al., 2006; Winocur et al., 2010).

The pioneering work on the circuitry of remote memory has involved lesion studies (physical, pharmacological and genetic), which are highly effective but involve a tradeoff between cellular and temporal precision. Elegant genetic interventions can be cell-type specific (McHugh et al., 2007; Nakashiba et al., 2008) but are slow—on the timescale of days. Pharmacological lesions enable higher temporal resolution on the timescale of minutes (Kitamura et al., 2009; Wiltgen et al., 2010) but are still slower than neurons and not typically cell specific. Using an optogenetic approach, we were able to silence CA1 in real time and show that precise *real-time* inhibition of the CA1 region, sparing other hippocampal regions such as dorsal DG and CA3 as well as ventral CA1, is sufficient to impair remote recall, suggesting permanent role of the hippocampus in memory recall as long as a memory trace exist—even months after acquisition (Goshen et al., 2011). Specifically, we expressed NpHR3.1 in CA1 glutamatergic neurons under the CaMKIIα promoter, and showed that CA1 inhibition during recall blocks fear memory when administered 1 day to 12 weeks after conditioning. These results point to ongoing involvement of the hippocampus in remote contextual fear memories, suggesting that the intact hippocampus can still act as the default activator of the memory trace. However, we were able to obtain pharmacological data consistent with prior physical, pharmacological or genetic lesions to the hippocampus, in which the interval between lesion and recall-test ranges from tens of minutes to several weeks (Anagnostaras et al., 1999; Goshen et al., 2011; Kim and Fanselow, 1992; Shimizu et al., 2000; Wiltgen et al., 2010). Indeed, we showed that pharmacological inhibition of hippocampus using TTX and CNQX, as previously reported (Kitamura et al., 2009), disturbed only recent but not remote fear recall in our own hands as well. One hypothesis that may explain this discrepancy between optogenetic and pharmacological findings is that the temporal precision of optogenetic inhibition permits necessity-testing without allowing expression of compensatory mechanisms. We have proved this hypothesis by repeating the remote optogenetic experiment with precise illumination during the test or prolonged illumination for 30 min before testing and during the test, to mimic a slower intervention and allow time for putative compensatory mechanisms to be engaged. Precise optogenetic inhibition impaired remote memory, whereas prolonged inhibition had no detectable effect (Goshen et al., 2011). This is true for remote memory, after presumptive extrahippocampal consolidation, but not for recent memory, which may rely solely on hippocampal memory traces, and thus was not rescued by prolonged illumination.

We further showed that the ACC is one of the brain areas that participate in compensating for hippocampal inactivation: First, we observed an increase in ACC activity with remote recall (inferring activity with cFos levels measurement). We also showed that CA1 inhibition during remote recall reduced this neuronal activity in ACC. However, when given enough time to compensate for the absence of hippocampal activity, ACC activity not only returned to but exceeded control levels, suggesting active compensation for hippocampal inactivation. Second, we showed that optogenetic ACC inhibition at a remote (but not recent) time point impaired contextual fear memory (Goshen et al., 2011), as was previously suggested using other methods (Frankland et al., 2004). We found that precise and prolonged optogenetic inhibition of ACC similarly impaired remote memory but had no effect on recent memory (Goshen et al., 2011). Together, these findings support the remote-memory importance of neocortex, and also illustrate that even following cortical reorganization, there may exist a default requirement for the hippocampus in recalling remote memory traces. The contribution of the ACC appears to be important enough that the hippocampus alone cannot independently support the full remote memory in contrast to the recent timepoint, but relies on the ACC at least partially, as seen by the impaired remote memory in the presence of ACC inhibition. Our finding that both CA1 and ACC inhibition interfere with remote recall could also support the multiple trace theory, suggesting that in the process of systemwide consolidation the memory is not merely copied from hippocampus to cortex, but rather transformed, possibly saved in different variations in several cortical regions, and that all memory copies remain available, with continuous interplay (Nadel and Moscovitch, 1997; Winocur et al., 2009, 2010, 2007). Further support for this idea was recently reported by Wheeler et al. using a brainwide global mapping of cFos expression, which identified networks of brain regions activated following recall of long-term fear memories in mice (Wheeler et al., 2013). They report that the functional connectivity of the hippocampus with other brain regions is not decreased at the remote time point, but rather strengthened. Indeed, long-term memory recall engages a network that has a distinct thalamic-hippocampal-cortical signature (Wheeler et al., 2013).

MEMORY GENERATION AND MEMORY ENHANCEMENT USING OPTOGENETICS

A better temporal and spatial understanding of the complex mechanisms underlying memory is an essential basis for possible memory enhancement in the future. A major hypothesis in neuroscience is that sparse discrete neuronal populations underlie any specific memory trace. The existence of such populations in the lateral amygdala was indeed demonstrated (Han et al., 2007; Reijmers et al., 2007), and their necessity for the support of the memory trace was also established by ablating these neurons and thus erasing a specific memory trace without affecting other traces (Han et al., 2009; Zhou et al., 2009). However, until recently, no demonstration that these neuronal ensembles are not only necessary but also sufficient to encode a specific memory trace was available. Liu et al. (2012) provided the first proof that the stimulation of a specific memory engram in the hippocampus can in fact support the memory of a specific context, by using a combination of genetic and optogenetic tools: ChR2 was specifically expressed in a neuronal population in the DG, activated in response to a specific context as follows: The context-specific expression of ChR2 was achieved by using the cFos-tTA mouse line, expressing the tetracycline transactivator (tTA) under the promoter for cFos, an immediate-early gene serving as a marker for neuronal activity (Kubik et al., 2007; Reijmers et al., 2007). Thus, tTA is expressed in cells that were recently active following a specific task. The cFos-tTA mice were injected with a virus encoding for ChR2, driven by tetracycline responsive element (TRE) into their DG. Accordingly, in the injected mice activity drives the expression of tTA in the cells that participate in a specific engram, which subsequently induces the expression of ChR2. This expression is persistent (lasts for several days), and thus in order to restrict ChR2 expression to a specific context, and not to every context encountered by the mouse, mice are kept on a doxycycline (Dox)-containing diet, which prevents tTA from binding to TRE (Shockett and Schatz, 1996). Consequently, only when Dox is *not* present is ChR2 expressed.

In an elegant experiment, Liu et al. (2012) used this system to express ChR2 only in the DG neurons activated in a specific context B, during FC, by taking the mice off Dox for 2 days prior to exposure to this context. The mice were later returned to a Dox-supplemented diet, and introduced into a different context A, while the expressing neurons were illuminated. Despite the fact that no aversive stimulus was ever present in context A during testing or in the past, the ChR2 expressing mice demonstrated fear. The interpretation of these results is that the light activation of the memory engram of context B resulted in fear response even though the mice were actually in the neutral context A (Liu et al., 2012). This effect was even bigger when mice were allowed only 1 day with no Dox (thus increasing the specificity of the neuronal tagging by tTA), and even more when the virus injection and illumination were performed bilaterally (Liu et al., 2012). When no association is formed between the tagged neurons and an aversive stimulus (i.e., the mice are off-Dox in context B with no shock, and then exposed to a shock in context C under Dox), no light-induced fear is observed in context A (Liu et al., 2012). Thus, it is possible to elicit the behavioral output of a specific memory by directly activating the population of neurons in the DG that were active during its acquisition, proving that activation of a specific sparse neuronal ensemble is sufficient for the recall of a contextual memory.

In a follow-up study, Ramirez et al. (2013) took this idea one step further, and instead of activating an existing memory trace, created a false memory trace by first tagging a specific neuronal ensemble in context B, and then activating this population with light while administering a foot shock in context A, thus creating an offline association between the engram of B and an aversive stimulus, that resulted in fear of the previously neutral context B upon reintroduction to this context with no light (Ramirez et al., 2013). The recall of the false memory is context specific, that is, even after the offline conditioning, freezing is not observed in either a newly presented context C or a formerly presented (but not tagged or conditioned) context D. However, similar to the fear induced by the light activation of a real memory in a neutral environment (Liu et al., 2012), light activation of a false memory trace in a neutral environment also resulted in a fear response (Ramirez et al., 2013). The generation of a false fear memory was also demonstrated in the conditioned place avoidance paradigm: in the classic version of this behavioral test mice experience an aversive experience in a specific compartment in a three-chamber arena and later avoid entering this compartment and exploring it (Cunningham et al., 2006). To create a false fear memory of one of the cambers (chamber X), mice were allowed to explore it off Dox, thus allowing the expression of ChR2 in the DG neurons that encode this context. Mice were then placed back on Dox and 2 days later received a foot shock in a different cage with light stimulation, thus creating an association between the foot shock and the neuronal ensemble encoding the specific chamber X. Consequently, these mice showed a clear avoidance of chamber X that was associated offline with an aversive stimulus, and strongly preferred the other two chambers (Ramirez et al., 2013). Interestingly, the generation of a false memory trace interfered with the memory of the real conditioning context itself upon introduction to this context with no light (Ramirez et al., 2013). The authors interpret this finding as an example for competitive conditioning—that is, the availability of two conditioned stimuli impairs the strength of each one of them by itself (Brandon et al., 2000). This theory is further supported by the fact that when the false memory is activated upon reintroduction to the conditioning context by light, fear levels increase back to normal levels, based on the combined recall of both the tagged context and the conditioning context engrams (Ramirez et al., 2013).

Finally, this paper provides a well-designed demonstration of the importance of the sparse coding in the DG compared to CA1 (Ramirez et al., 2013). The researchers exposed mice to a novel context when off Dox (thus enabling the expression of ChR2), and then 24 h later exposed them while on Dox to either the same context or to a different context, and stained for cFos activity. In the DG, an overlap of only about 1% of the cells was found between the new and old context—demonstrating the sparse coding in this area, whereas in the CA1 a 30% overlap was found between the cells active in the different contexts (Ramirez et al., 2013). The functional consequence of the high selectivity of neuronal representation in the DG compared to CA1 was that a false memory trace could be generated by DG neuronal light activation, but not by activation of the neurons activated in CA1 in response to a specific context. The same was true for conditioned place aversion—mice showed avoidance of the falsely aversive chamber only upon tagging and activation of DG, but not CA1, neurons (Ramirez et al., 2013).

An interesting demonstration of the advantages provided by optogenetics compared to other methods is provided by comparing an optogenetic false memory trace that is able to support a behavioral output (Ramirez et al., 2013), to a pharmacogenetic false trace, which does not provide the same robustness (Garner et al., 2012). Specifically, Garner et al. (2012) expressed the designer receptor hM_3D_q in activated neurons and later activated it by its specific ligand clozapine-N-oxide (CNO) as follows: Double-transgenic mice expressing tTA under the activity-regulated cFos promoter, *and* hM_3D_q under the tet Operator (tetO), activated by tTA in the absence of Dox. Consequently, hM_3D_q is expressed in the brains of these mice in an activity-dependent manner when not treated with Dox (Alexander et al., 2009; Garner et al., 2012; Reijmers et al., 2007). The hM_3D_q receptor can then be activated by injecting its specific ligand CNO and produces strong depolarization and spiking in pyramidal neurons (Alexander et al., 2009). The researchers tagged the ensemble of neurons encoding a specific context by taking the mice off Dox and introduce them to a novel context A. They then activated this ensemble during FC in context B by injecting the mice with CNO, thus creating a false memory trace connecting the tagged neurons encoding context A with the aversive unconditioned stimulus. They found that this by itself *cannot* support a behavioral expression of fear, but can only interfere with the "real" memory of the conditioning context (Garner et al., 2012). Both the pharmacogenetic and the optogenetic techniques offer an activity-dependent expression of a protein that can later be activated at will. Two reasons may explain the robustness of the optogenetic false trace (directly eliciting a behavioral response) compared to the pharmacogenetic false trace: (1) Temporal precision: Light activation can be administered in a millisecond precision, whereas drug administration is orders-of-magnitude slower, activating the false trace for a long duration. (2) Spatial precision: The optogenetic false memory trace was efficient only when the manipulation was performed on DG neurons, where each context is sparsely represented, but not when performed in CA1, where the ensembles encoding different contexts are more overlapping. The pharmacogenetic trace includes neurons brainwide, thus diluting the pure representation of the context in the DG.

The generation of a false memory in a sophisticatedly targeted group of neurons is a remarkable achievement, but in practical terms for near-future memory enhancement it will be technically complicated to apply to complex memories or higher species. However, a previous work had managed to both create fear memory, and even more remarkably, an appetitive behavior, in response to nonspecific neuronal targeting (Choi et al., 2011). The researchers from the Axel group targeted ChR2 to neurons in the piriform cortex in three ways—expression in all neurons (excitatory and inhibitory, under the hSynapsin1 promoter), in excitatory neurons only (under the Emx1 promoter), or sparsely in all neurons (in hSynapsin1::Cre:EGFP mice) (Choi et al., 2011). They first used the active avoidance paradigm, in which the mouse is exposed to a shock (US) in one side of a specific context, paired to a previously neutral CS (e.g., smell) and can terminate the shock by fleeing to the other side of the arena. After several pairings, the CS itself will generate a flight response (Yan et al., 2008). They used light stimulation of piriform cortex neurons by ChR2 as the CS. During testing, mice were placed in the context, and the flight response to piriform stimulation alone (with no shock) was recorded. They found that, using all three expression methods, the conditioning resulted in a strong escape behavior in response to the light stimulation (Choi et al., 2011). Importantly, a randomly targeted group of piriform neurons could also drive appetitive behavior when paired to a socially rewarding stimulus (a female mouse). When a random piriform neurons ensemble in male mice is activated in a cage compartment in which a female is present, they will later prefer to be in a compartment that offers light stimulation even when no female is present (Choi et al., 2011). Similarly, light stimulation of somatosensory neurons can also serve as a cue for learning (Huber et al., 2008). Furthermore, mice can also be trained to associate light delivery with a water reward, and show increased licking in response to light delivery (Choi et al., 2011). Interestingly, the very same random population can be entrained to support both appetitive and aversive behavior.

In summary, the incorporation of optogenetics into the study of learning and memory led to a major leap in our understanding of the networks underlying complex cognitive processes. All of the mentioned experiments were performed over a period of less than 5 years, and further advances in this field are sure to arise in the very near future. The power of this tool already enabled the generation of light-induced memory traces (either real or false) and may be used to enhance existing memories in years to come. Such development will rely on deeper understanding of the contribution of specific neuronal populations, and the complex connections between them, first to relatively simple learning tasks like FC, and then to more elaborate memory challenges.

REFERENCES

Adamantidis, A.R., Zhang, F., Aravanis, A.M., Deisseroth, K., de Lecea, L., 2007. Neural substrates of awakening probed with optogenetic control of hypocretin neurons. Nature 450, 420–424.

Aimone, J.B., Deng, W., Gage, F.H., 2011. Resolving new memories: a critical look at the dentate gyrus, adult neurogenesis, and pattern separation. Neuron 70, 589–596.

Airan, R.D., Thompson, K.R., Fenno, L.E., Bernstein, H., Deisseroth, K., 2009. Temporally precise in vivo control of intracellular signalling. Nature 458, 1025–1029.

Alexander, G.M., Rogan, S.C., Abbas, A.I., Armbruster, B.N., Pei, Y., Allen, J.A., et al., 2009. Remote control of neuronal activity in transgenic mice expressing evolved G protein-coupled receptors. Neuron 63, 27–39.

Anagnostaras, S.G., Maren, S., Fanselow, M.S., 1999. Temporally graded retrograde amnesia of contextual fear after hippocampal damage in rats: within-subjects examination. J. Neurosci. 19, 1106–1114.

Apicella, P., 2007. Leading tonically active neurons of the striatum from reward detection to context recognition. Trends Neurosci. 30, 299–306.

Apicella, P., Ravel, S., Deffains, M., Legallet, E., 2011. The role of striatal tonically active neurons in reward prediction error signaling during instrumental task performance. J. Neurosci. 31, 1507–1515.

Aravanis, A.M., Wang, L.P., Zhang, F., Meltzer, L.A., Mogri, M.Z., Schneider, M.B., et al., 2007. An optical neural interface: in vivo control of rodent motor cortex with integrated fiberoptic and optogenetic technology. J. Neural Eng. 4, S143–S156.

Arenkiel, B.R., Peca, J., Davison, I.G., Feliciano, C., Deisseroth, K., Augustine, G.J., et al., 2007. In vivo light-induced activation of neural circuitry in transgenic mice expressing channelrhodopsin-2. Neuron 54, 205–218.

Atasoy, D., Aponte, Y., Su, H.H., Sternson, S.M., 2008. A FLEX switch targets Channelrhodopsin-2 to multiple cell types for imaging and long-range circuit mapping. J. Neurosci. 28, 7025–7030.

Baeg, E.H., Kim, Y.B., Jang, J., Kim, H.T., Mook-Jung, I., Jung, M.W., 2001. Fast spiking and regular spiking neural correlates of fear conditioning in the medial prefrontal cortex of the rat. Cereb. Cortex 11, 441–451.

Bangasser, D.A., Waxler, D.E., Santollo, J., Shors, T.J., 2006. Trace conditioning and the hippocampus: the importance of contiguity. J. Neurosci. 26, 8702–8706.

Bannerman, D.M., Deacon, R.M., Offen, S., Friswell, J., Grubb, M., Rawlins, J.N., 2002. Double dissociation of function within the hippocampus: spatial memory and hyponeophagia. Behav. Neurosci. 116, 884–901.

Bannerman, D.M., Rawlins, J.N., McHugh, S.B., Deacon, R.M., Yee, B.K., Bast, T., et al., 2004. Regional dissociations within the hippocampus–memory and anxiety. Neurosci. Biobehav. Rev. 28, 273–283.

Bannerman, D.M., Yee, B.K., Good, M.A., Heupel, M.J., Iversen, S.D., Rawlins, J.N., 1999. Double dissociation of function within the hippocampus: a comparison of dorsal, ventral, and complete hippocampal cytotoxic lesions. Behav. Neurosci. 113, 1170–1188.

Berndt, A., Yizhar, O., Gunaydin, L.A., Hegemann, P., Deisseroth, K., 2009. Bi-stable neural state switches. Nat. Neurosci. 12, 229–234.

Bernstein, J.G., Boyden, E.S., 2011. Optogenetic tools for analyzing the neural circuits of behavior. Trends Cogn. Sci. 15, 592–600.

Bock, R., Shin, J.H., Kaplan, A.R., Dobi, A., Markey, E., Kramer, P.F., et al., 2013. Strengthening the accumbal indirect pathway promotes resilience to compulsive cocaine use. Nat. Neurosci. 16, 632–638.

Bontempi, B., Laurent-Demir, C., Destrade, C., Jaffard, R., 1999. Time-dependent reorganization of brain circuitry underlying long-term memory storage. Nature 400, 671–675.

Boyden, E.S., Zhang, F., Bamberg, E., Nagel, G., Deisseroth, K., 2005. Millisecond-timescale, genetically targeted optical control of neural activity. Nat. Neurosci. 8, 1263–1268.

Brandon, S.E., Vogel, E.H., Wagner, A.R., 2000. A componential view of configural cues in generalization and discrimination in Pavlovian conditioning. Behav. Brain Res. 110, 67–72.

Brown, M.T., Tan, K.R., O'Connor, E.C., Nikonenko, I., Muller, D., Luscher, C., 2012. Ventral tegmental area GABA projections pause accumbal cholinergic interneurons to enhance associative learning. Nature 492, 452–456.

Chawla, M.K., Guzowski, J.F., Ramirez-Amaya, V., Lipa, P., Hoffman, K.L., Marriott, L.K., et al., 2005. Sparse, environmentally selective expression of Arc RNA in the upper blade of the rodent fascia dentata by brief spatial experience. Hippocampus 15, 579–586.

Choi, G.B., Stettler, D.D., Kallman, B.R., Bhaskar, S.T., Fleischmann, A., Axel, R., 2011. Driving opposing behaviors with ensembles of piriform neurons. Cell 146, 1004–1015.

Chow, B.Y., Han, X., Dobry, A.S., Qian, X., Chuong, A.S., Li, M., et al., 2010. High-performance genetically targetable optical neural silencing by light-driven proton pumps. Nature 463, 98–102.

Ciocchi, S., Herry, C., Grenier, F., Wolff, S.B., Letzkus, J.J., Vlachos, I., et al., 2010. Encoding of conditioned fear in central amygdala inhibitory circuits. Nature 468, 277–282.

Cipolotti, L., Bird, C.M., 2006. Amnesia and the hippocampus. Curr. Opin. Neurol. 19, 593–598.

Crick, F.H., 1979. Thinking about the brain. Sci. Am. 241, 219–232.

Cunningham, C.L., Gremel, C.M., Groblewski, P.A., 2006. Drug-induced conditioned place preference and aversion in mice. Nat. Protoc. 1, 1662–1670.

Debiec, J., LeDoux, J.E., Nader, K., 2002. Cellular and systems reconsolidation in the hippocampus. Neuron 36, 527–538.

Deisseroth, K., 2010. Controlling the brain with light. Sci. Am. 303, 48–55.

Deisseroth, K., 2011. Optogenetics. Nat. Methods 8, 26–29.

Deisseroth, K., Feng, G., Majewska, A.K., Miesenbock, G., Ting, A., Schnitzer, M.J., 2006. Next-generation optical technologies for illuminating genetically targeted brain circuits. J. Neurosci. 26, 10380–10386.

Deisseroth, K., Schnitzer, M.J., 2013. Engineering approaches to illuminating brain structure and dynamics. Neuron 80, 568–577.

Everitt, B.J., Parkinson, J.A., Olmstead, M.C., Arroyo, M., Robledo, P., Robbins, T.W., 1999. Associative processes in addiction and reward. The role of amygdala-ventral striatal subsystems. Ann. N. Y. Acad. Sci. 877, 412–438.

Fanselow, M.S., 2000. Contextual fear, gestalt memories, and the hippocampus. Behav. Brain Res. 110, 73–81.

Fanselow, M.S., Dong, H.W., 2010. Are the dorsal and ventral hippocampus functionally distinct structures? Neuron 65, 7–19.

Fanselow, M.S., LeDoux, J.E., 1999. Why we think plasticity underlying Pavlovian fear conditioning occurs in the basolateral amygdala. Neuron 23, 229–232.

Fenno, L., Yizhar, O., Deisseroth, K., 2011. The development and application of optogenetics. Annu. Rev. Neurosci. 34, 389–412.

Frankland, P.W., Bontempi, B., 2005. The organization of recent and remote memories. Nat. Rev. Neurosci. 6, 119–130.

Frankland, P.W., Bontempi, B., Talton, L.E., Kaczmarek, L., Silva, A.J., 2004. The involvement of the anterior cingulate cortex in remote contextual fear memory. Science 304, 881–883.

Garner, A.R., Rowland, D.C., Hwang, S.Y., Baumgaertel, K., Roth, B.L., Kentros, C., et al., 2012. Generation of a synthetic memory trace. Science 335, 1513–1516.

Gilmartin, M.R., Miyawaki, H., Helmstetter, F.J., Diba, K., 2013. Prefrontal activity links nonoverlapping events in memory. J. Neurosci. 33, 10910–10914.

Goosens, K.A., Maren, S., 2003. Pretraining NMDA receptor blockade in the basolateral complex, but not the central nucleus, of the amygdala prevents savings of conditional fear. Behav. Neurosci. 117, 738–750.

Goshen, I., Brodsky, M., Prakash, R., Wallace, J., Gradinaru, V., Ramakrishnan, C., et al., 2011. Dynamics of retrieval strategies for remote memories. Cell 147, 678–689.

Gradinaru, V., Thompson, K.R., Zhang, F., Mogri, M., Kay, K., Schneider, M.B., et al., 2007. Targeting and readout strategies for fast optical neural control in vitro and in vivo. J. Neurosci. 27, 14231–14238.

Gradinaru, V., Zhang, F., Ramakrishnan, C., Mattis, J., Prakash, R., Diester, I., et al., 2010. Molecular and cellular approaches for diversifying and extending optogenetics. Cell 141, 154–165.

Gu, Y., Arruda-Carvalho, M., Wang, J., Janoschka, S.R., Josselyn, S.A., Frankland, P.W., et al., 2012. Optical controlling reveals time-dependent roles for adult-born dentate granule cells. Nat. Neurosci. 15, 1700–1706.

Gunaydin, L.A., Yizhar, O., Berndt, A., Sohal, V.S., Deisseroth, K., Hegemann, P., 2010. Ultrafast optogenetic control. Nat. Neurosci. 13, 387–392.

Hagglund, M., Borgius, L., Dougherty, K.J., Kiehn, O., 2010. Activation of groups of excitatory neurons in the mammalian spinal cord or hindbrain evokes locomotion. Nat. Neurosci. 13, 246–252.

Han, J.H., Kushner, S.A., Yiu, A.P., Cole, C.J., Matynia, A., Brown, R.A., et al., 2007. Neuronal competition and selection during memory formation. Science 316, 457–460.

Han, J.H., Kushner, S.A., Yiu, A.P., Hsiang, H.L., Buch, T., Waisman, A., et al., 2009. Selective erasure of a fear memory. Science 323, 1492–1496.

Haubensak, W., Kunwar, P.S., Cai, H., Ciocchi, S., Wall, N.R., Ponnusamy, R., et al., 2010. Genetic dissection of an amygdala microcircuit that gates conditioned fear. Nature 468, 270–276.

Huber, D., Petreanu, L., Ghitani, N., Ranade, S., Hromadka, T., Mainen, Z., et al., 2008. Sparse optical microstimulation in barrel cortex drives learned behaviour in freely moving mice. Nature 451, 61–64.

Huber, D., Veinante, P., Stoop, R., 2005. Vasopressin and oxytocin excite distinct neuronal populations in the central amygdala. Science 308, 245–248.

Jasnow, A.M., Ehrlich, D.E., Choi, D.C., Dabrowska, J., Bowers, M.E., McCullough, K.M., et al., 2013. Thy1-expressing neurons in the basolateral amygdala may mediate fear inhibition. J. Neurosci. 33, 10396–10404.

Johansen, J.P., Hamanaka, H., Monfils, M.H., Behnia, R., Deisseroth, K., Blair, H.T., et al., 2010. Optical activation of lateral amygdala pyramidal cells instructs associative fear learning. Proc. Natl. Acad. Sci. U.S.A. 107, 12692–12697.

Kempermann, G., Gast, D., Gage, F.H., 2002. Neuroplasticity in old age: sustained fivefold induction of hippocampal neurogenesis by long-term environmental enrichment. Ann. Neurol. 52, 135–143.

Kempermann, G., Wiskott, L., Gage, F.H., 2004. Functional significance of adult neurogenesis. Curr. Opin. Neurobiol. 14, 186–191.

Kheirbek, M.A., Drew, L.J., Burghardt, N.S., Costantini, D.O., Tannenholz, L., Ahmari, S.E., et al., 2013. Differential control of learning and anxiety along the dorsoventral axis of the dentate gyrus. Neuron 77, 955–968.

Kim, J.J., Fanselow, M.S., 1992. Modality-specific retrograde amnesia of fear. Science 256, 675–677.

Kitamura, T., Saitoh, Y., Takashima, N., Murayama, A., Niibori, Y., Ageta, H., et al., 2009. Adult neurogenesis modulates the hippocampus-dependent period of associative fear memory. Cell 139, 814–827.

Kjelstrup, K.G., Tuvnes, F.A., Steffenach, H.A., Murison, R., Moser, E.I., Moser, M.B., 2002. Reduced fear expression after lesions of the ventral hippocampus. Proc. Natl. Acad. Sci. U.S.A. 99, 10825–10830.

Kleinlogel, S., Feldbauer, K., Dempski, R.E., Fotis, H., Wood, P.G., Bamann, C., et al., 2011. Ultra light-sensitive and fast neuronal activation with the Ca^{2+}-permeable channelrhodopsin CatCh. Nat. Neurosci. 14, 513–518.

Kravitz, A.V., Freeze, B.S., Parker, P.R., Kay, K., Thwin, M.T., Deisseroth, K., et al., 2010. Regulation of parkinsonian motor behaviours by optogenetic control of basal ganglia circuitry. Nature 466, 622–626.

Krettek, J.E., Price, J.L., 1978. A description of the amygdaloid complex in the rat and cat with observations on intra-amygdaloid axonal connections. J. Comp. Neurol. 178, 255–280.

Kubik, S., Miyashita, T., Guzowski, J.F., 2007. Using immediate-early genes to map hippocampal subregional functions. Learn. Mem. 14, 758–770.

LeDoux, J.E., 2000. Emotion circuits in the brain. Annu. Rev. Neurosci. 23, 155–184.

LeDoux, J.E., Iwata, J., Cicchetti, P., Reis, D.J., 1988. Different projections of the central amygdaloid nucleus mediate autonomic and behavioral correlates of conditioned fear. J. Neurosci. 8, 2517–2529.

Lee, J.H., Durand, R., Gradinaru, V., Zhang, F., Goshen, I., Kim, D.S., et al., 2010. Global and local fMRI signals driven by neurons defined optogenetically by type and wiring. Nature 465, 788–792.

Letzkus, J.J., Wolff, S.B., Meyer, E.M., Tovote, P., Courtin, J., Herry, C., et al., 2011. A disinhibitory microcircuit for associative fear learning in the auditory cortex. Nature 480, 331–335.

Leutgeb, J.K., Leutgeb, S., Moser, M.B., Moser, E.I., 2007. Pattern separation in the dentate gyrus and CA3 of the hippocampus. Science 315, 961–966.

Levitz, J., Pantoja, C., Gaub, B., Janovjak, H., Reiner, A., Hoagland, A., et al., 2013. Optical control of metabotropic glutamate receptors. Nat. Neurosci. 16, 507–516.

Lin, J.Y., Lin, M.Z., Steinbach, P., Tsien, R.Y., 2009. Characterization of engineered channelrhodopsin variants with improved properties and kinetics. Biophys. J. 96, 1803–1814.

Liu, X., Ramirez, S., Pang, P.T., Puryear, C.B., Govindarajan, A., Deisseroth, K., et al., 2012. Optogenetic stimulation of a hippocampal engram activates fear memory recall. Nature 484, 381–385.

Maren, S., 2001. Neurobiology of Pavlovian fear conditioning. Annu. Rev. Neurosci. 24, 897–931.

Maren, S., Aharonov, G., Fanselow, M.S., 1997. Neurotoxic lesions of the dorsal hippocampus and Pavlovian fear conditioning in rats. Behav. Brain Res. 88, 261–274.

Maren, S., Holt, W., 2000. The hippocampus and contextual memory retrieval in Pavlovian conditioning. Behav. Brain Res. 110, 97–108.

Maren, S., Phan, K.L., Liberzon, I., 2013. The contextual brain: implications for fear conditioning, extinction and psychopathology. Nat. Rev. Neurosci. 14, 417–428.

Maren, S., Quirk, G.J., 2004. Neuronal signalling of fear memory. Nat. Rev. Neurosci. 5, 844–852.

Masseck, O.A., Spoida, K., Dalkara, D., Maejima, T., Rubelowski, J.M., Wallhorn, L., et al., 2014. Vertebrate cone opsins enable sustained and highly sensitive rapid control of Gi/o signaling in anxiety circuitry. Neuron 81, 1263–1273.

Mattis, J., Tye, K.M., Ferenczi, E.A., Ramakrishnan, C., O'Shea, D.J., Prakash, R., et al., 2012. Principles for applying optogenetic tools derived from direct comparative analysis of microbial opsins. Nat. Methods 9, 159–172.

Maviel, T., Durkin, T.P., Menzaghi, F., Bontempi, B., 2004. Sites of neocortical reorganization critical for remote spatial memory. Science 305, 96–99.

McHugh, T.J., Jones, M.W., Quinn, J.J., Balthasar, N., Coppari, R., Elmquist, J.K., et al., 2007. Dentate gyrus NMDA receptors mediate rapid pattern separation in the hippocampal network. Science 317, 94–99.

Moscovitch, M., Nadel, L., Winocur, G., Gilboa, A., Rosenbaum, R.S., 2006. The cognitive neuroscience of remote episodic, semantic and spatial memory. Curr. Opin. Neurobiol. 16, 179–190.

Moser, M.B., Moser, E.I., 1998. Functional differentiation in the hippocampus. Hippocampus 8, 608–619.

Moser, M.B., Moser, E.I., Forrest, E., Andersen, P., Morris, R.G., 1995. Spatial learning with a minislab in the dorsal hippocampus. Proc. Natl. Acad. Sci. U.S.A. 92, 9697–9701.

Nadel, L., Moscovitch, M., 1997. Memory consolidation, retrograde amnesia and the hippocampal complex. Curr. Opin. Neurobiol. 7, 217–227.

Nakashiba, T., Young, J.Z., McHugh, T.J., Buhl, D.L., Tonegawa, S., 2008. Transgenic inhibition of synaptic transmission reveals role of CA3 output in hippocampal learning. Science 319, 1260–1264.

Narayanan, N.S., Land, B.B., Solder, J.E., Deisseroth, K., DiLeone, R.J., 2012. Prefrontal D1 dopamine signaling is required for temporal control. Proc. Natl. Acad. Sci. U.S.A. 109, 20726–20731.

Ramirez, S., Liu, X., Lin, P.A., Suh, J., Pignatelli, M., Redondo, R.L., et al., 2013. Creating a false memory in the hippocampus. Science 341, 387–391.

Rapp, P.R., Gallagher, M., 1996. Preserved neuron number in the hippocampus of aged rats with spatial learning deficits. Proc. Natl. Acad. Sci. U.S.A. 93, 9926–9930.

Raybuck, J.D., Lattal, K.M., 2013. Bridging the interval: theory and neurobiology of trace conditioning. Behav. Processes 101, 103–111.

Reijmers, L.G., Perkins, B.L., Matsuo, N., Mayford, M., 2007. Localization of a stable neural correlate of associative memory. Science 317, 1230–1233.

Reiner, A., Isacoff, E.Y., 2013. The Brain Prize 2013: the optogenetics revolution. Trends Neurosci. 36, 557–560.

Richmond, M.A., Yee, B.K., Pouzet, B., Veenman, L., Rawlins, J.N., Feldon, J., et al., 1999. Dissociating context and space within the hippocampus: effects of complete, dorsal, and ventral excitotoxic hippocampal lesions on conditioned freezing and spatial learning. Behav. Neurosci. 113, 1189–1203.

Shimizu, E., Tang, Y.P., Rampon, C., Tsien, J.Z., 2000. NMDA receptor-dependent synaptic reinforcement as a crucial process for memory consolidation. Science 290, 1170–1174.

Shockett, P.E., Schatz, D.G., 1996. Diverse strategies for tetracycline-regulated inducible gene expression. Proc. Natl. Acad. Sci. U.S.A. 93, 5173–5176.

Sohal, V.S., Zhang, F., Yizhar, O., Deisseroth, K., 2009. Parvalbumin neurons and gamma rhythms enhance cortical circuit performance. Nature 459, 698–702.

Squire, L.R., Bayley, P.J., 2007. The neuroscience of remote memory. Curr. Opin. Neurobiol. 17, 185–196.

Steinberg, E.E., Keiflin, R., Boivin, J.R., Witten, I.B., Deisseroth, K., Janak, P.H., 2013. A causal link between prediction errors, dopamine neurons and learning. Nat. Neurosci. 16, 966–973.

Stuber, G.D., Sparta, D.R., Stamatakis, A.M., van Leeuwen, W.A., Hardjoprajitno, J.E., Cho, S., et al., 2011. Excitatory transmission from the amygdala to nucleus accumbens facilitates reward seeking. Nature 475, 377–380.

Sun, N., Yi, H., Cassell, M.D., 1994. Evidence for a GABAergic interface between cortical afferents and brainstem projection neurons in the rat central extended amygdala. J. Comp. Neurol. 340, 43–64.

Sutherland, R.J., O'Brien, J., Lehmann, H., 2008. Absence of systems consolidation of fear memories after dorsal, ventral, or complete hippocampal damage. Hippocampus 18, 710–718.

Swanson, L.W., Cowan, W.M., 1977. An autoradiographic study of the organization of the efferent connections of the hippocampal formation in the rat. J. Comp. Neurol. 172, 49–84.

Tan, K.R., Yvon, C., Turiault, M., Mirzabekov, J.J., Doehner, J., Labouebe, G. et al., 2012. GABA neurons of the VTA drive conditioned place aversion. Neuron 73, 1173–1183.

Tsai, H.C., Zhang, F., Adamantidis, A., Stuber, G.D., Bonci, A., de Lecea, L., et al., 2009. Phasic firing in dopaminergic neurons is sufficient for behavioral conditioning. Science 324, 1080–1084.

Tye, K.M., Mirzabekov, J.J., Warden, M.R., Ferenczi, E.A., Tsai, H.C., Finkelstein, J., et al., 2013. Dopamine neurons modulate neural encoding and expression of depression-related behaviour. Nature 493, 537–541.

Tye, K.M., Prakash, R., Kim, S.Y., Fenno, L.E., Grosenick, L., Zarabi, H., et al., 2011. Amygdala circuitry mediating reversible and bidirectional control of anxiety. Nature 471, 358–362.

van Zessen, R., Phillips, J.L., Budygin, E.A., Stuber, G.D., 2012. Activation of VTA GABA neurons disrupts reward consumption. Neuron 73, 1184–1194.

Wang, H., Shimizu, E., Tang, Y.P., Cho, M., Kyin, M., Zuo, W., et al., 2003. Inducible protein knockout reveals temporal requirement of CaMKII reactivation for memory consolidation in the brain. Proc. Natl. Acad. Sci. U.S.A. 100, 4287–4292.

Wang, S.H., Teixeira, C.M., Wheeler, A.L., Frankland, P.W., 2009. The precision of remote context memories does not require the hippocampus. Nat. Neurosci. 12, 253–255.

Wheeler, A.L., Teixeira, C.M., Wang, A.H., Xiong, X., Kovacevic, N., Lerch, J.P., et al., 2013. Identification of a functional connectome for long-term fear memory in mice. PLoS Comput. Biol. 9, e1002853.

Wilensky, A.E., Schafe, G.E., Kristensen, M.P., LeDoux, J.E., 2006. Rethinking the fear circuit: the central nucleus of the amygdala is required for the acquisition, consolidation, and expression of Pavlovian fear conditioning. J. Neurosci. 26, 12387–12396.

Wiltgen, B.J., Zhou, M., Cai, Y., Balaji, J., Karlsson, M.G., Parivash, S.N., et al., 2010. The hippocampus plays a selective role in the retrieval of detailed contextual memories. Curr. Biol. 20, 1336–1344.

Winocur, G., Frankland, P.W., Sekeres, M., Fogel, S., Moscovitch, M., 2009. Changes in context-specificity during memory reconsolidation: selective effects of hippocampal lesions. Learn. Mem. 16, 722–729.

Winocur, G., Moscovitch, M., Bontempi, B., 2010. Memory formation and long-term retention in humans and animals: convergence towards a transformation account of hippocampal-neocortical interactions. Neuropsychologia 48, 2339–2356.

Winocur, G., Moscovitch, M., Sekeres, M., 2007. Memory consolidation or transformation: context manipulation and hippocampal representations of memory. Nat. Neurosci. 10, 555–557.

Witten, I.B., Lin, S.C., Brodsky, M., Prakash, R., Diester, I., Anikeeva, P., et al., 2010. Cholinergic interneurons control local circuit activity and cocaine conditioning. Science 330, 1677–1681.

Witten, I.B., Steinberg, E.E., Lee, S.Y., Davidson, T.J., Zalocusky, K.A., Brodsky, M., et al., 2011. Recombinase-driver rat lines: tools, techniques, and optogenetic application to dopamine-mediated reinforcement. Neuron 72, 721–733.

Xu, W., Sudhof, T.C., 2013. A neural circuit for memory specificity and generalization. Science 339, 1290–1295.

Yan, Z., Tan, J., Qin, C., Lu, Y., Ding, C., Luo, M., 2008. Precise circuitry links bilaterally symmetric olfactory maps. Neuron 58, 613–624.

Yizhar, O., Fenno, L.E., Davidson, T.J., Mogri, M., Deisseroth, K., 2011a. Optogenetics in neural systems. Neuron 71, 9–34.

Yizhar, O., Fenno, L.E., Prigge, M., Schneider, F., Davidson, T.J., O'Shea, D.J., et al., 2011b. Neocortical excitation/inhibition balance in information processing and social dysfunction. Nature 477, 171–178.

Zhang, F., Gradinaru, V., Adamantidis, A.R., Durand, R., Airan, R.D., de Lecea, L., et al., 2010. Optogenetic interrogation of neural circuits: technology for probing mammalian brain structures. Nat. Protoc. 5, 439–456.

Zhang, F., Wang, L.P., Boyden, E.S., Deisseroth, K., 2006. Channelrhodopsin-2 and optical control of excitable cells. Nat. Methods 3, 785–792.

Zhang, F., Wang, L.P., Brauner, M., Liewald, J.F., Kay, K., Watzke, N., et al., 2007. Multimodal fast optical interrogation of neural circuitry. Nature 446, 633–639.

Zhou, Y., Won, J., Karlsson, M.G., Zhou, M., Rogerson, T., Balaji, J., et al., 2009. CREB regulates excitability and the allocation of memory to subsets of neurons in the amygdala. Nat. Neurosci. 12, 1438–1443.

Chapter 8

Can Stem Cells Be Used to Enhance Cognition?

Natalie R.S. Goldberg[1] and Mathew Blurton-Jones[1,2,3]

[1]*Department of Neurobiology & Behavior, University of California Irvine, Irvine, CA, USA;*
[2]*Sue and Bill Gross Stem Cell Research Center, University of California Irvine, Irvine, CA, USA;*
[3]*Institute for Memory Impairments and Neurological Disorders, University of California Irvine, Irvine, CA, USA*

INTRODUCTION

Stem cells are defined by two key attributes: (i) they can self-renew, dividing to create near-perfect copies of themselves; and (ii) can also differentiate to produce distinct mature cell types. Many different types of stem cells exist and can be classified based on their source and capacity for differentiation. For example, embryonic stem cells are derived from the inner cell mass of an early stage blastocyst and are considered pluripotent because they are able to create every cell type within the body. In contrast, within the adult body, multipotent stem cells exist in virtually every organ system and can create a far more limited repertoire of cell types associated with that given organ. A growing body of work continues to demonstrate the importance of multipotent stem cells in maintaining normal tissue function and homeostasis, as well as playing critical roles in tissue repair following injury or disease (reviewed by Fuchs et al., 2004).

The equilibrium between cell loss and replacement is well maintained by stem cells in most adult tissues, with the exceptions of the pancreas, heart, and brain. With maturation and age, the brain's capacity to produce new neurons is significantly diminished (Rossi et al., 2008). In addition to a reduction in stem cell turnover, the function of mature differentiated cells also is often diminished with age because of both intrinsic and environmental factors such as DNA damage, oxidative stress, or the accumulation of misfolded proteins (Shetty et al., 2013; Welihinda et al., 1999). These changes result in reduced tissue integrity and age-associated impairments in organ function. As discussed in this chapter, one of the greatest functional correlates to the loss of cell homeostasis in the brain is a decline in cognitive function.

Cognitive Enhancement. http://dx.doi.org/10.1016/B978-0-12-417042-1.00008-5

THE ROLE OF ENDOGENOUS NEUROGENESIS IN COGNITION

Nearly 50 years ago, Altman and Das (1965) provided the first evidence that neurogenesis could occur in the adult mammalian brain (Figures 8.1 and 8.2). Only decades later did the first reports of adult human neurogenesis first emerge. In a seminal study, Eriksson et al. (1998) demonstrated that

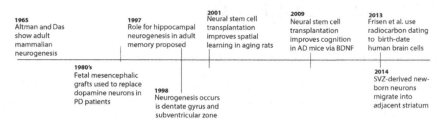

FIGURE 8.1   Timeline of seminal studies in neurogenesis and stem cell transplantation.

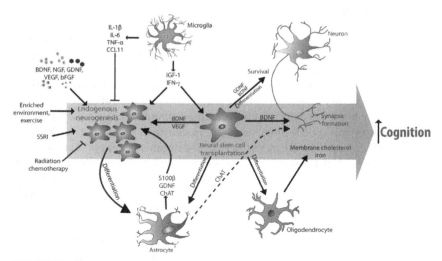

FIGURE 8.2   Stem cells can influence cognition via multiple mechanisms. Considerable evidence supports the notion that both adult neurogenesis and neural stem cell transplantation can contribute to cognition. Factors such as exercise, selective serotonin reuptake inhibitors (SSRIs), and inflammation can modulate adult neurogenesis, leading to enhanced or impaired cognition. Likewise, transplantation of neural stem cells can improve cognition in animal models of aging and neurodegenerative disease. While neurotrophic effects of stem cells are strongly implicated in this process, it is likely that many of the mechanisms shown here interact to modulate cognition. BDNF, brain-derived neurotrophic factor; bFGF, basic fibroblast growth factor; ChAT, choline acetyltransferase; GDNF, glial cell–derived neurotrophic factor; IFN, interferon; IGF, insulin-like growth factor; IL, interleukin; TNF, tumor necrosis factor; NGF, nerve growth factor. (This figure is reproduced in color in the color plate section.)

neurogenesis occurs in adult humans by tracing the incorporation of the thymidine analog bromodeoxyuridine (BrdU) into DNA within the brains of deceased cancer patients. These patients had previously received BrdU to assess tumor progression during treatment. The studies by Eriksson et al. (1998) revealed that humans do indeed exhibit adult neurogenesis in two key areas: the dentate gyrus of the hippocampus and the subventricular zone (SVZ) of the lateral ventricles. A more recent series of studies led by Dr. Jonas Frisen and colleagues used an inventive new approach to measure adult human neurogenesis (Ernst et al., 2014; Spalding et al., 2013). Between 1955 and 1963, above-ground nuclear bomb testing led to high atmospheric levels of ^{14}C that exponentially decreased after adoption of the Test Ban Treaty in 1963. Frisen and colleagues found that levels of ^{14}C within DNA at the time of birth closely paralleled atmospheric levels. Radiocarbon dating could therefore be used to retrospectively birth-date brain cells. Together, these studies confirmed that adult neurogenesis occurs within the hippocampus and SVZ of humans throughout life. Furthermore, adult hippocampal neurogenesis seems to be substantial; roughly 700 new neurons are generated in each hippocampus per day and up to one third of all hippocampal granule cell neurons are replaced during one's adult life. Ernst et al. (2014) most recently used the radiocarbon dating approach to provide compelling new data that SVZ-derived newborn neurons can also migrate into the adjacent striatum in humans, giving rise to cholinergic interneurons. These profound discoveries continue to provoke the question, What are the functional consequences of adult neurogenesis?

The functional role of neurogenesis in the adult brain has been studied in its germinative pools of the SVZ adjacent to the striatum (Alvarez-Buylla et al., 2000; Cheng et al., 2009), but our greatest understanding of the role of adult neurogenesis in cognition comes from studies of the dentate gyrus of the hippocampus. The hippocampus plays a critical role in encoding and retrieving memories (Izquierdo and Medina, 1997). A potential role for hippocampal neurogenesis in adult memory was first proposed by Shors et al. (2001). Support for this finding came in 2006, when studies showed that newborn granule cells of the dentate gyrus are more highly activated by a novel exploration task compared with mature neurons of the same region (Ramirez-Amaya et al., 2006). Possibly as a result of this increased excitability, newborn granule neurons also integrate more readily into memory-associated engrams than mature granule cells (Ge et al., 2007; Tashiro et al., 2006). Indeed, new granule cells have been shown to be preferentially integrated into spatial and temporal memory networks of the hippocampus compared with mature cells.

Over the past few years, several groups have adapted inducible transgenic approaches to test directly the necessity of adult hippocampal neurogenesis in learning and memory. For example, Imayoshi et al. (2008) used tamoxifen-inducible Cre-LoxP technology to generate a mouse model in which newborn neurons could be selectively ablated. Using this approach, the group demonstrated that adult newborn neurons were critical for long-term spatial memory and performance in the Barnes maze. In a similar study, Zhang et al. (2008) deleted the neurogenic gene *Tlx* (Tailess) in adult mice, leading to a dramatic reduction in hippocampal neurogenesis and impaired learning and memory in the Morris water maze. The dentate gyrus has increasingly been implicated in pattern separation, the process of transforming similar overlapping memories into distinct nonoverlapping representations (Aimone et al., 2011). It follows that recent studies have shown an important role for adult neurogenesis in pattern separation. For example, deletion of the *Bax* gene leads to increased adult neurogenesis, and mice exhibit an improved capacity to distinguish between two similar contexts, suggesting enhanced pattern separation (Sahay et al., 2011). Taken together, these studies and others continue to show that procedures that abolish newborn neurons or progenitors such as γ- and X-ray radiation or genetic ablation eliminate or significantly decrease learning, suggesting that these new neurons are indeed crucial to this form of memory encoding (Imayoshi et al., 2008; Garcia et al., 2004; Saxe et al., 2006; Santarelli et al., 2003; Yeung et al., 2014) (Figures 8.1 and 8.2).

While there is significant evidence supporting a role for endogenous neurogenesis in rodent cognitive function, it has been far more challenging to study such relationships in humans. However, recent data suggest that hippocampal neurogenesis likely plays a similar role in the adult human brain. The phenomenon of "chemo brain" is one of the first observable correlations between human cognitive function and adult neurogenesis. During and following cancer chemotherapy and radiotherapy, patients commonly experience difficulty with memory, executive function, attention, and visuospatial function (Raffa et al., 2006; Staat and Segatore, 2005). In 2007, the hippocampi of four patients who had undergone cranial radiotherapy for various malignancies were examined postmortem and showed significantly decreased neurogenesis (Monje et al., 2007). In this case study, one patient who experienced greater radiation exposure in one hemisphere than the other had more severely decreased newborn neurons on that side compared with the less exposed hippocampus. Such correlations can, of course, be much more readily examined in animal models; indeed, multiple recent studies have supported a link between chemotherapy-related cognitive impairment and hippocampal neurogenesis in murine models (Hou et al., 2013; Yang et al., 2010) (Table 8.1 and Figure 8.3). As new potentially quantitative measures of adult neurogenesis are developed (Ernst et al., 2014; Manganas et al., 2007; Spalding et al., 2013), it is likely that our understanding of the role of adult neurogenesis in human cognition will continue to improve and evolve.

TABLE 8.1 Factors that Influence In vivo Neurogenesis and Their Association with Cognitive Function

	Factor/Pharmacological Agent	Effect on Neurogenesis	Correlation with Cognitive Function
Trophic Factors	S100B	↑	☑
	IGF-1	↑↑	☑
	BDNF	↑↑	☑
	VEGF	↑	☑
Anti-Depressants	SSRI	↑	☑
	SNI	↑	☑
	MAOI	↑	☑
Cytokines	IFN-γ	↑	☑
	IL1-β	↓	☑
	IL6	↓	☑
	TNF-α	↓	☑
	CCL11	↓↓	☑

↑ = Increase in in vivo neurogenesis; ↓ = Decrease in in vivo neurogenesis. Checkmarks indicate that a change in that signaling factor has also been associated with improved cognitive function.

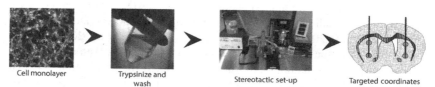

Cell monolayer   Trypsinize and wash   Stereotactic set-up   Targeted coordinates

FIGURE 8.3   Stem cell preparation and transplantation into the brain. Neural stem cells (NSCs) are derived at postnatal day 1 (P1) from green fluorescent protein–expressing transgenic mice. NSCs are expanded for 15 passages, at which time cells are dissociated with trypsin and neutralized in antibiotic-free growth media. NSCs then are resuspended and washed twice with transplantation vehicle (Hank's buffered saline solution, 20 ng/mL epidermal growth factor), then counted. Only cell populations with ≥90% viability are used, and concentration is adjusted to yield 50,000 cells/μL. NSCs or vehicle are then transplanted bilaterally into the striatum using a 30-gauge Hamilton microsyringe and stereotaxic apparatus (1 uL/site; anterior/posterior = +0.02; medial/lateral = ±2.00; dorsal/ventral = −3.0 and −3.5). (This figure is reproduced in color in the color plate section.)

ENDOGENOUS STEM CELLS IN AGING AND DISEASE

The balance between neurogenesis and the elimination of cells seems to be subject to alterations with age and disease. Aged mice, for example, show reductions in the number of olfactory bulb neurons arising from the SVZ. This diminished neurogenesis is in turn associated with impaired olfactory discrimination (Enwere et al., 2004). Similarly, there is an age-related decrease in neural progenitors in the hippocampus of both rodents and canines (Kuhn et al., 1996). The loss of these newborn cells also is associated with declining cognitive function in these animal models (Siwak-Tapp et al., 2007). One powerful demonstration of this phenomenon and the role of chemokines in age-related reduction in neurogenesis was provided by Villeda et al. (2011). To examine the interaction between peripheral signals and age-associated declines in neurogenesis, this group used parabiosis, a paradigm in which the circulatory system of two mice are connected to allow exchange of blood. By introducing the "systemic milieu" of blood from aged mice to young adult mice via parabiosis, Villeda et al. (2011) showed that aged blood could reduce both neurogenesis and cognitive function in young mice. Furthermore, aged mice injected with the plasma of young mice exhibited increased hippocampal neurogenesis. Interestingly, the effects of old and young plasma seem to be mediated via specific chemokines such as CCL11: injection of this chemokine alone into young mice impaired both neurogenesis and cognition. Thus the peripheral immune system and changes in inflammatory state that occur with age seem to play a critical role in age-associated changes in neurogenesis (Table 8.1 and Figure 8.3).

In addition to aging, disease-associated changes in neurogenesis also occur and likely contribute to cognitive decline. For example, reduction in hippocampal neurogenesis has been demonstrated in animal models of several neurodegenerative disorders including Alzheimer's disease (AD), Parkinson's disease (PD), Huntington's disease (HD), and frontotemporal dementia (Donovan et al., 2006; Fedele et al., 2011; Haughey et al., 2002; Hoglinger et al., 2004; Phillips et al., 2005; Ransome et al., 2012; Varela-Nallar et al., 2010; Wen et al., 2004). A recent radiocarbon dating study further confirmed the association between HD and reduced neurogenesis, showing significant reduction in newborn cholinergic interneurons within the striatum of patients with HD (Ernst et al., 2014). Disease-associated reductions in neurogenesis seem to be greater than those that occur during normal human aging (Simic et al., 1997). However, conflicting reports have led to speculation that neurogenesis may actually increase during earlier stages of disease (Jin et al., 2004). This phenomenon is thought to represent a compensatory response to initial manifestations of pathology and supports the potential of enhancing neurogenesis as a therapeutic approach. Yet by the time these disorders progress to later stages, there seems to be a consistent and significant reduction in adult neurogenesis (Donovan et al., 2006; Fedele et al., 2011; Haughey et al., 2002; Hoglinger et al., 2004; Phillips et al., 2005; Ransome et al., 2012; Varela-Nallar et al., 2010; Wen et al., 2004).

IMPROVING COGNITION BY ENHANCING NEUROGENESIS

Given the strong association between declining neurogenesis and worsening cognitive function, there is a growing interest in elucidating the mechanisms that drive adult neurogenesis and developing therapies that could be used to enhance it.

Immune Modulation of Neurogenesis

One area of very active research focuses on the role of the immune system in adult neurogenesis. Growing evidence shows that both microglia and astrocytes actively participate in the generation and functional integration of newborn neurons (see "The Role of Endogenous Neurogenesis in Cognition"). It is generally agreed that acute microglial activation interferes with adult neurogenesis in both healthy and pathological states (Hanisch and Kettenmann, 2007). The work of Belarbi et al. (2012) demonstrates that chronic proinflammatory signaling can also be detrimental to the integration of newborn neurons into hippocampal circuitry and the hippocampal processing of contextual memory in rats. The proinflammatory cytokines interleukin-1β, interleukin-6 and tumor necrosis factor (TNF)-α are thought to be responsible for this negative effect of microglial activation on neurogenesis (Monje et al., 2003). In contrast, chronic low levels of the microglial-derived insulin-like growth factor 1 (IGF-1) and interferon-γ have been correlated with increased adult hippocampal neurogenesis and concomitant improved spatial cognitive performance in rats (Beck et al., 1995; Choi et al., 2008; Aberg et al., 2003). While these findings underscore the clear importance of the immune system in adult neurogenesis, they also highlight the need for a better understanding of the type of microglial activation states that either hinder or enhance adult neurogenesis.

Astrocytes also seem to play a critical role in adult neurogenesis. In addition, radial glia, the primary neural progenitors of the developing nervous system, also play an important role in adult neurogenesis (Mori et al., 2005). Radial glia were initially considered to be scaffolds and supporting cells during early neurogenesis (Kunze et al., 2009). However, Hartfuss et al. (2003) were among the first to show that radial glia also divide and may actively contribute to neurogenesis during development (Noctor et al., 2002). Later, it was shown that radial glia maintain proliferative activity and may promote the generation, differentiation, and survival of newborn neurons in adult teleost fish and in mice (Merkle et al., 2004; Zupanc, 2001; Zupanc and Clint, 2003). In addition to their direct involvement in neurogenesis, astrocyte-derived molecules also seem to make distinct contributions. An example of this is the effect of S100B, a protein involved in astrocytic signaling that exhibits both mitogenic and neurotrophic activity (Kleindienst et al., 2005). In this study, the authors examined the effect of intraventricular infusion of S100B in a rat model of traumatic brain injury. Infusion of S100B for 7 days led to a significant increase in both neurogenesis and hippocampal-dependent cognitive function. Thus age- and injury-associated changes in astrocytic activity likely influence adult neurogenesis and cognition. Other immune-associated cells also seem to play a role in adult neurogenesis and cognition. Reports have suggested, for example, that (CNS) central nervous system–specific T cells are required for spatial learning and the maintenance of hippocampal neurogenesis in adulthood (Ziv et al., 2006). Depending on their state of activation and functional phenotype, immune system components clearly have great potential as therapeutic targets to enhance adult neurogenesis in both the intact and injured brain. Please refer to Chapter 6 for a brief review of inflammation and cognitive function.

The Effects of Antidepressants on Neurogenesis and Cognition

The potential influence of antidepressant drugs on adult neurogenesis has been widely studied but remains a contentious area of research. In the late 1990s, researchers began to suggest that both antidepressants and stress might modulate adult hippocampal neurogenesis (Duman et al., 1999; McEwen, 2001). Since then, numerous reports have shown that antidepressant treatments, including selective serotonin reuptake inhibitors (SSRIs) and even electroconvulsive therapy, can increase hippocampal neurogenesis (Madsen et al., 2000; Perera et al., 2007; Li et al., 2009; Peng et al., 2008). Several of these groups also proposed that the antidepressant benefit of SSRIs was dependent on increased neurogenesis. However, evidence that the mood-improving effects of antidepressants did not depend on neurogenesis, but rather neuronal remodeling, arose in 2008; the blockade of neurogenesis failed to diminish the antidepressant activity of several SSRIs (Bessa et al., 2009). Furthermore, the decline of neurogenesis caused by natural aging does not seem to be effected by fluoxetine, a commonly prescribed SSRI (Couillard-Despres et al., 2009). Despite these findings and the persistent debate regarding the role of neurogenesis in depression, the effect of SSRIs on adult neurogenesis and cognition in disease models remains clear: SSRI treatment can enhance neurogenesis and improve cognitive performance in murine models of Down syndrome (Bianchi et al., 2010; Clark et al., 2006), HD (Grote et al., 2005), anxiety, depression (David et al., 2009), PD (Ubhi et al., 2012), stroke (Li et al., 2009), and AD (Nelson et al., 2007).

Trophic Factors, Neurogenesis, and Cognition

The speculated involvement of growth factors in the mechanism underlying the effect of antidepressants and neuromodulators shifted therapeutic focus to the direct administration of these factors (Siuciak et al., 1997; Lee, 2009 #95). Antidepressant drugs such as selective SSRIs, selective norepinephrine reuptake inhibitors and monoamine oxidase inhibitors have been shown to enhance the expression of brain-derived neurotrophic factor (BDNF), vascular endothelial growth factor (VEGF), and IGF-1 (Huang et al., 2008; Warner-Schnidt and Duman, 2007). Treatment with basic fibroblast growth factor or VEGF was found to increase both hippocampal and SVZ neurogenesis in rats following traumatic brain injury (TBI), and this increase contributed to cognitive recovery (Sun et al., 2009; Lee and Agoston, 2010). Intrahippocampal infusion of BDNF also has been reported to increase neurogenesis in adult rats (Scharfman et al., 2005), and other studies have shown that BDNF infusion can improve cognition (Blurton-Jones et al., 2009). However, the precise mechanistic relationship between BDNF, neurogenesis, and cognition has yet to be directly examined. Nevertheless, this growth factor has been heavily implicated in exercise-mediated effects on neurogenesis and cognition (reviewed by Cotman et al. (2007), Cotman and Berchtold (2002), van Praag (2008, van Praag et al. (2005)).

Noninvasive Approaches to Enhance Neurogenesis and Cognition

Over the years, noninvasive lifestyle therapies such as exercise and environmental enrichment have shown robust effects on neurogenesis in aging animal models (van Praag et al., 1999; Cotman and Berchtold, 2002; van Praag et al., 2005; Kempermann et al., 1998) (Table 8.1 and Figure 8.2). The positive effect of exercises such as free or forced running on neurogenesis and cognition is consistent in models of disease and in young mice following irradiation-induced loss of newborn cells (Harrison et al., 2013). This effect has even been partially translated to studies of human aging; aerobic exercise has been shown to reduce brain tissue loss (Colcombe et al., 2003).

Environmental enrichment (EE) also has been associated with increased adult neurogenesis in animal models. Rodents are typically placed in a large cage with 6–10 cage mates, and stimulating new toys and climbing apparatuses are regularly exchanged. Young adult rats and mice housed in enriched environments for at least 4 weeks showed both increased hippocampal neurogenesis as well as heightened performance on spatial memory tests compared with rats housed in standard conditions or isolation (Nilsson et al., 1999). Interestingly, multiple studies have reported that EE can also improve cognition and enhance neurogenesis in transgenic models of AD without altering the deposition of pathological amyloid-β (Jankowsky et al., 2005; Nichol et al., 2007). However, occasional studies also suggest that this may not be the case in models of more severe AD (Cotel et al., 2012). Over the past few years it has been argued that the effect of an EE on neurogenesis is largely due to the aerobic exercise available via a running wheel within the cage, a common component of an EE (Mustroph et al., 2012). However, the contribution of various aspects of EE to neurogenesis and cognition remains controversial; other studies have shown a benefit of EE without running wheels, in comparison to running alone or socially enriched environments without toys (Wolf et al., 2006; Madronal et al., 2010).

The potential role of growth factors in exercise and EE-induced changes in neurogenesis and cognition is not new. At present, BDNF and IGF-1 are thought to be the principle factors modulating the effects of exercise on learning and mood disorders, where IGF-1 and VEGF are more strongly implicated in hippocampal neurogenesis (Ding et al., 2006; Nichol, 2009). Both *BDNF* and *IGF-1* gene expression are elevated after only a few days of exercise in rats and are crucial to the cognitive benefits of exercise because blockade of growth factor signaling prevents exercise-induced improvements (Berchtold et al., 2005; Trejo et al., 2001). For example, intrahippocampal injection of function-blocking antibodies to the BDNF receptor TrkB attenuates the effects of exercise on spatial learning (Vaynman et al., 2004). Similarly, intrahippocampal injection of anti-IGF-1 prevents enhancement of spatial recall as well as neurogenesis (Ding et al., 2006).

Collectively, these findings suggest that antidepressants and lifestyle factors such as exercise both have a beneficial effect on adult neurogenesis and cognition. A growing number of studies suggest that both immune-related and trophic-related mechanisms likely play a critical role in this process. Ongoing prospective clinical studies examining the effect of exercise on AD and cognition will likely further enhance our understanding of the effects of lifestyle and neurogenesis on cognition.

IMPROVING COGNITION WITH STEM CELL TRANSPLANTATION

Our growing understanding of neurogenic mechanisms and their involvement in cognition could lead to novel therapeutic strategies for preserving or enhancing cognition. While many groups and several biotechnology companies are focused on the development of drugs that increase endogenous neurogenesis, stem cell transplantation may offer an alternative approach to either replace degenerated cells or provide support for dysfunctional neurons. This prospect has important clinical implications for numerous neurological disorders that are characterized by significant neuronal loss and cognitive impairment. Yet this is a daunting task, given the seemingly infinite variation of structural and neurochemical phenotypes that comprise the neurons and synapses of the adult human brain. Fortunately, recent studies suggest that stem cell transplantation may provide meaningful benefit in animal models of neurodegeneration. Interestingly, these effects occur not necessarily via neuronal replacement, but rather by more indirect neuroprotective and plasticity-promoting mechanisms. In the remaining sections of this chapter, we describe some of the key findings in this active area of neuroscience research and make an argument for the continued pursuit of research into the effects of stem cell transplantation on cognition.

Neural Stem Cell Transplantation in Aging

There is growing evidence that neural stem cell (NSC) transplantation can improve cognition in both aging and pathologically effected brains. There is even some indication that NSC transplantation can enhance performance in healthy brains. The mechanisms by which stem cells achieve these benefits likely vary across each of these three microenvironmental conditions, which speaks to the flexibility of these cells as a potential therapy. One of the first studies to examine the potential effect of NSC transplantation in aging injected human NSCs into the lateral ventricle of aged rats, leading to improved performance in spatial learning and memory as measured in the Morris water maze task (Qu et al., 2001). Interestingly, NSC transplantation can itself enhance endogenous hippocampal neurogenesis, suggesting that this likely plays a role in the effects of transplantation on cognition (Hattiangady et al., 2007). Because of the minimal neurodegeneration that takes place in the aging brain relative to the diseased brain, it was important to determine whether such results could also be translated into animal models of brain injury and disease. Consequently, in the past decade multiple studies demonstrating that stem cell transplantation can provide cognitive benefits in a wide variety of disease states have emerged.

Neural Stem Cell Transplantation in Neurological Disease

Numerous preclinical studies have shown that stem cell transplantation can improve motor function in models of HD, PD, stroke, and TBI (Lee et al., 2012). Until recently, however, few studies assessed the potential effect of NSCs on cognitive function. One study did explore the combined effects of NSC transplantation and BDNF infusion in a unilateral fimbria–fornix transection model, finding improved performance in a Y-maze with BDNF and NSC treatment (Xuan et al., 2008). Our own studies also strongly implicate BDNF in stem cell–mediated effects on cognition. For example, we found that murine NSC transplantation in the triple transgenic (3xTg-AD) model of AD improves cognition in Morris water maze and novel object recognition tasks via a BDNF-dependent mechanism (Blurton-Jones et al., 2009). To confirm the importance of NSC-derived BDNF in functional recovery, we genetically modified NSCs with a small hairpin RNA to stably knock down BDNF expression by 87%. Treatment of transgenic mice with AD with these BDNF-depleted NSCs no longer improved cognition, demonstrating the necessity of BDNF signaling in NSC-mediated recovery.

While most stem cell transplantation studies report some evidence of functional improvement, several note that transplantation improved some behaviors but not others. For example, Hoane et al. (2004) reported that embryonic stem cell–derived neuronal and glial precursor transplantation could improve sensorimotor deficits in a model of TBI but failed to restore cognitive function. Gao et al. (2006) found contrasting results, reporting that human fetal NSCs could improve cognitive function in a rat model of TBI. Differences between these findings likely result from a number of factors, including variability in the severity of TBI and the resulting neuronal loss. One potential way to avoid such variability is to use a genetic ablation approach. By pairing neuronal expression of the diphtheria toxin A-chain with tetracycline-regulated expression, one can, for example, produce a much more consistent hippocampal injury. For example, we previously found that tetracycline-regulated expression of diphtheria toxin A-chain under control of the Cam kinase 2α promoter can be induced for varying durations, allowing more vulnerable CA1 neurons to be ablated while sparing dentate granule and cortical neurons. Using such an approach, we showed that NSC transplantation can improve cognitive function following ablation of CA1 hippocampal neurons (Yamasaki et al., 2007).

Most recently, we observed a similar capacity of NSCs to improve memory in a transgenic model of PD (Goldberg and Blurton-Jones, unpublished data) (Figure 8.3). To perform these studies we used a transgenic model of PD that overexpresses wild-type human α-synuclein, a protein that accumulates in PD-associated Lewy bodies. These mice exhibit dysfunctional production and transmission of dopamine in primary motor pathways, leading to deficits not only in motor function but also in multiple cognitive domains (Lam et al., 2011). Syngeneic NSCs were transplanted bilaterally into the striatum of aged α-synuclein mice, and 1 month later motor and cognitive behavior was examined. NSCs survive in the striatum and begin to differentiate into glia (glial fibrillary acidic protein) and neurons (doublecortin) (Figure 8.4). In these initial studies we found robust improvements not only in motor function

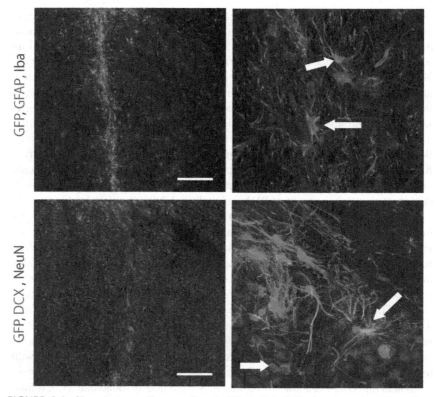

FIGURE 8.4 Neural stem cells engraft and differentiate following transplantation. One month after transplantation, neural stem cells (NSCs) begin to differentiate into astrocytes (GFAP; white arrows, bottom right), neurons (DCX; white arrows, bottom left), or oligodendrocytes (not shown). In recent unpublished studies we found that striatal transplantation of NSCs can improve cognitive function in a transgenic model of Parkinson's disease. Scale bar = 300 μm. (This figure is reproduced in color in the color plate section.)

but also in cognitive function, and, again, BDNF seems to be central to these improvements.

Stem Cell Transplantation in the Healthy Adult Brain

Until very recently, no studies reported an enhanced benefit of stem cell transplantation in the intrinsically functioning adult brain. However, in 2013, Han et al. (2013) showed that human glial progenitor transplantation into the frontal cortex of immune-deficient neonatal mice led to significant enhancements in the cognitive function of adult and aged mice. In contrast, transplantation of murine glial progenitors had no such effect. These researchers suggested that one potential explanation for the differential effect between human and murine progenitors may relate to species-specific differences in calcium wave propagation, a mechanism by which astrocytes communicate. Human glial progenitor calcium waves propagated at least threefold faster than did mouse cells, which may be attributable to their much larger size and structural complexity. These differences also likely contributed to the heightened basal level of excitatory transmission and enhanced long-term potentiation that also were observed in this study. Another recent study examined the effect of NSCs that were modified to overexpress choline acetyltransferase (ChAT), an enzyme responsible for acetylcholine synthesis (Park et al., 2013). In this report, Park and colleagues transplanted these modified NSCs into the lateral ventricle of young and aged mice, and learning and physical activity were assessed 1 month later. Interestingly, this group found significant improvements in passive avoidance, Morris water maze performance, and spontaneous locomotor activity in aged mice receiving ChAT-expressing stem cells. The group suggests that the benefit of these ChAT-enhanced stem cells may be the secretion of either produced acetylcholine or the growth factors BDNF or nerve growth factor, which are commonly reported to be secreted from human stem cells. Although the studies by both Han and Park studies as well as others, return to the hypothesis of neurotrophin-based mechanisms of stem cell–induced change, the immune system also continues to be implicated. Both studies transplanted human cells into immunodeficient mouse models; however, Han et al. acknowledged the role of the cytokine TNF-α in glial progenitor transplant signaling, reporting that transplantation increased hippocampal TNF-α levels, leading to increased expression of the AMPA receptor GluR1, suggesting an important role for cytokine-regulated alteration of excitatory transmission. This is, however, in contrast to other studies that argue that the proinflammatory nature of TNF-α likely makes it detrimental to endogenous NSC proliferation. The relative effect of TNF-α and other cytokines on both endogenous and exogenous-derived NSCs and their influence on cognition clearly warrants further study.

As detailed above, several studies have now examined the effects of NSCs on cognition in various animal models of injury, aging, and disease. Likewise, some studies have explored the potential effects of glial precursors on cognition. To date, however, no reports have directly compared these varying cell sources. It therefore remains unclear whether a specific stem cell type is more appropriate for enhancing cognition and whether the ability of given stem cell population to improve cognition varies with age or disease.

CONTRIBUTION OF DIFFERENT TRANSPLANTED CELL TYPES TO COGNITION

Neuronal Replacement

The traditional goal of stem cell transplantation in the CNS was to replace dead or dysfunctional cells. In the substantial history of transplantation for PD, this has meant trying to replace the dopamine-producing neurons of the substantia nigra, where the disease pathology manifests in extensive neurodegeneration. To achieve this, studies focused on the engraftment of fetal mesencephalic stem cells, which commonly develop a dopaminergic neuronal phenotype. Since the early 1980s, dopaminergic precursor or dopamine-producing stem cells have been transplanted into the striatum of human patients, with some initial evidence of moderately improved motor control and decreased rigidity and tremor. However, there has been little to no reported effect of this approach on PD-associated cognitive deficits. In murine studies, transplantation of these cells into the substantia nigra often results in short-term restoration of motor control, although effects on cognition have not been examined or reported (Barker et al., 2013). Neuronal replacement clearly holds promise, but arguments can also be made for the transplantation of NSCs and progenitors of other specific cells types, such as astrocytes, that might influence cognition via more indirect mechanisms (Figure 8.2).

Glial Precursor and Astrocyte Transplantation

The previously mentioned human glial progenitor transplantation study conducted by Han et al. (2013) takes advantage of the supportive role of glia in the regulation of synaptic plasticity and neuronal function. Surprisingly, there have been few such studies exploring the effects of glial stem cell transplantation on cognition or other brain function. Instead, most studies of glial progenitor transplantation focused on conditions that affect the spinal cord, including amyotrophic lateral sclerosis and spinal cord injury (Suzuki et al., 2007; reviewed by Toft et al., 2013 and Nout et al., 2011). One exception is a study from over two decades ago that compared the capacity of fetal brain tissue and purified astrocytes to improve ethanol-induced cognitive deficits (Bruckner and Arendt, 1992). This group found that astrocytes, but not fetal brain tissue grafts, could restore memory as assessed by the radial arm maze. Intracortical astrocyte grafts were associated with increased ChAT in the basal forebrain, which was thought likely to result from astrocyte-induced neurotrophic activity on cholinergic efferents. A few years later Bradbury et al. (1995) reported that astrocyte transplantation into the cortex and hippocampus could also improve spatial memory in rats with basal forebrain lesions. However, this group suggested that the effect of astrocytes were independent of cholinergic neurotransmission because fetal brain tissue grafts were able to elevate ChAT activity but failed to improve memory. Instead, they proposed that astrocyte-induced cognitive improvements likely resulted from altered immune and trophic activity. Finally, recent developments in cell reprogramming research have identified that astrocytes may be a more useful parent cell type than the commonly used skin fibroblast (Tian et al., 2011). Tian and colleagues showed that reprogrammed mouse astrocytes retained a "memory" of their tissue origin and a greater potential for neuronal differentiation compared to fibroblasts. This same potential was identified in human astrocytes that were reprogrammed to NSCs and neurons (Corti et al., 2012). Given the strong mechanistic evidence for the potential of transplanted astrocytes to improve cognition, astrocyte reprogramming may make these cells ideal candidates for studies of induced pluripotent stem cell (iPSC) transplantation (Table 8.2). Regardless of the precise mechanism by which astrocyte and glial precursor transplantation improves cognition, it seems that astrocyte and progenitor cells may provide a powerful approach to enhance cognition (Figure 8.2).

NSCs and glial progenitors can also differentiate into oligodendrocytes, which generate myelin to insulate neuronal axons in the brain and promote the conduction of action potentials. The loss of oligodendrocyte precursor cells has been implicated in cognitive decline following ischemic injury in rats (Chida et al., 2011; Huang et al., 2009) and radiation therapy in humans (Monje and Dietrich, 2012). Oligodendrocytes also have been proposed as a potential biomarker and therapeutic target for preventing cognitive decline in AD (Bartzokis, 2004). Specifically, it has been noted that oligodendrocytic regulation of iron and membrane cholesterol in the brain may be disrupted by AD pathology and predict cognitive decline (Kadish et al., 2009). Although no oligodendrocyte fate-restricted transplant studies have been performed in the brain, several NSC

TABLE 8.2 Contribution of Different Stem Cell Lineages to Cognitive Function

Transplanted Stem Cell Lineage	Identified Signaling Mechanisms	Correlation with Cognitive Function	Circuitry Integration
Neural stem cell	☑	☑	n/d
Astrocyte progenitor	☑	☑	n/d
Fetal mesencephalic	☑	n/d	☑
Embryonic stem cell	☑	☑	☑
IPSC	n/d	n/d	n/d

For several stem cell lineages, affected molecular mechanisms that correlate to changes in cognitive function have been reported. For only some of these cell lineages has integration with endogenous circuitry been established. Checkmarks indicate that changes in the parallel signaling factors have been shown to correlate with cognitive function. ND = not determined.

and glial progenitor transplant studies report that a large portion of these cells become oligodendrocytes, which may contribute significantly to cell-mediated cognitive improvement (Blurton-Jones et al., 2009; Kelly et al., 2004). Therefore it is likely that these cells could also play an important role in enhancing cognition (Figure 8.2).

REMAINING CHALLENGES

Tumorigenesis

Stem cell–based strategies clearly offer a novel approach to enhance cognition in normal, aged, and diseased brains. Yet these strategies are certainly not without risk. By definition, one of the key properties of stem cells is that they can replicate to create near-perfect copies of themselves. This property is inherent not only to stem cells but also to cancer cells. Indeed, there is growing evidence that cancer stem cells play a major role in tumorigenesis, metastasis, and recurrence (Baccelli and Trumpp, 2012). Transplantation of stem cells or enhancement of endogenous stem cell populations therefore presents some risk of tumorigenesis. Once transplanted into the microenvironment of the brain, some stem cell populations seem to be unable to fully differentiate and instead continue to proliferate unchecked (Knoepfler, 2009). This risk of tumorigenesis seems to be quite dependent on the type and maturation of a given stem cell. Pluripotent stem cells, for example, can readily form teratomas when transplanted into an immune-deficient host (Gutierrez-Aranda, 2010). Embryonic stem cell–derived NSCs can also form tumors, although this is dramatically influenced by their maturation state, and more extensive predifferentiation protocols reduce tumorigenesis (Fukuda et al., 2006; Seminatore et al., 2010). In contrast, there are very few reports of tumorigenesis following fetal-derived NSC transplantation (Geny et al., 1994). Transplantation therapies that use more fully differentiated and restricted progenitors are therefore likely to provide a safer approach.

Takahashi and Yamanaka's (2006) groundbreaking work establishing methods to generate iPSCs provided a novel source of pluripotent stem cells that circumvented many of the ethical concerns regarding fetal and embryonic stem cell research. It seems, however, that iPSCs may be more prone to tumorigenesis than other stem cells. Many of the genes used to induce pluripotency are either established oncogenes (i.e., Myc and KLF4) (Yamanaka, 2007; Wei et al., 2006) or are variably associated with tumorigenesis (i.e., Sox2, Nanog, and Oct3/4) (Chen et al., 2008; Chiou et al., 2008; Palma et al., 2008). The rapid adoption of nonintegrating approaches for iPSC generation will likely resolve many of these issues (Table 8.2). However, iPSCs derived from aged cell sources will carry increased numbers of de novo DNA mutations that could still promote tumorigenesis. The majority of stem cell transplant studies reporting occasional teratoma formation leave the issue largely unresolved. However, there are many strategies that could likely mitigate the risk of tumorigenesis (reviewed by Knoepfler (2009)). For example, introduction of a stem cell–specific suicide gene or specifically targeted chemotherapeutic agent could be used to eliminate stem cells that fail to terminally differentiate. Predifferentiation of cells toward more mature lineages likely will also greatly diminish risk.

Delivering Stem Cells to the Brain

One of the major challenges to the potential use of stem cell–based therapies for neurological conditions is the difficulty of delivering stem cells to the brain. Several approaches have been examined, including intravenous, intra-arterial, intranasal, and direct intraparenchemal injection. Yet the great majority of data suggests that of these, only direct intraparenchemal transplantation achieves meaningful engraftment of stem cells within the brain (Andres et al., 2011; Blurton-Jones et al., 2009; Ebert et al., 2008; Redmond et al., 2013; Yamasaki et al., 2007). Venous delivery, for example, leads primarily to an accumulation of injected stem cells within the lungs, with no cells reaching the brain (Pendharkar et al., 2010). As one might expect, injection into the carotid artery can increase the number of cells reaching the brain, although only a few cells transmigrate across the endothelial blood–brain barrier into the brain parenchema (Pendharkar et al., 2010). Intranasal delivery offers an intriguing noninvasive approach to delivering stem cells to the brain. In theory, cells might be able to pass through the foramina within the cribriform plate, a part of the skull that allows olfactory nerves to pass into the nasal epithelium. A few reports have tested this approach, and while some stem cells may reach the brain via intranasal delivery, the numbers are extremely low (Danielyan et al., 2009; Reitz et al., 2012). One promising new approach is to couple carotid artery stem cell injection with magnetic resonance imaging–guided focused ultrasound. The ultrasound temporarily disrupts the blood–brain barrier within a specific brain region, allowing NSCs to pass from a local cerebral artery into the brain parenchema (Burgess et al., 2011). These new methods may one day provide a promising, less invasive approach to deliver stem cells to the brain. Thus far, however, direct stereotactic intraparenchemal injection remains the optimal approach to achieve robust stem cell engraftment within the brain (Andres et al., 2011; Blurton-Jones et al., 2009; Ebert et al., 2008; Redmond et al., 2013; Yamasaki et al., 2007).

CONCLUSIONS

From decades of research across many subfields, key molecular mechanisms involved in the cognitive benefits of stem cells have been identified. Interestingly, one fairly consistent finding is that stem cells often influence cognition and disease via multiple mechanisms (Figure 8.2). Clearly, a great deal of additional research is needed to determine whether increasing endogenous neurogenesis or directly transplanting stem cells into the brain can be safely adapted to clinical use. Exactly which aspects of human cognition may or may not be influenced by stem cell–based therapies also remain to be determined. Nevertheless, stem cell research may one day uncover promising new approaches to enhance human cognition.

ACKNOWLEDGMENTS

This work was supported by AG029378, AG16573, CIRM RT1-01108, Alzheimer's Association NIRG (MBJ), and NSF Graduate Research Fellowship Program #2011117469 (NRSG).

REFERENCES

Aberg, M.A., Aberg, N.D., Palmer, T.D., Alborn, A.M., Carlsson-Skwirut, C., Bang, P., Eriksson, P.S., 2003. IGF-I has a direct proliferative effect in adult hippocampal progenitor cells. Mol. Cell Neurosci. 24 (1), 23–40.

Aimone, J.B., Deng, W., Gage, F.H., 2011. Resolving new memories: a critical look at the dentate gyrus, adult neurogenesis, and pattern separation. Neuron 70 (4), 589–596.

Altman, J., Das, G.D., 1965. Autoradiographic and histological evidence of postnatal hippocampal neurogenesis in rats. J. Comp. Neurol. 124 (3), 319–335.

Alvarez-Buylla, A., Herrera, D.G., Wichterle, H., 2000. The subventricular zone: source of neuronal precursors for brain repair. Prog. Brain Res. 127, 1–11.

Andres, R.H., Horie, N., Slikker, W., Keren-Gill, H., Zhan, K., Sun, G., Steinberg, G.K., 2011. Human neural stem cells enhance structural plasticity and axonal transport in the ischaemic brain. Brain 134 (Pt 6), 1777–1789.

Baccelli, I., Trumpp, A., 2012. The evolving concept of cancer and metastasis stem cells. J. Cell Biol. 198 (3), 281–293.

Barker, R.A., Barrett, J., Mason, S.L., Bjorklund, A., 2013. Fetal dopaminergic transplantation trials and the future of neural grafting in Parkinson's disease. Lancet Neurol. 12 (1), 84–91.

Bartzokis, G., 2004. Age-related myelin breakdown: a developmental model of cognitive decline and Alzheimer's disease. Neurobiol. Aging 25 (1), 5–18; author reply 49–62.

Beck, K.D., Powell-Braxton, L., Widmer, H.R., Valverde, J., Hefti, F., 1995. Igf1 gene disruption results in reduced brain size, CNS hypomyelination, and loss of hippocampal granule and striatal parvalbumin-containing neurons. Neuron 14 (4), 717–730.

Belarbi, K., Arellano, C., Ferguson, R., Jopson, T., Rosi, S., 2012. Chronic neuroinflammation impacts the recruitment of adult-born neurons into behaviorally relevant hippocampal networks. Brain Behav. Immun. 26 (1), 18–23.

Berchtold, N.C., Chinn, G., Chou, M., Kesslak, J.P., Cotman, C.W., 2005. Exercise primes a molecular memory for brain-derived neurotrophic factor protein induction in the rat hippocampus. Neuroscience 133 (3), 853–861.

Bessa, J.M., Ferreira, D., Melo, I., Marques, F., Cerqueira, J.J., Palha, J.A., Sousa, N., 2009. The mood-improving actions of antidepressants do not depend on neurogenesis but are associated with neuronal remodeling. Mol. Psychiatry 14 (8), 739, 764–773.

Bianchi, P., Ciani, E., Guidi, S., Trazzi, S., Felice, D., Grossi, G., Bartesaghi, R., 2010. Early pharmacotherapy restores neurogenesis and cognitive performance in the Ts65Dn mouse model for Down syndrome. J. Neurosci. 30 (26), 8769–8779.

Blurton-Jones, M., Kitazawa, M., Martinez-Coria, H., Castello, N.A., Muller, F.J., Loring, J.F., LaFerla, F.M., 2009. Neural stem cells improve cognition via BDNF in a transgenic model of Alzheimer disease. Proc. Natl. Acad. Sci. U.S.A. 106 (32), 13594–13599.

Bradbury, E.J., Kershaw, T.R., Marchbanks, R.M., Sinden, J.D., 1995. Astrocyte transplants alleviate lesion induced memory deficits independently of cholinergic recovery. Neuroscience 65 (4), 955–972.

Bruckner, M.K., Arendt, T., 1992. Intracortical grafts of purified astrocytes ameliorate memory deficits in rat induced by chronic treatment with ethanol. Neurosci. Lett. 141 (2), 251–254.

Burgess, A., Ayala-Grosso, C.A., Ganguly, M., Jordao, J.F., Aubert, I., Hynynen, K., 2011. Targeted delivery of neural stem cells to the brain using MRI-guided focused ultrasound to disrupt the blood–brain barrier. PLoS One 6 (11), e27877.

Chen, Y., Shi, L., Zhang, L., Li, R., Liang, J., Yu, W., Shang, Y., 2008. The molecular mechanism governing the oncogenic potential of SOX2 in breast cancer. J. Biol. Chem. 283 (26), 17969–17978.

Cheng, L.C., Pastrana, E., Tavazoie, M., Doetsch, F., 2009. miR-124 regulates adult neurogenesis in the subventricular zone stem cell niche. Nat. Neurosci. 12 (4), 399–408.

Chida, Y., Kokubo, Y., Sato, S., Kuge, A., Takemura, S., Kondo, R., Kayama, T., 2011. The alterations of oligodendrocyte, myelin in corpus callosum, and cognitive dysfunction following chronic cerebral ischemia in rats. Brain Res. 1414, 22–31.

Chiou, S.H., Yu, C.C., Huang, C.Y., Lin, S.C., Liu, C.J., Tsai, T.H., Lo, J.F., 2008. Positive correlations of Oct-4 and Nanog in oral cancer stem-like cells and high-grade oral squamous cell carcinoma. Clin. Cancer Res. 14 (13), 4085–4095.

Choi, Y.S., Cho, H.Y., Hoyt, K.R., Naegele, J.R., Obrietan, K., 2008. IGF-1 receptor-mediated ERK/MAPK signaling couples status epilepticus to progenitor cell proliferation in the subgranular layer of the dentate gyrus. Glia 56 (7), 791–800.

Clark, S., Schwalbe, J., Stasko, M.R., Yarowsky, P.J., Costa, A.C., 2006. Fluoxetine rescues deficient neurogenesis in hippocampus of the Ts65Dn mouse model for Down syndrome. Exp. Neurol. 200 (1), 256–261.

Colcombe, S.J., Erickson, K.I., Raz, N., Webb, A.G., Cohen, N.J., McAuley, E., Kramer, A.F., 2003. Aerobic fitness reduces brain tissue loss in aging humans. J. Gerontol. A Biol. Sci. Med. Sci. 58 (2), 176–180.

Corti, S., Nizzardo, M., Simone, C., Falcone, M., Donadoni, C., Salani, S., Comi, G.P., 2012. Direct reprogramming of human astrocytes into neural stem cells and neurons. Exp. Cell Res. 318 (13), 1528–1541.

Cotel, M.C., Jawhar, S., Christensen, D.Z., Bayer, T.A., Wirths, O., 2012. Environmental enrichment fails to rescue working memory deficits, neuron loss, and neurogenesis in APP/PS1KI mice. Neurobiol. Aging 33 (1), 96–107.

Cotman, C.W., Berchtold, N.C., 2002. Exercise: a behavioral intervention to enhance brain health and plasticity. Trends Neurosci. 25 (6), 295–301.

Cotman, C.W., Berchtold, N.C., Christie, L.A., 2007. Exercise builds brain health: key roles of growth factor cascades and inflammation. Trends Neurosci. 30 (9), 464–472.

Couillard-Despres, S., Wuertinger, C., Kandasamy, M., Caioni, M., Stadler, K., Aigner, R., Aigner, L., 2009. Ageing abolishes the effects of fluoxetine on neurogenesis. Mol. Psychiatry 14 (9), 856–864.

Danielyan, L., Schafer, R., von Ameln-Mayerhofer, A., Buadze, M., Geisler, J., Klopfer, T., Frey 2nd, W.H., 2009. Intranasal delivery of cells to the brain. Eur. J. Cell Biol. 88 (6), 315–324.

David, D.J., Samuels, B.A., Rainer, Q., Wang, J.W., Marsteller, D., Mendez, I., Hen, R., 2009. Neurogenesis-dependent and -independent effects of fluoxetine in an animal model of anxiety/depression. Neuron 62 (4), 479–493.

Ding, Q., Vaynman, S., Akhavan, M., Ying, Z., Gomez-Pinilla, F., 2006. Insulin-like growth factor I interfaces with brain-derived neurotrophic factor-mediated synaptic plasticity to modulate aspects of exercise-induced cognitive function. Neuroscience 140 (3), 823–833.

Donovan, M.H., Yazdani, U., Norris, R.D., Games, D., German, D.C., Eisch, A.J., 2006. Decreased adult hippocampal neurogenesis in the PDAPP mouse model of Alzheimer's disease. J. Comp. Neurol. 495 (1), 70–83.

Duman, R.S., Malberg, J., Thome, J., 1999. Neural plasticity to stress and antidepressant treatment. Biol. Psychiatry 46 (9), 1181–1191.

Ebert, A.D., Beres, A.J., Barber, A.E., Svendsen, C.N., 2008. Human neural progenitor cells over-expressing IGF-1 protect dopamine neurons and restore function in a rat model of Parkinson's disease. Exp. Neurol. 209 (1), 213–223.

Enwere, E., Shingo, T., Gregg, C., Fujikawa, H., Ohta, S., Weiss, S., 2004. Aging results in reduced epidermal growth factor receptor signaling, diminished olfactory neurogenesis, and deficits in fine olfactory discrimination. J. Neurosci. 24 (38), 8354–8365.

Eriksson, P.S., Perfilieva, E., Bjork-Eriksson, T., Alborn, A.M., Nordborg, C., Peterson, D.A., Gage, F.H., 1998. Neurogenesis in the adult human hippocampus. Nat. Med. 4 (11), 1313–1317.

Ernst, A., Alkass, K., Bernard, S., Salehpour, M., Perl, S., Tisdale, J., Frisen, J., 2014. Neurogenesis in the striatum of the adult human brain. Cell 156 (5), 1072–1083.

Fedele, V., Roybon, L., Nordstrom, U., Li, J.Y., Brundin, P., 2011. Neurogenesis in the R6/2 mouse model of Huntington's disease is impaired at the level of NeuroD1. Neuroscience 173, 76–81.

Fuchs, E., Tumbar, T., Guasch, G., 2004. Socializing with the neighbors: stem cells and their niche. Cell 116 (6), 769–778.

Fukuda, H., Takahashi, J., Watanabe, K., Hayashi, H., Morizane, A., Koyanagi, M., Hashimoto, N., 2006. Fluorescence-activated cell sorting-based purification of embryonic stem cell-derived neural precursors averts tumor formation after transplantation. Stem Cells 24 (3), 763–771.

Gao, J., Prough, D.S., McAdoo, D.J., Grady, J.J., Parsley, M.O., Ma, L., Wu, P., 2006. Transplantation of primed human fetal neural stem cells improves cognitive function in rats after traumatic brain injury. Exp. Neurol. 201 (2), 281–292.

Garcia, A.D., Doan, N.B., Imura, T., Bush, T.G., Sofroniew, M.V., 2004. GFAP-expressing progenitors are the principal source of constitutive neurogenesis in adult mouse forebrain. Nat. Neurosci. 7 (11), 1233–1241.

Ge, S., Yang, C.H., Hsu, K.S., Ming, G.L., Song, H., 2007. A critical period for enhanced synaptic plasticity in newly generated neurons of the adult brain. Neuron 54 (4), 559–566.

Geny, C., Naimi-Sadaoui, S., Jeny, R., Belkadi, A.M., Juliano, S.L., Peschanski, M., 1994. Long-term delayed vascularization of human neural transplants to the rat brain. J. Neurosci. 14 (12), 7553–7562.

Grote, H.E., Bull, N.D., Howard, M.L., van Dellen, A., Blakemore, C., Bartlett, P.F., Hannan, A.J., 2005. Cognitive disorders and neurogenesis deficits in Huntington's disease mice are rescued by fluoxetine. Eur. J. Neurosci. 22 (8), 2081–2088.

Gutierrez-Aranda, I., Ramos-Mejia, V., Munoz-Lopez, M., Real, P.J., Macia, A., Sanchez, L., Ligero, G., Garcia-Parez, J.L., Menendez, P., 2010. Human induced pluripotent stem cells develop teratoma more efficiently and faster than human embryonic stem cells regardless the site of injection. Stem Cells 28 (9), 1568–1570.

Han, X., Chen, M., Wang, F., Windrem, M., Wang, S., Shanz, S., Nedergaard, M., 2013. Forebrain engraftment by human glial progenitor cells enhances synaptic plasticity and learning in adult mice. Cell Stem Cell 12 (3), 342–353.

Hanisch, U.K., Kettenmann, H., 2007. Microglia: active sensor and versatile effector cells in the normal and pathologic brain. Nat. Neurosci. 10 (11), 1387–1394.

Harrison, D.J., Busse, M., Openshaw, R., Rosser, A.E., Dunnett, S.B., Brooks, S.P., 2013. Exercise attenuates neuropathology and has greater benefit on cognitive than motor deficits in the R6/1 Huntington's disease mouse model. Exp. Neurol. 248, 457–469.

Hartfuss, E., Forster, E., Bock, H.H., Hack, M.A., Leprince, P., Luque, J.M., Gotz, M., 2003. Reelin signaling directly affects radial glia morphology and biochemical maturation. Development 130 (19), 4597–4609.

Hattiangady, B., Shuai, B., Cai, J., Coksaygan, T., Rao, M.S., Shetty, A.K., 2007. Increased dentate neurogenesis after grafting of glial restricted progenitors or neural stem cells in the aging hippocampus. Stem Cells 25 (8), 2104–2117.

Haughey, N.J., Nath, A., Chan, S.L., Borchard, A.C., Rao, M.S., Mattson, M.P., 2002. Disruption of neurogenesis by amyloid beta-peptide, and perturbed neural progenitor cell homeostasis, in models of Alzheimer's disease. J. Neurochem. 83 (6), 1509–1524.

Hoane, M.R., Becerra, G.D., Shank, J.E., Tatko, L., Pak, E.S., Smith, M., Murashov, A.K., 2004. Transplantation of neuronal and glial precursors dramatically improves sensorimotor function but not cognitive function in the traumatically injured brain. J. Neurotrauma 21 (2), 163–174.

Hoglinger, G.U., Rizk, P., Muriel, M.P., Duyckaerts, C., Oertel, W.H., Caille, I., Hirsch, E.C., 2004. Dopamine depletion impairs precursor cell proliferation in Parkinson disease. Nat. Neurosci. 7 (7), 726–735.

Hou, J.G., Xue, J.J., Lee, M.R., Sun, M.Q., Zhao, X.H., Zheng, Y.N., Sung, C.K., 2013. Compound K is able to ameliorate the impaired cognitive function and hippocampal neurogenesis following chemotherapy treatment. Biochem. Biophys. Res. Commun. 436 (1), 104–109.

Huang, T.L., Lee, C.T., Liu, Y.L., 2008. Serum brain-derived neurotrophic factor levels in patients with major depression: effects of antidepressants. J. Psychiatry Res. 42 (7), 521–525.

Huang, Z., Liu, J., Cheung, P.Y., Chen, C., 2009. Long-term cognitive impairment and myelination deficiency in a rat model of perinatal hypoxic-ischemic brain injury. Brain Res. 1301, 100–109.

Imayoshi, I., Sakamoto, M., Ohtsuka, T., Takao, K., Miyakawa, T., Yamaguchi, M., Kageyama, R., 2008. Roles of continuous neurogenesis in the structural and functional integrity of the adult forebrain. Nat. Neurosci. 11 (10), 1153–1161.

Izquierdo, I., Medina, J.H., 1997. Memory formation: the sequence of biochemical events in the hippocampus and its connection to activity in other brain structures. Neurobiol. Learn. Mem. 68 (3), 285–316.

Jankowsky, J.L., Melnikova, T., Fadale, D.J., Xu, G.M., Slunt, H.H., Gonzales, V., Savonenko, A.V., 2005. Environmental enrichment mitigates cognitive deficits in a mouse model of Alzheimer's disease. J. Neurosci. 25 (21), 5217–5224.

Jin, K., Galvan, V., Xie, L., Mao, X.O., Gorostiza, O.F., Bredesen, D.E., Greenberg, D.A., 2004. Enhanced neurogenesis in Alzheimer's disease transgenic (PDGF-APPSw,Ind) mice. Proc. Natl. Acad. Sci. U.S.A. 101 (36), 13363–13367.

Kadish, I., Thibault, O., Blalock, E.M., Chen, K.C., Gant, J.C., Porter, N.M., Landfield, P.W., 2009. Hippocampal and cognitive aging across the lifespan: a bioenergetic shift precedes and increased cholesterol trafficking parallels memory impairment. J. Neurosci. 29 (6), 1805–1816.

Kelly, S., Bliss, T.M., Shah, A.K., Sun, G.H., Ma, M., Foo, W.C., Steinberg, G.K., 2004. Transplanted human fetal neural stem cells survive, migrate, and differentiate in ischemic rat cerebral cortex. Proc. Natl. Acad. Sci. U.S.A. 101 (32), 11839–11844.

Kempermann, G., Brandon, E.P., Gage, F.H., 1998. Environmental stimulation of 129/SvJ mice causes increased cell proliferation and neurogenesis in the adult dentate gyrus. Curr. Biol. 8 (16), 939–942.

Kleindienst, A., McGinn, M.J., Harvey, H.B., Colello, R.J., Hamm, R.J., Bullock, M.R., 2005. Enhanced hippocampal neurogenesis by intraventricular S100B infusion is associated with improved cognitive recovery after traumatic brain injury. J. Neurotrauma 22 (6), 645–655.

Knoepfler, P.S., 2009. Deconstructing stem cell tumorigenicity: a roadmap to safe regenerative medicine. Stem Cells 27 (5), 1050–1056.

Kuhn, H.G., Dickinson-Anson, H., Gage, F.H., 1996. Neurogenesis in the dentate gyrus of the adult rat: age-related decrease of neuronal progenitor proliferation. J. Neurosci. 16 (6), 2027–2033.

Kunze, A., Congreso, M.R., Hartmann, C., Wallraff-Beck, A., Huttmann, K., Bedner, P., Steinhauser, C., 2009. Connexin expression by radial glia-like cells is required for neurogenesis in the adult dentate gyrus. Proc. Natl. Acad. Sci. U.S.A. 106 (27), 11336–11341.

Lam, H.A., Wu, N., Cely, I., Kelly, R.L., Hean, S., Richter, F., Maidment, N.T., 2011. Elevated tonic extracellular dopamine concentration and altered dopamine modulation of synaptic activity precede dopamine loss in the striatum of mice overexpressing human alpha-synuclein. J. Neurosci. Res. 89 (7), 1091–1102.

Lee, E., Son, H., 2009. Adult hippocampal neurogenesis and related neurotrophic factors. BMB Rep. 42 (5), 239–244.

Lee, C., Agoston, D.V., 2010. Vascular endothelial growth factor is involved in mediating increased de novo hippocampal neurogenesis in response to traumatic brain injury. J. Neurotrauma 27 (3), 541–553.

Lee, H.J., Lee, J.K., Lee, H., Carter, J.E., Chang, J.W., Oh, W., Bae, J.S., 2012. Human umbilical cord blood-derived mesenchymal stem cells improve neuropathology and cognitive impairment in an Alzheimer's disease mouse model through modulation of neuroinflammation. Neurobiol. Aging 33 (3), 588–602.

Li, W.L., Cai, H.H., Wang, B., Chen, L., Zhou, Q.G., Luo, C.X., Zhu, D.Y., 2009. Chronic fluoxetine treatment improves ischemia-induced spatial cognitive deficits through increasing hippocampal neurogenesis after stroke. J. Neurosci. Res. 87 (1), 112–122.

Madronal, N., Lopez-Aracil, C., Rangel, A., del Rio, J.A., Delgado-Garcia, J.M., Gruart, A., 2010. Effects of enriched physical and social environments on motor performance, associative learning, and hippocampal neurogenesis in mice. PLoS One 5 (6), e11130.

Madsen, T.M., Treschow, A., Bengzon, J., Bolwig, T.G., Lindvall, O., Tingstrom, A., 2000. Increased neurogenesis in a model of electroconvulsive therapy. Biol. Psychiatry 47 (12), 1043–1049.

Manganas, L.N., Zhang, X., Li, Y., Hazel, R.D., Smith, S.D., Wagshul, M.E., Maletic-Savatic, M., 2007. Magnetic resonance spectroscopy identifies neural progenitor cells in the live human brain. Science 318 (5852), 980–985.

McEwen, B.S., 2001. Plasticity of the hippocampus: adaptation to chronic stress and allostatic load. Ann. N Y Acad. Sci. 933, 265–277.

Merkle, F.T., Tramontin, A.D., Garcia-Verdugo, J.M., Alvarez-Buylla, A., 2004. Radial glia give rise to adult neural stem cells in the subventricular zone. Proc. Natl. Acad. Sci. U.S.A. 101 (50), 17528–17532.

Monje, M., Dietrich, J., 2012. Cognitive side effects of cancer therapy demonstrate a functional role for adult neurogenesis. Behav. Brain Res. 227 (2), 376–379.

Monje, M.L., Toda, H., Palmer, T.D., 2003. Inflammatory blockade restores adult hippocampal neurogenesis. Science 302 (5651), 1760–1765.

Monje, M.L., Vogel, H., Masek, M., Ligon, K.L., Fisher, P.G., Palmer, T.D., 2007. Impaired human hippocampal neurogenesis after treatment for central nervous system malignancies. Ann. Neurol. 62 (5), 515–520.

Mori, T., Buffo, A., Gotz, M., 2005. The novel roles of glial cells revisited: the contribution of radial glia and astrocytes to neurogenesis. Curr. Top. Dev. Biol. 69, 67–99.

Mustroph, M.L., Chen, S., Desai, S.C., Cay, E.B., DeYoung, E.K., Rhodes, J.S., 2012. Aerobic exercise is the critical variable in an enriched environment that increases hippocampal neurogenesis and water maze learning in male C57BL/6J mice. Neuroscience 219, 62–71.

Nelson, R.L., Guo, Z., Halagappa, V.M., Pearson, M., Gray, A.J., Matsuoka, Y., Mattson, M.P., 2007. Prophylactic treatment with paroxetine ameliorates behavioral deficits and retards the development of amyloid and tau pathologies in 3xTgAD mice. Exp. Neurol. 205 (1), 166–176.

Nichol, K.E., Parachikova, A.I., Cotman, C.W., 2007. Three weeks of running wheel exposure improves cognitive performance in the aged Tg2576 mouse. Behav. Brain Res. 184 (2), 124–132.

Nichol, K., Deeny, S.P., Seif, J., Camaclang, K., Cotman, C.W., 2009. Exercise improves cognition and hippocampal plasticity in APOE epsilon4 mice. Alzheimers Dement 5 (4), 287–294.

Nilsson, M., Perfilieva, E., Johansson, U., Orwar, O., Eriksson, P.S., 1999. Enriched environment increases neurogenesis in the adult rat dentate gyrus and improves spatial memory. J. Neurobiol. 39 (4), 569–578.

Noctor, S.C., Flint, A.C., Weissman, T.A., Wong, W.S., Clinton, B.K., Kriegstein, A.R., 2002. Dividing precursor cells of the embryonic cortical ventricular zone have morphological and molecular characteristics of radial glia. J. Neurosci. 22 (8), 3161–3173.

Nout, Y.S., Culp, E., Schmidt, M.H., Tovar, C.A., Proschel, C., Mayer-Proschel, M., Bresnahan, J.C., 2011. Glial restricted precursor cell transplant with cyclic adenosine monophosphate improved some autonomic functions but resulted in a reduced graft size after spinal cord contusion injury in rats. Exp. Neurol. 227 (1), 159–171.

Palma, I., Pena, R.Y., Contreras, A., Ceballos-Reyes, G., Coyote, N., Erana, L., Queipo, G., 2008. Participation of OCT3/4 and beta-catenin during dysgenetic gonadal malignant transformation. Cancer Lett. 263 (2), 204–211.

Park, D., Yang, Y.H., Bae, D.K., Lee, S.H., Yang, G., Kyung, J., Kim, Y.B., 2013. Improvement of cognitive function and physical activity of aging mice by human neural stem cells over-expressing choline acetyltransferase. Neurobiol. Aging 34 (11), 2639–2646.

Pendharkar, A.V., Chua, J.Y., Andres, R.H., Wang, N., Gaeta, X., Wang, H., Guzman, R., 2010. Biodistribution of neural stem cells after intravascular therapy for hypoxic-ischemia. Stroke 41 (9), 2064–2070.

Peng, Q., Masuda, N., Jiang, M., Li, Q., Zhao, M., Ross, C.A., Duan, W., 2008. The antidepressant sertraline improves the phenotype, promotes neurogenesis and increases BDNF levels in the R6/2 Huntington's disease mouse model. Exp. Neurol. 210 (1), 154–163.

Perera, T.D., Coplan, J.D., Lisanby, S.H., Lipira, C.M., Arif, M., Carpio, C., Dwork, A.J., 2007. Antidepressant-induced neurogenesis in the hippocampus of adult nonhuman primates. J. Neurosci. 27 (18), 4894–4901.

Phillips, W., Morton, A.J., Barker, R.A., 2005. Abnormalities of neurogenesis in the R6/2 mouse model of Huntington's disease are attributable to the in vivo microenvironment. J. Neurosci. 25 (50), 11564–11576.

van Praag, H., 2008. Neurogenesis and exercise: past and future directions. Neuromolecular Med. 10 (2), 128–140.

van Praag, H., Christie, B.R., Sejnowski, T.J., Gage, F.H., 1999. Running enhances neurogenesis, learning, and long-term potentiation in mice. Proc. Natl. Acad. Sci. U.S.A. 96 (23), 13427–13431.

van Praag, H., Shubert, T., Zhao, C., Gage, F.H., 2005. Exercise enhances learning and hippocampal neurogenesis in aged mice. J. Neurosci. 25 (38), 8680–8685.

Qu, T., Brannen, C.L., Kim, H.M., Sugaya, K., 2001. Human neural stem cells improve cognitive function of aged brain. Neuroreport 12 (6), 1127–1132.

Raffa, R.B., Duong, P.V., Finney, J., Garber, D.A., Lam, L.M., Mathew, S.S., Jen Weng, H.F., 2006. Is 'chemo-fog'/'chemo-brain' caused by cancer chemotherapy? J. Clin. Pharm. Ther. 31 (2), 129–138.

Ramirez-Amaya, V., Marrone, D.F., Gage, F.H., Worley, P.F., Barnes, C.A., 2006. Integration of new neurons into functional neural networks. J. Neurosci. 26 (47), 12237–12241.

Ransome, M.I., Renoir, T., Hannan, A.J., 2012. Hippocampal neurogenesis, cognitive deficits and affective disorder in Huntington's disease. Neural Plast. 2012, 874387.

Redmond Jr., D.E., McEntire, C.R., Kingsbery, J.P., Leranth, C., Elsworth, J.D., Bjugstad, K.B., Sladek Jr., J.R., 2013. Comparison of fetal mesencephalic grafts, AAV-delivered GDNF, and both combined in an MPTP-induced nonhuman primate Parkinson's model. Mol. Ther. 21 (12), 2160–2168.

Reitz, M., Demestre, M., Sedlacik, J., Meissner, H., Fiehler, J., Kim, S.U., Schmidt, N.O., 2012. Intranasal delivery of neural stem/progenitor cells: a noninvasive passage to target intracerebral glioma. Stem Cells Transl. Med. 1 (12), 866–873.

Rossi, D.J., Jamieson, C.H., Weissman, I.L., 2008. Stems cells and the pathways to aging and cancer. Cell 132 (4), 681–696.

Sahay, A., Scobie, K.N., Hill, A.S., O'Carroll, C.M., Kheirbek, M.A., Burghardt, N.S., Hen, R., 2011. Increasing adult hippocampal neurogenesis is sufficient to improve pattern separation. Nature 472 (7344), 466–470.

Santarelli, L., Saxe, M., Gross, C., Surget, A., Battaglia, F., Dulawa, S., Hen, R., 2003. Requirement of hippocampal neurogenesis for the behavioral effects of antidepressants. Science 301 (5634), 805–809.

Saxe, M.D., Battaglia, F., Wang, J.W., Malleret, G., David, D.J., Monckton, J.E., Drew, M.R., 2006. Ablation of hippocampal neurogenesis impairs contextual fear conditioning and synaptic plasticity in the dentate gyrus. Proc. Natl. Acad. Sci. U.S.A. 103 (46), 17501–17506.

Scharfman, H., Goodman, J., Macleod, A., Phani, S., Antonelli, C., Croll, S., 2005. Increased neurogenesis and the ectopic granule cells after intrahippocampal BDNF infusion in adult rats. Exp. Neurol. 192 (2), 348–356.

Seminatore, C., Polentes, J., Ellman, D., Kozubenko, N., Itier, V., Tine, S., Onteniente, B., 2010. The postischemic environment differentially impacts teratoma or tumor formation after transplantation of human embryonic stem cell-derived neural progenitors. Stroke 41 (1), 153–159.

Shetty, G.A., Hattiangady, B., Shetty, A.K., 2013. Neural stem cell- and neurogenesis-related gene expression profiles in the young and aged dentate gyrus. Age (Dordr) 35 (6), 2165–2176.

Shors, T.J., Miesegaes, G., Beylin, A., Zhao, M., Rydel, T., Gould, E., 2001. Neurogenesis in the adult is involved in the formation of trace memories. Nature 410 (6826), 372–376.

Simic, G., Kostovic, I., Winblad, B., Bogdanovic, N., 1997. Volume and number of neurons of the human hippocampal formation in normal aging and Alzheimer's disease. J. Comp. Neurol. 379 (4), 482–494.

Siuciak, J.A., Lewis, D.R., Wiegand, S.J., Lindsay, R.M., 1997. Antidepressant-like effect of brain-derived neurotrophic factor (BDNF). Pharmacol. Biochem. Behav. 56 (1), 131–137.

Siwak-Tapp, C.T., Head, E., Muggenburg, B.A., Milgram, N.W., Cotman, C.W., 2007. Neurogenesis decreases with age in the canine hippocampus and correlates with cognitive function. Neurobiol. Learn. Mem. 88 (2), 249–259.

Spalding, K.L., Bergmann, O., Alkass, K., Bernard, S., Salehpour, M., Huttner, H.B., Frisen, J., 2013. Dynamics of hippocampal neurogenesis in adult humans. Cell 153 (6), 1219–1227.

Staat, K., Segatore, M., 2005. The phenomenon of chemo brain. Clin. J. Oncol. Nurs. 9 (6), 713–721.

Sun, D., Bullock, M.R., McGinn, M.J., Zhou, Z., Altememi, N., Hagood, S., Colello, R.J., 2009. Basic fibroblast growth factor-enhanced neurogenesis contributes to cognitive recovery in rats following traumatic brain injury. Exp. Neurol. 216 (1), 56–65.

Suzuki, M., McHugh, J., Tork, C., Shelley, B., Klein, S.M., Aebischer, P., Svendsen, C.N., 2007. GDNF secreting human neural progenitor cells protect dying motor neurons, but not their projection to muscle, in a rat model of familial ALS. PLoS One 2 (8), e689.

Takahashi, K., Yamanaka, S., 2006. Induction of pluripotent stem cells from mouse embryonic and adult fibroblast cultures by defined factors. Cell 126 (4), 663–676.

Tashiro, A., Sandler, V.M., Toni, N., Zhao, C., Gage, F.H., 2006. NMDA-receptor-mediated, cell-specific integration of new neurons in adult dentate gyrus. Nature 442 (7105), 929–933.

Tian, C., Wang, Y., Sun, L., Ma, K., Zheng, J.C., 2011. Reprogrammed mouse astrocytes retain a "memory" of tissue origin and possess more tendencies for neuronal differentiation than reprogrammed mouse embryonic fibroblasts. Protein Cell 2 (2), 128–140.

Toft, A., Tome, M., Barnett, S.C., Riddell, J.S., 2013. A comparative study of glial and non-neural cell properties for transplant-mediated repair of the injured spinal cord. Glia 61 (4), 513–528.

Trejo, J.L., Carro, E., Torres-Aleman, I., 2001. Circulating insulin-like growth factor I mediates exercise-induced increases in the number of new neurons in the adult hippocampus. J. Neurosci. 21 (5), 1628–1634.

Ubhi, K., Inglis, C., Mante, M., Patrick, C., Adame, A., Spencer, B., Masliah, E., 2012. Fluoxetine ameliorates behavioral and neuropathological deficits in a transgenic model mouse of alpha-synucleinopathy. Exp. Neurol. 234 (2), 405–416.

Varela-Nallar, L., Aranguiz, F.C., Abbott, A.C., Slater, P.G., Inestrosa, N.C., 2010. Adult hippocampal neurogenesis in aging and Alzheimer's disease. Birth Defects Res. C Embryo Today 90 (4), 284–296.

Vaynman, S., Ying, Z., Gomez-Pinilla, F., 2004. Hippocampal BDNF mediates the efficacy of exercise on synaptic plasticity and cognition. Eur. J. Neurosci. 20 (10), 2580–2590.

Villeda, S.A., Luo, J., Mosher, K.I., Zou, B., Britschgi, M., Bieri, G., Wyss-Coray, T., 2011. The ageing systemic milieu negatively regulates neurogenesis and cognitive function. Nature 477 (7362), 90–94.

Warner-Schmidt, J.L., Duman, R.S., 2007. VEGF is an essential mediator of the neurogenic and behavioral actions of antidepressants. Proc. Natl. Acad. Sci. U. S. A. 104 (11), 4647–4652.

Wei, D., Kanai, M., Huang, S., Xie, K., 2006. Emerging role of KLF4 in human gastrointestinal cancer. Carcinogenesis 27 (1), 23–31.

Welihinda, A.A., Tirasophon, W., Kaufman, R.J., 1999. The cellular response to protein misfolding in the endoplasmic reticulum. Gene Expr. 7 (4–6), 293–300.

Wen, P.H., Hof, P.R., Chen, X., Gluck, K., Austin, G., Younkin, S.G., Elder, G.A., 2004. The presenilin-1 familial Alzheimer disease mutant P117L impairs neurogenesis in the hippocampus of adult mice. Exp. Neurol. 188 (2), 224–237.

Wolf, S.A., Kronenberg, G., Lehmann, K., Blankenship, A., Overall, R., Staufenbiel, M., Kempermann, G., 2006. Cognitive and physical activity differently modulate disease progression in the amyloid precursor protein (APP)-23 model of Alzheimer's disease. Biol. Psychiatry 60 (12), 1314–1323.

Xuan, A.G., Long, D.H., Gu, H.G., Yang, D.D., Hong, L.P., Leng, S.L., 2008. BDNF improves the effects of neural stem cells on the rat model of Alzheimer's disease with unilateral lesion of fimbria-fornix. Neurosci. Lett. 440 (3), 331–335.

Yamanaka, S., 2007. Strategies and new developments in the generation of patient-specific pluripotent stem cells. Cell Stem Cell 1 (1), 39–49.

Yamasaki, T.R., Blurton-Jones, M., Morrissette, D.A., Kitazawa, M., Oddo, S., LaFerla, F.M., 2007. Neural stem cells improve memory in an inducible mouse model of neuronal loss. J. Neurosci. 27 (44), 11925–11933.

Yang, M., Kim, J.S., Song, M.S., Kim, S.H., Kang, S.S., Bae, C.S., Moon, C., 2010. Cyclophosphamide impairs hippocampus-dependent learning and memory in adult mice: possible involvement of hippocampal neurogenesis in chemotherapy-induced memory deficits. Neurobiol. Learn. Mem. 93 (4), 487–494.

Yeung, S.T., Myczek, K., Kang, A.P., Chabrier, M.A., Baglietto-Vargas, D., Laferla, F.M., 2014. Impact of hippocampal neuronal ablation on neurogenesis and cognition in the aged brain. Neuroscience 259, 214–222.

Zhang, C.L., Zou, Y., He, W., Gage, F.H., Evans, R.M., 2008. A role for adult TLX-positive neural stem cells in learning and behaviour. Nature 451 (7181), 1004–1007.

Ziv, Y., Ron, N., Butovsky, O., Landa, G., Sudai, E., Greenberg, N., Schwartz, M., 2006. Immune cells contribute to the maintenance of neurogenesis and spatial learning abilities in adulthood. Nat. Neurosci. 9 (2), 268–275.

Zupanc, G.K., 2001. Adult neurogenesis and neuronal regeneration in the central nervous system of teleost fish. Brain Behav. Evol. 58 (5), 250–275. doi: 57569.

Zupanc, G.K., Clint, S.C., 2003. Potential role of radial glia in adult neurogenesis of teleost fish. Glia 43 (1), 77–86.

Chapter 9

Alzheimer's Disease and Mechanism-Based Attempts to Enhance Cognition

Jonathan E. Draffin,[1] Shira Knafo[2,3] and Michael T. Heneka[4,5]

[1]*Centro de Biología Molecular Severo Ochoa, Consejo Superior de Investigaciones Científicas/ Universidad Autónoma de Madrid, Madrid, Spain;* [2]*Unidad de Biofísica, CSIC, UPV/EHU, Universidad del País Vasco, Leioa, Spain;* [3]*Ikerbasque, Basque Foundation for Science;* [4]*Department of Neurology, Clinical Neuroscience Unit, Universitätsklinikum Bonn, Bonn, Germany;* [5]*German Center for Neurodegenerative Disease (DZNE), Bonn, Germany*

INTRODUCTION

Alzheimer's disease (AD) is the most common dementing illness of our society and currently affects approximately 150 million patients worldwide. Clinically, AD is characterized by progressive short-term memory failure and dysfunction of higher cognitive domains, including but not restricted to speech processing, orientation, executive functions and attention. Recent evidence suggests that there is a disconnect between the clinical appearance of first symptoms and the actual beginning of the underlying neurodegenerative processes in the brain, which may be initiated several decades before (Jack et al., 2013). During this clinically silent period, various life-style factors have been found to influence the overall AD risk. Thus, mid-life obesity, hypertension, reduced physical or cognitive activity, and brain trauma can increase the risk to develop AD (Barnes and Yaffe, 2011). Since current treatment options are limited to symptomatic treatment with acetylcholinesterase inhibitors and memantine, both being effective only for a limited period of time, the control of these risk factors has recently emerged as an important preventive measure.

Histopathologically, AD is characterized by the deposition of extracellular misfolded beta-amyloid peptides (Aβ), neurofibrillary tangles, and a widespread neuroinflammatory component (Figure 9.1). Aβ is generated through the sequential cleavage of the amyloid precursor protein (APP) by two aspartyl proteases: β-secretase 1 and γ-secretase. A balanced Aβ concentration appears to be crucial for the maintenance of the peptide's structure, because the tissue concentration of peptides of variable length as well as several posttranslational modifications increase

Cognitive Enhancement. http://dx.doi.org/10.1016/B978-0-12-417042-1.00009-7

193

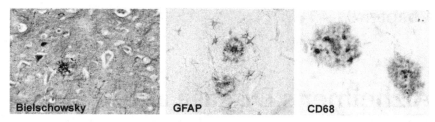

FIGURE 9.1 **Bielschowsky staining revealing the classical hallmarks of Alzheimer's disease: neurofibrillary tangle formation, dendritic damage and extracellular deposition of misfolded beta-amyloid peptides (Aβ).** Glial fibrillary acidic protein (GFAP) positive astrocytes surround the sites of Aβ deposition. CD68 positive microglia residing at the Aβ plaque show a round-to-oval morphological phenotype, which indicates an activated, inflammatory state of these cells.

the propensity of Aβ to misfold and aggregate. Soluble oligomers of Aβ may be directly toxic to neurons and accumulate prior to Aβ deposition. Phosphorylation of the tau protein is a second pathological hallmark and occurs within the neuron itself. Involved mechanisms are the activation of the phosphokinases, CDK5 and GSK3β (Yoshiyama et al., 2013), alone or in concert with reduced phosphatase activity of PPA2 (Torrent and Ferrer, 2012). Disturbed neuronal function and degeneration as well as the accumulation of misfolded proteins elicit an inflammatory activation of micro- and astroglia, which results in the generation and release of inflammatory mediators. These mediators directly affect neuronal function and survival thereby contributing to disease progression (Heneka et al., 2014).

Memory impairment associated with AD and mild cognitive impairment (MCI) involves the selective loss of the ability to consolidate new memories; the capacity to recall information from the distant past is preserved. This impairment of recent, but not distant, memory together with the rapid decay of newly acquired information is reminiscent of the deficits seen in patients with bilateral hippocampal damage (Scoville and Milner, 1957; Zola-Morgan et al., 1986). The prominent pathology observed in the perforant pathway in the early stages of AD (Hyman et al., 1986) and the well-characterized role of the hippocampus in encoding the memory of recent events (Geinisman, n.d.; Martin and Morris, 2002) affirm that degeneration of the hippocampal formation is likely to underlie the progressive memory decline characteristic of AD.

The inherited form of this neurodegenerative disease, which accounts for approximately 1–3% of all AD cases, is due to Aβ overproduction caused by mutations of genes encoding proteins involved in the APP processing pathway including APP, presenilin 1 and presenilin 2. In contrast, the vast majority of AD cases, which are of sporadic nature, seem to arise from a compromised clearance of Aβ peptides from the brain (Mawuenyega et al., 2010).

Based on this described pathology, animal models of cerebral amyloidosis or tau accumulation have been generated by introducing human gene mutations into the murine genome. Preclinical studies have largely used these models to develop therapeutic approaches and have been primarily focused on modifying the respective pathological substrate. The translation of these (to some extent very successful) treatment strategies into patient therapy, however, has largely failed. One underlying reason for this failure may be the fact that the respective animal models do not reflect the entire disease pathology and patient treatment was initiated at time points that did not correspond to the respective treatment times in the mouse models.

Synapse loss and hippocampal atrophy in the early stages of AD mark an important step in the progression of the disease and represent drivers of cognitive decline. Preservation of synapse integrity and function, however, has only very recently been targeted, and by nutritional rather than pharmacological means. Cognitive preservation or enhancement will require protection of synaptic function, which is key to memory processing and cognition.

SYNAPTIC DYSFUNCTION IS A CENTRAL FEATURE OF ALZHEIMER'S PATHOLOGY

The notion that altered neuronal connectivity may account for pathological cognitive decline was eloquently expressed over 80 years ago by Santiago Ramón y Cajal when he suggested that "dementia could result when synapses between neurons are weakened as a result of a more or less pathological condition, that is, when processes atrophy and no longer form contacts, when cortical mnemonic or association areas suffer partial disorganization" (Cajal, 1928). A variety of the neuropathological alterations observed in AD have been considered as candidates for the physical basis of the cognitive and memory impairments characteristic of the disease: several studies have demonstrated an association between tangle counts and severity of dementia (Arriagada et al., 1992; Bierer et al., 1995; Giannakopoulos et al., 2003; Gómez-Isla et al., 1997; Ingelsson et al., 2004), whereas amyloid plaque burden appears to be a poor predictor of cognitive decline (Arriagada et al., 1992; Bierer et al., 1995; Giannakopoulos et al., 2003; Gómez-Isla et al., 1997; Hyman et al., 1993; Ingelsson et al., 2004). Of all alterations, however, loss of synapses is most closely tied to the progression of AD symptoms (e.g., Coleman, 2003; DeKosky and Scheff, 1990; Terry et al., 1991). Electron microscopy and immunohistochemical staining for synaptic markers have revealed dramatic decreases in synaptic density in the AD brain, most notably in the association cortices and hippocampus (Bertoni-Freddari et al., 1989; Davies et al., 1987; DeKosky and Scheff, 1990; Ingelsson et al., 2004; Masliah et al., 1994, 2001, 1990; Scheff et al., 1990; Scheff and Price, 1993; Sze et al., 1997; Terry et al., 1991). Revealingly, this reduction in synapse number and density is not proportional to neuronal death (Bertoni-Freddari et al., 1989; Davies et al., 1987; DeKosky and Scheff, 1990), which suggests that alterations of synapses occur independently of the loss of the cells of which they are part. Indeed, synaptic degeneration appears to be an early event in pathogenesis: synapse loss is evident in patients with early AD and MCI (Masliah et al., 2001; Scheff et al.,

2006, 2007) and the extent of loss is greater than could be accounted for by neuronal death alone.

Aβ MOUNTS THE SYNAPTIC ASSAULT

The discovery that AD could be inherited in an autosomal dominant fashion (Goate et al., 1991) led to the articulation of the "amyloid hypothesis" of AD (Hardy and Allsop, 1991; Hardy and Higgins, 1992; Hardy and Selkoe, 2002; Selkoe, 1991). A wealth of evidence has now accumulated that suggests that Aβ plays a central role in the pathogenesis of neuronal dysfunction in AD, the main lines of which can be summarized briefly as follows. First, Aβ is the amyloid subunit that constitutes neuritic plaques found in the AD brain (Glenner and Wong, 1984; Masters et al., 1985). Second, the *APP* gene is located on chromosome 21 (Goldgaber et al., 1987; Kang et al., 1987; Robakis et al., 1987; Tanzi et al., 1987), whose duplication in Down syndrome invariably leads to AD (Mann, 1988; Mann et al., 1984). In support of this link, a Down syndrome patient with partial trisomy in which the gene sequence for *APP* was present in only two copies failed to develop any signs of the disease (Prasher et al., 1998). In the corollary situation, patients with duplication of a small portion of chromosome 21 containing the *APP* gene developed early-onset AD (Rovelet-Lecrux et al., 2006). Third, inherited mutations in the *APP* gene within or immediately adjacent to the Aβ region increase Aβ levels and/or its propensity to polymerize (Clements et al., 1993; De Jonghe et al., 1998; Fraser et al., 1992; Nilsberth et al., 2001; Van Nostrand et al., 2001; Watson et al., 1999) and are sufficient to cause early-onset AD (Goate et al., 1991; Levy et al., 1990). Similarly, mutations in presenilin 1 (*PS1*) and presenilin 2 (*PS2*) genes, which cause particularly aggressive forms of early-onset AD, selectively increase the production of Aβ terminating at amino acid 42 (Aβ42; Borchelt et al., 1996; Citron et al., 1997; Duff et al., 1996; Scheuner et al., 1996), a form more prone to oligomerization than the more abundant Aβ40 peptide (Bitan et al., 2003; Burdick et al., 1992; Jarrett et al., 1993). Importantly, presenilin is the catalytic site component of γ-secretase, which is one of the enzymes involved in the generation of Aβ from APP (Osenkowski et al., 2008; Selkoe and Wolfe, 2000; Wolfe et al., 1999). Fourth, the inheritance of one or two ε4 alleles of apolipoprotein E (*ApoE*) is a prominent genetic risk factor for AD (Corder et al., 1993; Saunders et al., 1993; Strittmatter et al., 1993) and increases Aβ deposition in the brain (Rebeck et al., 1993; Schmechel et al., 1993). Consistent with this effect, ApoE has recently been found to negatively regulate Aβ clearance (Verghese et al., 2013). Fifth, transgenic mice that express human *APP* and/or *PSEN* genes with familial AD mutations exhibit an age-dependent increase in extracellular Aβ (Games et al., 1995; Hsia et al., 1999; Johnson-Wood et al., 1997; Sturchler-Pierrat et al., 1997) and develop morphological (e.g., synaptic alterations; Games et al., 1995; Hsia et al., 1999; Lesné et al., 2006; Mucke et al., 2000) and behavioral changes (Ashe, 2001; Chapman et al., 1999; Hsiao et al., 1996) associated with

AD. Sixth, immunization of AD transgenic mice with Aβ or anti-Aβ antibodies prevents or reduces Aβ accumulation (Bard et al., 2000; Oddo et al., 2004; Schenk et al., 1999; Sigurdsson et al., 2001) and ameliorates cognitive deficits in transgenic mice (Dodart et al., 2002; Janus et al., 2000; Morgan et al., 2000). Finally, Aβ is toxic to neurons, both in vitro and in vivo (e.g., Geula et al., 1998; Hartley et al., 1999; Klein et al., 2001; Lambert et al., 1998; Lashuel et al., 2002). Both synthetic and natural oligomers of Aβ induce behavioral deficits and hyperphosphorylation of tau when injected into rodent brains at concentrations comparable to those observed in the brains of AD patients (Meyer-Luehmann et al., 2006). In summary, all four confirmed genetic factors underlying inherited forms of AD increase the production and/or accelerate the aggregation of Aβ, and this can be detected in humans well before the onset of clinical symptoms. Although some controversy continues to surround the Aβ hypothesis, transgenic mice and in vitro and ex vivo studies with natural and synthetic Aβ have elucidated the means by which Aβ compromises synaptic function and lent credence to the idea that Aβ is the cause of Alzheimer's pathology.

ANIMAL MODELS OF AD

The barriers to interactive investigation of all aspects of AD in humans have led to a concerted effort to reproduce its characteristics in a mouse model of the disease. The identification of Aβ (Glenner and Wong, 1984), the cloning of APP and the elucidation of its role in generating of Aβ (Goldgaber et al., 1987; Kang et al., 1987; Robakis et al., 1987; Tanzi et al., 1987), and the discovery of FAD-linked mutations in *APP* (Goate et al., 1991) led to the creation of the first transgenic mouse with AD-like pathology (Games et al., 1995). A panoply of such mice have now been created, in which mutant genes for human *APP, PS1, PS2,* and tau are present, often in combination. Most of these models recapitulate some, but not all, of the neuropathological features of the human disease. For example, in APP mice, APP overexpression of four- to five-fold is typically sufficient to induce the formation of detectable amyloid plaques similar to those observed in AD, with Aβ42/40 peptide ratio apparently being the critical determinant (Mucke et al., 2000). Overexpression levels depend on the strain of the mouse (Hsiao, 1998), although an age-dependent increase in plaque density is consistently observed (Games et al., 1995; Hsia et al., 1999; Hsiao et al., 1996; Johnson-Wood et al., 1997; Sturchler-Pierrat et al., 1997). Notably, most APP transgenic mice appear to show no loss of neurons (Irizarry et al., 1997a,b) and do not develop paired helical filaments (PHF) or tangles (Games et al., 1995; Hsia et al., 1999; Hsiao et al., 1996; Moechars et al., 1999; Sturchler-Pierrat et al., 1997), in contrast to AD patients. However, coexpression in APP mice of human tau bearing the P301L mutation that causes frontotemporal dementia (bigenic mice), or in triple transgenic mice that also express mutant PS1, causes PHF and tangle deposition (Lewis et al., 2001; Oddo et al., 2003) at an accelerated rate to that seen in mice expressing P301L tau alone.

In addition to overproducing Aβ, most transgenic AD mice also overexpress APP and APP fragments, which has given rise to concerns that the phenotypes of these animals are artificial. This has been recently addressed with the generation of *APP* knock-in mice in which the *APP* gene is replaced with the murine *APP* sequence containing a humanized Aβ region with familial Alzheimer's Disease (FAD)-linked mutations (Saito et al., 2014). In these mice, the Aβ42/40 ratio is increased and the mice show amyloid plaques in the cortex and hippocampus, microgliosis, and astrocytosis, especially in the vicinity of plaques, and synapse loss, suggesting that Aβ, and not another APP cleavage product, is indeed the primary causative agent in AD pathology. AD transgenic mice are characterized by a number of specific cognitive deficits (for review, see Spires-Jones and Knafo, 2012) compatible with AD, which makes them imperative for the testing of new AD therapeutics. The plastic nature of synapses and their central involvement in both early and late stages of cognitive decline in these AD models underscore the importance of synaptic targets for therapeutic approaches.

EXPERIMENTAL PARADIGMS CAN INFORM US ABOUT ALZHEIMER'S-RELATED PATHOPHYSIOLOGY

Hebb's postulate states that "when an Axon of cell A is near enough to excite a cell B and repeatedly or persistently takes part in firing it, some growth process or metabolic change takes place in one or both cells such that A's efficiency, as one of the cells firing B, is increased" (Hebb, 1949). Accordingly, two forms of such synaptic plasticity, long-term potentiation (LTP) and long-term depression (LTD), are widely used as cellular and synaptic models of learning and memory, and are believed to play a role in a variety of long-lasting forms of plasticity in the brain, with effects lasting for hours, days, or longer (Lynch, 2004; Malenka and Bear, 2004; Morris, 2003). Although demonstrating that the mechanisms of LTP and LTD underlie experience-dependent changes in synaptic activity and serve functional roles in vivo has been a formidable challenge, the near-universal ability of excitatory synapses in the mammalian brain to undergo such changes has been amply described and analogous modifications occur during learning in different regions of the brain (Pastalkova et al., 2006; Rioult-Pedotti et al., 2000; Ziemann et al., 2004). A balance in the ability of populations of synapses to undergo LTP or LTD ensures that the opposing threats of excitotoxicity and failure of networks to discriminate events and store information are quelled. Both LTP and LTD can occur at a given synapse, in response to different patterns of activation of N-methyl-D-aspartate (NMDA) and/or metabotropic glutamate receptors (mGluRs), depending on the experimental conditions (reviewed in Citri and Malenka, 2008; Kemp and Bashir, 2001). Mechanistically, the balance between synapse potentiation and depression is thought to depend on alterations in cytosolic Ca^{2+} concentration and the differential activation of certain kinases and phosphatases, such as calcium/calmodulin-dependent kinase II, calcineurin, and cyclic AMP response element binding protein (CREB). Ultimately, this balance in intraneuronal signaling appears to regulate the stability of the postsynaptic density and the trafficking of AMPA receptors to and from the postsynapse (Esteban et al., 2003; Kessels et al., 2009; Kessels and Malinow, 2009). Together, these changes dynamically modulate the magnitude of neurotransmission at the synaptic level. Synapse-level changes in receptor content during long-term plasticity are accompanied by changes at the level of the neuron, such as spine formation and increases in spine volume during LTP, and spine elimination and decreases in spine volume during LTD (Bastrikova et al., 2008; Engert and Bonhoeffer, 1999; Kopec et al., 2006; Maletic-Savatic et al., 1999; Matsuzaki et al., 2004; Zhou et al., 2004). It appears that changes in excitability are intimately linked to structural changes, such that glutamate-dependent insertion of AMPA receptors leads to an increase in spine stability (Lamprecht and LeDoux, 2004). Consistent with a role for these processes in learning and memory, learning induces spine formation (Fu et al., 2012; Xu et al., 2009) and the stability of dendritic spines is associated with the maintenance of lifelong memories (Xu et al., 2009; Yang, Pan, and Gan, 2009).

SYNAPTIC PLASTICITY AND MEMORY IS IMPAIRED IN TRANSGENIC MOUSE MODELS OF AD

Molecular and structural changes underlying modulation of neuronal excitability are consequential for cognition, and the dysregulation of this balance leads to excitotoxicity or degradation of stored memory. For these reasons, studies of synaptic plasticity employing both electrophysiological and morphological measures are essential for developing an understanding of how memory mechanisms are disrupted in disease. APP and its derivatives, as well as components of the APP-processing enzymes β-secretase and γ-secretase, have been detected in axons and dendrites by biochemical, immunostaining, and electron-microscopy studies (Buxbaum et al., 1998; Ferreira et al., 1993; Kaether et al., 2000; Koo et al., 1990; Lazarov et al., 2002; Sisodia et al., 1993; Xia et al., 2009). Evidence has accumulated that the introduction in transgenic mice of genes for one more of these familial AD-linked mutant proteins is sufficient to produce defects in functional and structural synaptic plasticity, as well as in cognitive function. These defects are often observed early relative to plaque development, thereby implicating soluble Aβ in the disruption. Early studies furnished evidence that defects in synaptic plasticity preceded the onset of amyloid deposition. Transgenic mice for human APP bearing the V717F mutation develop plaques after 12 months, but were found to exhibit impaired LTP at 3 (Moechars et al., 1999) and 4–5 months of age (Larson et al., 1999). Further support for a role of soluble Aβ species in neuronal dysfunction comes from the occurrence of progressive learning deficits, along with declines in synaptic transmission and synaptic density in the hippocampal CA1 region of APP V717F transgenic mice at times well before any amyloid plaques are observed (Hsia et al., 1999; Mucke et al., 2000; Palop et al.,

2003). These deficits increased with age but did not correlate with plaque number. A reduction of LTP has also been reported in mice that overexpress either the London (V642I; Moechars et al., 1999) or Swedish (APP$_{695}$SWE; Chapman et al., 1999; Jacobsen et al., 2006) mutations in APP, and similar impairments have been observed in mice expressing mutations in both APP and PS1 (Gengler et al., 2010; Trinchese et al., 2004). It should be noted, however, that a number of studies have failed to find impairment of LTP in several transgenic models overexpressing FAD mutant proteins (Brown et al., 2005; Fitzjohn et al., 2001; Gureviciene et al., 2004; Volianskis et al., 2010). These variations among studies could result from discrepancies in experimental design. Of particular relevance are differences in the ages at which the mice were tested and strain differences, as it is known that susceptibility to neuronal injury can vary widely across mouse strains (Schauwecker and Steward, 1997).

In addition to functional deficits in synaptic plasticity, animal models of AD often display structural dendritic and synaptic perturbations. The widely used Tg2576 mouse model expresses mutant human APP and shows decreased spine density in the CA1 and dentate gyrus well before the development of amyloid plaques (Jacobsen et al., 2006; Lanz et al., 2003; Perez-Cruz et al., 2011). Notably, cognitive impairments are detected in these mice at the time when spines become depleted, suggesting that synapse loss can drive cognitive decline. Transgenic mice bearing mutations in *APP* and *PS1* show large decreases in the density of large spines in the dentate gyrus (Knafo et al., 2009). Importantly, large spines may be physical traces of long-term memory (Bourne and Harris, 2007; Kasai et al., 2003, 2010). These mice display further dendritic abnormalities: dendrites near amyloid deposits experience shaft atrophy, neurite breakage, and greater reductions in spine density (Tsai et al., 2004). Together, results from AD animal models support the idea that synaptic degeneration is a central component of the AD pathology that leads to memory impairment. Encouragingly for the prospect of treatment of AD, structural alterations may be amenable to pharmacological improvement (Smith et al., 2009).

SOLUBLE, BUT NOT INSOLUBLE, Aβ DISRUPTS PLASTICITY AND MEMORY

Controversy surrounding the amyloid hypothesis has centered around the indirect relationship between the development of insoluble amyloid plaques and the clinical progression of AD (Braak and Braak, 1998; Knopman et al., 2003). However, evidence has since emerged that explains this apparent paradox. Early studies of the AD brain found robust correlations between cortical levels of soluble Aβ and the extent of synaptic loss and severity of cognitive impairment (Lue et al., 1999; McLean et al., 1999; Wang et al., 1999) and significant synapse loss also occurs in patients with MCI, a portent of future AD (Scheff et al., 2007). In order to investigate the effects of different Aβ species on memory and related synaptic mechanisms, acute treatment with Aβ provides a relatively simple but very attractive and manipulable model system, compared with transgenic APP animal models (Chambon et al., 2011). This acute approach gives the researcher the opportunity to control and characterize the biophysical state of Aβ preparations before use, which is likely to be relevant for AD therapy. Aβ is a product of normal neuronal metabolism (Haass et al., 1992; Seubert et al., 1992; Shoji et al., 1992) and is produced by sequential proteolysis of APP by β- and γ-secretases (De Strooper and Annaert, 2000). Aβ is a highly heterogeneous mixture of peptides, with different solubility, stability, and biological and toxic properties. C-terminal heterogeneity is generated by γ-secretase cleavage, which variably results in the production of 38- to 43-amino-acid Aβ peptides, of which Aβ40 is the dominant species (Benilova et al., 2012). The biophysical and biochemical properties of Aβ, such as its propensity to aggregate, vary strongly according to its length. In particular, Aβ42, which is overabundant in AD brain (Lemere et al., 1996), exhibits an increased tendency to aggregate compared to shorter forms of the peptide (Jarrett et al., 1993). Interestingly, Aβ42 more potently disrupts synaptic plasticity (Cullen et al., 1997; Nomura et al., 2012), and historically, the Aβ42/40 ratio has been used as an index of the neurotoxicity of a heterogeneous population of Aβ peptides (Hasegawa et al., 1999; Kuperstein et al., 2010). However, it is likely that aggregation and toxic properties of Aβ are influenced by the presence of other species. For example, Aβ43 is enriched in AD brain (Sandebring et al., 2013) and similarly supports an association between aggregation-proneness and disruption of learning and memory (Saito et al., 2011; Stéphan et al., 2001), and shorter peptides such as Aβ37 and Aβ38 are decreased (Portelius et al., 2010). In addition to variation in length, differences in primary sequence (Klyubin et al., 2004; Tomiyama et al., 2008) and post-translational modification (Jawhar et al., 2011; Kummer et al., 2011; Schlenzig et al., 2012; Youssef et al., 2008) of Aβ affect aggregation and potency of LTP inhibition. Despite the natural ability of Aβ, especially the human sequence, to form aggregates, the majority of natural or synthetically prepared Aβ usually contains a sizable fraction of Aβ monomers. However, preparations enriched in monomeric Aβ have little or no ability to disrupt synaptic functioning: such preparations fail to inhibit LTP (Hu et al., 2008; Klyubin et al., 2005, 2008; Ono et al., 2012; Shankar et al., 2008), facilitate LTD (Ono et al., 2012), or affect learned behavior (Cleary et al., 2005).

Dimers and beyond. Given the findings that Aβ monomers *per se* do not appear to impair synaptic function, the question arises as to which soluble Aβ aggregates are disruptive. Several lines of evidence suggest that small (2- to 20-mer) highly diffusible Aβ aggregates may be responsible for memory impairment in AD. The group led by D. Selkoe, having shown the presence of various Aβ assemblies in AD brain, suggested that soluble Aβ dimers are the smallest synaptotoxic species (Shankar et al., 2008) and are capable of compromising behavioral performance, inhibiting LTP and facilitating LTD in rodents (Barry et al., 2011; Li et al., 2009, 2011; Shankar et al., 2008). In contrast, the larger Aβ*56 12-mers extracted from APP transgenic mouse brain (Lesné et al., 2006) appear to be much less potent than cell-derived low-n oligomers or human brain Aβ dimer-containing soluble extracts at causing deficits in cognitive tasks (Reed et al., 2011; Shankar et al., 2008). However, although synthetic Aβ1-40 dimers blocked LTP both in vivo and in vitro when acutely applied at a concentration approximately 50-fold lower than unmodified Aβ1-40 (Hu et al., 2008; Shankar et al., 2008), it appears that these dimers need to assemble into larger aggregates before being able to potently inhibit LTP (O'Nuallain et al., 2010).

The aggregate zoo. Aβ forms oligomers whose conformations span several orders, although the mechanism by which this process occurs remains unknown. Soluble dimers, trimers, dodecamers, and higher order oligomers (Aβ-derived diffusible ligands and AβO spherical vesicles), protofibrils, annular protofibrils, and fibrils exist alongside monomeric Aβ (Harper et al., 1997; Hartley et al., 1999; Lambert et al., 1998; Lashuel et al., 2002; Walsh et al., 1999) and have all been found to impair LTP and induce cognitive impairment in mice, in combination with synaptotoxic effects (Cleary et al., 2005; Demuro et al., 2005; Deshpande et al., 2006; Hartley et al., 2008; Jin et al., 2011; Kayed et al., 2003; Kuperstein et al., 2010; Lambert et al., 1998; Lasagna-Reeves et al., 2011b; Lesné et al., 2006; Li et al., 2009; Noguchi et al., 2009; Podlisny et al., 1995; Reed et al., 2011; Roher et al., 1996; Sandberg et al., 2010; Shankar et al., 2008; Walsh et al., 2002; Wang et al., 2010; Xia et al., 1997; Zempel et al., 2010). In addition, "exotic" Aβ structures such as the amylospheroids, which are spherical assemblies of 10–15 nm, have been isolated from AD brain and found to show neurotoxicity and activate several pathways implicated in synaptic impairment (Hoshi et al., 2003; Matsumura et al., 2011; Noguchi et al., 2009). Regardless of the relationship between size of soluble Aβ aggregates and synaptic dysfunction, insoluble fibrils *per se* are unlikely candidates for memory impairment in AD. Rather, plaque-containing insoluble fibrils are likely to provide a major source and sink of memory disrupting soluble Aβ (Martins et al., 2008; Shankar et al., 2008). Synapse loss in AD is most evident in the immediate vicinity of senile plaques (Lanz et al., 2003; Moolman et al., 2004; Spires and Hannan, 2005; Tsai et al., 2004), and recent studies using multiphoton *in vivo* imaging revealed a halo of oligomeric Aβ around plaques in the brain of AD transgenic mice (Koffie et al., 2009), suggesting that oligomeric Aβ may exist in equilibrium with plaques in AD. Like Aβ, many other amyloidogenic proteins form aqueous soluble oligomers that are neurotoxic (Caughey and Lansbury, 2003; Haass and Selkoe, 2007). Intriguingly, many of these neurotoxic oligomers adopt similar conformations to Aβ, recognized by conformation-selective antibodies (Glabe, 2008; Kayed et al., 2003, 2004; Lambert et al., 2009; Yamin et al., 2008). Oligomers of proteins implicated in several neurodegenerative diseases, including tau (Lasagna-Reeves et al., 2011a; frontotemporal dementia), α-synuclein (Emmanouilidou et al., 2010; Hüls et al., 2011; Martin et al., 2012; Parkinson's disease), PrP106-126 (Klyubin et al., 2012; transmissible spongiform encephalopathies), and ADan (Schlenzig et al., 2012; familial Danish dementia) exhibit neurotoxic properties and impair synaptic plasticity, often in contrast to less aggregated forms of the protein. Given the shared ability of these aggregates to inhibit LTP, it has been suggested that a common conformation is critical for the disruptive actions on synaptic plasticity (and hence, on memory) of these very different peptides (Kayed et al., 2003). The mechanisms by which this disruption occurs in AD have begun to be dissected.

MECHANISMS OF Aβ-MEDIATED DISRUPTION OF SYNAPTIC PLASTICITY

Cleavage of APP by β- and γ-secretases liberates Aβ into the extracellular space, which accumulates in extracellular amyloid plaques. Classically, therefore, Aβ has been thought to exert its toxic effects by acting on neurons from the outside through one, or multiple, cell surface receptor(s), although intracellular Aβ is observed in cell and animal models and appears to be pathologically relevant (reviewed in LaFerla et al., 2007). A number of molecules have been proposed to act as Aβ receptors (Cissé et al., 2011; Diarra et al., 2009; Laurén et al., 2009; Lee and Landreth, 2010; Parri and Dineley, 2010; Yan et al., 1996), although the "stickiness" of Aβ suggests it is most pertinent to ask whether the interaction between Aβ and a molecule plays a role in the deleterious effects of Aβ.

Aβ inhibits a well-characterized form of LTP that depends on the activation of NMDA receptors (Hsieh et al., 2006; Shankar et al., 2007), and this inhibition is blocked by 2-amino-5-phosphonopentanoic acid (APV) an NMDA receptor antagonist. Using such antagonists to rescue LTP from the effects of Aβ is somewhat counterintuitive, since LTP itself requires the function of NMDA receptors, although the finding that Aβ acts through excessive activation of extrasynaptic NR2B-containing NMDA receptors provides a potential explanation for this result (Li et al., 2011). Accordingly, NR2B-selective antagonists are able to block Aβ inhibition of LTP (Hu et al., 2009; Rammes et al., 2011; Rönicke et al., 2011).

In addition to the inhibition of LTP, Aβ produces depression of glutamatergic synaptic transmission when overexpressed in hippocampal CA1 pyramidal neurons, either virally (after 16 h) (Kamenetz et al., 2003) or transgenically (after 3 weeks) (Hsia et al., 1999). The effect is seen both electrophysiologically (by a decrease in both AMPA receptor- and NMDA receptor-mediated transmission in CA1 region, with a selective reduction in NMDA receptor-mediated transmission in the dentate gyrus; Harris et al., 2010; Kamenetz et al., 2003), as well as structurally (by a reduction in dendritic spine density; Calabrese et al., 2007; Hsieh et al., 2006; Lacor et al., 2007; Lanz et al., 2003; Shankar et al., 2007; Shrestha et al., 2006). Intriguingly, this depression appears to exploit a recently described metabotropic function of NMDA receptors (Kessels et al., 2013), a function similarly implicated in mediating NMDA receptor-dependent LTD (Nabavi et al., 2013), although this latter claim has been contested (Babiec et al., 2014). The depressive effect of Aβ on excitatory transmission appears to use signaling pathways used by LTD (Hsieh et al., 2006; Jo et al., 2011; Shankar et al., 2007). For example, the activity of calcineurin, a calcium-activated phosphatase, is required for LTD and Aβ-induced synaptic depression (Dineley et al., 2010; Mulkey et al., 1994). Studies have also found that caspase-3, an element of the apoptotic pathway, and GSK3β, participate in both Aβ-induced synaptic depression and LTD (D'Amelio et al., 2011; Jo et al., 2011; Li et al., 2010; Peineau et al., 2007). Recent studies link these actions of Aβ, in finding that caspase-3 and GSK3β are also involved in the Aβ-inhibition of LTP (Jo et al., 2011) and that NMDA receptor-dependent LTD can be facilitated by Aβ (Li et al., 2009), suggesting that normal synaptic activity patterns in the brain may lead to an LTD-like synaptic weakening in the presence of Aβ.

Tau knockout mice have shed light on the mechanism by which Aβ induces cognitive deficits in APP transgenic models. Tau protein becomes hyperphosphorylated during the progression of AD and aggregates to form the neurofibrillary tangles characteristic of the disease. Although the primacy of Aβ or tau in the pathogenesis of AD was once a point of controversy in the field (βAptists vs. tauists), it appears that tau expression is necessary for Aβ-mediated inhibition of LTP (Shipton et al., 2011) and that tau alteration occurs downstream of Aβ accumulation in AD. Notably, APP transgenic mice do not develop extensive tau pathologies on their own. Rather, although tau is hyperphosphorylated, it remains soluble and does not resemble the neurofibrillary tangles found in the human disease. Analogous to Aβ, therefore, soluble tau may be more important to the AD process than its aggregated form. Another intriguing parallel with endogenous plasticity mechanisms was provided in a recent study showing that tau is required for NMDA receptor-dependent LTD, and that LTD is associated with the GSK3β-dependent phosphorylation of tau on the PHF epitope (Kimura et al., 2014). Collectively, therefore, these results suggest that Aβ alters the balance of activation of pathways integral to the physiological expression of NMDA receptor-dependent synaptic plasticity to lower the threshold for LTD and inhibit LTP. The commonality of the pathways involved indicates that these actions are two sides of the same coin.

Similarly, a central role for mGluRs in the dual action of Aβ has recently been uncovered. Aβ facilitates an mGluR-dependent form of LTD (Li et al., 2009; Shankar et al., 2008) and inhibits mGluR-dependent LTP (Hu et al., 2014)—two forms of synaptic plasticity independent of the activation of NMDA receptors. Remarkably, mGluRs are also required for the Aβ-mediated facilitation of NMDA receptor-dependent LTD and cellular prion protein (PrP^C), a receptor for certain synaptotoxic Aβ assemblies that associates with mGluRs at the postsynaptic density (Laurén et al., 2009; Nicoll et al., 2013; Ordóñez-Gutiérrez et al., 2013; Um et al., 2013), is a necessary cofactor (Hu et al., 2014). PrP^C may also be required for Aβ-mediated inhibition of LTP (Laurén et al., 2009), although there is some controversy surrounding this result (Balducci et al., 2010; Kessels et al., 2010). Regardless, the involvement of the protagonists of distinct neurodegenerative diseases, including tau and PrP^C, in the actions of Aβ at the synapse is an exciting frontier in AD research, the understanding of which will be important for identifying appropriate targets for the enhancement of cognition in AD.

Finally, the physiological role of Aβ may involve the regulation of neuronal activity at the circuit and network levels (reviewed in Palop and Mucke, 2010). Alteration of this function as a result of dysregulation of Aβ levels may be responsible for the increased incidence of epileptic seizures in individuals bearing FAD mutations (e.g., in ~83% of pedigrees with very early-onset AD (<40 years); Snider et al., 2005). Therefore, the preservation of physiological functions of Aβ will be an important consideration in the design of treatment strategies for AD.

In summary, Aβ appears to alter the balance of neuronal activity through the inhibition of LTP and facilitation of LTD. Mechanism-based therapy will require a greater understanding of these complex processes in order to effectively treat the symptoms of AD while minimizing side effects.

TREATMENT STRATEGIES

In general, there is a need for at least three distinct treatment strategies for AD: preventive therapeutics, given years ahead of clinical onset, course-modifying therapies, for patients at the beginning of the disease, and acute treatments for AD patients, who have developed the full clinical disease. Currently approved and clinically used drugs are symptomatic in nature and are of only transient benefit to the patient. Therefore, there is a pressing need to develop more efficient therapeutic interventions. To date, most drug development strategies have focused on substances that interfere with pathogenic mechanisms leading to the major pathological hallmarks: Aβ deposition and tau hyperphosphorylation. Inhibition of APP processing, activation of nonamyloidogenic APP cleavage, and vaccination against Aβ epitopes are key strategies.

Current Treatments

Both memantine (Chen et al., 2010; Martinez-Coria et al., 2010; Minkeviciene et al., 2004; Scholtzova et al., 2008), an NMDA receptor antagonist, and cholinesterase inhibitors (Dong et al., 2005; Van Dam et al., 2005, 2008; Van Dam and De Deyn, 2006) have been shown to be effective at improving cognition in AD mouse models. However, there is little evidence that either of these treatments significantly alter the progression of the disease in AD patients (Schneider et al., 2011). For a more detailed overview on the current treatment for AD, the reader is referred to Chapter 11.

Preventing Cleavage: γ- and β-Secretase Inhibitors

In addition to transgenic mouse models, which overproduce and recapitulate the Aβ and tau pathologies that are associated with AD, numerous genetically modified mice have been produced that lack genes associated with this disorder. For example, knockout mice have been created of the APP secretases (β-secretase (BACE), presenilin (1 and 2), and α-secretase (ADAM10 and 17) (Hartmann et al., 2002; Herreman et al., 1999; Lee et al., 2003; Luo et al., 2001; Shen et al., 1997)). These animals have furnished insights that have led to treatments for AD. When presenilin 1 was shown to be necessary for the production of Aβ, the presenilins and the γ-secretase complex became the primary small molecular drug target for AD. Early evidence suggested that the γ-secretase complex had vital roles beyond the production of Aβ: presenilin 1 knockout in mice was found to be lethal (Shen et al., 1997), and evidence for specific roles later emerged, including suppression of skin cancer (Zhang et al., 2007), calcium dyshomeostasis (Green and LaFerla, 2008) and autophagy (Lee et al., 2010; Neely et al., 2011). Despite the early warnings, subsequent efforts progressed towards the development of a smorgasbord of highly specific γ-secretase inhibitors. Several of these inhibitors were shown to improve cognition in transgenic mouse models of AD (Comery et al., 2005; Imbimbo et al., 2009; Martone et al., 2009), and, invariably, to decrease Aβ levels. A major setback in AD therapeutics came with the halting of a phase III clinical trial of semagacestat, which was found to cause increased cognitive decline, and increase the incidence of skin cancer (Schor, 2011). Consequently, these inhibitor programs have largely been abandoned in favor of more APP selective γ-secretase inhibitors, or γ-secretase modulators, which alter the site of APP cleavage to generate species of Aβ less prone to aggregation.

BACE1 is the sole β-secretase enzyme, and its activity is also crucial for the production of Aβ (Hussain et al., 2007; Sinha et al., 1999; Vassar et al., 1999). In contrast to γ-secretase, elimination of β-secretase activity by gene deletion essentially abolished the production of Aβ, yet resulted only in minor phenotypic abnormality in mice (Cai et al., 2001; Luo et al., 2001; Ohno et al., 2004; Roberds et al., 2001). Thus, BACE1 appears a much more attractive drug target than the γ-secretase complex. Indeed, the crossing of BACE1 knockout mice with Tg2576 mice prevented cognitive decline in these animals and dramatically reduced Aβ levels (Ohno et al., 2004). Careful further analysis has revealed several alterations in BACE1 knockout mice, including reduced myelination, subtle deficits in prepulse inhibition, hypersensitivity to a glutamatergic psychostimulant, cognitive impairments, and reduced dendritic spine density (Hu et al., 2006; Laird et al., 2005; Savonenko et al., 2008; Willem et al., 2006). Collectively, therefore, BACE1 knockout mice have established BACE1 as a primary target for the treatment of AD, although some deleterious side effects may result from the inhibition of BACE1 in the mature brain. Regardless, BACE1 remains a far safer target than γ-secretase, and work on its therapeutic manipulation is in progress. BACE1 has a large active site, and developing a compound large enough to inhibit it and yet small enough to cross the blood–brain barrier has proved challenging (Huang et al., 2009). However, some promising compounds have been reported to lower Aβ levels (Chang et al.,

2004; Eketjäll et al., 2013; Fukumoto et al., 2010a; Huang et al., 2009; Hussain et al., 2007; Lerchner et al., 2010; Mori et al., 2012) and improve cognition (Chang et al., 2007) in transgenic mice and human clinical trials are under way. A recent trial of LY2886721 failed in the phase II stage (see June 2013 Eli Lilly press release), although the liver toxicity associated with the drug is likely to be independent of BACE1 inhibition.

α-Secretase Activation

The α-secretase, which is the metalloprotease ADAM10, cleaves APP within the Aβ domain, thereby preventing generation of Aβ. For this reason, activation of α-secretase has been proposed as a treatment strategy for AD. Proof-of-concept for this strategy was furnished by work showing that overexpression of ADAM10 mice lowered brain Aβ levels and rescued LTP inhibition and spatial learning defects in APP transgenic mice (Postina et al., 2004). Interestingly, deprenyl, an anti-dementia drug, appears to promote the α-secretase-mediated cleavage of APP (Yang et al., 2007). ADAM10 can be activated by various cell-surface receptors, which activate PKC, mitogen-activated protein kinases, phosphoinositide 3-kinase, and calcium signaling (reviewed in Postina, 2012)—well-characterized pathways amenable to pharmacological manipulation. However, consideration of the potential side effects of α-secretase is warranted, since it possesses several substrates. In keeping with this cautionary sentiment, α-secretase cleavage targeted for activation should occur in brain areas affected in AD.

Sequestering Aβ: Immunotherapy

Aβ immunotherapy is elegant in its simplicity: the AD brain is exposed to anti-Aβ antibodies, either by "active" immunization (injection of an Aβ-containing immunogen to stimulate a host response) or "passive" immunization (administration of a recombinant monoclonal antibody) to stimulate the body's defenses to neutralize and clear Aβ as it would other invasive entities. Initial experimentation with active Aβ immunotherapy in a transgenic model of AD showed a remarkable reduction in amyloid-associated pathologies (Schenk et al., 1999). Importantly, in addition to clearance of amyloid plaques, synapses were preserved, neuritic dystrophy was reduced and inflammation subsided. Further studies in animal models showed cognitive improvements and improvements in Aβ pathology (Asuni et al., 2006; Bard et al., 2000; DeMattos et al., 2001; Janus et al., 2000; Lemere et al., 2001; Morgan et al., 2000; Sigurdsson et al., 2001, 2004). In addition, plaque reduction was observed post-mortem in the brain of an actively immunized patient (Nicoll et al., 2003) and a phase II trial of passive immunotherapy with bapineuzumab was also shown to reduce amyloid burden, as visualized by positron emission tomography (PET)/Pittsburgh compound B (PiB) methodology (Rinne et al., 2010). However, large-scale phase III clinical trials of bapineuzumab in patients with mild to moderate AD were halted in August 2012 when the drug failed to arrest cognitive decline (Salloway et al., 2014), and a similar fate awaited solanezumab, another anti-$A\beta$ antibody (Doody et al., 2014). Considered alongside the observation that bapineuzumab was effective in stabilizing amyloid plaque burden and lowering phosphorylated-tau levels in cerebrospinal fluid, two biomarkers of AD pathology, these results raised concerns about the propriety of $A\beta$ as a target without consideration of aggregation state. The original amyloid cascade hypothesis (Hardy and Higgins, 1992), which emphasized the role of the amyloid plaques characteristic of AD, has now evolved to include the important role of soluble $A\beta$-oligomers in synaptic dysfunction and toxicity (Benilova et al., 2012; De Felice et al., 2008; Jin et al., 2011; Sakono and Zako, 2010; Walsh and Selkoe, 2007; Zempel et al., 2010). Recent studies have shown that the concentration of soluble $A\beta$ oligomers in AD brain is several orders of magnitude lower than levels of monomeric or fibrillar $A\beta$ (Delacourte et al., 2002; Fukumoto et al., 2010b; Georganopoulou et al., 2005; Mehta et al., 2000), which bodes well for the feasibility of elimination strategies. Soluble $A\beta$ oligomers therefore represent a particularly attractive therapeutic target, and antibodies have been developed that effectively and selectively bind to soluble $A\beta$ oligomers, neutralizing their synaptotoxic potential in cell cultures and reducing memory deficits in transgenic AD mice (Hillen et al., 2010; Zago et al., 2012). In addition to immunotherapeutic strategies targeting soluble $A\beta$, inhibitors of $A\beta$ aggregation are currently being developed (Nie et al., 2011).

Tau

Tau protein appears to mediate $A\beta$-induced toxicity, and phosphorylation of tau is considerably increased in the brains of patients with AD (Hasegawa et al., 1992; Matsuo et al., 1994). Accordingly, tau has been the recent focus of several AD treatment strategies, directly targeting phosphorylation state or aggregation of tau protein.

Reducing hyperphosphorylation. Hyperphosphorylation of tau could lead to a loss- or gain-of-function, depending on the specific sites involved, and, therefore, identifying inhibitors of the appropriate kinases has considerable therapeutic appeal. Kinase inhibitors are in active development for the treatment of a variety of conditions, including cancer, and the endeavor has seen some success. However, the process has encountered difficulties germane to the strategy of inhibition of tau hyperphosphorylation. The shared mechanism of action of most kinase inhibitors, which compete for the ATP-binding site common to all tau kinases, makes selectivity difficult to achieve (Ghoreschi et al., 2009). Further, although several kinases have been shown to phosphorylate tau in vitro, including MAPK1, MARK1 GSK3β, and CDK5 (Gong and Iqbal, 2008; Hanger et al., 2009; Mazanetz and Fischer, 2007), the relative contribution of each kinase to tau phosphorylation in AD remains unclear. Nevertheless, there is substantial evidence that both GSK3 and CDK5 are relevant in tau pathologies: both kinases colocalize with NFTs (Augustinack et al., 2002; Imahori and Uchida, 1997; Pei et al., 1998; Yamaguchi et al., 1996), overexpression of GSK3β, or p25 (a cleavage product of an activator of CDK5) with mutant human tau, in transgenic mice increased tau hyperphosphorylation and caused neurodegeneration and cognitive deficits (Hernández et al., 2002; Lucas et al., 2001; Noble et al., 2003). However, the observation that inhibition of CDK5 in mice overexpressing p25 produced an increase of tau phosphorylation by GSK3β (Wen et al., 2008) has led to an increased focus on GSK3β inhibition as a treatment strategy for AD. Inhibition of GSK3β reduces tau phosphorylation and ameliorates memory impairments and neuropathology in transgenic mouse models of AD (Caccamo et al., 2007; Qing et al., 2008; Sereno et al., 2009; Toledo and Inestrosa, 2010), although given that a role for GSK3β in Aβ processing has been reported, it remains unclear to what extent these improvements can be attributed to a reduction in tau phosphorylation *per se* (Phiel et al., 2003; Rockenstein et al., 2007; Su et al., 2004). The notably promiscuous nature of GSK3β (Doble and Woodgett, 2003) raises concerns over target-related side effects; although inhibitors of other multifunctioning kinases have been used successfully in oncology. Small clinical trials of lithium, which also inhibits CDK5, proved inconclusive, although the aforementioned interaction between CDK5 and GSK3β raises the possibility of a lessened effect on GSK3β activity. A more selective inhibitor of GSK3β, TDZD, is currently being examined in a phase II trial.

Inhibiting aggregation. The conversion of soluble tau into oligomeric and fibrillar species could result in loss- and gain-of-function tau toxicities. Inhibiting the assembly of tau into multimeric structures might therefore prevent the formation of toxic species and increase levels of monomeric tau, which could contribute to microtubule stabilization. The dye methylene blue was the first compound reported to inhibit tau–tau interactions, and the compound was also shown to alter the structure of existing PHFs isolated from AD brain (Wischik et al., 1996). Recent studies have found evidence for potentially beneficial effects of methylene blue on fibrilization in vitro, autophagy and neuroprotection (Congdon et al., 2012; Crowe et al., 2013; Wen et al., 2011). Methylene blue increased clearance of Aβ in a transgenic mouse model of AD (Medina et al., 2011) and improved spatial learning and brain metabolism in rats (Deiana et al., 2009; Riha et al., 2011). Reports of a phase II trial of the compound described dramatic improvements in disease progression, and phase III trials for the treatment of AD and frontotemporal dementia are under way.

THE DRUGS DO NOT WORK: WHAT IS FAILING IN AD THERAPIES?

The story of Dimebon, a repurposed antihistamine drug shown to protect neurons, but which later failed to demonstrate efficacy in phase III clinical trials, serves as a reminder of the expediency of mechanism-based drug development. However, despite an increasing understanding of the mechanisms underlying AD pathology, recent drug development efforts have been followed by a series of clinical failures. It has become common to explain the results from failed AD therapeutic trials with assumptive anti-Aβ therapies as evidence that the Aβ hypothesis is wrong. However, such trials have not been definitive tests of the cascade hypothesis, but rather opportune means to test potentially disease-modifying AD therapies. Rather, the failure of mechanism-based treatments that showed promise in animal models of AD may be more parsimoniously explained in the following ways:

First, for many of the clinical trials that have been carried out on AD patients, it is unclear that the treatment was operative in the relevant brain regions and subcellular compartments (e.g., synapses), or that there was sufficient knowledge of the pathobiology of the target to predict whether an effect was to be expected with the degree of modulation that the intervention achieved.

Second, to the extent to which they allow for reliable predictions of drug efficacy and safety in clinical trials, transgenic animal models of AD are likely to be imperfect. However, aforementioned differences in the presentation of aspects of AD pathology, including neuronal death and tangle development, are likely to be differences in outcomes well downstream of Aβ and therefore of limited consequence to treatment translation. Aside from these differences, a frequently mentioned discrepancy is that cognitive deficits can be detected in transgenic mice before plaque formation but in humans presumably only after plaque formation. However, this difference may be accounted for by several reasons, including differences in the sensitivity of cognitive tests used, in numerous variables that affect the deposition of Aβ into amyloid plaques or the formation of Aβ oligomers, and in the ability of mice and humans to compensate for hippocampal deficits (cognitive reserve). Indeed, given that there is significant variation in cognitive reserve even among AD patients, it may be that cognitive measures are inadequate as an index of AD progression and clinical outcome.

Third, and perhaps most significantly, it is likely that current treatments are too little, too late. Treatment in transgenic mouse models of AD is typically begun either before the onset of amyloid pathology or in mice with very modest Aβ loads. Therefore, treatments successful in mouse models of AD may be failing in patients because such models simulate the asymptomatic phase of the disease, implying that the results of treatment interventions should be considered in the context of disease prevention, not of clinical treatment. Given the manifold nature of the pathology of AD, targeting the cause of disease once the pathogenic cascade has been triggered is unlikely to be successful. In support of this idea, treatments given to transgenic mice when amyloid deposition and associated pathology are established are generally less effective (Abramowski et al., 2008; Das et al., 2001).

THE FUTURE OF COGNITIVE ENHANCEMENT IN AD

The long presymptomatic phase of AD, which may precede the development of clinical symptoms by decades, and complex pathology in the clinical phase mean that two drug-based strategies have the potential to be successful in the treatment of the disease:

First, a multipronged approach, such as that used in the treatment of coronary heart disease, in which specific downstream pathologies are targeted (e.g., tau and microglial activation), in the hope that proximal effects of these pathologies are more easily reversed in the clinical stage than those of the cause of the disease (Aβ).

Second, preventative treatment in patients at risk of developing the disease. These patients may be identified using biomarkers such as brain shrinkage as viewed by magnetic resonance imaging and PET scans; PET-based detection in the brain of markers of Aβ, such as PiB; and measurements of Aβ and tau in the cerebrospinal fluid—markers whose relationship to the progression of AD is being mapped with increasing fidelity. Promising efforts are under way to identify more sensitive and specific biomarkers that might allow for the earlier identification of people at risk for developing the disease (Jack and Holtzman, 2013). The planning of preclinical trials of existing and novel compounds will be aided by at-risk patient networks such as the Dominantly Inherited Alzheimer's Network (DIAN; Bateman et al., 2011) and the Alzheimer's Prevention Initiative (API; Reiman et al., 2011).

CONCLUDING REMARKS

Despite intense efforts at the basic science, preclinical and clinical levels, we have not yet succeeded in providing new therapies to AD patients. Setbacks, as experienced in the development of anti-Aβ vaccination, are to be expected and should not discourage us from driving this further. New insights about pathogenesis and mechanisms need to be translated into therapeutics, and improvement of preclinical models should be sought to ease the translation of results into the clinic.

REFERENCES

Abramowski, D., Wiederhold, K.-H., Furrer, U., Jaton, A.-L., Neuenschwander, A., Runser, M.-J., Staufenbiel, M., 2008. Dynamics of Abeta turnover and deposition in different beta-amyloid precursor protein transgenic mouse models following gamma-secretase inhibition. J. Pharmacol. Exp. Ther. 327 (2), 411–424.

Arriagada, P.V., Growdon, J.H., Hedley-Whyte, E.T., Hyman, B.T., 1992. Neurofibrillary tangles but not senile plaques parallel duration and severity of Alzheimer's disease. Neurology 42 (3 Pt 1), 631–639.

Ashe, K.H., 2001. Learning and memory in transgenic mice modeling Alzheimer's disease. Learn. Mem. 8 (6), 301–308.

Asuni, A.A., Boutajangout, A., Scholtzova, H., Knudsen, E., Li, Y.S., Quartermain, D., Sigurdsson, E.M., 2006. Vaccination of Alzheimer's model mice with Abeta derivative in alum adjuvant reduces Abeta burden without microhemorrhages. Eur. J. Neurosci. 24 (9), 2530–2542.

Augustinack, J.C., Sanders, J.L., Tsai, L.-H., Hyman, B.T., 2002. Colocalization and fluorescence resonance energy transfer between cdk5 and AT8 suggests a close association in pre-neurofibrillary tangles and neurofibrillary tangles. J. Neuropathol. Exp. Neurol. 61 (6), 557–564.

Babiec, W.E., Guglietta, R., Jami, S.A., Morishita, W., Malenka, R.C., O'Dell, T.J., 2014. Ionotropic NMDA receptor signaling is required for the induction of long-term depression in the mouse hippocampal CA1 region. J. Neurosci. 34 (15), 5285–5290.

Balducci, C., Beeg, M., Stravalaci, M., Bastone, A., Sclip, A., Biasini, E., Forloni, G., 2010. Synthetic amyloid-beta oligomers impair long-term memory independently of cellular prion protein. Proc. Natl. Acad. Sci. U.S.A. 107 (5), 2295–2300.

Bard, F., Cannon, C., Barbour, R., Burke, R.L., Games, D., Grajeda, H., Yednock, T., 2000. Peripherally administered antibodies against amyloid beta-peptide enter the central nervous system and reduce pathology in a mouse model of Alzheimer disease. Nat. Med. 6 (8), 916–919.

Barry, A.E., Klyubin, I., Mc Donald, J.M., Mably, A.J., Farrell, M.A., Scott, M., Rowan, M.J., 2011. Alzheimer's disease brain-derived amyloid-β-mediated inhibition of LTP in vivo is prevented by immunotargeting cellular prion protein. J. Neurosci. 31 (20), 7259–7263.

Barnes, D.E., Yaffe, K., 2011. The projected effect of risk factor reduction on Alzheimer's disease prevalence. Lancet Neurol 10, 819–828.

Bastrikova, N., Gardner, G.A., Reece, J.M., Jeromin, A., Dudek, S.M., 2008. Synapse elimination accompanies functional plasticity in hippocampal neurons. Proc. Natl. Acad. Sci. U.S.A. 105 (8), 3123–3127.

Bateman, R.J., Aisen, P.S., De Strooper, B., Fox, N.C., Lemere, C.A., Ringman, J.M., Xiong, C., 2011. Autosomal-dominant Alzheimer's disease: a review and proposal for the prevention of Alzheimer's disease. Alzheimers Res. Ther. 3 (1), 1.

Benilova, I., Karran, E., De Strooper, B., 2012. The toxic Aβ oligomer and Alzheimer's disease: an emperor in need of clothes. Nat. Neurosci. 15 (3), 349–357.

Bertoni-Freddari, C., Fattoretti, P., Meier-Ruge, W., Ulrich, J., 1989. Computer-assisted morphometry of synaptic plasticity during aging and dementia. Pathol. Res. Pract. 185 (5), 799–802.

Bierer, L.M., Hof, P.R., Purohit, D.P., Carlin, L., Schmeidler, J., Davis, K.L., Perl, D.P., 1995. Neocortical neurofibrillary tangles correlate with dementia severity in Alzheimer's disease. Arch. Neurol. 52 (1), 81–88.

Bitan, G., Kirkitadze, M.D., Lomakin, A., Vollers, S.S., Benedek, G.B., Teplow, D.B., 2003. Amyloid beta -protein (Abeta) assembly: Abeta 40 and Abeta 42 oligomerize through distinct pathways. Proc. Natl. Acad. Sci. U.S.A. 100 (1), 330–335.

Borchelt, D.R., Thinakaran, G., Eckman, C.B., Lee, M.K., Davenport, F., Ratovitsky, T., Sisodia, S.S., 1996. Familial Alzheimer's disease–linked presenilin 1 variants elevate Aβ1–42/1–40 ratio in vitro and in vivo. Neuron 17 (5), 1005–1013.

Bourne, J., Harris, K.M., 2007. Do thin spines learn to be mushroom spines that remember? Curr. Opin. Neurobiol. 17 (3), 381–386.

Braak, H., Braak, E., 1998. Evolution of neuronal changes in the course of Alzheimer's disease. J. Neural Transm. Suppl. 53, 127–140.

Brown, J.T., Richardson, J.C., Collingridge, G.L., Randall, A.D., Davies, C.H., 2005. Synaptic transmission and synchronous activity is disrupted in hippocampal slices taken from aged TAS10 mice. Hippocampus 15 (1), 110–117.

Burdick, D., Soreghan, B., Kwon, M., Kosmoski, J., Knauer, M., Henschen, A., Glabe, C., 1992. Assembly and aggregation properties of synthetic Alzheimer's A4/beta amyloid peptide analogs. J. Biol. Chem. 267 (1), 546–554.

Buxbaum, J.D., Thinakaran, G., Koliatsos, V., O'Callahan, J., Slunt, H.H., Price, D.L., Sisodia, S.S., 1998. Alzheimer amyloid protein precursor in the rat hippocampus: transport and processing through the perforant path. J. Neurosci. 18 (23), 9629–9637.

Caccamo, A., Oddo, S., Tran, L.X., LaFerla, F.M., 2007. Lithium reduces tau phosphorylation but not A beta or working memory deficits in a transgenic model with both plaques and tangles. Am. J. Pathol. 170 (5), 1669–1675.

Cai, H., Wang, Y., McCarthy, D., Wen, H., Borchelt, D.R., Price, D.L., Wong, P.C., 2001. BACE1 is the major beta-secretase for generation of Abeta peptides by neurons. Nat. Neurosci. 4 (3), 233–234.

Cajal, S. R. y, 1928. Degeneration and Regeneration of the Nervous System. Oxford Press, London.

Calabrese, B., Shaked, G.M., Tabarean, I.V., Braga, J., Koo, E.H., Halpain, S., 2007. Rapid, concurrent alterations in pre- and postsynaptic structure induced by naturally-secreted amyloid-beta protein. Mol. Cell. Neurosci. 35 (2), 183–193.

Caughey, B., Lansbury, P.T., 2003. Protofibrils, pores, fibrils, and neurodegeneration: separating the responsible protein aggregates from the innocent bystanders. Annu. Rev. Neurosci. 26, 267–298.

Chambon, C., Wegener, N., Gravius, A., Danysz, W., 2011. Behavioural and cellular effects of exogenous amyloid-β peptides in rodents. Behav. Brain Res. 225 (2), 623–641.

Chang, W.-P., Downs, D., Huang, X.-P., Da, H., Fung, K.-M., Tang, J., 2007. Amyloid-beta reduction by memapsin 2 (beta-secretase) immunization. FASEB J. 21 (12), 3184–3196.

Chang, W.-P., Koelsch, G., Wong, S., Downs, D., Da, H., Weerasena, V., Tang, J., 2004. In vivo inhibition of Abeta production by memapsin 2 (beta-secretase) inhibitors. J. Neurochem. 89 (6), 1409–1416.

Chapman, P.F., White, G.L., Jones, M.W., Cooper-Blacketer, D., Marshall, V.J., Irizarry, M., Hsiao, K.K., 1999. Impaired synaptic plasticity and learning in aged amyloid precursor protein transgenic mice. Nat. Neurosci. 2 (3), 271–276.

Chen, T.-F., Huang, R.-F.S., Lin, S.-E., Lu, J.-F., Tang, M.-C., Chiu, M.-J., 2010. Folic acid potentiates the effect of memantine on spatial learning and neuronal protection in an Alzheimer's disease transgenic model. J. Alzheimers Dis. 20 (2), 607–615.

Cissé, M., Halabisky, B., Harris, J., Devidze, N., Dubal, D.B., Sun, B., Mucke, L., 2011. Reversing EphB2 depletion rescues cognitive functions in Alzheimer model. Nature 469 (7328), 47–52.

Citri, A., Malenka, R.C., 2008. Synaptic plasticity: multiple forms, functions, and mechanisms. Neuropsychopharmacology 33 (1), 18–41.

Citron, M., Westaway, D., Xia, W., Carlson, G., Diehl, T., Levesque, G., Selkoe, D.J., 1997. Mutant presenilins of Alzheimer's disease increase production of 42-residue amyloid β-protein in both transfected cells and transgenic mice. Nat. Med. 3 (1), 67–72.

Cleary, J.P., Walsh, D.M., Hofmeister, J.J., Shankar, G.M., Kuskowski, M.A., Selkoe, D.J., Ashe, K.H., 2005. Natural oligomers of the amyloid-beta protein specifically disrupt cognitive function. Nat. Neurosci. 8 (1), 79–84.

Clements, A., Walsh, D.M., Williams, C.H., Allsop, D., 1993. Effects of the mutations Glu22 to Gln and Ala21 to Gly on the aggregation of a synthetic fragment of the Alzheimer's amyloid β/A4 peptide. Neurosci. Lett. 161 (1), 17–20.

Coleman, P., 2003. Synaptic slaughter in Alzheimer's disease. Neurobiol. Aging 24 (8), 1023–1027.

Comery, T.A., Martone, R.L., Aschmies, S., Atchison, K.P., Diamantidis, G., Gong, X., Marquis, K.L., 2005. Acute gamma-secretase inhibition improves contextual fear conditioning in the Tg2576 mouse model of Alzheimer's disease. J. Neurosci. 25 (39), 8898–8902.

Congdon, E.E., Wu, J.W., Myeku, N., Figueroa, Y.H., Herman, M., Marinec, P.S., Duff, K.E., 2012. Methylthioninium chloride (methylene blue) induces autophagy and attenuates tauopathy in vitro and in vivo. Autophagy 8 (4), 609–622.

Corder, E.H., Saunders, A.M., Strittmatter, W.J., Schmechel, D.E., Gaskell, P.C., Small, G.W., Pericak-Vance, M.A., 1993. Gene dose of apolipoprotein E type 4 allele and the risk of Alzheimer's disease in late onset families. Science 261 (5123), 921–923.

Crowe, A., James, M.J., Lee, V.M.-Y., Smith, A.B., Trojanowski, J.Q., Ballatore, C., Brunden, K.R., 2013. Aminothienopyridazines and methylene blue affect Tau fibrillization via cysteine oxidation. J. Biol. Chem. 288 (16), 11024–11037.

Cullen, W.K., Suh, Y.H., Anwyl, R., Rowan, M.J., 1997. Block of LTP in rat hippocampus in vivo by beta-amyloid precursor protein fragments. Neuroreport 8 (15), 3213–3217.

D'Amelio, M., Cavallucci, V., Middei, S., Marchetti, C., Pacioni, S., Ferri, A., Cecconi, F., 2011. Caspase-3 triggers early synaptic dysfunction in a mouse model of Alzheimer's disease. Nat. Neurosci. 14 (1), 69–76.

Das, P., Murphy, M.P., Younkin, L.H., Younkin, S.G., Golde, T.E., 2001. Reduced effectiveness of Abeta1-42 immunization in APP transgenic mice with significant amyloid deposition. Neurobiol. Aging 22 (5), 721–727.

Davies, C.A., Mann, D.M.A., Sumpter, P.Q., Yates, P.O., 1987. A quantitative morphometric analysis of the neuronal and synaptic content of the frontal and temporal cortex in patients with Alzheimer's disease. J. Neurol. Sci. 78 (2), 151–164.

De Felice, F.G., Wu, D., Lambert, M.P., Fernandez, S.J., Velasco, P.T., Lacor, P.N., Klein, W.L., 2008. Alzheimer's disease-type neuronal tau hyperphosphorylation induced by A beta oligomers. Neurobiol. Aging 29 (9), 1334–1347.

De Jonghe, C., Zehr, C., Yager, D., Prada, C.M., Younkin, S., Hendriks, L., Eckman, C.B., 1998. Flemish and Dutch mutations in amyloid beta precursor protein have different effects on amyloid beta secretion. Neurobiol. Dis. 5 (4), 281–286.

De Strooper, B., Annaert, W., 2000. Proteolytic processing and cell biological functions of the amyloid precursor protein. J. Cell Sci. 113 (Pt 1), 1857–1870.

Deiana, S., Harrington, C.R., Wischik, C.M., Riedel, G., 2009. Methylthioninium chloride reverses cognitive deficits induced by scopolamine: comparison with rivastigmine. Psychopharmacology 202 (1–3), 53–65.

DeKosky, S.T., Scheff, S.W., 1990. Synapse loss in frontal cortex biopsies in Alzheimer's disease: correlation with cognitive severity. Ann. Neurol. 27 (5), 457–464.

Delacourte, A., Sergeant, N., Champain, D., Wattez, A., Maurage, C.-A., Lebert, F., David, J.-P., 2002. Nonoverlapping but synergetic tau and APP pathologies in sporadic Alzheimer's disease. Neurology 59 (3), 398–407.

DeMattos, R.B., Bales, K.R., Cummins, D.J., Dodart, J.C., Paul, S.M., Holtzman, D.M., 2001. Peripheral anti-A beta antibody alters CNS and plasma A beta clearance and decreases brain A beta burden in a mouse model of Alzheimer's disease. Proc. Natl. Acad. Sci. U.S.A. 98 (15), 8850–8855.

Demuro, A., Mina, E., Kayed, R., Milton, S.C., Parker, I., Glabe, C.G., 2005. Calcium dysregulation and membrane disruption as a ubiquitous neurotoxic mechanism of soluble amyloid oligomers. J. Biol. Chem. 280 (17), 17294–17300.

Deshpande, A., Mina, E., Glabe, C., Busciglio, J., 2006. Different conformations of amyloid beta induce neurotoxicity by distinct mechanisms in human cortical neurons. J. Neurosci. 26 (22), 6011–6018.

Diarra, A., Geetha, T., Potter, P., Babu, J.R., 2009. Signaling of the neurotrophin receptor p75 in relation to Alzheimer's disease. Biochem. Biophys. Res. Commun. 390 (3), 352–356.

Dineley, K.T., Kayed, R., Neugebauer, V., Fu, Y., Zhang, W., Reese, L.C., Taglialatela, G., 2010. Amyloid-beta oligomers impair fear conditioned memory in a calcineurin-dependent fashion in mice. J. Neurosci. Res. 88 (13), 2923–2932.

Doble, B.W., Woodgett, J.R., 2003. GSK-3: tricks of the trade for a multi-tasking kinase. J. Cell Sci. 116 (Pt 7), 1175–1186.

Dodart, J.-C., Bales, K.R., Gannon, K.S., Greene, S.J., DeMattos, R.B., Mathis, C., Paul, S.M., 2002. Immunization reverses memory deficits without reducing brain Abeta burden in Alzheimer's disease model. Nat. Neurosci. 5 (5), 452–457.

Dong, H., Csernansky, C.A., Martin, M.V., Bertchume, A., Vallera, D., Csernansky, J.G., 2005. Acetylcholinesterase inhibitors ameliorate behavioral deficits in the Tg2576 mouse model of Alzheimer's disease. Psychopharmacology 181 (1), 145–152.

Doody, R.S., Thomas, R.G., Farlow, M., Iwatsubo, T., Vellas, B., Joffe, S., Mohs, R., 2014. Phase 3 trials of solanezumab for mild-to-moderate Alzheimer's disease. N. Engl. J. Med. 370 (4), 311–321.

Duff, K., Eckman, C., Zehr, C., Yu, X., Prada, C.M., Perez-tur, J., Younkin, S., 1996. Increased amyloid-beta42(43) in brains of mice expressing mutant presenilin 1. Nature 383 (6602), 710–713.

Eketjäll, S., Janson, J., Jeppsson, F., Svanhagen, A., Kolmodin, K., Gustavsson, S., Fälting, J., 2013. AZ-4217: a high potency BACE inhibitor displaying acute central efficacy in different in vivo models and reduced amyloid deposition in Tg2576 mice. J. Neurosci. 33 (24), 10075–10084.

Emmanouilidou, E., Melachroinou, K., Roumeliotis, T., Garbis, S.D., Ntzouni, M., Margaritis, L.H., Vekrellis, K., 2010. Cell-produced alpha-synuclein is secreted in a calcium-dependent manner by exosomes and impacts neuronal survival. J. Neurosci. 30 (20), 6838–6851.

Engert, F., Bonhoeffer, T., 1999. Dendritic spine changes associated with hippocampal long-term synaptic plasticity. Nature 399 (6731), 66–70.

Esteban, J.A., Shi, S.-H., Wilson, C., Nuriya, M., Huganir, R.L., Malinow, R., 2003. PKA phosphorylation of AMPA receptor subunits controls synaptic trafficking underlying plasticity. Nat. Neurosci. 6 (2), 136–143.

Ferreira, A., Caceres, A., Kosik, K.S., 1993. Intraneuronal compartments of the amyloid precursor protein. J. Neurosci. 13 (7), 3112–3123.

Fitzjohn, S.M., Morton, R.A., Kuenzi, F., Rosahl, T.W., Shearman, M., Lewis, H., Seabrook, G.R., 2001. Age-related impairment of synaptic transmission but normal long-term potentiation in transgenic mice that overexpress the human APP695SWE mutant form of amyloid precursor protein. J. Neurosci. 21 (13), 4691–4698.

Fraser, P.E., Nguyen, J.T., Inouye, H., Surewicz, W.K., Selkoe, D.J., Podlisny, M.B., Kirschner, D.A., 1992. Fibril formation by primate, rodent, and Dutch-hemorrhagic analogs of Alzheimer amyloid beta-protein. Biochemistry 31 (44), 10716–10723.

Fu, M., Yu, X., Lu, J., Zuo, Y., 2012. Repetitive motor learning induces coordinated formation of clustered dendritic spines in vivo. Nature 483 (7387), 92–95.

Fukumoto, H., Takahashi, H., Tarui, N., Matsui, J., Tomita, T., Hirode, M., Miyamoto, M., 2010a. A noncompetitive BACE1 inhibitor TAK-070 ameliorates Abeta pathology and behavioral deficits in a mouse model of Alzheimer's disease. J. Neurosci. 30 (33), 11157–11166.

Fukumoto, H., Tokuda, T., Kasai, T., Ishigami, N., Hidaka, H., Kondo, M., Nakagawa, M., 2010b. High-molecular-weight beta-amyloid oligomers are elevated in cerebrospinal fluid of Alzheimer patients. FASEB J. 24 (8), 2716–2726.

Games, D., Adams, D., Alessandrini, R., Barbour, R., Berthelette, P., Blackwell, C., Gillespie, F., 1995. Alzheimer-type neuropathology in transgenic mice overexpressing V717F beta-amyloid precursor protein. Nature 373 (6514), 523–527.

Geinisman, Y., n.d. Age-related decline in memory function: is it associated with a loss of synapses? Neurobiol. Aging 20 (3), 353–356. Discussion 359–60.

Gengler, S., Hamilton, A., Hölscher, C., 2010. Synaptic plasticity in the hippocampus of a APP/PS1 mouse model of Alzheimer's disease is impaired in old but not young mice. PloS One 5 (3), e9764.

Georganopoulou, D.G., Chang, L., Nam, J.-M., Thaxton, C.S., Mufson, E.J., Klein, W.L., Mirkin, C.A., 2005. Nanoparticle-based detection in cerebral spinal fluid of a soluble pathogenic biomarker for Alzheimer's disease. Proc. Natl. Acad. Sci. U.S.A. 102 (7), 2273–2276.

Geula, C., Wu, C.K., Saroff, D., Lorenzo, A., Yuan, M., Yankner, B.A., 1998. Aging renders the brain vulnerable to amyloid beta-protein neurotoxicity. Nat. Med. 4 (7), 827–831.

Ghoreschi, K., Laurence, A., O'Shea, J.J., 2009. Selectivity and therapeutic inhibition of kinases: to be or not to be? Nat. Immunol. 10 (4), 356–360.

Giannakopoulos, P., Herrmann, F.R., Bussière, T., Bouras, C., Kövari, E., Perl, D.P., Hof, P.R., 2003. Tangle and neuron numbers, but not amyloid load, predict cognitive status in Alzheimer's disease. Neurology 60 (9), 1495–1500.

Glabe, C.G., 2008. Structural classification of toxic amyloid oligomers. J. Biol. Chem. 283 (44), 29639–29643.

Glenner, G.G., Wong, C.W., 1984. Alzheimer's disease: Initial report of the purification and characterization of a novel cerebrovascular amyloid protein. Biochem. Biophys. Res. Commun. 120 (3), 885–890.

Goate, A., Chartier-Harlin, M.C., Mullan, M., Brown, J., Crawford, F., Fidani, L., James, L., 1991. Segregation of a missense mutation in the amyloid precursor protein gene with familial Alzheimer's disease. Nature 349 (6311), 704–706.

Goldgaber, D., Lerman, M.I., McBride, O.W., Saffiotti, U., Gajdusek, D.C., 1987. Characterization and chromosomal localization of a cDNA encoding brain amyloid of Alzheimer's disease. Science 235 (4791), 877–880.

Gómez-Isla, T., Hollister, R., West, H., Mui, S., Growdon, J.H., Petersen, R.C., Hyman, B.T., 1997. Neuronal loss correlates with but exceeds neurofibrillary tangles in Alzheimer's disease. Ann. Neurol. 41 (1), 17–24.

Gong, C.-X., Iqbal, K., 2008. Hyperphosphorylation of microtubule-associated protein tau: a promising therapeutic target for Alzheimer disease. Curr. Med. Chem. 15 (23), 2321–2328.

Green, K.N., LaFerla, F.M., 2008. Linking calcium to Abeta and Alzheimer's disease. Neuron 59 (2), 190–194.

Gureviciene, I., Ikonen, S., Gurevicius, K., Sarkaki, A., van Groen, T., Pussinen, R., Tanila, H., 2004. Normal induction but accelerated decay of LTP in APP+PS1 transgenic mice. Neurobiol. Dis. 15 (2), 188–195.

Haass, C., Schlossmacher, M.G., Hung, A.Y., Vigo-Pelfrey, C., Mellon, A., Ostaszewski, B.L., Teplow, D.B., 1992. Amyloid beta-peptide is produced by cultured cells during normal metabolism. Nature 359 (6393), 322–325.

Haass, C., Selkoe, D.J., 2007. Soluble protein oligomers in neurodegeneration: lessons from the Alzheimer's amyloid beta-peptide. Nat. Rev. Mol. Cell Biol. 8 (2), 101–112.

Hanger, D.P., Anderton, B.H., Noble, W., 2009. Tau phosphorylation: the therapeutic challenge for neurodegenerative disease. Trends Mol. Med. 15 (3), 112–119.

Hardy, J.A., Higgins, G.A., 1992. Alzheimer's disease: the amyloid cascade hypothesis. Science 256 (5054), 184–185.

Hardy, J., Allsop, D., 1991. Amyloid deposition as the central event in the aetiology of Alzheimer's disease. Trends Pharmacol. Sci. 12 (10), 383–388.

Hardy, J., Selkoe, D.J., 2002. The amyloid hypothesis of Alzheimer's disease: progress and problems on the road to therapeutics. Science 297 (5580), 353–356.

Harper, J.D., Wong, S.S., Lieber, C.M., Lansbury, P.T., 1997. Observation of metastable Abeta amyloid protofibrils by atomic force microscopy. Chem. Biol. 4 (2), 119–125.

Harris, J.A., Devidze, N., Halabisky, B., Lo, I., Thwin, M.T., Yu, G.-Q., Mucke, L., 2010. Many neuronal and behavioral impairments in transgenic mouse models of Alzheimer's disease are independent of caspase cleavage of the amyloid precursor protein. J. Neurosci. 30 (1), 372–381.

Hartley, D.M., Walsh, D.M., Ye, C.P., Diehl, T., Vasquez, S., Vassilev, P.M., Selkoe, D.J., 1999. Protofibrillar intermediates of amyloid beta-protein induce acute electrophysiological changes and progressive neurotoxicity in cortical neurons. J. Neurosci. 19 (20), 8876–8884.

Hartley, D.M., Zhao, C., Speier, A.C., Woodard, G.A., Li, S., Li, Z., Walz, T., 2008. Transglutaminase induces protofibril-like amyloid beta-protein assemblies that are protease-resistant and inhibit long-term potentiation. J. Biol. Chem. 283 (24), 16790–16800.

Hartmann, D., de Strooper, B., Serneels, L., Craessaerts, K., Herreman, A., Annaert, W., Saftig, P., 2002. The disintegrin/metalloprotease ADAM 10 is essential for notch signalling but not for alpha-secretase activity in fibroblasts. Hum. Mol. Genet. 11 (21), 2615–2624.

Hasegawa, K., Yamaguchi, I., Omata, S., Gejyo, F., Naiki, H., 1999. Interaction between A beta (1-42) and A beta(1-40) in Alzheimer's beta-amyloid fibril formation in vitro. Biochemistry 38 (47), 15514–15521.

Hasegawa, M., Morishima-Kawashima, M., Takio, K., Suzuki, M., Titani, K., Ihara, Y., 1992. Protein sequence and mass spectrometric analyses of tau in the Alzheimer's disease brain. J. Biol. Chem. 267 (24), 17047–17054.

Hebb, D.O., 1949. A Neuropsychological Theory. Lawrence Erlbaum Associates, Mahwah NJ.

Heneka, M.T., Kummer, M.P., Latz, E., 2014. Innate immune activation in neurodegenerative disease. Nat. Rev. Immunol. 14, 463–477.

Hernández, F., Borrell, J., Guaza, C., Avila, J., Lucas, J.J., 2002. Spatial learning deficit in transgenic mice that conditionally over-express GSK-3beta in the brain but do not form tau filaments. J. Neurochem. 83 (6), 1529–1533.

Herreman, A., Hartmann, D., Annaert, W., Saftig, P., Craessaerts, K., Serneels, L., De Strooper, B., 1999. Presenilin 2 deficiency causes a mild pulmonary phenotype and no changes in amyloid precursor protein processing but enhances the embryonic lethal phenotype of presenilin 1 deficiency. Proc. Natl. Acad. Sci. U.S.A. 96 (21), 11872–11877.

Hillen, H., Barghorn, S., Striebinger, A., Labkovsky, B., Müller, R., Nimmrich, V., Ebert, U., 2010. Generation and therapeutic efficacy of highly oligomer-specific beta-amyloid antibodies. J. Neurosci. 30 (31), 10369–10379.

Hoshi, M., Sato, M., Matsumoto, S., Noguchi, A., Yasutake, K., Yoshida, N., Sato, K., 2003. Spherical aggregates of beta-amyloid (amylospheroid) show high neurotoxicity and activate tau protein kinase I/glycogen synthase kinase-3beta. Proc. Natl. Acad. Sci. U.S.A. 100 (11), 6370–6375.

Hsia, A.Y., Masliah, E., McConlogue, L., Yu, G.Q., Tatsuno, G., Hu, K., Mucke, L., 1999. Plaque-independent disruption of neural circuits in Alzheimer's disease mouse models. Proc. Natl. Acad. Sci. U.S.A. 96 (6), 3228–3233.

Hsiao, K., 1998. Transgenic mice expressing Alzheimer amyloid precursor proteins. Experimental Gerontology 33 (7–8), 883–889.

Hsiao, K., Chapman, P., Nilsen, S., Eckman, C., Harigaya, Y., Younkin, S., Cole, G., 1996. Correlative memory deficits, Abeta elevation, and amyloid plaques in transgenic mice. Science 274 (5284), 99–102.

Hsieh, H., Boehm, J., Sato, C., Iwatsubo, T., Tomita, T., Sisodia, S., Malinow, R., 2006. AMPAR removal underlies Abeta-induced synaptic depression and dendritic spine loss. Neuron 52 (5), 831–843.

Hu, N.-W., Klyubin, I., Anwyl, R., Anwy, R., Rowan, M.J., 2009. GluN2B subunit-containing NMDA receptor antagonists prevent Abeta-mediated synaptic plasticity disruption in vivo. Proc. Natl. Acad. Sci. U.S.A. 106 (48), 20504–20509.

Hu, N.-W., Nicoll, A.J., Zhang, D., Mably, A.J., O'Malley, T., Purro, S.A., Rowan, M.J., 2014. mGlu5 receptors and cellular prion protein mediate amyloid-β-facilitated synaptic long-term depression in vivo. Nat. Commun. 5, 3374.

Hu, N.-W., Smith, I.M., Walsh, D.M., Rowan, M.J., 2008. Soluble amyloid-beta peptides potently disrupt hippocampal synaptic plasticity in the absence of cerebrovascular dysfunction in vivo. Brain 131 (Pt 9), 2414–2424.

Hu, X., Hicks, C.W., He, W., Wong, P., Macklin, W.B., Trapp, B.D., Yan, R., 2006. Bace1 modulates myelination in the central and peripheral nervous system. Nat. Neurosci. 9 (12), 1520–1525.

Huang, W.-H., Sheng, R., Hu, Y.-Z., 2009. Progress in the development of nonpeptidomimetic BACE 1 inhibitors for Alzheimer's disease. Curr. Med. Chem. 16 (14), 1806–1820.

Hüls, S., Högen, T., Vassallo, N., Danzer, K.M., Hengerer, B., Giese, A., Herms, J., 2011. AMPA-receptor-mediated excitatory synaptic transmission is enhanced by iron-induced α-synuclein oligomers. J. Neurochem. 117 (5), 868–878.

Hussain, I., Hawkins, J., Harrison, D., Hille, C., Wayne, G., Cutler, L., Davis, J.B., 2007. Oral administration of a potent and selective non-peptidic BACE-1 inhibitor decreases beta-cleavage of amyloid precursor protein and amyloid-beta production in vivo. J. Neurochem. 100 (3), 802–809.

Hyman, B.T., Marzloff, K., Arriagada, P.V., 1993. The lack of accumulation of senile plaques or amyloid burden in Alzheimer's disease suggests a dynamic balance between amyloid deposition and resolution. J. Neuropathol. Exp. Neurol. 52 (6), 594–600.

Hyman, B.T., Van Hoesen, G.W., Kromer, L.J., Damasio, A.R., 1986. Perforant pathway changes and the memory impairment of Alzheimer's disease. Ann. Neurol. 20 (4), 472–481.

Imahori, K., Uchida, T., 1997. Physiology and pathology of tau protein kinases in relation to Alzheimer's disease. J. Biochem. 121 (2), 179–188.

Imbimbo, B.P., Hutter-Paier, B., Villetti, G., Facchinetti, F., Cenacchi, V., Volta, R., Windisch, M., 2009. CHF5074, a novel gamma-secretase modulator, attenuates brain beta-amyloid pathology and learning deficit in a mouse model of Alzheimer's disease. Br. J. Pharmacol. 156 (6), 982–993.

Ingelsson, M., Fukumoto, H., Newell, K.L., Growdon, J.H., Hedley-Whyte, E.T., Frosch, M.P., Irizarry, M.C., 2004. Early Abeta accumulation and progressive synaptic loss, gliosis, and tangle formation in AD brain. Neurology 62 (6), 925–931.

Irizarry, M.C., McNamara, M., Fedorchak, K., Hsiao, K., Hyman, B.T., 1997a. APPSw transgenic mice develop age-related A beta deposits and neuropil abnormalities, but no neuronal loss in CA1. J. Neuropathol. Exp. Neurol. 56 (9), 965–973.

Irizarry, M.C., Soriano, F., McNamara, M., Page, K.J., Schenk, D., Games, D., Hyman, B.T., 1997b. Abeta deposition is associated with neuropil changes, but not with overt neuronal loss in the human amyloid precursor protein V717F (PDAPP) transgenic mouse. J. Neurosci. 17 (18), 7053–7059.

Jack, C.R., Holtzman, D.M., 2013. Biomarker modeling of Alzheimer's disease. Neuron 80 (6), 1347–1358.

Jack Jr, C.R., Knopman, D.S., Jagust, W.J., et al., 2013. Tracking pathophysiological processes in Alzheimer's disease: an updated hypothetical model of dynamic biomarkers. Lancet Neurol 12, 207–216.

Jacobsen, J.S., Wu, C.-C., Redwine, J.M., Comery, T.A., Arias, R., Bowlby, M., Bloom, F.E., 2006. Early-onset behavioral and synaptic deficits in a mouse model of Alzheimer's disease. Proc. Natl. Acad. Sci. U.S.A. 103 (13), 5161–5166.

Janus, C., Pearson, J., McLaurin, J., Mathews, P.M., Jiang, Y., Schmidt, S.D., Westaway, D., 2000. A beta peptide immunization reduces behavioural impairment and plaques in a model of Alzheimer's disease. Nature 408 (6815), 979–982.

Jarrett, J.T., Berger, E.P., Lansbury, P.T., 1993. The carboxy terminus of the beta amyloid protein is critical for the seeding of amyloid formation: implications for the pathogenesis of Alzheimer's disease. Biochemistry 32 (18), 4693–4697.

Jawhar, S., Wirths, O., Bayer, T.A., 2011. Pyroglutamate amyloid-β (Aβ): a hatchet man in Alzheimer disease. J. Biol. Chem. 286 (45), 38825–38832.

Jin, M., Shepardson, N., Yang, T., Chen, G., Walsh, D., Selkoe, D.J., 2011. Soluble amyloid beta-protein dimers isolated from Alzheimer cortex directly induce Tau hyperphosphorylation and neuritic degeneration. Proc. Natl. Acad. Sci. U.S.A. 108 (14), 5819–5824.

Jo, J., Whitcomb, D.J., Olsen, K.M., Kerrigan, T.L., Lo, S.-C., Bru-Mercier, G., Cho, K., 2011. Aβ(1-42) inhibition of LTP is mediated by a signaling pathway involving caspase-3, Akt1 and GSK-3β. Nat. Neurosci. 14 (5), 545–547.

Johnson-Wood, K., Lee, M., Motter, R., Hu, K., Gordon, G., Barbour, R., McConlogue, L., 1997. Amyloid precursor protein processing and A 42 deposition in a transgenic mouse model of Alzheimer disease. Proc. Natl. Acad. Sci. U.S.A. 94 (4), 1550–1555.

Kaether, C., Skehel, P., Dotti, C.G., 2000. Axonal membrane proteins are transported in distinct carriers: a two-color video microscopy study in cultured hippocampal neurons. Mol. Biol. Cell 11 (4), 1213–1224.

Kamenetz, F., Tomita, T., Hsieh, H., Seabrook, G., Borchelt, D., Iwatsubo, T., Malinow, R., 2003. APP processing and synaptic function. Neuron 37 (6), 925–937.

Kang, J., Lemaire, H.G., Unterbeck, A., Salbaum, J.M., Masters, C.L., Grzeschik, K.H., Müller-Hill, B., 1987. The precursor of Alzheimer's disease amyloid A4 protein resembles a cell-surface receptor. Nature 325 (6106), 733–736.

Kasai, H., Fukuda, M., Watanabe, S., Hayashi-Takagi, A., Noguchi, J., 2010. Structural dynamics of dendritic spines in memory and cognition. Trends Neurosci. 33 (3), 121–129.

Kasai, H., Matsuzaki, M., Noguchi, J., Yasumatsu, N., Nakahara, H., 2003. Structure-stability-function relationships of dendritic spines. Trends Neurosci. 26 (7), 360–368.

Kayed, R., Head, E., Thompson, J.L., McIntire, T.M., Milton, S.C., Cotman, C.W., Glabe, C.G., 2003. Common structure of soluble amyloid oligomers implies common mechanism of pathogenesis. Science 300 (5618), 486–489.

Kayed, R., Sokolov, Y., Edmonds, B., McIntire, T.M., Milton, S.C., Hall, J.E., Glabe, C.G., 2004. Permeabilization of lipid bilayers is a common conformation-dependent activity of soluble amyloid oligomers in protein misfolding diseases. J. Biol. Chem. 279 (45), 46363–46366.

Kemp, N., Bashir, Z.I., 2001. Long-term depression: a cascade of induction and expression mechanisms. Prog. Neurobiol. 65 (4), 339–365.

Kessels, H.W., Kopec, C.D., Klein, M.E., Malinow, R., 2009. Roles of stargazin and phosphorylation in the control of AMPA receptor subcellular distribution. Nat. Neurosci. 12 (7), 888–896.

Kessels, H.W., Malinow, R., 2009. Synaptic AMPA receptor plasticity and behavior. Neuron 61 (3), 340–350.

Kessels, H.W., Nabavi, S., Malinow, R., 2013. Metabotropic NMDA receptor function is required for β-amyloid-induced synaptic depression. Proc. Natl. Acad. Sci. U.S.A. 110 (10), 4033–4038.

Kessels, H.W., Nguyen, L.N., Nabavi, S., Malinow, R., 2010. The prion protein as a receptor for amyloid-beta. Nature 466 (7308), E3–E4. Discussion E4–5.

Kimura, T., Whitcomb, D.J., Jo, J., Regan, P., Piers, T., Heo, S., Cho, K., 2014. Microtubule-associated protein tau is essential for long-term depression in the hippocampus. Philos. Trans. R. Soc. Lond. B Biol. Sci. 369 (1633), 20130144.

Klein, W.L., Krafft, G.A., Finch, C.E., 2001. Targeting small Abeta oligomers: the solution to an Alzheimer's disease conundrum? Trends Neurosci. 24 (4), 219–224.

Klyubin, I., Betts, V., Welzel, A.T., Blennow, K., Zetterberg, H., Wallin, A., Rowan, M.J., 2008. Amyloid beta protein dimer-containing human CSF disrupts synaptic plasticity: prevention by systemic passive immunization. J. Neurosci. 28 (16), 4231–4237.

Klyubin, I., Cullen, W.K., Hu, N.-W., Rowan, M.J., 2012. Alzheimer's disease Aβ assemblies mediating rapid disruption of synaptic plasticity and memory. Mol. Brain 5 (1), 25.

Klyubin, I., Walsh, D.M., Cullen, W.K., Fadeeva, J.V., Anwyl, R., Selkoe, D.J., Rowan, M.J., 2004. Soluble Arctic amyloid beta protein inhibits hippocampal long-term potentiation in vivo. Eur. J. Neurosci. 19 (10), 2839–2846.

Klyubin, I., Walsh, D.M., Lemere, C.A., Cullen, W.K., Shankar, G.M., Betts, V., Rowan, M.J., 2005. Amyloid beta protein immunotherapy neutralizes Abeta oligomers that disrupt synaptic plasticity in vivo. Nat. Med. 11 (5), 556–561.

Knafo, S., Alonso-Nanclares, L., Gonzalez-Soriano, J., Merino-Serrais, P., Fernaud-Espinosa, I., Ferrer, I., DeFelipe, J., 2009. Widespread changes in dendritic spines in a model of Alzheimer's disease. Cereb. Cortex 19 (3), 586–592.

Knopman, D.S., Parisi, J.E., Salviati, A., Floriach-Robert, M., Boeve, B.F., Ivnik, R.J., Petersen, R.C., 2003. Neuropathology of cognitively normal elderly. J. Neuropathol. Exp. Neurol. 62 (11), 1087–1095.

Koffie, R.M., Meyer-Luehmann, M., Hashimoto, T., Adams, K.W., Mielke, M.L., Garcia-Alloza, M., Spires-Jones, T.L., 2009. Oligomeric amyloid beta associates with postsynaptic densities and correlates with excitatory synapse loss near senile plaques. Proc. Natl. Acad. Sci. U.S.A. 106 (10), 4012–4017.

Koo, E.H., Sisodia, S.S., Archer, D.R., Martin, L.J., Weidemann, A., Beyreuther, K., Price, D.L., 1990. Precursor of amyloid protein in Alzheimer disease undergoes fast anterograde axonal transport. Proc. Natl. Acad. Sci. U.S.A. 87 (4), 1561–1565.

Kopec, C.D., Li, B., Wei, W., Boehm, J., Malinow, R., 2006. Glutamate receptor exocytosis and spine enlargement during chemically induced long-term potentiation. J. Neurosci. 26 (7), 2000–2009.

Kummer, M.P., Hermes, M., Delekarte, A., Hammerschmidt, T., Kumar, S., Terwel, D., Heneka, M.T., 2011. Nitration of tyrosine 10 critically enhances amyloid β aggregation and plaque formation. Neuron 71 (5), 833–844.

Kuperstein, I., Broersen, K., Benilova, I., Rozenski, J., Jonckheere, W., Debulpaep, M., De Strooper, B., 2010. Neurotoxicity of Alzheimer's disease Aβ peptides is induced by small changes in the Aβ42 to Aβ40 ratio. EMBO J. 29 (19), 3408–3420.

Lacor, P.N., Buniel, M.C., Furlow, P.W., Clemente, A.S., Velasco, P.T., Wood, M., Klein, W.L., 2007. Abeta oligomer-induced aberrations in synapse composition, shape, and density provide a molecular basis for loss of connectivity in Alzheimer's disease. J. Neurosci. 27 (4), 796–807.

LaFerla, F.M., Green, K.N., Oddo, S., 2007. Intracellular amyloid-beta in Alzheimer's disease. Nat. Rev. Neurosci. 8 (7), 499–509.

Laird, F.M., Cai, H., Savonenko, A.V., Farah, M.H., He, K., Melnikova, T., Wong, P.C., 2005. BACE1, a major determinant of selective vulnerability of the brain to amyloid-beta amyloidogenesis, is essential for cognitive, emotional, and synaptic functions. J. Neurosci. 25 (50), 11693–11709.

Lambert, M.P., Barlow, A.K., Chromy, B.A., Edwards, C., Freed, R., Liosatos, M., Klein, W.L., 1998. Diffusible, nonfibrillar ligands derived from A 1-42 are potent central nervous system neurotoxins. Proc. Natl. Acad. Sci. U.S.A. 95 (11), 6448–6453.

Lambert, M.P., Velasco, P.T., Viola, K.L., Klein, W.L., 2009. Targeting generation of antibodies specific to conformational epitopes of amyloid beta-derived neurotoxins. CNS Neurol. Disord. Drug Targets 8 (1), 65–81.

Lamprecht, R., LeDoux, J., 2004. Structural plasticity and memory. Nat. Rev. Neurosci. 5 (1), 45–54.

Lanz, T.A., Carter, D.B., Merchant, K.M., 2003. Dendritic spine loss in the hippocampus of young PDAPP and Tg2576 mice and its prevention by the ApoE2 genotype. Neurobiol. Dis. 13 (3), 246–253.

Larson, J., Lynch, G., Games, D., Seubert, P., 1999. Alterations in synaptic transmission and long-term potentiation in hippocampal slices from young and aged PDAPP mice. Brain Res. 840 (1–2), 23–35.

Lasagna-Reeves, C.A., Castillo-Carranza, D.L., Sengupta, U., Clos, A.L., Jackson, G.R., Kayed, R., 2011a. Tau oligomers impair memory and induce synaptic and mitochondrial dysfunction in wild-type mice. Molecular Neurodegeneration 6, 39.

Lasagna-Reeves, C.A., Glabe, C.G., Kayed, R., 2011b. Amyloid-β annular protofibrils evade fibrillar fate in Alzheimer disease brain. J. Biol. Chem. 286 (25), 22122–22130.

Lashuel, H.A., Hartley, D., Petre, B.M., Walz, T., Lansbury, P.T., 2002. Neurodegenerative disease: amyloid pores from pathogenic mutations. Nature 418 (6895), 291.

Laurén, J., Gimbel, D.A., Nygaard, H.B., Gilbert, J.W., Strittmatter, S.M., 2009. Cellular prion protein mediates impairment of synaptic plasticity by amyloid-beta oligomers. Nature 457 (7233), 1128–1132.

Lazarov, O., Lee, M., Peterson, D.A., Sisodia, S.S., 2002. Evidence that synaptically released beta-amyloid accumulates as extracellular deposits in the hippocampus of transgenic mice. J. Neurosci. 22 (22), 9785–9793.

Lee, C.Y.D., Landreth, G.E., 2010. The role of microglia in amyloid clearance from the AD brain. J. Neural Transm. 117 (8), 949–960.

Lee, D.C., Sunnarborg, S.W., Hinkle, C.L., Myers, T.J., Stevenson, M.Y., Russell, W.E., Jackson, L.F., 2003. TACE/ADAM17 processing of EGFR ligands indicates a role as a physiological convertase. Ann. N.Y. Acad. Sci. 995, 22–38.

Lee, J.-H., Yu, W.H., Kumar, A., Lee, S., Mohan, P.S., Peterhoff, C.M., Nixon, R.A., 2010. Lysosomal proteolysis and autophagy require presenilin 1 and are disrupted by Alzheimer-related PS1 mutations. Cell 141 (7), 1146–1158.

Lemere, C.A., Lopera, F., Kosik, K.S., Lendon, C.L., Ossa, J., Saido, T.C., Arango, V.J.C., 1996. The E280A presenilin 1 Alzheimer mutation produces increased Aβ42 deposition and severe cerebellar pathology. Nat. Med. 2 (10), 1146–1150.

Lemere, C.A., Maron, R., Selkoe, D.J., Weiner, H.L., 2001. Nasal vaccination with beta-amyloid peptide for the treatment of Alzheimer's disease. DNA Cell Biol. 20 (11), 705–711.

Lerchner, A., Machauer, R., Betschart, C., Veenstra, S., Rueeger, H., McCarthy, C., Neumann, U., 2010. Macrocyclic BACE-1 inhibitors acutely reduce Abeta in brain after po application. Bioorg. Med. Chem. Lett. 20 (2), 603–607.

Lesné, S., Koh, M.T., Kotilinek, L., Kayed, R., Glabe, C.G., Yang, A., Ashe, K.H., 2006. A specific amyloid-beta protein assembly in the brain impairs memory. Nature 440 (7082), 352–357.

Levy, E., Carman, M.D., Fernandez-Madrid, I.J., Power, M.D., Lieberburg, I., van Duinen, S.G., Frangione, B., 1990. Mutation of the Alzheimer's disease amyloid gene in hereditary cerebral hemorrhage, Dutch type. Science 248 (4959), 1124–1126.

Lewis, J., Dickson, D.W., Lin, W.L., Chisholm, L., Corral, A., Jones, G., McGowan, E., 2001. Enhanced neurofibrillary degeneration in transgenic mice expressing mutant tau and APP. Science 293 (5534), 1487–1491.

Li, S., Hong, S., Shepardson, N.E., Walsh, D.M., Shankar, G.M., Selkoe, D., 2009. Soluble oligomers of amyloid beta protein facilitate hippocampal long-term depression by disrupting neuronal glutamate uptake. Neuron 62 (6), 788–801.

Li, S., Jin, M., Koeglsperger, T., Shepardson, N.E., Shankar, G.M., Selkoe, D.J., 2011. Soluble Aβ oligomers inhibit long-term potentiation through a mechanism involving excessive activation of extrasynaptic NR2B-containing NMDA receptors. J. Neurosci. 31 (18), 6627–6638.

Li, Z., Jo, J., Jia, J.-M., Lo, S.-C., Whitcomb, D.J., Jiao, S., Sheng, M., 2010. Caspase-3 activation via mitochondria is required for long-term depression and AMPA receptor internalization. Cell 141 (5), 859–871.

Lucas, J.J., Hernández, F., Gómez-Ramos, P., Morán, M.A., Hen, R., Avila, J., 2001. Decreased nuclear beta-catenin, tau hyperphosphorylation and neurodegeneration in GSK-3beta conditional transgenic mice. EMBO J. 20 (1–2), 27–39.

Lue, L.-F., Kuo, Y.-M., Roher, A.E., Brachova, L., Shen, Y., Sue, L., Rogers, J., 1999. Soluble amyloid β peptide concentration as a predictor of synaptic change in Alzheimer's disease. Am. J. Pathol. 155 (3), 853–862.

Luo, Y., Bolon, B., Kahn, S., Bennett, B.D., Babu-Khan, S., Denis, P., Vassar, R., 2001. Mice deficient in BACE1, the Alzheimer's beta-secretase, have normal phenotype and abolished beta-amyloid generation. Nat. Neurosci. 4 (3), 231–232.

Lynch, M.A., 2004. Long-term potentiation and memory. Physiol. Rev. 84 (1), 87–136.

Malenka, R.C., Bear, M.F., 2004. LTP and LTD: an embarrassment of riches. Neuron 44 (1), 5–21.

Maletic-Savatic, M., Malinow, R., Svoboda, K., 1999. Rapid dendritic morphogenesis in CA1 hippocampal dendrites induced by synaptic activity. Science 283 (5409), 1923–1927.

Mann, D.M., 1988. Alzheimer's disease and Down's syndrome. Histopathology 13 (2), 125–137.

Mann, D.M., Yates, P.O., Marcyniuk, B., 1984. Alzheimer's presenile dementia, senile dementia of Alzheimer type and Down's syndrome in middle age form an age related continuum of pathological changes. Neuropathol. Appl. Neurobiol. 10 (3), 185–207.

Martin, S.J., Morris, R.G.M., 2002. New life in an old idea: the synaptic plasticity and memory hypothesis revisited. Hippocampus 12 (5), 609–636.

Martin, Z.S., Neugebauer, V., Dineley, K.T., Kayed, R., Zhang, W., Reese, L.C., Taglialatela, G., 2012. α-Synuclein oligomers oppose long-term potentiation and impair memory through a calcineurin-dependent mechanism: relevance to human synucleopathic diseases. J. Neurochem. 120 (3), 440–452.

Martinez-Coria, H., Green, K.N., Billings, L.M., Kitazawa, M., Albrecht, M., Rammes, G., LaFerla, F.M., 2010. Memantine improves cognition and reduces Alzheimer's-like neuropathology in transgenic mice. Am. J. Pathol. 176 (2), 870–880.

Martins, I.C., Kuperstein, I., Wilkinson, H., Maes, E., Vanbrabant, M., Jonckheere, W., Rousseau, F., 2008. Lipids revert inert Abeta amyloid fibrils to neurotoxic protofibrils that affect learning in mice. EMBO J. 27 (1), 224–233.

Martone, R.L., Zhou, H., Atchison, K., Comery, T., Xu, J.Z., Huang, X., Jacobsen, J.S., 2009. Begacestat (GSI-953): a novel, selective thiophene sulfonamide inhibitor of amyloid precursor protein gamma-secretase for the treatment of Alzheimer's disease. J. Pharmacol. Exp. Ther. 331 (2), 598–608.

Masliah, E., Mallory, M., Alford, M., DeTeresa, R., Hansen, L.A., McKeel, D.W., Morris, J.C., 2001. Altered expression of synaptic proteins occurs early during progression of Alzheimer's disease. Neurology 56 (1), 127–129.

Masliah, E., Mallory, M., Hansen, L., DeTeresa, R., Alford, M., Terry, R., 1994. Synaptic and neuritic alterations during the progression of Alzheimer's disease. Neurosci. Lett. 174 (1), 67–72.

Masliah, E., Terry, R.D., Mallory, M., Alford, M., Hansen, L.A., 1990. Diffuse plaques do not accentuate synapse loss in Alzheimer's disease. Am. J. Pathol. 137 (6), 1293–1297.

Masters, C.L., Simms, G., Weinman, N.A., Multhaup, G., McDonald, B.L., Beyreuther, K., 1985. Amyloid plaque core protein in Alzheimer disease and Down syndrome. Proc. Natl. Acad. Sci. U.S.A. 82 (12), 4245–4249.

Matsumura, S., Shinoda, K., Yamada, M., Yokojima, S., Inoue, M., Ohnishi, T., Hoshi, M., 2011. Two distinct amyloid beta-protein (Abeta) assembly pathways leading to oligomers and fibrils identified by combined fluorescence correlation spectroscopy, morphology, and toxicity analyses. J. Biol. Chem. 286 (13), 11555–11562.

Matsuo, E.S., Shin, R.W., Billingsley, M.L., Van deVoorde, A., O'Connor, M., Trojanowski, J.Q., Lee, V.M., 1994. Biopsy-derived adult human brain tau is phosphorylated at many of the same sites as Alzheimer's disease paired helical filament tau. Neuron 13 (4), 989–1002.

Matsuzaki, M., Honkura, N., Ellis-Davies, G.C.R., Kasai, H., 2004. Structural basis of long-term potentiation in single dendritic spines. Nature 429 (6993), 761–766.

Mawuenyega, K.G., Sigurdson, W., Ovod, V., Munsell, L., Kasten, T., Morris, J.C., Yarasheski, K.E., Bateman, R.J., 2010. Decreased clearance of CNS beta-amyloid in Alzheimer's disease. Science 330, 1774.

Mazanetz, M.P., Fischer, P.M., 2007. Untangling tau hyperphosphorylation in drug design for neurodegenerative diseases. Nat. Rev. Drug Discov. 6 (6), 464–479.

McLean, C.A., Cherny, R.A., Fraser, F.W., Fuller, S.J., Smith, M.J., Beyreuther, K., Masters, C.L., 1999. Soluble pool of Abeta amyloid as a determinant of severity of neurodegeneration in Alzheimer's disease. Ann. Neurol. 46 (6), 860–866.

Medina, D.X., Caccamo, A., Oddo, S., 2011. Methylene blue reduces aβ levels and rescues early cognitive deficit by increasing proteasome activity. Brain Pathol. 21 (2), 140–149.

Mehta, P.D., Pirttilä, T., Mehta, S.P., Sersen, E.A., Aisen, P.S., Wisniewski, H.M., 2000. Plasma and cerebrospinal fluid levels of amyloid beta proteins 1-40 and 1-42 in Alzheimer disease. Arch. Neurol. 57 (1), 100–105.

Meyer-Luehmann, M., Coomaraswamy, J., Bolmont, T., Kaeser, S., Schaefer, C., Kilger, E., Jucker, M., 2006. Exogenous induction of cerebral beta-amyloidogenesis is governed by agent and host. Science 313 (5794), 1781–1784.

Minkeviciene, R., Banerjee, P., Tanila, H., 2004. Memantine improves spatial learning in a transgenic mouse model of Alzheimer's disease. J. Pharmacol. Exp. Ther. 311 (2), 677–682.

Moechars, D., Dewachter, I., Lorent, K., Reversé, D., Baekelandt, V., Naidu, A., Van Leuven, F., 1999. Early phenotypic changes in transgenic mice that overexpress different mutants of amyloid precursor protein in brain. J. Biol. Chem. 274 (10), 6483–6492.

Moolman, D.L., Vitolo, O.V., Vonsattel, J.-P.G., Shelanski, M.L., 2004. Dendrite and dendritic spine alterations in Alzheimer models. J. Neurocytol. 33 (3), 377–387.

Morgan, D., Diamond, D.M., Gottschall, P.E., Ugen, K.E., Dickey, C., Hardy, J., Arendash, G.W., 2000. A beta peptide vaccination prevents memory loss in an animal model of Alzheimer's disease. Nature 408 (6815), 982–985.

Mori, T., Rezai-Zadeh, K., Koyama, N., Arendash, G.W., Yamaguchi, H., Kakuda, N., Town, T., 2012. Tannic acid is a natural β-secretase inhibitor that prevents cognitive impairment and mitigates Alzheimer-like pathology in transgenic mice. J. Biol. Chem. 287 (9), 6912–6927.

Morris, R.G.M., 2003. Long-term potentiation and memory. Philos. Trans. R. Soc. Lond. B Biol. Sci. 358 (1432), 643–647.

Mucke, L., Masliah, E., Yu, G.Q., Mallory, M., Rockenstein, E.M., Tatsuno, G., McConlogue, L., 2000. High-level neuronal expression of abeta 1-42 in wild-type human amyloid protein precursor transgenic mice: synaptotoxicity without plaque formation. J. Neurosci. 20 (11), 4050–4058.

Mulkey, R.M., Endo, S., Shenolikar, S., Malenka, R.C., 1994. Involvement of a calcineurin/inhibitor-1 phosphatase cascade in hippocampal long-term depression. Nature 369 (6480), 486–488.

Nabavi, S., Kessels, H.W., Alfonso, S., Aow, J., Fox, R., Malinow, R., 2013. Metabotropic NMDA receptor function is required for NMDA receptor-dependent long-term depression. Proc. Natl. Acad. Sci. U.S.A. 110 (10), 4027–4032.

Neely, K.M., Green, K.N., LaFerla, F.M., 2011. Presenilin is necessary for efficient proteolysis through the autophagy-lysosome system in a γ-secretase-independent manner. J. Neurosci. 31 (8), 2781–2791.

Nicoll, A.J., Panico, S., Freir, D.B., Wright, D., Terry, C., Risse, E., Collinge, J., 2013. Amyloid-β nanotubes are associated with prion protein-dependent synaptotoxicity. Nat. Commun. 4, 2416.

Nicoll, J.A.R., Wilkinson, D., Holmes, C., Steart, P., Markham, H., Weller, R.O., 2003. Neuropathology of human Alzheimer disease after immunization with amyloid-beta peptide: a case report. Nat. Med. 9 (4), 448–452.

Nie, Q., Du, X., Geng, M., 2011. Small molecule inhibitors of amyloid β peptide aggregation as a potential therapeutic strategy for Alzheimer's disease. Acta Pharmacol. Sin. 32 (5), 545–551.

Nilsberth, C., Westlind-Danielsson, A., Eckman, C.B., Condron, M.M., Axelman, K., Forsell, C., Lannfelt, L., 2001. The "Arctic" APP mutation (E693G) causes Alzheimer's disease by enhanced Abeta protofibril formation. Nat. Neurosci. 4 (9), 887–893.

Noble, W., Olm, V., Takata, K., Casey, E., Mary, O., Meyerson, J., Duff, K., 2003. Cdk5 is a key factor in tau aggregation and tangle formation in vivo. Neuron 38 (4), 555–565.

Noguchi, A., Matsumura, S., Dezawa, M., Tada, M., Yanazawa, M., Ito, A., Hoshi, M., 2009. Isolation and characterization of patient-derived, toxic, high mass amyloid beta-protein (Abeta) assembly from Alzheimer disease brains. J. Biol. Chem. 284 (47), 32895–32905.

Nomura, I., Takechi, H., Kato, N., 2012. Intraneuronally injected amyloid β inhibits long-term potentiation in rat hippocampal slices. J. Neurophysiol. 107 (9), 2526–2531.

O'Nuallain, B., Freir, D.B., Nicoll, A.J., Risse, E., Ferguson, N., Herron, C.E., Walsh, D.M., 2010. Amyloid beta-protein dimers rapidly form stable synaptotoxic protofibrils. J. Neurosci. 30 (43), 14411–14419.

Oddo, S., Billings, L., Kesslak, J.P., Cribbs, D.H., LaFerla, F.M., 2004. Abeta immunotherapy leads to clearance of early, but not late, hyperphosphorylated tau aggregates via the proteasome. Neuron 43 (3), 321–332.

Oddo, S., Caccamo, A., Shepherd, J.D., Murphy, M.P., Golde, T.E., Kayed, R., LaFerla, F.M., 2003. Triple-transgenic model of Alzheimer's disease with plaques and tangles: intracellular Abeta and synaptic dysfunction. Neuron 39 (3), 409–421.

Ohno, M., Sametsky, E.A., Younkin, L.H., Oakley, H., Younkin, S.G., Citron, M., Disterhoft, J.F., 2004. BACE1 deficiency rescues memory deficits and cholinergic dysfunction in a mouse model of Alzheimer's disease. Neuron 41 (1), 27–33.

Ono, K., Li, L., Takamura, Y., Yoshiike, Y., Zhu, L., Han, F., Yamada, M., 2012. Phenolic compounds prevent amyloid β-protein oligomerization and synaptic dysfunction by site-specific binding. J. Biol. Chem. 287 (18), 14631–14643.

Ordóñez-Gutiérrez, L., Torres, J.M., Gavín, R., Antón, M., Arroba-Espinosa, A.I., Espinosa, J.-C., Wandosell, F., 2013. Cellular prion protein modulates β-amyloid deposition in aged APP/PS1 transgenic mice. Neurobiol. Aging 34 (12), 2793–2804.

Osenkowski, P., Ye, W., Wang, R., Wolfe, M.S., Selkoe, D.J., 2008. Direct and potent regulation of gamma-secretase by its lipid microenvironment. J. Biol. Chem. 283 (33), 22529–22540.

Palop, J.J., Jones, B., Kekonius, L., Chin, J., Yu, G.-Q., Raber, J., Mucke, L., 2003. Neuronal depletion of calcium-dependent proteins in the dentate gyrus is tightly linked to Alzheimer's disease-related cognitive deficits. Proc. Natl. Acad. Sci. U.S.A. 100 (16), 9572–9577.

Palop, J.J., Mucke, L., 2010. Amyloid-beta-induced neuronal dysfunction in Alzheimer's disease: from synapses toward neural networks. Nat. Neurosci. 13 (7), 812–818.

Parri, R.H., Dineley, T.K., 2010. Nicotinic acetylcholine receptor interaction with beta-amyloid: molecular, cellular, and physiological consequences. Curr. Alzheimer Res. 7 (1), 27–39.

Pastalkova, E., Serrano, P., Pinkhasova, D., Wallace, E., Fenton, A.A., Sacktor, T.C., 2006. Storage of spatial information by the maintenance mechanism of LTP. Science 313 (5790), 1141–1144.

Pei, J.J., Grundke-Iqbal, I., Iqbal, K., Bogdanovic, N., Winblad, B., Cowburn, R.F., 1998. Accumulation of cyclin-dependent kinase 5 (cdk5) in neurons with early stages of Alzheimer's disease neurofibrillary degeneration. Brain Res. 797 (2), 267–277.

Peineau, S., Taghibiglou, C., Bradley, C., Wong, T.P., Liu, L., Lu, J., Collingridge, G.L., 2007. LTP inhibits LTD in the hippocampus via regulation of GSK3beta. Neuron 53 (5), 703–717.

Perez-Cruz, C., Nolte, M.W., van Gaalen, M.M., Rustay, N.R., Termont, A., Tanghe, A., Ebert, U., 2011. Reduced spine density in specific regions of CA1 pyramidal neurons in two transgenic mouse models of Alzheimer's disease. J. Neurosci. 31 (10), 3926–3934.

Phiel, C.J., Wilson, C.A., Lee, V.M.-Y., Klein, P.S., 2003. GSK-3alpha regulates production of Alzheimer's disease amyloid-beta peptides. Nature 423 (6938), 435–439.

Podlisny, M.B., Ostaszewski, B.L., Squazzo, S.L., Koo, E.H., Rydell, R.E., Teplow, D.B., Selkoe, D.J., 1995. Aggregation of secreted amyloid beta-protein into sodium dodecyl sulfate-stable oligomers in cell culture. J. Biol. Chem. 270 (16), 9564–9570.

Portelius, E., Andreasson, U., Ringman, J.M., Buerger, K., Daborg, J., Buchhave, P., Zetterberg, H., 2010. Distinct cerebrospinal fluid amyloid beta peptide signatures in sporadic and PSEN1 A431E-associated familial Alzheimer's disease. Mol. Neurodegener. 5, 2.

Postina, R., 2012. Activation of α-secretase cleavage. J. Neurochem. 120 (Suppl.), 46–54.

Postina, R., Schroeder, A., Dewachter, I., Bohl, J., Schmitt, U., Kojro, E., Fahrenholz, F., 2004. A disintegrin-metalloproteinase prevents amyloid plaque formation and hippocampal defects in an Alzheimer disease mouse model. J. Clin. Invest. 113 (10), 1456–1464.

Prasher, V.P., Farrer, M.J., Kessling, A.M., Fisher, E.M., West, R.J., Barber, P.C., Butler, A.C., 1998. Molecular mapping of Alzheimer-type dementia in Down's syndrome. Ann. Neurol. 43 (3), 380–383.

Qing, H., He, G., Ly, P.T.T., Fox, C.J., Staufenbiel, M., Cai, F., Song, W., 2008. Valproic acid inhibits Abeta production, neuritic plaque formation, and behavioral deficits in Alzheimer's disease mouse models. J. Exp. Med. 205 (12), 2781–2789.

Rammes, G., Hasenjäger, A., Sroka-Saidi, K., Deussing, J.M., Parsons, C.G., 2011. Therapeutic significance of NR2B-containing NMDA receptors and mGluR5 metabotropic glutamate receptors in mediating the synaptotoxic effects of β-amyloid oligomers on long-term potentiation (LTP) in murine hippocampal slices. Neuropharmacology 60 (6), 982–990.

Rebeck, G.W., Reiter, J.S., Strickland, D.K., Hyman, B.T., 1993. Apolipoprotein E in sporadic Alzheimer's disease: allelic variation and receptor interactions. Neuron 11 (4), 575–580.

Reed, M.N., Hofmeister, J.J., Jungbauer, L., Welzel, A.T., Yu, C., Sherman, M.A., Cleary, J.P., 2011. Cognitive effects of cell-derived and synthetically derived Aβ oligomers. Neurobiol. Aging 32 (10), 1784–1794.

Reiman, E.M., Langbaum, J.B.S., Fleisher, A.S., Caselli, R.J., Chen, K., Ayutyanont, N., Tariot, P.N., 2011. Alzheimer's prevention initiative: a plan to accelerate the evaluation of presymptomatic treatments. J. Alzheimers Dis. 26 (Suppl. 3), 321–329.

Riha, P.D., Rojas, J.C., Gonzalez-Lima, F., 2011. Beneficial network effects of methylene blue in an amnestic model. NeuroImage 54 (4), 2623–2634.

Rinne, J.O., Brooks, D.J., Rossor, M.N., Fox, N.C., Bullock, R., Klunk, W.E., Grundman, M., 2010. 11C-PiB PET assessment of change in fibrillar amyloid-beta load in patients with Alzheimer's disease treated with bapineuzumab: a phase 2, double-blind, placebo-controlled, ascending-dose study. Lancet Neurol. 9 (4), 363–372.

Rioult-Pedotti, M.S., Friedman, D., Donoghue, J.P., 2000. Learning-induced LTP in neocortex. Science 290 (5491), 533–536.

Robakis, N.K., Ramakrishna, N., Wolfe, G., Wisniewski, H.M., 1987. Molecular cloning and characterization of a cDNA encoding the cerebrovascular and the neuritic plaque amyloid peptides. Proc. Natl. Acad. Sci. U.S.A. 84 (12), 4190–4194.

Roberds, S.L., Anderson, J., Basi, G., Bienkowski, M.J., Branstetter, D.G., Chen, K.S., McConlogue, L., 2001. BACE knockout mice are healthy despite lacking the primary beta-secretase activity in brain: implications for Alzheimer's disease therapeutics. Hum. Mol. Genet. 10 (12), 1317–1324.

Rockenstein, E., Torrance, M., Adame, A., Mante, M., Bar-on, P., Rose, J.B., Masliah, E., 2007. Neuroprotective effects of regulators of the glycogen synthase kinase-3beta signaling pathway in a transgenic model of Alzheimer's disease are associated with reduced amyloid precursor protein phosphorylation. J. Neurosci. 27 (8), 1981–1991.

Roher, A.E., Chaney, M.O., Kuo, Y.-M., Webster, S.D., Stine, W.B., Haverkamp, L.J., Emmerling, M.R., 1996. Morphology and toxicity of A{beta}-(1-42) dimer derived from neuritic and vascular amyloid deposits of Alzheimer's disease. J. Biol. Chem. 271 (34), 20631–20635.

Rönicke, R., Mikhaylova, M., Rönicke, S., Meinhardt, J., Schröder, U.H., Fändrich, M., Reymann, K.G., 2011. Early neuronal dysfunction by amyloid β oligomers depends on activation of NR2B-containing NMDA receptors. Neurobiol. Aging 32 (12), 2219–2228.

Rovelet-Lecrux, A., Hannequin, D., Raux, G., Le Meur, N., Laquerrière, A., Vital, A., Campion, D., 2006. APP locus duplication causes autosomal dominant early-onset Alzheimer disease with cerebral amyloid angiopathy. Nature Genetics 38 (1), 24–26.

Saito, T., Matsuba, Y., Mihira, N., Takano, J., Nilsson, P., Itohara, S., Saido, T.C., 2014. Single App knock-in mouse models of Alzheimer's disease. Nat. Neurosci.

Saito, T., Suemoto, T., Brouwers, N., Sleegers, K., Funamoto, S., Mihira, N., Saido, T.C., 2011. Potent amyloidogenicity and pathogenicity of Aβ43. Nat. Neurosci. 14 (8), 1023–1032.

Sakono, M., Zako, T., 2010. Amyloid oligomers: formation and toxicity of Abeta oligomers. FEBS J. 277 (6), 1348–1358.

Salloway, S., Sperling, R., Fox, N.C., Blennow, K., Klunk, W., Raskind, M., Brashear, H.R., 2014. Two phase 3 trials of bapineuzumab in mild-to-moderate Alzheimer's disease. N. Engl. J. Med. 370 (4), 322–333.

Sandberg, A., Luheshi, L.M., Söllvander, S., Pereira de Barros, T., Macao, B., Knowles, T.P.J., Härd, T., 2010. Stabilization of neurotoxic Alzheimer amyloid-beta oligomers by protein engineering. Proc. Natl. Acad. Sci. U.S.A. 107 (35), 15595–15600.

Sandebring, A., Welander, H., Winblad, B., Graff, C., Tjernberg, L.O., 2013. The pathogenic aβ43 is enriched in familial and sporadic Alzheimer disease. PloS One 8 (2), e55847.

Saunders, A.M., Strittmatter, W.J., Schmechel, D., George-Hyslop, P.H., Pericak-Vance, M.A., Joo, S.H., Alberts, M.J., 1993. Association of apolipoprotein E allele epsilon 4 with late-onset familial and sporadic Alzheimer's disease. Neurology 43 (8), 1467–1472.

Savonenko, A.V., Melnikova, T., Laird, F.M., Stewart, K.-A., Price, D.L., Wong, P.C., 2008. Alteration of BACE1-dependent NRG1/ErbB4 signaling and schizophrenia-like phenotypes in BACE1-null mice. Proc. Natl. Acad. Sci. U.S.A. 105 (14), 5585–5590.

Schauwecker, P.E., Steward, O., 1997. Genetic determinants of susceptibility to excitotoxic cell death: implications for gene targeting approaches. Proc. Natl. Acad. Sci. U.S.A. 94 (8), 4103–4108.

Scheff, S.W., DeKosky, S.T., Price, D.A., 1990. Quantitative assessment of cortical synaptic density in Alzheimer's disease. Neurobiol. Aging 11 (1), 29–37.

Scheff, S.W., Price, D.A., 1993. Synapse loss in the temporal lobe in Alzheimer's disease. Ann. Neurol. 33 (2), 190–199.

Scheff, S.W., Price, D.A., Schmitt, F.A., DeKosky, S.T., Mufson, E.J., 2007. Synaptic alterations in CA1 in mild Alzheimer disease and mild cognitive impairment. Neurology 68 (18), 1501–1508.

Scheff, S.W., Price, D.A., Schmitt, F.A., Mufson, E.J., 2006. Hippocampal synaptic loss in early Alzheimer's disease and mild cognitive impairment. Neurobiol. Aging 27 (10), 1372–1384.

Schenk, D., Barbour, R., Dunn, W., Gordon, G., Grajeda, H., Guido, T., Seubert, P., 1999. Immunization with amyloid-beta attenuates Alzheimer-disease-like pathology in the PDAPP mouse. Nature 400 (6740), 173–177.

Scheuner, D., Eckman, C., Jensen, M., Song, X., Citron, M., Suzuki, N., Younkin, S., 1996. Secreted amyloid β–protein similar to that in the senile plaques of Alzheimer's disease is increased in vivo by the presenilin 1 and 2 and APP mutations linked to familial Alzheimer's disease. Nat. Med. 2 (8), 864–870.

Schlenzig, D., Rönicke, R., Cynis, H., Ludwig, H.-H., Scheel, E., Reymann, K., Demuth, H.-U., 2012. N-Terminal pyroglutamate formation of Aβ38 and Aβ40 enforces oligomer formation and potency to disrupt hippocampal long-term potentiation. J. Neurochem. 121 (5), 774–784.

Schmechel, D.E., Saunders, A.M., Strittmatter, W.J., Crain, B.J., Hulette, C.M., Joo, S.H., Roses, A.D., 1993. Increased amyloid beta-peptide deposition in cerebral cortex as a consequence of apolipoprotein E genotype in late-onset Alzheimer disease. Proc. Natl. Acad. Sci. U.S.A. 90 (20), 9649–9653.

Schneider, L.S., Insel, P.S., Weiner, M.W., 2011. Treatment with cholinesterase inhibitors and memantine of patients in the Alzheimer's disease neuroimaging initiative. Arch. Neurol. 68 (1), 58–66.

Scholtzova, H., Wadghiri, Y.Z., Douadi, M., Sigurdsson, E.M., Li, Y.-S., Quartermain, D., Wisniewski, T., 2008. Memantine leads to behavioral improvement and amyloid reduction in Alzheimer's-disease-model transgenic mice shown as by micromagnetic resonance imaging. J. Neurosci. Res. 86 (12), 2784–2791.

Schor, N.F., 2011. What the halted phase III γ-secretase inhibitor trial may (or may not) be telling us. Ann. Neurol. 69 (2), 237–239.

Scoville, W.B., Milner, B., 1957. Loss of recent memory after bilateral hippocampal lesions. J. Neurol. Neurosurg. Psychiatry 20 (1), 11–21.

Selkoe, D.J., 1991. The molecular pathology of Alzheimer's disease. Neuron 6 (4), 487–498.

Selkoe, D.J., Wolfe, M.S., 2000. In search of gamma-secretase: presenilin at the cutting edge. Proc. Natl. Acad. Sci. U.S.A. 97 (11), 5690–5692.

Serenó, L., Coma, M., Rodríguez, M., Sánchez-Ferrer, P., Sánchez, M.B., Gich, I., Gómez-Isla, T., 2009. A novel GSK-3beta inhibitor reduces Alzheimer's pathology and rescues neuronal loss in vivo. Neurobiol. Dis. 35 (3), 359–367.

Seubert, P., Vigo-Pelfrey, C., Esch, F., Lee, M., Dovey, H., Davis, D., Swindlehurst, C., 1992. Isolation and quantification of soluble Alzheimer's beta-peptide from biological fluids. Nature 359 (6393), 325–327.

Shankar, G.M., Bloodgood, B.L., Townsend, M., Walsh, D.M., Selkoe, D.J., Sabatini, B.L., 2007. Natural oligomers of the Alzheimer amyloid-beta protein induce reversible synapse loss by modulating an NMDA-type glutamate receptor-dependent signaling pathway. J. Neurosci. 27 (11), 2866–2875.

Shankar, G.M., Li, S., Mehta, T.H., Garcia-Munoz, A., Shepardson, N.E., Smith, I., Selkoe, D.J., 2008. Amyloid-beta protein dimers isolated directly from Alzheimer's brains impair synaptic plasticity and memory. Nat. Med. 14 (8), 837–842.

Shen, J., Bronson, R.T., Chen, D.F., Xia, W., Selkoe, D.J., Tonegawa, S., 1997. Skeletal and CNS defects in Presenilin-1-deficient mice. Cell 89 (4), 629–639.

Shipton, O.A., Leitz, J.R., Dworzak, J., Acton, C.E.J., Tunbridge, E.M., Denk, F., Vargas-Caballero, M., 2011. Tau protein is required for amyloid {beta}-induced impairment of hippocampal long-term potentiation. J. Neurosci. 31 (5), 1688–1692.

Shoji, M., Golde, T.E., Ghiso, J., Cheung, T.T., Estus, S., Shaffer, L.M., Frangione, B., 1992. Production of the Alzheimer amyloid beta protein by normal proteolytic processing. Science 258 (5079), 126–129.

Shrestha, B.R., Vitolo, O.V., Joshi, P., Lordkipanidze, T., Shelanski, M., Dunaevsky, A., 2006. Amy-loid beta peptide adversely affects spine number and motility in hippocampal neurons. Mol. Cell. Neurosci. 33 (3), 274–282.

Sigurdsson, E.M., Knudsen, E., Asuni, A., Fitzer-Attas, C., Sage, D., Quartermain, D., Wisniewski, T., 2004. An attenuated immune response is sufficient to enhance cognition in an Alzheimer's disease mouse model immunized with amyloid-beta derivatives. J. Neurosci. 24 (28), 6277–6282.

Sigurdsson, E.M., Scholtzova, H., Mehta, P.D., Frangione, B., Wisniewski, T., 2001. Immuniza-tion with a nontoxic/nonfibrillar amyloid-beta homologous peptide reduces Alzheimer's disease-associated pathology in transgenic mice. Am. J. Pathol. 159 (2), 439–447.

Sinha, S., Anderson, J.P., Barbour, R., Basi, G.S., Caccavello, R., Davis, D., John, V., 1999. Purifi-cation and cloning of amyloid precursor protein beta-secretase from human brain. Nature 402 (6761), 537–540.

Sisodia, S.S., Koo, E.H., Hoffman, P.N., Perry, G., Price, D.L., 1993. Identification and transport of full-length amyloid precursor proteins in rat peripheral nervous system. J. Neurosci. 13 (7), 3136–3142.

Smith, D.L., Pozueta, J., Gong, B., Arancio, O., Shelanski, M., 2009. Reversal of long-term den-dritic spine alterations in Alzheimer disease models. Proc. Natl. Acad. Sci. U.S.A. 106 (39), 16877–16882.

Snider, B.J., Norton, J., Coats, M.A., Chakraverty, S., Hou, C.E., Jervis, R., Morris, J.C., 2005. Novel presenilin 1 mutation (S170F) causing Alzheimer disease with Lewy bodies in the third decade of life. Arch. Neurol. 62 (12), 1821–1830.

Spires, T.L., Hannan, A.J., 2005. Nature, nurture and neurology: gene-environment interactions in neurodegenerative disease. FEBS anniversary prize lecture delivered on 27 June 2004 at the 29th FEBS Congress in Warsaw. FEBS J. 272 (10), 2347–2361.

Spires-Jones, T., Knafo, S., 2012. Spines, plasticity, and cognition in Alzheimer's model mice. Neu-ral Plast. 2012, 319836.

Stéphan, A., Laroche, S., Davis, S., 2001. Generation of aggregated beta-amyloid in the rat hippo-campus impairs synaptic transmission and plasticity and causes memory deficits. J. Neurosci. 21 (15), 5703–5714.

Strittmatter, W.J., Weisgraber, K.H., Huang, D.Y., Dong, L.M., Salvesen, G.S., Pericak-Vance, M., Roses, A.D., 1993. Binding of human apolipoprotein E to synthetic amyloid beta peptide: isoform-specific effects and implications for late-onset Alzheimer disease. Proc. Natl. Acad. Sci. U.S.A. 90 (17), 8098–8102.

Sturchler-Pierrat, C., Abramowski, D., Duke, M., Wiederhold, K.-H., Mistl, C., Rothacher, S., Sommer, B., 1997. Two amyloid precursor protein transgenic mouse models with Alzheimer disease-like pathology. Proc. Natl. Acad. Sci. U.S.A. 94 (24), 13287–13292.

Su, Y., Ryder, J., Li, B., Wu, X., Fox, N., Solenberg, P., Ni, B., 2004. Lithium, a common drug for bipolar disorder treatment, regulates amyloid-β precursor protein processing. Biochemistry 43 (22), 6899–6908.

Sze, C.I., Troncoso, J.C., Kawas, C., Mouton, P., Price, D.L., Martin, L.J., 1997. Loss of the pre-synaptic vesicle protein synaptophysin in hippocampus correlates with cognitive decline in Alzheimer disease. J. Neuropathol. Exp. Neurol. 56 (8), 933–944.

Tanzi, R.E., Gusella, J.F., Watkins, P.C., Bruns, G.A., St George-Hyslop, P., Van Keuren, M.L., Neve, R.L., 1987. Amyloid beta protein gene: cDNA, mRNA distribution, and genetic linkage near the Alzheimer locus. Science 235 (4791), 880–884.

Terry, R.D., Masliah, E., Salmon, D.P., Butters, N., DeTeresa, R., Hill, R., Katzman, R., 1991. Physical basis of cognitive alterations in Alzheimer's disease: synapse loss is the major cor-relate of cognitive impairment. Ann. Neurol. 30 (4), 572–580.

Toledo, E.M., Inestrosa, N.C., 2010. Activation of Wnt signaling by lithium and rosiglitazone reduced spatial memory impairment and neurodegeneration in brains of an APPswe/PSEN1D-eltaE9 mouse model of Alzheimer's disease. Mol. Psychiatry 15 (3), 272–285, 228.

Tomiyama, T., Nagata, T., Shimada, H., Teraoka, R., Fukushima, A., Kanemitsu, H., Mori, H., 2008. A new amyloid beta variant favoring oligomerization in Alzheimer's-type dementia. Ann. Neurol. 63 (3), 377–387.

Torrent, L., Ferrer, I., 2012. PP2A and Alzheimer disease. Curr Alzheimer Res. 9, 248–256.

Trinchese, F., Liu, S., Battaglia, F., Walter, S., Mathews, P.M., Arancio, O., 2004. Progressive age-related development of Alzheimer-like pathology in APP/PS1 mice. Ann. Neurol. 55 (6), 801–814.

Tsai, J., Grutzendler, J., Duff, K., Gan, W.-B., 2004. Fibrillar amyloid deposition leads to local synaptic abnormalities and breakage of neuronal branches. Nat. Neurosci. 7 (11), 1181–1183.

Um, J.W., Kaufman, A.C., Kostylev, M., Heiss, J.K., Stagi, M., Takahashi, H., Strittmatter, S.M., 2013. Metabotropic glutamate receptor 5 is a coreceptor for Alzheimer aβ oligomer bound to cellular prion protein. Neuron 79 (5), 887–902.

Van Dam, D., Abramowski, D., Staufenbiel, M., De Deyn, P.P., 2005. Symptomatic effect of donepezil, rivastigmine, galantamine and memantine on cognitive deficits in the APP23 model. Psychopharmacology 180 (1), 177–190.

Van Dam, D., Coen, K., De Deyn, P.P., 2008. Cognitive evaluation of disease-modifying efficacy of donepezil in the APP23 mouse model for Alzheimer's disease. Psychopharmacology 197 (1), 37–43.

Van Dam, D., De Deyn, P.P., 2006. Cognitive evaluation of disease-modifying efficacy of galantamine and memantine in the APP23 model. Eur. Neuropsychopharmacol. 16 (1), 59–69.

Van Nostrand, W.E., Melchor, J.P., Cho, H.S., Greenberg, S.M., Rebeck, G.W., 2001. Pathogenic effects of D23N Iowa mutant amyloid beta -protein. J. Biol. Chem. 276 (35), 32860–32866.

Vassar, R., Bennett, B.D., Babu-Khan, S., Kahn, S., Mendiaz, E.A., Denis, P., Citron, M., 1999. Beta-secretase cleavage of Alzheimer's amyloid precursor protein by the transmembrane aspartic protease BACE. Science 286 (5440), 735–741.

Verghese, P.B., Castellano, J.M., Garai, K., Wang, Y., Jiang, H., Shah, A., Holtzman, D.M., 2013. ApoE influences amyloid-β (Aβ) clearance despite minimal apoE/Aβ association in physiological conditions. Proc. Natl. Acad. Sci. U.S.A. 110 (19), E1807–E1816.

Volianskis, A., Køstner, R., Mølgaard, M., Hass, S., Jensen, M.S., 2010. Episodic memory deficits are not related to altered glutamatergic synaptic transmission and plasticity in the CA1 hippocampus of the APPswe/PS1ΔE9-deleted transgenic mice model of β-amyloidosis. Neurobiol. Aging 31 (7), 1173–1187.

Walsh, D.M., Hartley, D.M., Kusumoto, Y., Fezoui, Y., Condron, M.M., Lomakin, A., Teplow, D.B., 1999. Amyloid beta-protein fibrillogenesis. Structure and biological activity of protofibrillar intermediates. J. Biol. Chem. 274 (36), 25945–25952.

Walsh, D.M., Klyubin, I., Fadeeva, J.V., Cullen, W.K., Anwyl, R., Wolfe, M.S., Selkoe, D.J., 2002. Naturally secreted oligomers of amyloid beta protein potently inhibit hippocampal long-term potentiation in vivo. Nature 416 (6880), 535–539.

Walsh, D.M., Selkoe, D.J., 2007. A beta oligomers – a decade of discovery. J. Neurochem. 101 (5), 1172–1184.

Wang, J., Dickson, D.W., Trojanowski, J.Q., Lee, V.M., 1999. The levels of soluble versus insoluble brain Abeta distinguish Alzheimer's disease from normal and pathologic aging. Exp. Neurol. 158 (2), 328–337.

Wang, X., Perry, G., Smith, M.A., Zhu, X., 2010. Amyloid-beta-derived diffusible ligands cause impaired axonal transport of mitochondria in neurons. Neurodegener. Dis. 7 (1–3), 56–59.

Watson, D.J., Selkoe, D.J., Teplow, D.B., 1999. Effects of the amyloid precursor protein Glu693→Gln "Dutch" mutation on the production and stability of amyloid beta-protein. Biochem. J. 340 (Pt 3), 703–709.

Wen, Y., Li, W., Poteet, E.C., Xie, L., Tan, C., Yan, L.-J., Yang, S.-H., 2011. Alternative mitochondrial electron transfer as a novel strategy for neuroprotection. J. Biol. Chem. 286 (18), 16504–16515.

Wen, Y., Planel, E., Herman, M., Figueroa, H.Y., Wang, L., Liu, L., Duff, K.E., 2008. Interplay between cyclin-dependent kinase 5 and glycogen synthase kinase 3 beta mediated by neuregulin signaling leads to differential effects on tau phosphorylation and amyloid precursor protein processing. J. Neurosci. 28 (10), 2624–2632.

Willem, M., Garratt, A.N., Novak, B., Citron, M., Kaufmann, S., Rittger, A., Haass, C., 2006. Control of peripheral nerve myelination by the beta-secretase BACE1. Science 314 (5799), 664–666.

Wischik, C.M., Edwards, P.C., Lai, R.Y., Roth, M., Harrington, C.R., 1996. Selective inhibition of Alzheimer disease-like tau aggregation by phenothiazines. Proc. Natl. Acad. Sci. U.S.A. 93 (20), 11213–11218.

Wolfe, M.S., Xia, W., Ostaszewski, B.L., Diehl, T.S., Kimberly, W.T., Selkoe, D.J., 1999. Two transmembrane aspartates in presenilin-1 required for presenilin endoproteolysis and gamma-secretase activity. Nature 398 (6727), 513–517.

Xia, W., Yang, T., Shankar, G., Smith, I.M., Shen, Y., Walsh, D.M., Selkoe, D.J., 2009. A specific enzyme-linked immunosorbent assay for measuring beta-amyloid protein oligomers in human plasma and brain tissue of patients with Alzheimer disease. Arch. Neurol. 66 (2), 190–199.

Xia, W., Zhang, J., Kholodenko, D., Citron, M., Podlisny, M.B., Teplow, D.B., Selkoe, D.J., 1997. Enhanced production and oligomerization of the 42-residue amyloid beta-protein by Chinese hamster ovary cells stably expressing mutant presenilins. J. Biol. Chem. 272 (12), 7977–7982.

Xu, T., Yu, X., Perlik, A.J., Tobin, W.F., Zweig, J.A., Tennant, K., Zuo, Y., 2009. Rapid formation and selective stabilization of synapses for enduring motor memories. Nature 462 (7275), 915–919.

Yamaguchi, H., Ishiguro, K., Uchida, T., Takashima, A., Lemere, C.A., Imahori, K., 1996. Preferential labeling of Alzheimer neurofibrillary tangles with antisera for tau protein kinase (TPK) I/glycogen synthase kinase-3 beta and cyclin-dependent kinase 5, a component of TPK II. Acta Neuropathol. 92 (3), 232–241.

Yamin, G., Ono, K., Inayathullah, M., Teplow, D.B., 2008. Amyloid beta-protein assembly as a therapeutic target of Alzheimer's disease. Curr. Pharm. Des. 14 (30), 3231–3246.

Yan, S.D., Chen, X., Fu, J., Chen, M., Zhu, H., Roher, A., Schmidt, A.M., 1996. RAGE and amyloid-beta peptide neurotoxicity in Alzheimer's disease. Nature 382 (6593), 685–691.

Yang, G., Pan, F., Gan, W.-B., 2009. Stably maintained dendritic spines are associated with lifelong memories. Nature 462 (7275), 920–924.

Yang, H.-Q., Ba, M.-W., Ren, R.-J., Zhang, Y.-H., Ma, J.-F., Pan, J., Chen, S.-D., 2007. Mitogen activated protein kinase and protein kinase C activation mediate promotion of sAPPalpha secretion by deprenyl. Neurochem. Int. 50 (1), 74–82.

Yoshiyama, Y., Lee, V.M., Trojanowski, J.Q., 2013. Therapeutic strategies for tau mediated neurodegeneration. J Neurol Neurosurg Psychiatry 84, 784–795.

Youssef, I., Florent-Béchard, S., Malaplate-Armand, C., Koziel, V., Bihain, B., Olivier, J.-L., Pillot, T., 2008. N-truncated amyloid-beta oligomers induce learning impairment and neuronal apoptosis. Neurobiol. Aging 29 (9), 1319–1333.

Zago, W., Buttini, M., Comery, T.A., Nishioka, C., Gardai, S.J., Seubert, P., Kinney, G.G., 2012. Neutralization of soluble, synaptotoxic amyloid β species by antibodies is epitope specific. J. Neurosci. 32 (8), 2696–2702.

Zempel, H., Thies, E., Mandelkow, E., Mandelkow, E.-M., 2010. Abeta oligomers cause localized Ca(2+) elevation, missorting of endogenous Tau into dendrites, Tau phosphorylation, and destruction of microtubules and spines. J. Neurosci. 30 (36), 11938–11950.

Zhang, Y., Wang, R., Liu, Q., Zhang, H., Liao, F.-F., Xu, H., 2007. Presenilin/gamma-secretase-dependent processing of beta-amyloid precursor protein regulates EGF receptor expression. Proc. Natl. Acad. Sci. U.S.A. 104 (25), 10613–10618.

Zhou, Q., Homma, K.J., Poo, M., 2004. Shrinkage of dendritic spines associated with long-term depression of hippocampal synapses. Neuron 44 (5), 749–757.

Ziemann, U., Ilić, T.V., Iliać, T.V., Pauli, C., Meintzschel, F., Ruge, D., 2004. Learning modifies subsequent induction of long-term potentiation-like and long-term depression-like plasticity in human motor cortex. J. Neurosci. 24 (7), 1666–1672.

Zola-Morgan, S., Squire, L.R., Amaral, D.G., 1986. Human amnesia and the medial temporal region: enduring memory impairment following a bilateral lesion limited to field CA1 of the hippocampus. J. Neurosci. 6 (10), 2950–2967.

Chapter 10

Pharmacological Treatment of Cognitive Dysfunction in Neuropsychiatric Disorders

César Venero

Faculty of Psychology, Universidad Nacional de Educación a Distancia (UNED), Madrid, Spain

INTRODUCTION

Our understanding of the neurobiological alterations that underlie neuropsychiatric disorders has advanced sufficiently for us to develop and evaluate distinct pharmacotherapeutic approaches aimed at restoring cognitive function. There is now a large variety of pharmacological agents to treat specific mood-related symptoms and cognitive deficits in distinct neuropsychiatric disorders. Animal models have proved critical in basic neuroscience to identify neurobiological substrates that are altered in neuropsychiatric diseases and the mechanisms of actions of newly developed drugs. Nevertheless, when tested in clinical trials of humans these drugs do not always produce the expected therapeutic outcomes, and the conclusions drawn between studies are too often inconsistent. In addition, in addition to the possible differences in methodology (dose, duration, study design, etc.), many factors may influence the reliability and reproducibility of clinical findings in psychiatric studies, including biological heterogeneity, high attrition, poor adherence, and high response rates to the placebo.

This chapter highlights the advances made recently in neurobiological research and summarizes the information from clinical trials that offers evidence for the efficacy of medications on several domains of cognition in certain mood disorders: posttraumatic stress disorder (PTSD), attention deficit/hyperactivity disorder (ADHD), major depressive disorder, schizophrenia, and bipolar disorder.

POSTTRAUMATIC STRESS DISORDER

PTSD is an illness that can develop after a traumatic event. It is characterized by four distinct diagnostic clusters: (1) reexperience (spontaneous

Cognitive Enhancement. http://dx.doi.org/10.1016/B978-0-12-417042-1.00010-3
233

memories of the traumatic event, recurrent nightmares, and flashbacks); (2) avoidance; (3) negative cognitions and mood (feelings that range from a persistent and distorted sense of self-blame or blame of others to an inability to remember key aspects of an event); and (4) arousal (aggressive and irritable behavior, sleep disturbances, hypervigilance, etc.). These symptoms result from a maladaptation to a traumatic stressor, and they only develop in a subpopulation (10–15%) of people experiencing such a traumatic event (Kessler et al., 2005).

The cognitive domains predominantly affected in PTSD are sustained attention and executive function (the ability to plan, organize, follow through, direct, and manage thoughts and activities). In addition, explicit memory domains may also be moderately impaired, particularly verbal memory (Brewin et al., 2007). There is some controversy in the literature concerning the memory deficits in patients with PTSD; some authors indicate that hyperarousal and hypervigilance to threat in the environment displayed by patients with PTSD can distract their attention away from the important aspects of tasks that evaluate memory (Diamond et al., 2001). Nevertheless, a number of studies reliably observed explicit memory deficits in PTSD (reviewed by Isaac et al., 2006, and Brewin et al., 2007). The distinct symptoms observed in this disorder—flashbacks, nightmares, hyperarousal, anxiety, impulsivity, anger, avoidance, numbing, or aggression—are probably caused by alterations affecting several neurotransmitter systems (Goodman et al., 2012), as well as dysfunction and/or damage in several brain areas, including the orbitofrontal, prefrontal, and anterior cingulate cortices, hippocampus, and amygdala (Milad and Rauch, 2007; Quirk and Mueller, 2008; Figure 10.1).

A variety of medications to alleviate the anxiety symptoms of PTSD are available, including selective serotonin reuptake inhibitors (SSRIs), serotonin–norepinephrine reuptake inhibitors (SNRIs), monoamine oxidase inhibitors, tricyclic antidepressants, anticonvulsants, and atypical antipsychotics and benzodiazepines (Jeffreys et al., 2012). Although SSRIs have shown some efficiency in ameliorating the severity of symptoms and in preventing relapse in patients with PTSD (Steckler and Risbrough, 2012), a significant percentage of patients fail to respond to these and other pharmacological treatments and/or do not recover after being treated for several years (Ipser et al., 2006; Darves-Bornoz et al., 2008).

At present there are no approved medications to treat specifically the cognitive symptoms characteristic of PTSD. However, studies of laboratory animals have helped us to understand better the neurobiological basis of emotional memory and to develop new agents that are potentially useful for treating this disorder. Flashbacks, nightmares, or intrusive recollections are associated with the activation of an aversive memory trace of the traumatic event. Therefore, pharmacological treatments that prevent the retrieval of such memories might be beneficial to alleviate PTSD symptoms. The following agents are those that seem to best prevent the development of PTSD.

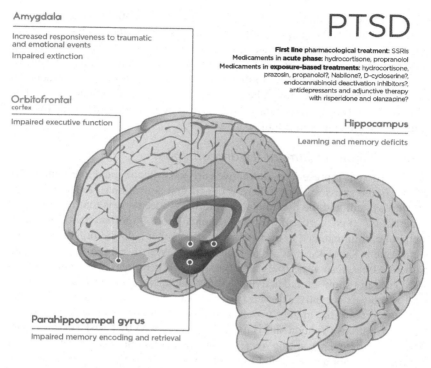

FIGURE 10.1   Cognitive symptoms in posttraumatic stress disorder (PTSD) and the brain areas involved. Medications administered during the acute phase should be given in the initial hours following the traumatic event to prevent the development of PTSD symptoms. The medications used with exposure-based therapies aim to improve the efficacy of such therapies in ameliorating the symptoms of patients suffering from PTSD. SSRI, selective serotonin reuptake inhibitor. (This figure is reproduced in color in the color plate section.)

Early Pharmacological Interventions

Adrenergic Receptor Antagonists

During exposure to the traumatic event, there is enhanced sympathetic activity and catecholamine release that can facilitate the exaggeration of emotional memories into traumatic memories (Pitman, 1989). Hence, one therapeutic intervention that may prevent the development of PTSD is blocking adrenergic receptors. Several clinical trials have reported that prazosin, an alpha-1 receptor antagonist, can reduce psychological distress, as well as sleep disturbances and nightmares, in patients with PTSD (Peskind et al., 2003; Taylor et al., 2008), although in other studies no differences in PTSD symptoms were found between those receiving prazosin or a placebo (Raskind et al., 2007).

Another therapeutic strategy to treat PTSD symptoms is to administrate propanolol, a β-receptor antagonist. Antagonism of this receptor reduces the activity of the sympathetic system, interfering with its ability to establish the traumatic memory. When propranolol is administered within hours after exposure to the traumatic experience it diminishes the probability of developing PTSD, probably because it interferes with the consolidation and reconsolidation of the traumatic memory (Pitman and Delahanty, 2005). The time delay of propranolol treatment seems to be critical in its therapeutic efficacy, and when administrated 2 days after trauma, it did not provide any benefits to the patients compared with a placebo (Stein et al., 2007).

Glucocorticoid Treatment (Hydrocortisone)

Glucocorticoids represent an alternative early pharmacological intervention for PTSD. In the stress response, there is concurrent activation of the sympathetic nervous system and the hypothalamic–pituitary–adrenal axis that releases glucocorticoids (i.e., cortisol). Glucocorticoids exert important cardiovascular, metabolic, immune, and neurobiological effects that help the organism to face a challenge (Sapolsky et al., 2000), and they may also restrain the acute sympathetic stress response (Joëls and Baram, 2009). Remarkably, patients with PTSD usually show altered activity in the hypothalamic–pituitary–adrenal axis, and in subjects recently exposed to a traumatic event, low plasma concentrations of cortisol (the main glucocorticoid) are related to a higher incidence of PTSD symptoms (Yehuda and Harvey, 1997; reviewed by Hruska et al., 2014). Indeed, if there is a strong increase in catecholamine concentrations after trauma that is not accompanied by a significant increase in cortisol concentrations, consolidation of that emotional memory may be altered and symptoms of PTSD will probably develop (Yehuda and Harvey, 1997; Yehuda et al., 1998). According to this theory, it was hypothesized that glucocorticoid administration soon after trauma may prevent PTSD symptoms from developing. In fact, it was observed that administering hydrocortisone (a glucocorticoid) immediately after trauma reduced the frequency of PTSD symptoms weeks and months later in patients with distinct traumatic profiles (Delahanty et al., 2013, Zohar et al., 2011; Figure 10.1).

Exposure-Based Pharmacological Therapies in PTSD

Exposure-based psychotherapies are commonly used to treat PTSD and are considered the most appropriate type of psychotherapy for this condition (Ballenger et al., 2000). These therapies involve repeated and controlled exposure to the trauma memory, and their success is based on a fear extinction model (Foa and Kozak, 1986). A common characteristic of patients suffering from PTSD is that they display difficulties in the extinction of learned fear (Guthrie and Bryant, 2006). Therefore, the use of adjunctive agents that may enhance extinction and avoid fear retrieval during exposure-based therapies could potentially be interesting in treating patients with PTSD.

Glucocorticoids

Exposure-based psychotherapy treatments are commonly used to treat PTSD, and they are considered the most appropriate type of psychotherapy for PTSD (Ballenger et al., 2000). Indeed, glucocorticoid administration during exposure was found to enhance the success of exposure-based psychotherapy in PTSD (Soravia et al., 2006; de Quervain et al., 2011). Although the precise mechanisms of action of glucocorticoids as exposure therapy are not well understood, they seem to restrain fear retrieval and disturb the cycle of retrieval, reexperience, and reconsolidation that is thought to underlie traumatic memories in PTSD (de Quervain and Margraf, 2008).

Propanolol

In addition to glucocorticoids, propanolol treatment has recently been proposed as an effective therapeutic option for PTSD, mainly in military personnel (Tawa and Murphy, 2013). However, more studies are needed to confirm the efficacy of this treatment in conjunction with exposure-based treatments.

Cannabinoids

It has been recently postulated that the endocannabinoid system might be a good therapeutic target to reverse the emotional and cognitive dysfunctions that characterize PTSD (Neumeister, 2013). The endocannabinoid system consists of a group of neuromodulatory lipids (endocannabinoids), two cannabinoid receptors (CB1 and CB2), and the enzymes that synthesize and degrade endocannabinoids (Piomelli, 2003). In the brain, cannabinoid receptors are mainly expressed in limbic structures, and they are involved in the modulation of emotions and cognition (Hill and Gorzalka, 2009). Interestingly, patients with PTSD show altered plasma concentrations of endocannabinoid and enhanced CB1 receptor availability in limbic brain regions, including the amygdala and hippocampus (Neumeister, 2013). Because studies in animals have demonstrated that cannabinoid ligands can enhance memory extinction and impair memory retrieval (Lutz, 2007; Atsak et al., 2012), it was postulated that cannabinoids might reduce the persistent retrieval of traumatic memories and facilitate the extinction process in patients with PTSD. In fact, cannabis was reported to diminish PTSD symptoms among Vietnam veterans (Bremner et al., 1996), and nabilone, a synthetic cannabinoid, significantly reduced the number and intensity of nightmares (Fraser, 2009). Cannabinoid ligands have a high potential for abuse, and hence other therapeutic agents have been developed. One novel therapeutic approach is to use endocannabinoid deactivation inhibitors, which may enhance the availability of endogenous agonists of cannabinoid receptors, such as anandamide (Varvel et al., 2007; Figure 10.1). Given that the administration of cannabinoid agonists to animals immediately after aversive training enhances memory consolidation (Campolongo et al., 2009), it has been speculated that agonists of endocannabinoid deactivation inhibitors are not appropriate for administration in the early phases after trauma.

D-Cycloserine

The *N*-methyl-D-aspartate (NMDA) receptor is known to play a key role in extinction; in fact, D-cycloserine, an agonist of the glycine site at the NMDA receptor, improves fear extinction (Myers et al., 2011). Given that patients suffering from PTSD also display impaired extinction of learned fear (Blechert et al., 2007), it was hypothesized that D-cycloserine may exert beneficial effects on fear extinction in patients with PTSD. However, few clinical studies have investigated the potential efficacy of D-cycloserine administration concomitant with exposure therapy, and its effects remain controversial because although mild positive effects were reported in some studies, no significant effects of treatment with D-cycloserine were found in others (Difede et al., 2014; Rothbaum et al., 2014; Scheeringa and Weems, 2014).

ATTENTION DEFICIT/HYPERACTIVITY DISORDER

ADHD is a developmental disorder characterized by inappropriate levels of attention, hyperactivity, and impulsivity (Biederman and Faraone, 2005). Heritability of ADHD is estimated to be greater than 60%, although environmental risk factors also have been identified, including maternal alcohol or tobacco use during pregnancy, lead exposure, or familial conflict. Notably, ADHD is the most prevalent childhood psychiatric disorder, affecting 6–7% of children (Getahun et al., 2013), and it has important consequences on educational achievement and social relationships during adolescence. Unfortunately, the cognitive impairment that occurs during childhood or adolescence persists into adulthood (Vaidya and Stollstorff, 2008).

Cognitive Domains Affected in ADHD

In ADHD, attention is not the only cognitive domain affected; impairment in working memory, processing speed, and fluency may also be observed (Barkley, 1997; Boonstra et al., 2005; Vaidya and Stollstorff, 2008). Clinical research data from neuropsychological, neurochemical, and neuroimaging studies indicate that patients with ADHD have some dysfunction in the dorsolateral prefrontal cortex, dorsal anterior midcingulate cortex, and the parietal cortex, which probably underlie the pathophysiological mechanisms of this illness (Bush et al., 1999; Mehta et al., 2000; Dickstein et al., 2006; Figure 10.2). Interestingly, several neuroimaging studies evidenced that children with ADHD show a delay in cortical maturation (Shaw et al., 2007), as well as functional and morphological abnormalities in the brain (Schulz et al., 2005; Castellanos et al., 2002; Mostofsky et al., 2002). In a recent meta-analysis of functional magnetic resonance imaging studies, the attention deficits observed in patients with ADHD were closely related to altered functional activation of the right prefrontal cortex (Hart et al., 2013).

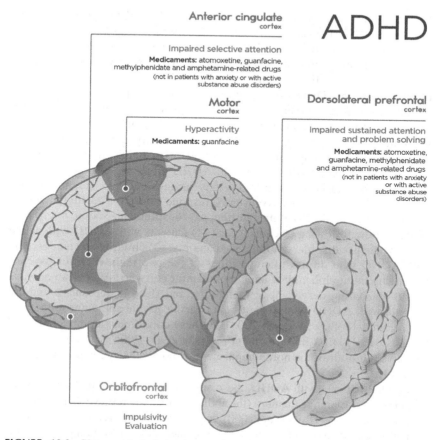

FIGURE 10.2   Pharmacological treatments for attention deficit/hyperactivity disorder (ADHD). Dysfunction in certain frontal brain areas is characteristic of ADHD. The main medications proven to be effective in improving attention and problem solving in patients suffering from ADHD are indicated. (This figure is reproduced in color in the color plate section.)

Psychostimulants

Because attention is a function that depends on the dopaminergic and noradrenergic systems, drugs that stimulate these systems, such as methylphenidate and several amphetamine-related drugs, have been used frequently to improve attention and processing speed in patients with ADHD (Pringsheim and Steeves, 2011). Interestingly, methylphenidate can improve impulsivity in children with ADHD (Losier et al., 1996; Riccio et al., 2001), and given that methylphenidate inhibits both dopamine and norepinephrine transport at synapses, its therapeutic actions are probably related to the increase of these neurotransmitters in the striatum and prefrontal cortex (Berridge and Devilbiss, 2011). In fact, a 6-week treatment with a methylphenidate hydrochloride osmotic-release oral system increased brain activity in the dorsal anterior midcingulate cortex during the Multi-Source Interference Task (Bush et al., 2008).

Despite the effectiveness of treatment with methylphenidate or amphetamine-related drugs in many patients with ADHD, psychostimulants are not recommended in patients with comorbid anxiety. Approximately 25–50% of children with ADHD suffer from at least one form of anxiety disorder, including separation anxiety and social and generalized anxiety, which can affect daily functioning and behavior and decrease quality of life (Jarrett and Ollendick, 2008; Sciberras et al., 2014). Importantly, children with ADHD and anxiety show stronger impairment of attention and heightened cognitive difficulties compared with those with ADHD alone (Bowen et al., 2008). This issue should be taken into account because children diagnosed with ADHD and comorbid anxiety usually respond poorly to methylphenidate (Ter-Stepanian et al., 2010). In addition, psychostimulants should not be prescribed in the following circumstances: (1) patients with ADHD with active substance abuse disorders or comorbid anxiety; (2) children and adolescents with ADHD who do not tolerate either of the two main types of psychostimulants (methylphenidate and amphetamine) or who suffer from adverse effects (including nervousness, irritability, and sleep disturbance); and (3) patients with ADHD who do not benefit from psychostimulant monotherapy (around 10–30%; Wilens, 2008). In these conditions, atomoxetine may be considered a first-line treatment (Pliszka et al., 2006); atomoxetine is a selective inhibitor of the norepinephrine transporter (Michelson et al., 2002; Figure 10.2).

In adult patients with ADHD, the main cognitive deficits include working memory and declarative memory (the ability to store and retrieve facts, plans, or ideas from memory) (Ross et al., 2000). In these patients, psychostimulants such as methylphenidate have been reported to enhance the functioning of working and declarative memories (Cooper et al., 2005; Mehta et al., 2000; Verster et al., 2010) and to improve sustained attention (Biederman et al., 2008a,b). Moreover, psychostimulants may enhance long-term academic performance among adolescents (Powers et al., 2008), an effect that seems to be restricted to undergraduate students who show a substantial deficit in episodic memory (Advokat and Scheithauer, 2013). Finally, it should be noted that recent reviews indicate that the nootropic effects of psychostimulants are inconclusive, not only in subjects with ADHD (Advokat and Vinci, 2012), but also in healthy people (Quednow, 2010).

Noradrenergic Drugs

Atomoxetine, an SNRI, was the first nonstimulant drug approved for the treatment of ADHD, and it enhances cognitive performance in people with ADHD (Wilens, 2008). In a recent neuroimaging study, treatment with atomoxetine for 6 weeks activated the cognitive attention network, including the right dorsolateral prefrontal cortex, parietal cortex, and caudate nucleus (Bush et al., 2013).

Other drugs that modulate noradrenergic activity were found to have a therapeutic effect on ADHD (Figure 10.2). Indeed, agonists of the noradrenergic system (e.g., guanfacine) also are effective in improving cognitive function in patients with ADHD (Hunt et al., 1995), mainly working memory deficits and behavioral inhibition (Wilens, 2008). Guanfacine binds preferentially to postsynaptic α-2 noradrenergic receptors in the prefrontal cortex, and it enhances the signal-to-noise ratio from environmental stimuli that may facilitate the maintenance of attention in patients with ADHD (Stahl, 2008). In fact, a recent meta-analysis of the effect of α-2 noradrenergic receptor agonist monotherapy for ADHD (including guanfacine) indicated that these drugs are helpful in treating the symptoms of hyperactivity and inattention in this illness (Hirota et al., 2014). Interestingly, in children 6–12 years old with ADHD, guanfacine was demonstrated to be an effective pharmacological option, not only as monotherapy, but also as an adjunct treatment to psychostimulants (Elbe and Reddy, 2014).

MAJOR DEPRESSIVE DISORDER

MDD involves a range of emotional, cognitive, and behavioral symptoms, including persistent poor mood and reduced interest or pleasure (Nelson and Charney, 1981; Boland and Keller, 2009). According to the World Health Organization Global Burden of Disease Study, depression accounts for 40% of the total disability-adjusted life years, and it is associated with morbidity and mortality (Whiteford et al., 2013). At present, there are a variety of therapeutic approaches available to treat depression, including psychotherapeutic management strategies, such as cognitive therapy, and pharmacological treatments that mainly modulate the monoamine neurotransmitter systems in the brain. However, only modest response (a 50% decrease in depression severity) and remission rate are observed with these treatments (Rush et al., 2006); moreover, more depressive patients relapse within 2 years of recovering from a depressive episode (Boland and Keller, 2009).

Cognitive Aspects of Depression

Attention is frequently affected early in the course of major depression (Lampe et al., 2004) and other domains often are subsequently compromised, including processing speed, executive functioning, working memory, verbal and visuo-spatial memory, and long-term memory (Porter et al., 2003; Vythilingam et al., 2004; Landro et al., 2001; Taylor Tavares et al., 2007; Castaneda et al., 2008; Hammar et al., 2003). According to neuropsychological and imaging studies, these cognitive deficits are related to structural changes and dysfunction in the frontal lobe and hippocampal brain areas (Bremner et al., 2004; Cornwell et al., 2010; Rogers et al., 2004; Figure 10.3).

In major depression, cognitive impairment is associated with the severity of depression (Millan et al., 2012), with poor psychosocial functioning and

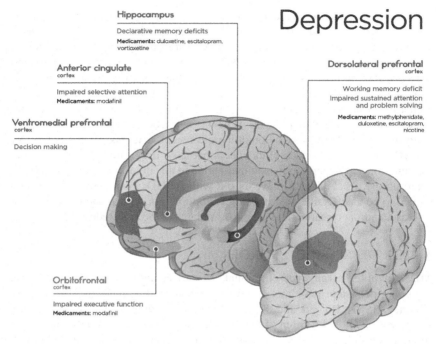

Hippocampus
Declarative memory deficits
Medicaments: duloxetine, escitalopram, vortioxetine

Depression

Anterior cingulate
cortex
Impaired selective attention
Medicaments: modafinil

Dorsolateral prefrontal
cortex
Working memory deficit
Impaired sustained attention and problem solving
Medicaments: methylphenidate, duloxetine, escitalopram, nicotine

Ventromedial prefrontal
cortex
Decision making

Orbitofrontal
cortex
Impaired executive function
Medicaments: modafinil

FIGURE 10.3   Cognitive deficits and brain dysfunction in major depressive disorder. The key medications proven to have clinical effects, or that are potentially beneficial, are indicated in each cognitive domain. (This figure is reproduced in color in the color plate section.)

disability (Rock et al., 2013). Moreover, individuals with severe depression and psychotic features, as well as elderly depressed patients, usually show more general and severe cognitive deficits (Castaneda et al., 2008). Therefore, interventions to alleviate depressive symptoms and cognitive impairment are thought to be important in improving functional outcome in depressed patients (Rock et al., 2013).

Whether cognitive impairment observed in major depression is due to mood symptoms or if it is a different feature of this disorder remains to be elucidated. After mood recovery, usually an improvement in certain cognitive deficits can be observed (psychomotor speed, verbal fluency, and verbal memory) (Herrera-Guzman et al., 2009). The fact that deficits in attention and executive function frequently persist after significant remission of mood symptoms (Paelecke-Habermann et al., 2005; Douglas and Porter, 2009) suggests that cognitive impairment is a trait rather than a state of major depression (Maalouf et al., 2011). Currently, cognitive impairment is widely accepted as representing a core feature of depression that cannot be considered totally secondary to symptoms of poor mood and that may be an important target for future interventions (Rock et al., 2013).

At present, there are a variety of antidepressants that, according to their mechanism of action, can be classified in eight distinct classes: SSRIs, SNRIs, noradrenaline dopamine reuptake inhibitors, noradrenergic specific serotonergic antidepressants, serotonin antagonist reuptake inhibitors, serotonin partial agonist reuptake inhibitors, tricyclic antidepressants, and monoamine oxidase inhibitors. In each patient, some antidepressants are more efficient than others, depending on the symptoms presented (anxiety, fatigue, insomnia, and pain) (Lin and Stevens, 2014).

Pharmacological Treatments for Depression that Can Improve Cognition

Antidepressants

Certain controversy regarding the beneficial or detrimental effects of antidepressants on cognitive function exists (Lee et al., 2012). Nevertheless, a meta-analysis of the response to antidepressant treatment in relation to cognitive performance before treatment indicated that patients who respond to antidepressant treatment also show improved cognitive deficits (McLennan and Mathias, 2010).

Among the pharmacological treatments that can improve mood and cognitive impairment in major depression are agents such as the SSRI escitalopram and duloxetine, an SNRI. These agents improve processing speed, working memory, and episodic memory, although duloxetine treatment produces greater benefits. However, even after treatment with antidepressants, some impairment could still be observed in depressed patients (Herrera-Guzman et al., 2009).

Glutamatergic Treatments

In treatment-resistant depression, acute intravenous administration of ketamine, a potent glutamatergic NMDA receptor antagonist, can rapidly (within hours) improve depressive behavior (Zarate et al., 2006; Murrough et al., 2013). Nevertheless, important side effects may occur after ketamine administration, including hypertension, psychotic symptoms, perceptual disturbance, and even short-term cognitive impairment (Krystal et al., 1994; Duncan et al., 2001). However, the increased risk of important side effects with ketamine has limited its clinical use.

An alternative glutamatergic treatment is the use of memantine, a noncompetitive, midaffinity NMDA receptor antagonist. This medicine has some advantages over ketamine: it is safer to use, can be orally administered, and it readily crosses the blood–brain barrier. At present, memantine is used to improve cognitive function in Alzheimer's disease (Kovács, 2009); interestingly, memantine may improve mood and cognition in depressed patients, probably by reducing glutamatergic transmission and normalizing NMDA functioning (Teng and Demetrio, 2006; Zarate et al., 2004; Dang et al., 2014). However, further studies are needed to elucidate whether memantine is efficient in restoring cognitive function in major depression.

Adjunctive Pharmacological Treatments to Improve Cognitive Impairment in Depression

Methylphenidate

In depression, methylphenidate can rapidly diminish tiredness and enhance attention and arousal (Orr and Taylor, 2007; Candy et al., 2008; Figure 10.3). While several studies have reported that methylphenidate can improve mood in melancholic and bipolar depression (Candy et al., 2008; Stahl, 2000), a randomized, double-blind, placebo-controlled trial did not find significant benefits of methylphenidate in treatment-resistant depression (Patkar et al., 2006). Hence, while the ability of methylphenidate to alleviate mood in depression remains uncertain, positive effects on attention and arousal are consistently observed.

Modafinil

Modafinil is a drug approved by the US Food and Drug Administration (FDA) for treating excessive sleepiness in narcolepsy, obstructive sleep apnea, and shift-work sleep disorder (Pack et al., 2001; Czeisler et al., 2005). It acts by inhibiting both the dopamine and the norepinephrine transporters; as a consequence, the extracellular levels of both transmitters are increased, provoking increased activation of α-adrenergic D1 and D2 receptors (Minzenberg and Carter, 2008; Müller et al., 2013). In contrast to conventional psychostimulants, modafinil has weaker side effects and less potential for abuse (Minzenberg and Carter, 2008). Interestingly, a recent meta-analysis of randomized controlled trials indicated that modafinil is a good drug of choice for augmentation therapy in acute depressive episodes, even for symptoms of fatigue (Goss et al., 2013). In major depression, adjuvant modafinil treatment administered to patients medicated with SSRIs was reported to improve depression and executive function (DeBattista et al., 2004; Menza et al., 2000; Figure 10.3).

Vortioxetine

Vortioxetine is a novel medication with a good safety and tolerance profile that has recently been approved by the FDA for the treatment of major depression. This medication is an orally administered molecule with distinct mechanisms of action, inhibiting the activity of serotonin transporters and acting as an agonist of the serotonin 5-HT1A receptor, a partial agonist of 5-HT1B and an antagonist of the 5-HT3A, 5-HT7, and 5-HT1D receptors. In a recent randomized, double-blind, placebo-controlled study, vortioxetine was reported to improve processing speed, verbal learning, and memory in patients with major depression (Katona et al., 2012; Dhir, 2013).

Treating Cognitive Deficits in Late-Life Depression

In late-life depression, cognitive deficits are evident through executive function, processing and motor speed, planning, and memory (Weisenbach et al., 2012). These impairments are associated with white matter alterations and atrophy in the frontal, cingulate, and temporal cortices that are evident in neuroimaging studies (Taylor et al., 2003, 2008). Interestingly, the severity of the cognitive deficits is associated not only with greater depression symptoms (Taylor et al., 2002) and functional decline (Johnson et al., 2007), but also with a weaker response to antidepressants (McLennan and Mathias, 2010) and a higher risk of recurrence (Alexopoulos et al., 2000). In fact, depressed people with high impairment of executive function usually show low remission rates (Potter et al., 2004). Unfortunately, antidepressants are not very efficient in alleviating mood and cognitive symptoms in most depressed older individuals (Beekman et al., 2002), and although cognitive impairments usually improve in responders to antidepressant treatment, they are still evident (Nebes et al., 2003; Bhalla et al., 2006).

Adjunctive Treatments to Antidepressants in Elderly Depressed Patients

To improve cognition in elderly depressed patients, different pharmacological adjunctive treatments have been tested along with antidepressants. Given that the cholinergic system plays a key role in the cognitive symptoms associated with normal aging and dementia (Dumas and Newhouse, 2011), pharmacotherapy approaches have been based on administering a cholinesterase inhibitor that increases extracellular acetylcholine by blocking its breakdown. Such cholinesterase inhibitors are to some degree efficacious in mild cognitive impairment and in several dementias (including Alzheimer's disease), as well as for memory function in depressed patients (Jacobsen and Comas-Diaz, 1999; Iosifescu et al., 2009). However, some cholinesterase inhibitors, such as donepezil, were found to exacerbate symptoms of depression and to increase the risk of the recurrence of depression (Reynolds et al., 2011). The causes for the worsening of symptoms of depression after donepezil treatment are not clear but they may be because in this illness there is hypersensitivity to the activation of muscarinic receptors (Sunderland et al., 1988; Drevets et al., 2012). In fact, activation of muscarinic receptors increases depressive symptoms, whereas their blockade improves mood in depressed patients (Furey and Drevets, 2006; Drevets et al., 2012).

Therefore, an alternative acetylcholine strategy to improve cognition without worsening mood symptoms is to activate nicotinic receptors. It was recently proposed that administering nicotinic agonists to elderly depressed patients would probably enhance brain activity in the frontal regions that are involved in attention and executive function (Jansari et al., 2013). Furthermore, nicotinic stimulation in other brain regions might also improve processing speed and memory. Future studies will indicate the efficacy of nicotinic agonists as a therapeutic approach to treat cognitive impairment in late-life depression.

SCHIZOPHRENIA

According to recent epidemiological data, schizophrenia affects 4 of every 1000 individuals around the world (Saha et al., 2005), and it can be considered the third leading cause of disability (Hyman, 2008). Schizophrenia is broadly characterized by three core symptoms: positive symptoms (hallucinations, delusions, grandiosity, paranoia, and suspiciousness); negative symptoms (blunted affect, social avoidance, poor rapport, lack of motivation, lack of spontaneity, and emotional withdrawal); and cognitive dysfunction (Tandon et al., 2009). Cognitive impairment is evident in around 85% of these patients (Keefe et al., 2003), and while working and declarative memory are strongly disrupted in schizophrenia (Mohs, 1995; Bilder et al., 2000; Weickert and Goldberg, 2005), other cognitive domains may also be impaired, including attention, executive function, language/fluency, processing speed, and social cognition (Heinrichs and Zakzanis, 1998; Hutton et al., 1998; Conkiln et al., 2000; Buchanan et al., 2005; Braw et al., 2008; Figure 10.4). The cognitive dysfunction observed in patients with schizophrenia has long been considered to be the result of altered cortical-cerebellar-thalamic-cortical circuit activity (Andreasen et al., 1998). Interestingly, cognitive deficits are present early in the course of schizophrenia, before psychosis (Lencz et al., 2006; Gonzalez-Blanch et al., 2008), and in patients without medication (Mohamed et al., 1999). At present, neurocognitive deficits found in schizophrenia are considered to constitute an endophenotype because they are stable and heritable (Green et al., 2004).

Beneficial and Detrimental Effects of Antipsychotic Treatments on Cognitive Function in Schizophrenic Patients

There are several antipsychotic medications approved by the FDA to alleviate the positive symptoms of schizophrenia. FDA-approved medications are typical and atypical antipsychotics that can treat positive symptoms with similar efficacy (Leucht et al., 2009). Typical antipsychotic drugs are antagonists or partial agonists of the dopamine D2 receptor, although they do not enhance cognitive function in patients with schizophrenia (Friedman et al., 2002; Peuskens et al., 2005). In fact, they may negatively affect cognition because of their anticholinergic activity (Minzenberg et al., 2004). However, atypical antipsychotic drugs that combine partial agonism of the dopamine D2 receptor with antagonism at the serotonin 5-HT2A receptor may have positive effects on cognitive function in schizophrenic patients (Sumiyoshi et al., 2013).

In patients with persistent negative and cognitive symptoms, an antipsychotic (usually clozapine) is frequently prescribed along with another atypical antipsychotic, although this combination therapy is not always beneficial

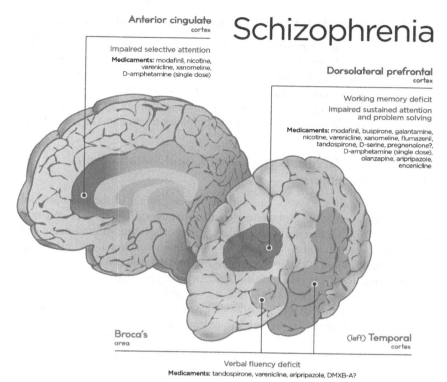

FIGURE 10.4   Brain areas altered in schizophrenia and those involved in cognitive impairment. The adjuvant pharmacotherapy for the different cognitive deficits observed in schizophrenic patients is indicated for each cognitive domain affected. DMXB-A, 3-[2,4-dimethoxybenzylidene] anabaseine. (This figure is reproduced in color in the color plate section.)

for improving negative or cognitive symptoms (Citrome, 2011). Given that the degree of magnitude and the extent of cognitive impairment is greater in schizophrenia than in bipolar disorder, even small improvements in cognition after pharmacological treatment can be readily detected. Thus, in contrast to what has been observed in bipolar disorder, the use of atypical antipsychotics (such as risperidone or quetiapine) in schizophrenia does not seem to negatively affect cognition (Keefe et al., 2007). Conversely, some atypical antipsychotics (particularly olanzapine or risperidone) may even improve some domains such as immediate memory, executive function, vigilance, verbal fluency, or visuo-spatial processing (Harvey and Keefe, 2001; Bilder et al., 2002; Lindenmayer et al., 2007; Houthoofd et al., 2008), although they do not restore cognitive function to normal levels (Peuskens et al., 2005; Keefe et al., 2007; Davidson et al., 2009; van Veelen et al., 2010). Hence, pursuing effective therapies for all cognitive deficits that occur in schizophrenia is the main focus of research into this disease.

Adjunct Treatments for Cognitive Dysfunction in Schizophrenia

At present, no medications have been approved by the FDA to treat cognitive impairments in schizophrenia. More than 50 clinical trials of patients with schizophrenia have been carried out, but the improvements in cognitive function achieved have been modest (Citrome, 2014). Given that the approaches to treat cognitive dysfunction in schizophrenia involve different types of drugs, we pay attention here to only the most relevant of these treatments (Figure 10.4).

Glutamatergic Targets: NMDA, AMPA, and Metabotropic Glutamate Receptors

Two neurotransmitter systems are believed to be critical in the pathophysiology of schizophrenia: the glutamatergic and dopaminergic systems (Kantrowitz and Javitt, 2010). Glutamate is an excitatory neurotransmitter found in the central nervous system, and it is critical in many brain functions, including cognition (Moghgaddam, 2003). Neuroimaging and pharmacological studies of schizophrenia have provided strong evidence of glutamatergic dysfunction; interestingly, blockers of NMDA receptors (such as ketamine or phencyclidine) reproduce many of the positive and negative symptoms of schizophrenia in healthy volunteers as well as induce cognitive impairment, whereas they exacerbate these symptoms in patients with schizophrenia (Javitt and Zukin, 1991; Krystal et al., 1994; Morgan and Curran, 2006). These findings led to the hypothesis that hypofunctional NMDA receptor signaling may explain the positive, negative, and cognitive symptoms of schizophrenia (Coyle and Tsai, 2004; Javitt, 2009; Gao, 2012).

Studies of experimental animals have examined the involvement of the ionotropic (AMPA, NMDA, and kainate) and metabotropic glutamate receptors in cognitive function. Moreover, because these receptors are important for learning and memory processes, clinical trials testing the efficacy of some agonists of these receptors on cognition have been performed.

Ionotropic and Metabotropic Glutamate Receptors

While several ampakines (positive modulators of AMPA-type glutamate receptors) have been found to improve learning and memory in animals, they were ineffective in enhancing cognition in patients with schizophrenia when given as adjuncts to antipsychotic drugs (Goff et al., 2008a,b). Kainate receptors also have been identified as a therapeutic target and tested by administering topiramate, an anticonvulsant, as an adjunct to atypical antipsychotics. However, adjunctive topiramate treatment produced cognitive dulling in a randomized controlled study (Muscatello et al., 2011).

In humans, NMDA glutamate receptors in the prefrontal cortex are involved in executive function, those in the visual cortex are important in detecting movement, and those in the hippocampus are critical for learning and memory.

Because such sensory and cognitive deficits are found in patients with schizophrenia (Kantrowitz and Javitt, 2011), most effort has concentrated on investigating the effects of drugs that could enhance NMDA receptor activity. NMDA receptors can only be activated in the presence of glutamate and glycine. Because glycine does not readily cross the blood–brain barrier, the effects of other drugs that act at the glycine coagonist site of the NMDA receptor, such as D-serine and D-cycloserine, have been tested. Although D-cycloserine was initially reported to improve executive function in patients with schizophrenia (Heresco-Levy et al., 2005), subsequent studies reported a low efficacy of D-cycloserine in ameliorating cognitive deficits in these patients (Buchanan et al., 2007). By contrast, D-serine has been reported to improve several symptom domains (Kantrowitz et al., 2010), and it was effective when administered as an adjunct with certain antipsychotics, such as risperidone or olanzapine, but not clozapine (Tsai and Lin, 2010; Figure 10.4).

Glycine Transporter-1 Inhibitors

At present, a novel therapeutic target for the treatment of schizophrenia is the use of glycine transporter-1 inhibitors, which may help increase the availability of glycine at the synapse (Chue, 2013). Indeed, clinical studies involving treatment with glycine transporter inhibitors such as sarcosine and bitopertin were found to improve some of the core symptoms associated with schizophrenia (Hashimoto, 2010; Javitt, 2012). Remarkably, sarcosine as an adjunctive treatment with different antipsychotics improved several symptoms in schizophrenic patients, yet not when combined with the antipsychotic clozapine (Tsai and Lin, 2010). This seems to be related to the glycine transport inhibitory activity of clozapine itself (Javitt et al., 2005). In two recent clinical trials, the glycine transporter inhibitor bitopertin was found to be well tolerated and to reduce positive and negative symptoms in patients with schizophrenia, although pro-cognitive effects were not investigated (Bugarski-Kirola et al., 2014; Umbricht et al., 2014).

The potential therapeutic utility of metabotropic receptors also has been investigated; initially, a selective agonist for the metabolic Glu2/3 receptor was found to effectively treat positive and negative symptoms of schizophrenia (Patil et al., 2007). However, further studies did not replicate these findings, and no more clinical trials using this agonist have been carried out.

Acetylcholinesterase Inhibitors

Given that acetylcholine is a critical neurotransmitter in learning and memory processes, several studies have investigated the potential benefits of using acetylcholinesterase inhibitors to improve cognitive function in schizophrenia (Buchanan et al., 2003). The use of donepezil, an acetylcholinesterase inhibitor, indirectly increases the levels of acetylcholine in the brain through reuptake blockade, as seen in case report studies, and a general improvement in attention, memory, coherent speech, and word fluency was reported in an open-label trial (MacEwan et al., 2001; Stryjer et al., 2002; Chung et al., 2009). By contrast, in other studies donepezil was not effective in improving cognitive function in patients with schizophrenia when added to risperidone (Fagerlund et al., 2007; Akhondzadeh et al., 2008), ziprasidone (Friedman et al., 2002), or other atypical antipsychotics (Keefe et al., 2008). Moreover, a recent prospective assessment of the benefits of donepezil on cognitive impairment in schizophrenia failed to support the use of this medication (Thakurathi et al., 2013). Inconclusive results were obtained with galantamine, another cholinesterase inhibitor. Thus, while there are indications that these drugs may be effective in treating cognitive impairments in people with schizophrenia (Schubert et al., 2006; Lee et al., 2007; Buchannan et al., 2008), these beneficial effects on cognition were been found in all these patients (Dyer et al., 2008; Sacco et al., 2008). In addition, other studies observed no benefits on cognition after treatment with rivastigmine, another acetylcholinesterase inhibitor (Sharma et al., 2006).

Nicotinic and Muscarinic Acetylcholine Receptors as Targets for Cognitive Enhancement in Schizophrenia

The fact that up to 88% of people with schizophrenia are smokers (Moss et al., 2009) led to the formulation of two hypotheses: (1) the self-mediation hypothesis, suggesting that patients smoke to alleviate their psychiatric symptomatology and the side effects of antipsychotics (Khantzian, 1985; Winterer, 2010); and (2) the addition vulnerability hypothesis (Chambers et al., 2001), which proposes that schizophrenia and tobacco addiction not only share genetic factors but also brain alterations (George, 2007). Nicotine is the main psychoactive element in tobacco, and after inhalation of tobacco smoke into the lungs, nicotine is rapidly delivered in the bloodstream, reaching the brain and activating nicotinic and muscarinic receptors. In addition, nicotine affects the release of other neurotransmitters including dopamine, glutamate, and γ-aminobutyric acid. Several studies have confirmed that nicotine administration to patients with schizophrenia enhances attention, reaction time, working memory, as well as verbal and spatial memory (Levin et al., 1996; Depatie et al., 2002; Smith et al., 2002; Harris et al., 2004; AhnAllen et al., 2008). Because patients with schizophrenia who smoke have low rates of quitting, different pharmacotherapies that act on central nicotinic receptors (nicotine replacement, bupropion, and varenicline) have been tested for smoking cessation (George and O'Malley, 2004). Interestingly, varenicline has not only proven to be effective for smoking cessation but also in improving attention, executive function, as well as verbal learning and memory (Smith et al., 2009; Hong et al., 2011; Shim et al., 2012). Furthermore, a recent meta-analysis highlighted the positive effects of using cholinergic receptor agonists as adjunct pharmacotherapy for cognitive deficits in schizophrenia (Choi et al., 2013). There is also recent evidence that xanomeline, an M1/M4 agonist, significantly restores cognitive deficits with repeated dosing (Melancon et al., 2013).

At present, several pharmaceutical companies are carrying out clinical trials to define the utility of different agonists of nicotinic receptors for treating cognitive impairments in patients with schizophrenia and Alzheimer's disease. Their research is mainly focused on the α7 nicotinic receptors (α7nAChR)—because these receptors are abundant in brain areas involved in attention and long-term and working memory—and testing several new nicotinic agonists. Thus, some anabaseine derivatives that are partial agonists of α7nAChR have been tested, but with different results. While some authors indicated that 3-[2,4-dimethoxy-benzylidene]anabaseine improved attention and working memory in non-smokers with schizophrenia (Olincy and Freedman, 2012), others reported that it did not ameliorate cognitive deficits in patients with schizophrenia (Freedman et al., 2008). TC-5619, a full agonist of α7nAChR, was recently reported to produce some cognitive benefits in schizophrenia (Lieberman et al., 2013). Moreover, encenicline (EVP-6124) is another agonist that is well tolerated; in addition to reducing negative symptoms, it also enhances cognitive function in schizophrenic patients taking antipsychotics (Mazurov et al., 2012; Preskorn et al., 2014; Figure 10.4).

Noradrenergic Drugs

Drugs that increase noradrenergic activity have been found to improve ADHD. Because attention functions are affected in patients with schizophrenia, several drugs that target the noradrenergic system have been tested in schizophrenia. Thus, treatment with guanfacine, a selective α2 adrenergic receptor agonist, was reported to improve not only attention (Friedman et al., 2001) but also cognition (McClure et al., 2007). However, other noradrenergic transport inhibitors that are used in ADHD, such as atomoxetine, did not enhance cognition (Friedman et al., 2008; Kelly et al., 2009).

5-HT1A Receptor Agonists

Because low dopamine concentrations in the prefrontal cortex are considered to be one of the main biological substrates underlying several of the cognitive impairments observed in schizophrenia, drugs that may enhance dopamine neurotransmission in this brain area may improve cognition in this psychiatric disease (Sawaguchi and Goldman-Rakic, 1991; Murphy et al., 1996). It was postulated that potential benefits could be obtained by administering atypical antipsychotics that act as D2/D5-HT2A receptor antagonists together with 5-HT1A receptor agonists that can also enhance dopamine release in the prefrontal cortex (Ichikawa et al., 2001). Interestingly, some atypical antipsychotics (e.g., clozapine, olanzapine, and ziprazidone) are also partial 5-HT1A receptor agonists what has been associated to their poor capability to improve negative and cognitive symptoms of schizophrenia (Li et al., 1998). Thus, administration of tandospirone, a 5-HT1A agonist, to patients with schizophrenia receiving stable doses of atypical antipsychotics improved executive function and verbal memory (Sumiyoshi et al., 2001). The same research group subsequently found that when administered with atypical antipsychotics, buspirone improved attention (Sumiyoshi et al., 2007).

Psychostimulants

Psychostimulants increase the release of dopamine and norepinephrine, and they are widely used to treat attention disorders (Mattay et al., 2000). In addition, some beneficial effects on processing speed, attention, executive function, working memory accuracy, and language production were reported when D-amphetamine was concomitantly administered with antipsychotics in single-dose trials (Barch and Carter, 2005; Pietrzak et al., 2010). However, long-term treatment with psychostimulants is not recommended because psychostimulants can worsen psychosis. Nevertheless, D-amphetamine improved the reaction times of spatial working memory and in Stroop tasks in both participants with schizophrenia and controls, and it increased language production and improved working memory accuracy in those with schizophrenia (Barch and Carter, 2005).

Modafinil is a wakefulness-promoting medication that was reported to improve attention and executive functions, as well as short-term verbal and visual memory, in patients with schizophrenia (Hunter et al., 2006; Turner et al., 2004; Sevy et al., 2005; Morein-Zamir et al., 2007; Figure 10.4). However, other studies demonstrated that modafinil had no positive effects on cognitive dysfunction in schizophrenia (Freudenreich et al., 2009; Kane et al., 2010; Lohr et al., 2013). Although the reasons remain unclear, there are case reports in the literature indicating that modafinil can worsen psychosis in patients with schizophrenia (Narendran et al., 2002). Therefore, the use of this medication to improve cognition in schizophrenia is more than questionable.

Why Is It Difficult to Restore Cognition in Schizophrenia?

The fact that most drugs assessed had only modest effects or failed to restore cognitive function in patients with schizophrenia has led researchers to postulate that the cognitive impairment observed in schizophrenic patients is caused by structural brain changes (including changes in cortical structure and the loss of gray matter) (DeLisi et al., 2006), modifications that are unlikely to be reverted by pharmacological methods. In addition, it is possible that concomitant treatment with antipsychotic medications may diminish the positive effects of nootropics on cognitive impairment in patients with schizophrenia. A significant blockade of dopamine D2 receptor is typically necessary to achieve a clinical response in schizophrenic patients (Laruelle et al., 1998), a fact that may alter neural plasticity. In addition, atypical antipsychotics can act through 5-HT2A receptors and affect the serotonergic system, which is known to play a critical role in the regulation of other neurotransmitter systems. In addition, it is possible that the use of antipsychotics impairs the pro-cognitive effects of other drugs, or that these drugs might increase the side effects of atypical antipsychotics. Finally, the appropriate dose of the nootropic drug may differ in schizophrenic patients taking antipsychotic medication. Thus, doses of procholinergic medications that are typically used in Alzheimer's disease, in which an extensive loss of cholinergic neurons occur, are probably not appropriate to treat schizophrenic patients who do not suffer from comparable cholinergic functional impairment.

BIPOLAR DISORDER

Bipolar disorder is characterized by severe changes in mood, with the occurrence of a clear manic episode, according to the criteria defined in the *Diagnostic and Statistical Manual of Mental Disorders, Fifth Edition*. Patients with bipolar disorder show deficits in many of the same cognitive domains previously described as altered in patients with schizophrenia (attention, executive function, processing speed, and verbal memory), although the extent and magnitude are generally less severe and insidious than in schizophrenia (Daban et al., 2006). By contrast, other cognitive functions such as visuospatial memory and verbal fluency are relatively well preserved in bipolar disorder (Buchanan et al., 2005). Interestingly, during periods of euthymia (a nondepressed period), deficits in working memory and visual memory usually remit, although the deficits in selective attention, response inhibition, strategic thinking, processing speed, or verbal memory persist (Dixon et al., 2004; Martinez- Aran et al., 2004). It is likely that the impairments in cognitive function observed in patients with bipolar disorder are related to the abnormalities in the activation of the frontal, subcortical, and limbic regions, as observed using functional magnetic resonance imaging during cognitive tasks (reviewed by Yurgelun-Todd and Ross (2006)).

Lithium and Other Medications to Treat Bipolar Disorder That May Affect Cognition

The treatment of bipolar disorder can involve different medications including mood stabilizers (e.g., lithium and valproic acid), atypical antipsychotics (e.g., aripiprazole), and antidepressants, such as SSRIs. Importantly, some of these medications can also influence cognitive function.

Lithium has long been considered the cornerstone for the treatment of bipolar disorder, not only during the acute and maintenance phase but also to prevent relapse and to reduce the risk of suicide (Farinde, 2013). However, lithium treatment can impair short- and long-term memory, speed of information processing, and verbal fluency (Pachet and Wisniewski, 2003; Goldberg, 2008). In general, typical antipsychotic medications and benzodiazepines have been found to affect working memory and processing speed (Mintzer and Griffiths, 2003), whereas atypical antipsychotic agents have been reported to induce neutral or adverse cognitive effects, mainly affecting executive function (Frangou et al., 2005; Altshuler et al., 2004; Goldberg, 2008; Goldberg and Young, 2008).

Anticonvulsants, another type of medication for bipolar disorder, can exert distinct effects on cognitive function. Thus, while topiramate can affect executive function and memory, thereby potentially disturbing daily and occupational activities (Salinsky et al., 2005; Goldberg, 2008), other medications, such as carbamazepine, lamotrigine, and gabapentine, have minimal effects on cognition (Stoll et al., 1996; Meador et al., 2001; Salinsky et al., 2005). Interestingly, in adolescent bipolar patients with comorbid ADHD, global improvement was reported in those taking divalproex, an anticonvulsant medication containing sodium valproate and valproic acid that is used in bipolar disorder as a mood-stabilizing drug (Scheffer et al., 2005). Finally, antidepressants, in particular SSRIs, seem to be neutral or beneficial in improving cognitive function in patients with bipolar disorder (Zobel et al., 2004).

Pharmacological Approaches to the Treatment of Cognitive Dysfunction in Bipolar Disorder

Procholinergics

In patients with bipolar disorder, there are reports of positive effects on cognitive function after adjuvant treatment with galantamine, a cholinesterase inhibitor (Dias et al., 2006; Schrauwen and Ghaemi, 2006). Moreover, galantamine treatment for 4 months was found to improve attention and episodic memory in 19 patients with bipolar disorder in remission (Iosifescu et al., 2009). However, the limitations associated with the latter study, including the small sample size and the open design with no placebo control, make it difficult to assess the true benefits patients with bipolar disorder may receive from galantamine administration.

Antiglutamatergic Agents

A few studies have investigated whether antiglutamatergic drugs can improve cognition in bipolar disorder. Several studies of cognitive deficits in bipolar patients provided evidence for the beneficial effects of memantine, a noncompetitive NMDA receptor antagonist with a medium affinity (Martínez-Arán et al., 2004; Koukopoulos et al., 2012; Sani et al., 2012). Interestingly, acute administration of memantine was reported to enhance cognition in patients with treatment-resistant bipolar disorder (Teng and Demetrio, 2006). Moreover, in one case report, memantine administration for 10 weeks improved mood, cognitive functioning, and quality of life without producing any side effects (Strzelecki et al., 2013).

Glucocorticoid Receptor Antagonists

Because bipolar disorder is associated with hypercortisolemia, the potential benefits of antiglucocorticoid drugs on mood and cognitive function have been tested. Administration of mifepristone (a glucocorticoid and progesterone antagonist) can reduce plasma cortisol concentrations in bipolar disorder (Gallagher et al., 2008). Interestingly, adjunct treatment combining mifepristone with antipsychotics not only improved the severity of depressive symptoms but also enhanced recognition memory (Young et al., 2004; Watson et al., 2012).

Psychostimulants

A few studies have investigated the effects of methylphenidate in bipolar disorder, demonstrating that it is well tolerated and has minimal risk for worsening the affective state (Carlson et al., 2004; Lydon and El-Mallakn, 2006). With continued use over time, psychostimulants can induce physiological dependence (Seiden et al., 1988), and hence they are not commonly prescribed. However, the use of psychostimulants has been reconsidered after the recent introduction of modafinil, a novel psychostimulant that was found to be effective in unipolar and bipolar disorders (Thase et al., 2006). Modafinil is a wakefulness-promoting agent that inhibits the reuptake of norepinephrine and dopamine, enhances glutamate release, and improves cognitive function in bipolar disorder (Feraro et al., 1999; Madras et al., 2006; Dell'Osso and Ketter, 2013). A recent meta-analysis found that modafinil treatment can be considered an effective augmentation strategy for acute depressive episodes, not only in bipolar disorder but also in MDD (Goss et al., 2013).

Concluding Remarks

In each neuropsychiatric disorder, cognitive impairment can be the consequence of dysfunction in distinct brain areas and neurotransmitter systems. Therefore, different pharmacological strategies to restore cognitive function in these disorders are needed. Current knowledge has allowed the use of medicaments that achieved some success in the treatment of cognitive deficits in different neuropsychiatric illnesses. However, additional research studies are needed to better understand the neurobiological substrates of neuropsychiatric disorders and to develop new drugs with better efficacy to restore cognitive function.

REFERENCES

Advokat, C., Scheithauer, M., 2013. Attention-deficit hyperactivity disorder (ADHD) stimulant medications as cognitive enhancers. Front. Neurosci. 7, 82.

Advokat, C., Vinci, C., 2012. Do stimulant medications for attention deficit/hyperactivity disorder (ADHD) enhance cognition? In: Norvilitis, J.M. (Ed.), Current Directions in ADHD and its Treatment. InTech, Rijeka, pp. 125–156.

AhnAllen, C.G., Nestor, P.G., Shenton, M.E., McCarley, R.W., Niznikiewicz, M.A., 2008. Early nicotine withdrawal and transdermal nicotine effects on neurocognitive performance in schizophrenia. Schizophr. Res. 100, 261–269.

Akhondzadeh, S., Gerami, M., Noroozian, M., et al., 2008. A 12-week, double-blind, placebo-controlled trial of donepezil adjunctive treatment to risperidone in chronic and stable schizophrenia. Prog. Neuropsychopharmacol. Biol. Psychiatry 32, 1810–1815.

Alexopoulos, G.S., Meyers, B.S., Young, R.C., Kalayam, B., Kakuma, T., Gabrielle, M., et al., 2000. Executive dysfunction and long-term outcomes of geriatric depression. Arch. Gen. Psychiatry 57, 285–290.

Altshuler, L.L., Ventura, J., van Gorp, W.G., Gree, M.F., Theberge, D.C., Mintz, J., 2004. Neurocognitive function in clinically stable men with bipolar I disorder or schizophrenia and normal control subjects. Biol. Psychiatry 56, 560–569.

Andreasen, N.C., Paradiso, S., O'Leary, D.S., 1998. "Cognitive dysmetria" as an integrative theory of schizophrenia: a dysfunction in cortical-subcortical-cerebellar circuitry? Schizophr. Bull. 24 (2), 203–218.

Atsak, P., Roozendaal, B., Campolongo, P., 2012. Role of the endocannabinoid system in regulating glucocorticoid effects on memory for emotional experiences. Neuroscience 204, 104–116.

Ballenger, J.C., Davidson, J.R.T., Lecrubier, Y., et al., 2000. Consensus statement on posttraumatic stress disorder from the international consensus group on depression and anxiety. J. Clin. Psychiatry 61 (Suppl. 5), 60–66.

Barch, D.M., Carter, C.S., 2005. Amphetamine improves cognitive function in medicated individuals with schizophrenia and in healthy volunteers. Schizophr. Res. 77 (1), 43–58.

Barkley, R.A., 1997. Behavioral inhibition, sustained attention, and executive functions: constructing a unifying theory of ADHD. Psychol. Bull. 121, 65–94.

Beekman, A.T., Geerlings, S.W., Deeg, D.J., Smit, J.H., Schoevers, R.S., de Beurs, E., et al., 2002. The natural history of late-life depression: a 6-year prospective study in the community. Arch. Gen. Psychiatry 59, 605–611.

Berridge, C.W., Devilbiss, D.M., 2011. Psychostimulants as cognitive enhancers: the prefrontal cortex, catecholamines, and attentiondeficit/hyperactivity disorder. Biol. Psychiatry 69, 101–111.

Bhalla, R.K., Butters, M.A., Mulsant, B.H., Begley, A.E., Zmuda, M.D., Schoderbek, B., et al., 2006. Persistence of neuropsychologic deficits in the remitted state of late-life depression. Am. J. Geriatr. Psychiatry 14, 419–427.

Biederman, J., Faraone, S.V., 2005. Attention-deficit hyperactivity disorder. Lancet 366, 237–248.

Biederman, J., Seidman, L.J., Petty, C.R., et al., 2008a. Effects of stimulant medication on neuropsychological functioning in young adults with attention-deficit/hyperactivity disorder. J. Clin. Psychiatry 69, 1150–1156.

Biederman, J., Seidman, L.J., Petty, C.R., et al., 2008b. Effects of stimulant medication on neuropsychological functioning in young adults with attention-deficit/hyperactivity disorder. J. Clin. Psychiatry 69, 1150–1156.

Bilder, R.M., Goldman, R.S., Robinson, D., Reiter, G., Bell, L., Bates, J.A., Pappadopulos, E., Willson, D.F., Alvir, J.M., Woerner, M.G., Geisler, S., Kane, J.M., Lieberman, J.A., 2000. Neuropsychology of first-episode schizophrenia: initial characterization and clinical correlates. Am. J. Psychiatry 157 (4), 549–559.

Bilder, R.M., Goldman, R.S., Volavka, J., et al., 2002. Neurocognitive effects of clozapine, olanzapine, risperidone, and haloperidol in patients with chronic schizophrenia or schizoaffective disorder. Am. J. Psychiatry 159, 1018–1028.

Blechert, J., Michael, T., Vriends, N., Markgraf, J., Wilhelm, F.H., 2007. Fear conditioning in posttraumatic stress disorder: evidence for delayed extinction of autonomic, experimental, and behavioural responses. Behav. Res. Ther. 45, 2019–2033.

Boland, R.J., Keller, M.B., 2009. Course and outcome of depression. In: Gotlib, I.H., Hammen, C.L. (Eds.), Handbook of Depression. Guilford, New York, pp. 23–43.

Boonstra, A.M., Oosterlaan, J., Sergeant, J.A., Buitelaar, J.K., 2005. Executive functioning in adult ADHD: a meta-analytic review. Psychol. Med. 35, 1097–1108.

Bowen, R., Chavira, D.A., Bailey, K., Stein, M.T., Stein, M.B., 2008. Nature of anxiety comorbid with attention deficit hyperactivity disorder in children from a pediatric primary care setting. Psychiatry Res. 157 (1–3), 201–209.

Braw, Y., Bloch, Y., Mendelovich, S., et al., 2008. Cognition in young schizophrenia outpatients: comparison of first-episode with multiepisode patients. Schizophr. Bull. 34 (3), 544–554.

Bremner, J.D., Southwick, S.M., Darnell, A., Charney, D.S., 1996. Chronic PTSD in Vietnam combat veterans: course of illness and substance abuse. Am. J. Psychiatry 53 (3), 369–375.

Bremner, J.D., Vythilingam, M., Vermetten, E., Vaccarino, V., Charney, D.S., 2004. Deficits in hippocampal and anterior cingulate functioning during verbal declarative memory encoding in midlife major depression. Am. J. Psychiatry 161 (4), 637–645.

Brewin, C.R., Kleiner, J.S., Vasterling, J.J., Field, A.P., 2007. Memory for emotionally neutral information in posttraumatic stress disorder: a meta-analytic investigation. J. Abnorm. Psychol. 116, 448–463.

Buchanan, R.W., Davis, M., Goff, D., et al., 2005. A summary of the FDA-NIMH-MATRICS workshop on clinical trial design for neurocognitive drugs for schizophrenia. Schizophr. Bull. 31, 5–19.

Buchanan, R.W., Javitt, D.C., Marder, S.R., et al., 2007. The cognitive and negative symptoms in Schizophrenia trial (CONSIST): the efficacy of glutamatergic agents for negative symptoms and cognitive impairment. Am. J. Psychiatry 164, 1593–1602.

Buchanan, R.W., Summerfelt, A., Tek, C., Gold, J., 2003. An open-labeled trial of adjunctive donepezil for cognitive impairments in patients with schizophrenia. Schizophr. Res. 59, 29–33.

Buchanan, R.W., Conley, R.R., Dickinson, D., Ball, M.P., Feldman, S., Gold, J.M., et al., 2008. Galantamine for the treatment of cognitive impairments in people with schizophrenia. Am. J. Psychiatry 165, 82–89.

Bugarski-Kirola, D., Wang, A., Abi-Saab, D., Blättler, T., 2014. A phase II/III trial of bitopertin monotherapy compared with placebo in patients with an acute exacerbation of schizophrenia – results from the CandleLyte study. Eur. Neuropsychopharmacol. 24 (7), 1024–1036.

Bush, G., Frazier, J.A., Rauch, S.L., Seidman, L.J., Whalen, P.J., Jenike, M.A., Rosen, B.R., Biederman, J., 1999. Anterior cingulate cortex dysfunction in attention-deficit/hyperactivity disorder revealed by fMRI and the counting stroop. Biol. Psychiatry 45 (12), 1542–1552.

Bush, G., Holmes, J., Shin, L.M., Surman, C., Makris, N., Mick, E., et al., 2013. Atomoxetine increases fronto-parietal functional MRI activation in attention-deficit/hyperactivity disorder: a pilot study. Psychiatry Res. 211, 88–91.

Bush, G., Spencer, T.J., Holmes, J., Shin, L.M., Valera, E.M., Seidman, L.J., Makris, N., Surman, C., Aleardi, M., Mick, E., Biederman, J., 2008. Functional magnetic resonance imaging of methylphenidate and placebo in attention-deficit/hyperactivity disorder during the multi-source interference task. Arch. Gen. Psychiatry 65 (1), 102–114.

Campolongo, P., Roozendaal, B., Trezza, V., Hauer, D., Schelling, G., McGaugh, J.L., et al., 2009. Endocannabinoids in the rat basolateral amygdale enhance memory consolidation and enable glucocorticoid modulation of memory. Proc. Natl. Acad. Sci. U.S.A. 106, 4888–4893.

Candy, M., Jones, L., Williams, R., et al., 2008. Psychostimulants for depression. Cochrane Database Syst. Rev. 16 (2), CD006722.

Carlson, P.J., Merlock, M.C., Suppes, T., 2004. Adjunctive stimulant use in patients with bipolar disorder: treatment of residual depression and sedation. Bipolar Disord. 2004 (6), 416–420.

Castaneda, A., Tuulio-Henriksson, A., Marttunen, M., Lonnqvist, J., Suvisaari, J., 2008. A review on cognitive impairments in depressive and anxiety disorders with a focus on young adults. J. Affect. Disord. 106, 1–27.

Castellanos, F.X., Lee, P.P., Sharp, W., Jeffries, N.O., Greenstein, D.K., et al., 2002. Developmental trajectories of brain volume abnormalities in children and adolescents with attention-deficit/hyperactivity disorder. J. Am. Med. Assoc. 288, 1740–1748.

Chambers, R.A., Krystal, J.H., Self, D.W., 2001. A neurobiological basis for substance abuse comorbidity in schizophrenia. Biol. Psychiatry 50, 71–83.

Choi, K.H., Wykes, T., Kurtz, M.M., 2013. Adjunctive pharmacotherapy for cognitive deficits in schizophrenia: meta-analytical investigation of efficacy. Br. J. Psychiatry 203 (3), 172–178.

Chung, Y.C.1, Lee, C.R., Park, T.W., Yang, K.H., Kim, K.W., 2009. Effect of donepezil added to atypical antipsychotics on cognition in patients with schizophrenia: an open-label trial. World J. Biol. Psychiatry 10 (2), 156–162.

Chue, P., 2013. Glycine reuptake inhibition as a new therapeutic approach in schizophrenia: focus on the glycine transporter 1 (GlyT1). Curr. Pharm. Des. 19 (7), 1311–1320.

Citrome, L., 2011. Treatment-resistant schizophrenia: what's next. Schizophr. Res. 133 (1–3), 1–2.

Citrome, L., 2014. Unmet needs in the treatment of schizophrenia: new targets to help different symptom domains. J. Clin. Psychiatry 75 (1), 21–26.

Conklin, H.M., Curtis, C.E., Katsanis, J., Iacono, W.G., 2000. Verbal working memory impairment in schizophrenia patients and their first-degree relatives: evidence from the digit span task. Am. J. Psychiatry 157 (2), 275–277.

Cooper, N.J., Keage, H., Hermens, D., Williams, L.M., Debrota, D., Clark, C.R., et al., 2005. The dose-dependent effect of methylphenidate on performance, cognition and psychophysiology. J. Integr. Neurosci. 4, 123–144.

Cornwell, B.R., Salvadore, G., Colon-Rosario, V., Latov, D.R., Holroyd, T., Carver, F.W., et al., 2010. Abnormal hippocampal functioning and impaired spatial navigation in depressed individuals: evidence from whole-head magnetoencephalography. Am. J. Psychiatry 167 (7), 836–844.

Coyle, J.T., Tsai, G., 2004. NMDA receptor function, neuroplasticity, and the pathophysiology of schizophrenia. Int. Rev. Neurobiol. 59, 491–515.

Czeisler, C.A., Walsh, J.K., Roth, T., Hughes, R.J., Wright, K.P., Kingsbury, L., Arora, S., Schwartz, J.R., Niebler, G.E., Dinges, D.F., 2005. US Modafinil in Shift Work Sleep Disorder Study Group: Modafinil for excessive sleepiness associated with shift-work sleep disorder. N. Engl. J. Med. 353, 476–486.

Daban, C., Martinez-Aran, A., Torrent, C., et al., 2006. Specificity of cognitive deficits in bipolar disorder versus schizophrenia: a systematic review. Psychother. Psychosom. 75, 72–84.

Dang, Y.H., Ma, X.C., Zhang, J.C., Ren, Q., Wu, J., Gao, C.G., Hashimoto, K., January 10, 2014. Targeting of NMDA receptors in the treatment of major depression. Curr. Pharm. Des. [Epub ahead of print].

Darves-Bornoz, J.M., Alonso, J., De Girolamo, G., DeGraaf, R., Haro, J.M., Kovess-Masfety, V., et al., 2008. Main traumatic events in Europe: PTSD in the European study of the epidemiology of mental disorders survey. J. Trauma. Stress 21, 455–462.

Davidson, M., Galderisi, S., Weiser, M., Werbeloff, N., Fleischhacker, W.W., Keefe, R.S., Boter, H., Keet, I.P., Prelipceanu, D., Rybakowski, J.K., Libiger, J., Hummer, M., Dollfus, S., Lopez-Ibor, J.J., Hranov, L.G., Gaebel, W., Peuskens, J., Lindefors, N., Riecher-Rossler, A., Kahn, R.S., 2009. Cognitive effects of antipsychotic drugs in first-episode schizophrenia and schizophreniform disorder: a randomized, open-label clinical trial (EUFEST). Am. J. Psychiatry 166, 675–682.

DeBattista, C., Lembke, A., Solvason, H.B., Ghebremichael, R., Poirier, J., 2004. A prospective trial of modafinil as an adjunctive treatment of major depression. J. Clin. Psychopharmacol. 24, 87–90.

DeLisi, L.E., Szulc, K.U., Bertisch, H.C., Majcher, M., Brown, K., 2006. Understanding structural brain changes in schizophrenia. Dialogues Clin. Neurosci. 8, 71–78.

Delahanty, D.L., Gabert-Quillen, C., Ostrowski, S.A., Nugent, N.R., Fischer, B., Morris, A., Pitman, R.K., Bon, J., Fallon, W., 2013. The efficacy of initial hydrocortisone administration at preventing posttraumatic distress in adult trauma patients: a randomized trial. CNS Spectr. 18 (2), 103–111.

Dell'Osso, B., Ketter, T.A., 2013. Use of adjunctive stimulants in adult bipolar depression. Int. J. Neuropsychopharmacol. 16 (1), 55–68.

Depatie, L., O'Driscoll, G.A., Holahan, A.L., Atkinson, V., Thavundayil, J.X., Kin, N.N., Lal, S., 2002. Nicotine and behavioral markers of risk for schizophrenia: a double-blind, placebo-controlled, cross-over study. Neuropsychopharmacology 27, 1056–1070.

Dhir, A., 2013. Vortioxetine for the treatment of major depression. Drugs Today (Barc.) 49 (12), 781–790.

Diamond, T., Muller, R., Rondeau, L.A., Rich, J.G., 2001. The relationships among PTSD symptomatology and cognitive functioning in adult survivors of child maltreatment. In: Columbus, F. (Ed.), Advances in psychology research, vol. V. Nova Science Publishers, Huntington, New York, pp. 253–279.

Dias, V.V., Brissos, S., Gorman, J.M., 2006. Adjuvant galantamine for cognitive dysfunction in a patient with bipolar disorder. J. Psychiatr. Pract. 12, 327–331.

Dickstein, S.G., Bannon, K., Castellanos, F.X., Milham, M.P., 2006. The neural correlates of attention deficit hyperactivity disorder: an ALE meta-analysis. J. Child Psychol. Psychiatry 47 (10), 1051–1062.

Difede, J., Cukor, J., Wyka, K., Olden, M., Hoffman, H., Lee, F.S., Altemus, M., 2014. D-cycloserine augmentation of exposure therapy for post-traumatic stress disorder: a pilot randomized clinical trial. Neuropsychopharmacology 39 (5), 1052–1058.

Dixon, T., Kravariti, E., Frith, C., Murray, R.M., McGuire, P.K., 2004. Effect of symptoms on executive function in bipolar illness. Psychol. Med. 34, 811–821.

Douglas, K.M., Porter, R.J., 2009. Longitudinal assessment of neuropsychological function in major depression. Aust N Z J Psychiatry 43 (12), 1105–1117.

Drevets, W.C., Zarate Jr., C.A., Furey, M.L., 2012. Antidepressant effects of the muscarinic cholinergic receptor antagonist scopolamine: a review. Biol. Psychiatry 73, 1156–1163.

Dumas, J.A., Newhouse, P.A., 2011. The cholinergic hypothesis of cognitive aging revisited again: cholinergic functional compensation. Pharmacol. Biochem. Behav. 99, 254–261.

Duncan, E.J., Madonick, S.H., Parwani, A., et al., 2001. Clinical and sensorimotor gating effects of ketamine in normals. Neuropsychopharmacology 25 (1), 72–83.

Dyer, M.A., Freudenreich, O., Culhane, M.A., et al., 2008. High-dose galantamine augmentation inferior to placebo on attention, inhibitory control and working memory performance in non-smokers with schizophrenia. Schizophr. Res. 102, 88–95.

Elbe, D., Reddy, D., 2014. Focus on guanfacine extended-release: a review of its use in child and adolescent psychiatry. J. Can. Acad. Child Adolesc. Psychiatry 23 (1), 48–60.

Fagerlund, B., Søholm, B., Fink-Jensen, A., Lublin, H., Glenthøj, B.Y., 2007. Effects of donepezil adjunctive treatment to ziprasidone on cognitive deficits in schizophrenia: a double-blind, placebo-controlled study. Clin. Neuropharmacol. 30, 3–12.

Farinde, A., 2013. Bipolar disorder: a brief examination of lithium therapy. J. Basic Clin. Pharm. 4 (4), 93–94.

Ferraro, L., Antonelli, T., Tanganelli, S., et al., 1999. The vigilance promoting drug modafinil increases extracellular glutamate levels in the medial preoptic area and the posterior hypothalamus of the conscious rat: prevention by local GABAA receptor blockade. Neuropsychopharmacology 20, 346–356.

Foa, E.B., Kozak, M.J., 1986. Emotional processing of fear: exposure to corrective information. Psychol. Bull. 99, 20–35.

Frangou, S., Donaldson, S., Hadjulis, M., Landau, S., Goldstein, L.H., 2005. The Maudsley bipolar disorder project: executive dysfunction in bipolar disorder I and its clinical correlates. Biol. Psychiatry 58, 859–864.

Fraser, G.A., 2009. The use of a synthetic cannabinoid in the management of treatment-resistant nightmares in posttraumatic stress disorder (PTSD). CNS Neurosci. Ther. Winter 15 (1), 84–88.

Freedman, R., Olincy, A., Buchanan, R.W., Harris, J.G., Gold, J.M., Johnson, L., et al., 2008. Initial phase 2 trial of a nicotinic agonist in schizophrenia. Am. J. Psychiatry 165, 1040–1047.

Freudenreich, O., Henderson, D.C., Macklin, E.A., Evins, A.E., Fan, X., Cather, C., Walsh, J.P., Goff, D.C., 2009. Modafinil for clozapine-treated schizophrenia patients: a double-blind, placebo-controlled pilot trial. J. Clin. Psychiatry 70 (12), 1674–1680.

Friedman, J.I., Adler, D.N., Howanitz, E., et al., 2002. A double blind placebo controlled trial of donepezil adjunctive treatment to risperidone for the cognitive impairment of schizophrenia. Biol. Psychiatry 51, 349–357.

Friedman, J.I., Adler, D.N., Temporini, H.D., Kemether, E., Harvey, P.D., White, L., et al., 2001. Guanfacine treatment of cognitive impairment in schizophrenia. Neuropsychopharmacology 25, 402–409.

Friedman, J.I., Carpenter, D., Lu, J., Fan, J., Tang, C.Y., White, L., Parrella, M., Bowler, S., Elbaz, Z., Flanagan, L., Harvey, P.D., 2008. A pilot study of adjunctive atomoxetine treatment to second-generation antipsychotics for cognitive impairment in schizophrenia. J. Clin. Psychopharmacol. 28 (1), 59–63.

Frye, M.A., Grunze, H., Suppes, T., McElroy, S.L., Keck Jr., P.E., Walden, J., Leverich, G.S., Altshuler, L.L., Nakelsky, S., Hwang, S., Mintz, J., Post, R.M., 2007. A placebo-controlled evaluation of adjunctive modafinil in the treatment of bipolar depression. Am. J. Psychiatry 164 (8), 1242–1249.

Furey, M.L., Drevets, W.C., 2006. Antidepressant efficacy of the antimuscarinic drug scopolamine: a randomized, placebo-controlled clinical trial. Arch. Gen. Psychiatry 63, 1121–1129.

Gallagher, P., Watson, S., Dye, C.E., Young, A.H., Nicol Ferrier, I., 2008. Persistent effects of mifepristone (RU-486) on cortisol levels in bipolar disorder and schizophrenia. J. Psychiatr. Res. 42, 1037–1041.

Gao, W.J., 2012. Dopaminergic and glutamatergic dysfunctions in the neuropathophysiology of schizophrenia. In: Kudo, Y., Fujii, Y. (Eds.), Dopamine: Functions, Regulation and Health Effects. Nova Science Publishers, New York, pp. 169–194.

George, T.P., O'Malley, S.S., 2004. Current pharmacological treatments for nicotine dependence. Trends Pharmacol. Sci. 25, 42–48.

George, T.P., 2007. Neurobiological links between nicotine addiction and schizophrenia. J. Dual Diagn. 3, 27–42.

Getahun, D., Jacobsen, S.J., Fassett, M.J., Chen, W., Demissie, K., Rhoads, G.G., 2013. Recent trends in childhood attention-deficit/hyperactivity disorder. JAMA Pediatr. 167 (3), 282–288.

Goff, D.C., Cather, C., Gottlieb, J.D., et al., 2008a. Once-weekly d-cycloserine effects on negative symptoms and cognition in schizophrenia: an exploratory study. Schizophr. Res. 106, 320–327.

Goff, D.C., Lamberti, J.S., Leon, A.C., et al., 2008b. A placebo-controlled add-on trial of the ampakine, CX516, for cognitive deficits in schizophrenia. Neuropsychopharmacology 33 (3), 465–472. 22.

Goldberg, J.F., Young, L.T., 2008. Pharmacologic strategies to enhance neurocognitive function. In: Goldberg, J.F., Burdick, K.E. (Eds.), Cognitive Dysfunction in Bipolar Disorder: A Guide for Clinicians. American Psychiatric Press, Washington, DC, pp. 159–194.

Goldberg, J.F., 2008. Adverse cognitive effects of psychotropic medications. In: Goldberg, J.F., Burdick, K.E. (Eds.), Cognitive Dysfunction in Bipolar Disorder: A Guide for Clinicians. American Psychiatric Press, Washington, DC, pp. 137–158.

Gonzalez-Blanch, C., Crespo-Facorro, B., Varez-Jimenez, M., Rodriguez-Sanchez, J.M., Pelayo-Teran, J.M., Perez-Iglesias, R., Vazquez-Barquero, J.L., 2008. Pretreatment predictors of cognitive deficits in early psychosis. Psychol. Med. 38, 737–746.

Goodman, J., Leong, K.C., Packard, M.G., 2012. Emotional modulation of multiple memory systems: implications for the neurobiology of post-traumatic stress disorder. Rev. Neurosci. 23, 627–643.

Goss, A.J., Kaser, M., Costafreda, S.G., Sahakian, B.J., Fu, C.H., 2013. Modafinil augmentation therapy in unipolar and bipolar depression: a systematic review and meta-analysis of randomized controlled trials. J. Clin. Psychiatry 74 (11), 1101–1107.

Green, M.F., Nuechterlein, K.H., Gold, J.M., Barch, D.M., Cohen, J., Essock, S., et al., 2004. Approaching a consensus cognitive battery for clinical trials in schizophrenia: the NIMH-MATRICS conference to select cognitive domains and test criteria. Biol. Psychiatry 56, 301–307.

Guthrie, R.M., Bryant, R.A., 2006. Extinction learning before trauma and subsequent posttraumatic stress. Psychosom. Med. 68 (2), 307–311.

Hammar, A., Lund, A., Hugdahl, K., 2003. Selective impairment in effortful information processing in major depression. J. Int. Neuropsychol. Soc. JINS 9, 954–959.

Harris, J.G., Kongs, S., Allensworth, D., Martin, L., Tregellas, J., Sullivan, B., et al., 2004. Effects of nicotine on cognitive deficits in schizophrenia. Neuropsychopharmacology 29, 1378–1385.

Hart, H., Radua, J., Nakao, T., Mataix-Cols, D., Rubia, K., 2013. Metaanalysis of functional magnetic resonance imaging studies of inhibition and attention in attention-deficit/hyperactivity disorder: exploring task-specific, stimulant medication, and age effects. JAMA Psychiatry 70, 185–198.

Harvey, P.D., Keefe, R.S., 2001. Studies of cognitive change in patients with schizophrenia following novel antipsychotic treatment. Am. J. Psychiatry 158, 176–184.

Hashimoto, K., 2010. Glycine transport inhibitors for the treatment of schizophrenia. Open Med. Chem. J. 4, 10–19.

Heinrichs, R.W., Zakzanis, K.K., 1998. Neurocognitive deficit in schizophrenia: a quantitative review of the evidence. Neuropsychology 12 (3), 426–445.

Heresco-Levy, U., Javitt, D.C., Ebstein, R., et al., 2005. D-serine efficacy as add-on pharmacotherapy to risperidone and olanzapine for treatment-refractory schizophrenia. Biol. Psychiatry 57, 577–585.

Herrera-Guzmán, I., Gudayol-Ferré, E., Herrera-Guzmán, D., Guàrdia-Olmos, J., Hinojosa-Calvo, E., Herrera-Abarca, J.E., 2009. Effects of selective serotonin reuptake and dual serotonergic-noradrenergic reuptake treatments on memory and mental processing speed in patients with major depressive disorder. J. Psychiatr. Res. 43, 855–863.

Hill, M.N., Gorzalka, B.B., 2009. The endocannabinoid system and the treatment of mood and anxiety disorders. CNS Neurol. Disord. Drug Targets 8, 451–458.

Hirota, T., Schwartz, S., Correll, C.U., 2014. Alpha-2 agonists for attention-deficit/hyperactivity disorder in youth: a systematic review and meta-analysis of monotherapy and add-on trials to stimulant therapy. J. Am. Acad. Child Adolesc. Psychiatry 53 (2), 153–173.

Hong, L.E., Thaker, G.K., McMahon, R.P., Summerfelt, A., Rachbeisel, J., Fuller, R.L., et al., 2011. Effects of moderate-dose treatment with varenicline on neurobiological and cognitive biomarkers in smokers and nonsmokers with schizophrenia or schizoaffective disorder. Arch. Gen. Psychiatry 68, 1195–1206.

Houthoofd, S.A., Morrens, M., Sabbe, B.G., 2008. Cognitive and psychomotor effects of risperidone in schizophrenia and schizoaffective disorder. Clin. Ther. 30, 1565–1589.

Hruska, B., Cullen, P.K., Delahanty, D.L., 2014. Pharmacological modulation of acute trauma memories to prevent PTSD: considerations from a developmental perspective. Neurobiol. Learn. Mem. 112, 122–129.

Hunt, R.D., Arnsten, A.F.T., Asbell, M.D., 1995. An open trial of guanfacine in the treatment of attention deficit hyperactivity disorder. J. Am. Acad. Child Adolesc. Psychiatry 34, 50–54.

Hunter, M.D., Ganesan, V., Wilkinson, I.D., Spence, S.A., 2006. Impact of modafinil on prefrontal executive function in schizophrenia. Am. J. Psychiatry 163, 2184–2186.

Hutton, S.B., Puri, B.K., Duncan, L.J., Robbins, T.W., Barnes, T.R.E., Joyce, E.M., 1998. Executive function in first-episode schizophrenia. Psychol. Med. 28 (2), 463–473.

Hyman, S.E., 2008. A glimmer of light for neuropsychiatric disorders. Nature 455, 890–893.

Ichikawa, J., Ishii, H., Bonaccorso, S., Fowler, W.L., O'laughlin, I.A., Meltzer, H.Y., 2001. 5-HT(2A) and D(2) receptor blockade increases cortical DA release via 5-HT(1A) receptor activation: a possible mechanism of atypical antipsychotic-induced cortical dopamine release. J. Neurochem. 76, 1521–1531.

Iosifescu, D.V., Moore, C.M., Deckersbach, T., Tilley, C.A., Ostacher, M.J., Sachs, G.S., et al., 2009. Galantamine-ER for cognitive dysfunction in bipolar disorder and correlation with hippocampal neuronal viability: a proof-of-concept study. CNS Neurosci. Ther. 15, 309–319.

Ipser, J., Seedat, S., Stein, D.J., 2006. Pharmacotherapy for post-traumatic stress disorder – a systematic review and meta-analysis. S. Afr. Med. J. 96 (10), 1088–1096.

Isaac, C.L., Cushway, D., Jones, G.V., 2006. Is posttraumatic stress disorder associated with specific deficits in episodic memory? Clin. Psychol. Rev. 26 (8), 939–955.

Jacobsen, F.M., Comas-Diaz, L., 1999. Donepezil for psychotropic-induced memory loss. J. Clin. Psychiatry 60, 698–704.

Jansari, A.S., Froggatt, D., Edginton, T., Dawkins, L., 2013. Investigating the impact of nicotine on executive functions using a novel virtual reality assessment. Addiction 108, 977–984.

Jarrett, M.A., Ollendick, T.H., 2008. A conceptual review of the comorbidity of attention-deficit/hyperactivity disorder and anxiety: implications for future research and practice. Clin. Psychol. Rev. 28 (7), 1266–1280.

Javitt, D.C., Duncan, L., Balla, A., Sershen, H., 2005. Inhibition of system A-mediated glycine transport in cortical synaptosomes by therapeutic concentrations of clozapine: implications for mechanisms of action. Mol. Psychiatry 10 (3), 275–287.

Javitt, D.C., 2009. Glycine transport inhibitors for the treatment of schizophrenia: symptom and disease modification. Curr. Opin. Drug Discov. Devel. 12, 468–478.

Javitt, D.C., 2012. Glycine transport inhibitors in the treatment of schizophrenia. Handb. Exp. Pharmacol. 213, 367–399.

Javitt, D.C., Zukin, S.R., 1991. Recent advances in the phencyclidine model of schizophrenia. Am. J. Psychiatry 148, 1301–1308.

Jeffreys, M., Capehart, B., Friedman, M.J., 2012. Pharmacotherapy for posttraumatic stress disorder: review with clinical applications. J. Rehabil. Res. Dev. 49 (5), 703–715.

Joels, M., Baram, T.Z., 2009. The neuro-symphony of stress. Nature Reviews Neuroscience 10, 459–466.

Johnson, J.K., Lui, L.Y., Yaffe, K., 2007. Executive function, more than global cognition, predicts functional decline and mortality in elderly women. Journals Gerontol. Ser. A Biol. Sci. Med. Sci. 62, 1134–1141.

Kane, J.M., D'Souza, D.C., Patkar, A.A., Youakim, J.M., Tiller, J.M., Yang, R., Keefe, R.S., 2010. Armodafinil as adjunctive therapy in adults with cognitive deficits associated with schizophrenia: a 4-week, double-blind, placebo-controlled study. J. Clin. Psychiatry 71 (11), 1475–1481.

Kantrowitz, J.T., Javitt, D.C., 2010. Thinking glutamatergically: changing concepts of schizophrenia based upon changing neurochemical models. Clin. Schizophr. Relat. Psychoses. 4 (3), 189–200.

Kantrowitz, J.T., Javitt, D.C., 2011. Glutamate: new hope for schizophrenia treatment. Curr. Psychiatry 10 (4), 69–74.

Kantrowitz, J.T., Malhotra, A.K., Cornblatt, B., Silipo, G., Balla, A., Suckow, R.F., D'Souza, C., Saksa, J., Woods, S.W., Javitt, D.C., 2010. High dose D-serine in the treatment of schizophrenia. Schizophr. Res. 121 (1–3), 125–130.

Katona, C., Hansen, T., Olsen, C.K., 2012. A randomized, doubleblind, placebo-controlled, duloxetine-referenced, fixed dose study comparing the efficacy and safety of Lu AA21004 in elderly patients with major depressive disorder. Int. Clin. Psychopharmacol. 27 (4), 215–223.

Keefe, R.S., Bilder, R.M., Davis, S.M., et al., 2007. Neurocognitive effects of antipsychotic medications in patients with chronic schizophrenia in the CATIE trial. Arch. Gen. Psychiatry 64, 633–647.

Keefe, R.S., Eesley, C.E., Poe, M.P., 2003. Defining a cognitive function decrement in schizophrenia. Biol. Psychiatry 57 (6), 688–691.

Keefe, R.S., Malhotra, A.K., Meltzer, H.Y., et al., 2008. Efficacy and safety of donepezil in patients with schizophrenia or schizoaffective disorder: significant placebo/practice effects in a 12-week, randomized, double-blind, placebocontrolled trial. Neuropsychopharmacol 33, 1217–1228.

Kelly, D.L., Buchanan, R.W., Boggs, D.L., McMahon, R.P., Dickinson, D., Nelson, M., Gold, J.M., Ball, M.P., Feldman, S., Liu, F., Conley, R.R., 2009. A randomized double-blind trial of atomoxetine for cognitive impairments in 32 people with schizophrenia. J. Clin. Psychiatry 70 (4), 518–525.

Kessler, R.C., Berglund, P., Demler, O., Jin, R., Merikangas, K.R., Walters, E.E., 2005. Lifetime prevalence and age-of-onset distributions of DSM-IV disorders in the national comorbidity survey replication. Arch. Gen. Psychiatry 62, 593–602.

Khantzian, E.J., 1985. The self-medication hypothesis of addictive disorders: focus on heroin and cocaine dependence. Am. J. Psychiatry 142, 1259–1264.

Koukopoulos, A., Serra, G., Koukopoulos, A.E., Reginaldi, D., Serra, G., 2012. The sustained mood-stabilizing effect of memantine in the management of treatment resistant bipolar disorders: findings from a 12-month naturalistic trial. J. Affect. Disord. 136, 163–166.

Kovacs, T., 2009. Therapy of Alzheimer disease. Neuropsychopharmacol. Hung. 11 (1), 27–33.

Krystal, J.H., Karper, L.P., Seibyl, J.P., Freeman, G.K., Delaney, R., Bremner, J.D., Heninger, G.R., Bowers Jr., M.B., Charney, D.S., 1994. Subanesthetic effects of the noncompetitive NMDA antagonist, ketamine, in humans. Psychotomimetic, perceptual, cognitive, and neuroendocrine responses. Arch. Gen. Psychiatry 51, 199–214.

Lampe, I.K., Sitskoorn, M.M., Heeren, T.J., 2004. Effects of recurrent major depressive disorder on behavior and cognitive function in female depressed patients. Psychiatry Res. 125, 73–79.

Landro, N.I., Stiles, T.C., Sletvold, H., 2001. Neuropsychological function in nonpsychotic unipolar major depression. Neuropsychiatry Neuropsychol. Behav. Neurol. 14, 233–240.

Laruelle, M., Gelernter, J., Innis, R.B., 1998. D2 receptors binding potential is not affected by Taq1 polymorphism at the D2 receptor gene. Mol. Psychiatry 3 (3), 261–265.

Lee, S.W., Lee, J.G., Lee, B.J., Kim, Y.H., 2007. A 12-week, doubleblind, placebo-controlled trial of galantamine adjunctive treatment to conventional antipsychotics for the cognitive impairments in chronic schizophrenia. Int. Clin. Psychopharmacol. 22, 63–68.

Lee, R.S.C., Hermens, D.F., Porter, M.A., Redoblado-Hodge, M.A., 2012. A meta-analysis of cognitive deficits in first-episode major depressive disorder. J. Affect. Disord. 140, 113–124.

Lencz, T., Smith, C.W., McLaughlin, D., Auther, A., Nakayama, E., Hovey, L., Cornblatt, B.A., 2006. Generalized and specific neurocognitive deficits in prodromal schizophrenia. Biol. Psychiatry 59, 863–871.

Leucht, S., Corves, C., Arbter, D., Engel, R.R., Li, C., Davis, J.M., 2009. Second-generation versus first-generation antipsychotic drugs for schizophrenia: a meta-analysis. Lancet 373 (9657), 31–41.

Levin, E.D., Wilson, W., Rose, J.E., McEvoy, J., 1996. Nicotine-haloperidol interactions and cognitive performance in schizophrenics. Neuropsychopharmacology 15, 429–436.

Li, X.M., Perry, K.W., Wong, D.T., Bymaster, F.P., 1998. Olanzapine increases *in vivo* dopamine and norepinephrine release in rat prefrontal cortex, nucleus accumbens and striatum. Psychopharmacology (Berl) 136 (2), 153–161.

Lieberman, J.A., Dunbar, G., Segreti, A.C., Girgis, R.R., Seoane, F., Beaver, J.S., Duan, N., Hosford, D.A., 2013. A randomized exploratory trial of an alpha-7 nicotinic receptor agonist (TC-5619) for cognitive enhancement in schizophrenia. Neuropsychopharmacology 38, 968–975.

Lin, S.Y., Stevens, M.B., 2014. The symptom cluster-based approach to individualize patient-centered treatment for major depression. J. Am. Board Fam. Med. 27 (1), 151–159.

Lindenmayer, J.P., Khan, A., Iskander, A., Abad, M.T., Parker, B., 2007. A randomized controlled trial of olanzapine versus haloperidol in the treatment of primary negative symptoms and neurocognitive deficits in schizophrenia. J. Clin. Psychiatry 68, 368–379.

Lohr, J.B., Liu, L., Caligiuri, M.P., Kash, T.P., May, T.A., Murphy, J.D., Ancoli-Israel, S., 2013. Modafinil improves antipsychotic-induced parkinsonism but not excessive daytime sleepiness, psychiatric symptoms or cognition in schizophrenia and schizoaffective disorder: a randomized, double-blind, placebo-controlled study. Schizophr. Res. 150 (1), 289–296.

Losier, B.J., McGrath, P.J., Klein, R.M., 1996. Error patterns on the continuous performance test in non-medicated and medicated samples of children with and without AD/HD: a meta-analytic review. J. Child Psychol. Psychiatry 37, 971–987.

Lu, P.H., Edland, S.D., Teng, E., Tingus, K., Petersen, R.C., Cummings, J.L., Alzheimer's disease cooperative study group, 2009. Donepezil delays progression to AD in MCI subjects with depressive symptoms. Neurology 72 (24), 2115–2121.

Lutz, B., 2007. The endocannabinoid system and extinction learning. Mol. Neurobiol. 36, 92–101.

Lydon, E., El-Mallakh, R.S., 2006. Naturalistic long-term use of methylphenidate in bipolar disorder. J. Clin. Psychopharmacol. 26, 516–518.

Maalouf, F.T., Brent, D., Clark, L., Tavitian, L., McHugh, R.M., Sahakian, B.J., Phillips, M.L., 2011. Neurocognitive impairment in adolescent major depressive disorder: state vs trait illness markers. J. Affect. Disord. 133, 625–632.

MacEwan, G.W., Ehmann, T.S., Khanbhai, I., Wrixon, C., 2001. Donepezil in schizophrenia–is it helpful? an experimental design case study. Acta Psychiatr. Scand. 104 (6), 469–472.

Madras, B.K., Xie, Z., Lin, Z., et al., 2006. Modafinil occupies dopamine and norepinephrine transporters in vivo and modulates the transporters and trace amine activity in vivo. J. Pharmacol. Exper. Ther. 319, 561–569.

Martínez-Arán, A., Vieta, E., Reinares, M., Colom, F., Torrent, C., Sánchez-Moreno, J., et al., 2004. Cognitive function across manic or hypomanic, depressed, and euthymic states in bipolar disorder. Am. J. Psychiatry 161, 262–270.

Mattay, V.S., Callicott, J.H., Bertolino, A., Heaton, I., Frank, J.A., Coppola, R., Berman, K.F., Goldberg, T.E., Weinberger, D.R., 2000. Effects of dextroamphetamine on cognitive performance and cortical activation. Neuroimage 12 (3), 268–275.

Mazurov, A.A., Kombo, D.C., Hauser, T.A., Miao, L., Dull, G., Genus, J.F., Fedorov, N.B., Benson, L., Sidach, S., Xiao, Y., Hammond, P.S., James, J.W., Miller, C.H., Yohannes, D., 2012. Discovery of (2S,3R)-N-[2-(pyridin-3-ylmethyl)-1-azabicyclo[2.2.2]oct-3-yl]benzo[b] furan-2-carboxamide (TC-5619), a selective α7 nicotinic acetylcholine receptor agonist, for the treatment of cognitive disorders. J. Med. Chem. 55 (22), 9793–9809.

McClure, M.M., Barch, D.M., Romero, M.J., Minzenberg, M.J., Triebwasser, J., Harvey, P.D., et al., 2007. The effects of guanfacine on context processing abnormalities in schizotypal personality disorder. Biol. Psychiatry 61, 1157–1160.

McLennan, S.N., Mathias, J.L., 2010. The depression-executive dysfunction (DED) syndrome and response to antidepressants: a meta-analytic review. Int. J. Geriatr. Psychiatry 25 (10), 933–944.

Meador, K.J., Loring, D.W., Ray, P.G., et al., 2001. Differential cognitive and behavioral effects of carbamazepine and lamotrigine. Neurology 56, 1177–1182.

Mehta, M.A., Owen, A.M., Sahakian, B.J., Mavaddat, N., Pickard, J.D., Robbins, T.W., 2000. Methylphenidate enhances working memory by modulating discrete frontal and parietal lobe regions in the human brain. J. Neurosci. 20, RC65.

Melancon, B.J., Tarr, J.C., Panarese, J.D., Wood, M.R., Lindsley, C.W., 2013. Allosteric modulation of the M1 muscarinic acetylcholine receptor: improving cognition and a potential treatment for schizophrenia and Alzheimer's disease. Drug Discov. Today 18, 23–24.

Menza, M.A., Kaufman, K.R., Castellanos, A., 2000. Modafinil augmentation of antidepressant treatment in depression. J. Clin. Psychiatry 61 (5), 378–381.

Michelson, D., Allen, A.J., Busner, J., Casat, C., Dunn, D., Kratochvil, C., et al., 2002. Once-daily atomoxetine treatment for children and adolescents with attention deficit hyperactivity disorder: a randomized, placebo-controlled study. Am. J. Psychiatry 159, 1896–1901.

Milad, M.R., Rauch, S.L., 2007. The role of the orbitofrontal cortex in anxiety disorders. Ann. N.Y. Acad. Sci. 1121, 546–561.

Millan, M.J., Agid, Y., Brune, M., Bullmore, E.T., Carter, C.S., Clayton, N.S., Connor, R., Davis, S., Deakin, B., DeRubeis, R.J., Dubois, B., Geyer, M.A., Goodwin, G.M., Gorwood, P., Jay, T.M., Joels, M., Mansuy, I.M., Meyer-Lindenberg, A., Murphy, D., Rolls, E., Saletu, B., Spedding, M., Sweeney, J., Whittington, M., Young, L.J., 2012. Cognitive dysfunction in psychiatric disorders: characteristics, causes and the quest for improved therapy. Nat. Rev. Drug Discov. 11, 141–168.

Mintzer, M.Z., Griffiths, R.R., 2003. Lorazepam and scopolamine: a single-dose comparison of effects on human memory and attentional processes. Exp. Clin. Psychopharmacol. 11, 56–72.

Minzenberg, M.J., Carter, C.S., 2008. Modafinil: a review of neurochemical actions and effects on cognition. Neuropsychopharmacology 33 (7), 1477–1502.

Minzenberg, M.J., Poole, J.H., Benton, C., Vinogradov, S., 2004. Association of anticholinergic load with impairment of complex attention and memory in schizophrenia. Am. J. Psychiatry 161, 116–124.

Moghaddam, B., 2003. Bringing order to the glutamate chaos in schizophrenia. Neuron 40 (5), 881–884.

Mohamed, S., Paulsen, J.S., O'Leary, D., Arndt, S., Andreasen, N., 1999. Generalized cognitive deficits in schizophrenia: a study of first-episode patients. Arch. Gen. Psychiatry 56, 749–754.

Mohs, R.C., 1995. Assessing cognitive function in schizophrenics and patients with Alzheimer's disease. Schizophr. Res. 17 (1), 115–121.

Morein-Zamir, S., Turner, D.C., Sahakian, B.J., 2007. A review of the effects of modafinil on cognition in schizophrenia. Schizophr. Bull. 33, 1298–1306.

Morgan, C.J., Curran, H.V., 2006. Acute and chronic effects of ketamine upon human memory: a review. Psychopharmacology 188, 408–424.

Moss, T.G., Sacco, K.A., Allen, T.M., Weinberger, A.H., Vessicchio, J.C., George, T.P., 2009. Prefrontal cognitive dysfunction is associated with tobacco dependence treatment failure in smokers with schizophrenia. Drug Alcohol Depend. 104, 94–99.

Mostofsky, S.H., Cooper, K.L., Kates, W.R., Denckla, M.B., Kaufmann, W.E., 2002. Smaller prefrontal and premotor volumes in boys with attention-deficit/hyperactivity disorder. Biol. Psychiatry 52, 785–794.

Müller, U., Rowe, J.B., Rittman, T., et al., 2013. Effects of modafinil on non-verbal cognition, task enjoyment and creative thinking in healthy volunteers. Neuropharmacology 64, 490–495.

Murphy, B.L., Arnsten, A.F.T., Goldman-Rakic, P.S., Roth, R.H., 1996. Increased dopamine turnover in the prefrontal cortex impairs spatial working memory performance in rats and monkeys. Proc. Natl. Acad. Sci. U.S.A. 93, 1325–1329.

Murrough, J.W., Iosifescu, D.V., Chang, L.C., et al., 2013. Antidepressant efficacy of ketamine in treatment-resistant major depression: a two-site randomized controlled trial. Am. J. Psychiatry 170 (10), 1134–1142.

Muscatello, M.R., Bruno, A., Pandolfo, G., Micò, U., Bellinghieri, P.M., Scimeca, G., Cacciola, M., Campolo, D., Settineri, S., Zoccali, R., 2011. Topiramate augmentation of clozapine in schizophrenia: a double-blind, placebo-controlled study. J. Psychopharmacol. 25 (5), 667–674.

Myers, K.M., Carlezon Jr, W.A., Davis, M., 2011. Glutamate receptors in extinction and extinction-based therapies for psychiatric illness. Neuropsychopharmacology 36 (1), 274–293.

Narendran, R., Young, C.M., Valenti, A.M., Nickolova, M.K., Pristach, C.A., 2002. Is psychosis exacerbated by modafinil? Arch. Gen. Psychiatry 59, 292–293.

Nebes, R.D., Pollock, B.G., Houck, P.R., Butters, M.A., Mulsant, B.H., Zmuda, M.D., et al., 2003. Persistence of cognitive impairment in geriatric patients following antidepressant treatment: a randomized, double-blind clinical trial with nortriptyline and paroxetine. J. Psychiatr. Res. 37, 99–108.

Nelson, J.C., Charney, D.S., 1981. The symptoms of major depressive illness. Am. J. Psychiatry 138, 1–13.

Neumeister, A., 2013. The endocannabinoid system provides an avenue for evidence-based treatment development for PTSD. Depress. Anxiety 30, 93–96.

Olincy, A., Freedman, R., 2012. Nicotinic mechanisms in the treatment of psychotic disorders: a focus on the α7 nicotinic receptor. Handb. Exp. Pharmacol. 213, 211–232.

Orr, K., Taylor, D., 2007. Psychostimulants in the treatment of depression: a review of the evidence. CNS Drugs 21, 239–257.

Pachet, A.K., Wisniewski, A.M., 2003. The effects of lithium on cognition: an updated review. Psychopharmacology 170, 225–234.

Pack, A.I., Black, J.E., Schwartz, J.R.L., Matheson, J.K., 2001. Modafinil as adjunct therapy for daytime sleepiness in obstructive sleep apnea. Am. J. Respir. Crit. Care. Med. 164, 1675–1681.

Paelecke-Habermann, Y., Pohl, J., Leplow, B., 2005. Attention and executive functions in remitted major depression patients. J. Affect. Disord. 89, 125–135.

Patil, S.T., Zhang, L., Martenyi, F., Patil, S.T., Zhang, L., Martenyi, F., Lowe, S.L., Jackson, K.A., Andreev, B.V., Avedisova, A.S., Bardenstein, L.M., et al., 2007. Activation of mGlu2/3 receptors as a new approach to treat schizophrenia: a randomized Phase 2 clinical trial. Nat. Med. 13 (9), 1102–1107.

Patkar, A.A., Masand, P.S., Pae, C.U., et al., 2006. A randomized, double-blind, placebo-controlled trial of augmentation with an extended release formulation of methylphenidate in outpatients with treatment-resistant depression. J. Clin. Psychopharmacol. 26, 653–656.

Peskind, E.R., Bonner, L.T., Hoff, D.J., Raskind, M.A., 2003. Prazosin reduces trauma-related nightmares in older men with chronic posttraumatic stress disorder. J. Geriatr. Psychiatry Neurol. 16 (3), 165–171.

Peuskens, J., Demily, C., Thibaut, F., 2005. Treatment of cognitive dysfunction in schizophrenia. Clin. Ther. 27 (1), S25–S37.

Pietrzak, R.H., Snyder, P.J., Maruff, P., 2010. Use of an acute challenge with d-amphetamine to model cognitive improvement in chronic schizophrenia. Hum. Psychopharmacol. 25 (4), 353–358.

Piomelli, D., 2003. The molecular logic of endocannabinoid signalling. Nat. Rev. Neurosci. 4, 873–884.

Pitman, R.K., 1989. Post-traumatic stress disorder, hormones, and memory. Biol. Psychiatry 26 (3), 221–223.

Pitman, R.K., Delahanty, D.L., 2005. Conceptually driven pharmacological approaches to acute trauma. CNS Spectr. 10, 99–106.

Pliszka, S.R., Crismon, M.L., Hughes, C.W., 2006. The Texas children's medication algorithm project: revision of the algorithm for pharmacotherapy of attention-deficit/hyperactivity disorder. J. Am. Acad. Child Adolesc. Psychiatry 45, 642–657.

Porter, R.J., Gallagher, P., Thompson, J.M., Young, A.H., 2003. Neurocognitive impairment in drug-free patients with major depressive disorder. Br. J. Psychiatry J. Ment. Sci. 182, 214–220.

Potter, G.G., Kittinger, J.D., Wagner, H.R., Steffens, D.C., Krishnan, K.R., 2004. Prefrontal neuro-psychological predictors of treatment remission in late-life depression. Neuropsychopharmacology, 2266–2271.

Powers, R.L., Marks, D.J., Miller, C.J., Newcorn, J.H., Halperin, J.M., 2008. Stimulant treatment in children with attention-deficit/hyperactivity disorder moderates adolescent academic outcome. J. Child Adolesc. Psychopharmacol. 18, 449–459.

Preskorn, S.H., Gawryl, M., Dgetluck, N., Palfreyman, M., Bauer, L.O., Hilt, D.C., 2014. Normalizing effects of EVP-6124, an alpha-7 nicotinic partial agonist, on event-related potentials and cognition: a proof of concept, randomized trial in patients with schizophrenia. J. Psychiatr. Pract. 20 (1), 12–24.

Pringsheim, T., Steeves, T., 2011. Pharmacological treatment for attention deficit hyperactivity disorder (ADHD) in children with comorbid tic disorders. Cochrane Database Syst. Rev. 4, CD007990.

Quednow, B.B., 2010. Ethics of neuroenhancement: a phantom debate. Biosocieties 5, 153–156.

de Quervain, D.J., Margraf, J., 2008. Glucocorticoids for the treatment of post-traumatic stress disorder and phobias: a novel therapeutic approach. Eur. J. Pharmacol. 583 (2–3), 365–371.

de Quervain, D.J., Bentz, D., Michael, T., Bolt, O.C., Wiederhold, B.K., Margraf, J., et al., 2011. Glucocorticoids enhance extinction-based psychotherapy. Proceedings of the National Academy of Sciences of the United States of America 108 (16), 6621–6625.

Quirk, G.J., Mueller, D., 2008. Neural mechanisms of extinction learning and retrieval. Neuropsychopharmacology 33, 56–72.

Raskind, M.A., Peskind, E.R., Hoff, D.J., Hart, K.L., Holmes, H.A., Warren, D., Shofer, J., O'Connell, J., Taylor, F., Gross, C., Rohde, K., McFall, M.E., 2007. A parallel group placebo controlled study of prazosin for trauma nightmares and sleep disturbance in combat veterans with post-traumatic stress disorder. Biol. Psychiatry. 561 (8), 928–934.

Reynolds 3rd, C.F., Butters, M.A., Lopez, O., Pollock, B.G., Dew, M.A., Mulsant, B.H., et al., 2011. Maintenance treatment of depression in old age: a randomized, double-blind, placebo-controlled evaluation of the efficacy and safety of donepezil combined with antidepressant pharmacotherapy. Arch. Gen. Psychiatry 68, 51–60.

Riccio, C.A., Waldrop, J.J., Reynolds, C.R., Lowe, P., 2001. Effects of stimulants on the continuous performance test (CPT): implications for CPT use and interpretation. J. Neuropsychiatry Clin. Neurosci. 13, 326–335.

Rock, P.L., Roiser, J.P., Riedel, W.J., Blackwell, A.D., 2013. Cognitive impairment in depression: a systematic review and meta-analysis. Psychol. Med. 29, 1–12.

Rogers, M.A., Kasai, K., Koji, M., Fukuda, R., Iwanami, A., Nakagome, K., Fukuda, M., Kato, N., 2004. Executive and prefrontal dysfunction in unipolar depression: a review of neuropsychological and imaging evidence. Neurosci. Res. 50 (1), 1–11.

Ross, R.G., Harris, J.G., Olincy, A., Radant, A., 2000. Eye movement task measures inhibition and spatial working memory in adults with schizophrenia, ADHD, and a normal comparison group. Psychiatry Res. 95, 35–42.

Rothbaum, B.O., Price, M., Jovanovic, T., Norrholm, S.D., Gerardi, M., Dunlop, B., Davis, M., Bradley, B., Duncan, E.J., Rizzo, A., Ressler, K.J., 2014. A randomized, double-blind evaluation of d-cycloserine or Alprazolam combined with virtual reality exposure therapy for posttraumatic stress disorder in Iraq and Afghanistan war veterans. Am. J. Psychiatry 171 (6), 640–648.

Rush, A.J., Trivedi, M.H., Wisniewski, S.R., Nierenberg, A.A., Stewart, J.W., Warden, D., et al., 2006. Acute and longer-term outcomes in depressed outpatients requiring one or several treatment steps: a STAR/D report. Am. J. Psychiatry 163, 1905–1917.

Sacco, K.A., Creeden, C., Reutenauer, E.L., George, T.P., 2008. Effects of galantamine on cognitive deficits in smokers and non-smokers with schizophrenia. Schizophr. Res. 103, 326–327.

Saha, S., Chant, D., Welham, J., McGrath, J., 2005. A systematic review of the prevalence of schizophrenia. PLoS Med. 2, e141.

Salinsky, M.C., Storzbach, D., Spencer, D.C., Oken, B.S., Landry, T., Dodrill, C.B., 2005. Effects of topiramate and gabapentin on cognitive abilities in healthy volunteers. Neurology 64, 792–798.

Sani, G., Serra, G., Kotzalidis, G.D., Romano, S., Tamorri, S.M., Manfredi, G., et al., 2012. The role of memantine in the treatment of psychiatric disorders other than the dementias: a review of current preclinical and clinical evidence. CNS Drugs 26, 663–690.

Sapolsky, R.M., Romero, L.M., Munck, A.U., 2000. How do glucocorticoids influence stress responses? Integrating permissive, suppressive, stimulatory, and preparative actions. Endocr. Rev. 21 (1), 55–89.

Sawaguchi, T., Goldman-Rakic, P.S., 1991. D1 dopamine receptors in prefrontal cortex: involvement in working memory. Science 251, 947–950.

Scheeringa, M.S., Weems, C.F., 2014. Randomized placebo-controlled D-cycloserine with cognitive behavior therapy for pediatric posttraumatic stress. J. Child Adolesc. Psychopharmacol. 24 (2), 69–77.

Scheffer, R.E., Kowatch, R.A., Carmody, T., Rush, A.J., 2005. Randomized, placebo-controlled trial of mixed amphetamine salts for symptoms of comorbid ADHD in pediatric bipolar disorder after mood destabilization with divalproex sodium. Am. J. Psychiatry 162, 58–64.

Schrauwen, E., Ghaemi, S.N., 2006. Galantamine treatment of cognitive impairment in bipolar disorder: four cases. Bipolar Disord. 8, 196–199.

Schubert, M.H., Young, K.A., Hicks, P.B., 2006. Galantamine improves cognition in schizophrenic patients stabilized on risperidone. Biol. Psychiatry 60, 530–533.

Schulz, K.P., Newcorn, J.H., Fan, J., Tang, C.Y., Halperin, J.M., 2005. Brain activation gradients in ventrolateral prefrontal cortex related to persistence of ADHD in adolescence. J. Am. Acad. Child Adolesc. Psychiatry 44, 47–54.

Sciberras, E., Lycett, K., Efron, D., Mensah, F., Gerner, B., Hiscock, H., April 21, 2014. Anxiety in children with attention-deficit/hyperactivity disorder. Pediatrics. [Epub ahead of print].

Seiden, L.S., Commins, D.L., Vosmer, G., Axt, K., Marek, G., 1988. Neurotoxicity in dopamine and 5-hydroxytryptamine terminal fields: a regional analysis in nigrostriatal and mesolimbic projections. Ann. N.Y. Acad. Sci. 537, 161–172.

Sevy, S., Rosenthal, M.H., Alvir, J., et al., 2005. Double-blind, placebo-controlled study of modafinil for fatigue and cognition in schizophrenia patients treated with psychotropic medications. J. Clin. Psychiatry 66 (7), 839–843.

Sharma, T., Reed, C., Aasen, I., Kumari, V., 2006. Cognitive effects of adjunctive 24-weeks Rivastigmine treatment to antipsychotics in schizophrenia: a randomized, placebo controlled, double-blind investigation. Schizophr. Res. 85, 73–83.

Shaw, P., Eckstrand, K., Sharp, W., Blumenthal, J., Lerch, J.P., et al., 2007. Attention-deficit/hyperactivity disorder is characterized by a delay in cortical maturation. Proc. Natl. Acad. Sci. U.S.A. 104, 19649–19654.

Shim, J.C., Jung, D.U., Jung, S.S., Seo, Y.S., Cho, D.M., Lee, J.H., et al., 2012. Adjunctive varenicline treatment with antipsychotic medications for cognitive impairments in people with schizophrenia: a randomized double-blind placebo-controlled trial. Neuropsychopharmacology 37, 660–668.

Smith, R.C., Lindenmayer, J.P., Davis, J.M., Cornwell, J., Noth, K., Gupta, S., et al., 2009. Cognitive and antismoking effects of varenicline in patients with schizophrenia or schizoaffective disorder. Schizophr. Res. 110, 149–155.

Smith, R.C., Singh, A., Infante, M., Khandat, A., Kloos, A., 2002. Effects of cigarette smoking and nicotine nasal spray on psychiatric symptoms and cognition in schizophrenia. Neuropsychopharmacology 27, 479–497.

Soravia, L.M., Heinrichs, M., Aerni, A., Maroni, C., Schelling, G., Ehlert, U., et al., 2006. Glucocorticoids reduce phobic fear in humans. Proceedings of the National Academy of Sciences of the United States of America 103 (14), 5585–5590.

Stahl, S.M., 2008. Stahl's Essential Psychopharmacology: Neuroscientific Basis and Practical Application, third ed. Cambridge University Press, New York, NY, USA.

Stahl, S.M., 2000. Essential Psychopharmacology of Depression and Bipolar Disorder. Cambridge University Press, Cambridge, UK.

Steckler, T., Risbrough, V., 2012. Pharmacological treatment of PTSD - established and new approaches. Neuropharmacology 62 (2), 617–627.

Stein, M.B., Kerridge, C., Dimsdale, J.E., Hoyt, D.B., 2007. Pharmacotherapy to prevent PTSD: results from a randomized controlled proof-of-concept trial in physically injured patients. J. Trauma. Stress 20, 923–932.

Stoll, A.L., Locke, C.A., Vuckovic, A., Mayer, P.V., 1996. Lithium associated cognitive and functional deficits reduced by a switch to divalproex: a case series. J. Clin. Psychiatry 57, 356–359.

Stryjer, R., Bar, F., Strous, R.D., Baruch, Y., Rabey, J.M., 2002. Donepezil management of schizophrenia with associated dementia. J. Clin. Psychopharmacol. 22 (2), 226–229.

Strzelecki, D., Tabaszewska, A., Barszcz, Z., Józefowicz, O., Kropiwnicki, P., Rabe-Jabłońska, J., 2013. A 10-week memantine treatment in bipolar depression: a case report. Focus on depressive symptomatology, cognitive parameters and quality of life. Psychiatry Investig. 10 (4), 421–424.

Sumiyoshi, T., Matsui, M., Nohara, S., et al., 2001. Enhancement of cognitive performance in schizophrenia by addition of tandospirone to neuroleptic treatment. Am. J. Psychiatry 158, 1722–1725.

Sumiyoshi, T., Park, S., Jayathilake, K., Roy, A., Ertugrul, A., Meltzer, H.Y., 2007. Effect of buspirone, a serotonin(1A) partial agonist, on cognitive function in schizophrenia: a randomized, double-blind, placebo-controlled study. Schizophr. Res. 95, 158–168.

Sumiyoshi, T., Higuchi, Y., Uehara, T., 2013. Neural basis for the ability of atypical antipsychotic drugs to improve cognition in schizophrenia. Front. Behav. Neurosci. 16 (7), 140.

Sunderland, T., Tariot, P.N., Newhouse, P.A., 1988. Differential responsivity of mood, behavior, and cognition to cholinergic agents in elderly neuropsychiatric populations. Brain Res. 472 (4), 371–389.

Tandon, R., Nasrallah, H.A., Keshavan, M.S., 2009. Schizophrenia, "just the facts" 4. Clinical features and conceptualization. Schizophr. Res. 110, 1–23.

Tawa, J., Murphy, S., 2013. Psychopharmacological treatment for military posttraumatic stress disorder: an integrative review. J. Am. Assoc. Nurse Pract. 25 (8), 419–423.

Taylor Tavares, J.V., Clark, L., Cannon, D.M., Erickson, K., Drevets, W.C., Sahakian, B.J., 2007. Distinct profiles of neurocognitive function in unmedicated unipolar depression and bipolar II depression. Biol. Psychiatry 62, 917–924.

Taylor, W.D., Kuchibhatla, M., Payne, M.E., Macfall, J.R., Sheline, Y.I., Krishnan, K.R., et al., 2008. Frontal white matter anisotropy and antidepressant remission in latelife depression. PLoS ONE 3, e3267.

Taylor, W.D., MacFall, J.R., Steffens, D.C., Payne, M.E., Provenzale, J.M., Krishnan, K.R., 2003. Localization of age-associated white matter hyperintensities in late-life depression. Prog. Neuropsychopharmacol. Biol. Psychiatry 27, 539–544.

Taylor, W.D., Wagner, H.R., Steffens, D.C., 2002. Greater depression severity associated with less improvement in depression-associated cognitive deficits in older subjects. Am. J. Geriatr. Psychiatry 10, 632–635.

Teng, C.T., Demetrio, F.N., 2006. Memantine may acutely improve cognition and have a mood stabilizing effect in treatment-resistant bipolar disorder. Rev. Bras. Psiquiatr. 28, 252–254.

Ter-Stepanian, M., Grizenko, N., Zappitelli, M., Joober, R., 2010. Clinical response to methylphenidate in children diagnosed with attention-deficit hyperactivity disorder and comorbid psychiatric disorders. Can J. Psychiatry 55 (5), 305–312.

Thakurathi, N., Vincenzi, B., Henderson, D.C., 2013. Assessing the prospect of donepezil in improving cognitive impairment in patients with schizophrenia. Expert Opin. Investig. Drugs 22 (2), 259–265.

Thase, M.E., Fava, M., DeBattista, C., Arora, S., Hughes, R.J., 2006. Modafinil augmentation of SSRI therapy in patients with major depressive disorder and excessive sleepiness and fatigue: a 12-week, open-label, extension study. CNS Spectr. 11 (2), 93–102

Tsai, G.E., Lin, P.Y., 2010. Strategies to enhance N-methyl-d-aspartate receptor- mediated neurotransmission in schizophrenia, a critical review and meta-analysis. Curr. Pharm. Des. 16 (5), 522–537.

Turner, D.C., Clark, L., Pomarol-Clotet, E., McKenna, P., Robbins, T.W., Sahakian, B.J., 2004. Modafinil improves cognition and attentional set shifting in patients with chronic schizophrenia. Neuropsychopharmacology 29 (7), 1363–1373.

Umbricht, D., Alberati, D., Martin-Facklam, M., Borroni, E., Youssef, E.A., Ostland, M., Wallace, T.L., Knoflach, F., Dorflinger, E., Wettstein, J.G., Bausch, A., Garibaldi, G., Santarelli, L., 2014. Effect of bitopertin, a glycine reuptake inhibitor, on negative symptoms of schizophrenia: a randomized, double-blind, proof-of-concept study. JAMA Psychiatry. http://dx.doi.org/10.1001/jamapsychiatry.2014.163.

Vaidya, C.J., Stollstorff, M., 2008. Cognitive neuroscience of attention deficit hyperactivity disorder: current status and working hypotheses. Dev. Disabil. Res. Rev. 14 (4), 261–267.

Varvel, S.A., Wise, L.E., Niyuhire, F., Cravatt, B.F., Lichtman, A.H., 2007. Inhibition of fatty-acid amide hydrolase accelerates acquisition and extinction rates in a spatial memory task. Neuropsychopharmacology 32, 1032–1041.

Verster, J.C., Bekker, E.M., Kooij, J.J., Buitelaar, J.K., Verbaten, M.N., Volkerts, E.R., Olivier, B., 2010. Methylphenidate significantly improves declarative memory functioning of adults with ADHD. Psychopharmacology (Berl.) 212 (2), 277–281.

van Veelen, N.M., Grootens, K.P., Peuskens, J., Sabbe, B.G., Salden, M.E., Verkes, R.J., Kahn, R.S., Sitskoorn, M.M., 2010. Short term neurocognitive effects of treatment with ziprasidone and olanzapine in recent onset schizophrenia. Schizophr. Res. 120 (1–3), 191–198.

Vythilingam, M., Vermetten, E., Anderson, G.M., Luckenbaugh, D., Anderson, E.R., Snow, J., et al., 2004. Hippocampal volume, memory, and cortisol status in major depressive disorder: effects of treatment. Biol. Psychiatry 56, 101–112.

Watson, S., Gallagher, P., Porter, R.J., Smith, M.S., Herron, L.J., Bulman, S., 2012. A randomized trial to examine the effect of mifepristone on neuropsychological performance and mood in patients with bipolar depression. Biol. Psychiatry 72, 943–949.

Weickert, T.W., Goldberg, T.E., 2005. First- and second-generation antipsychotic medication and cognitive processing in schizophrenia. Curr. Psychiatry Rep. 7 (4), 304–310.

Weisenbach, S.L., Boore, L.A., Kales, H.C., 2012. Depression and cognitive impairment in older adults. Curr. Psychiatry Rep. 14, 280–288.

Whiteford, H.A., Degenhardt, L., Rehm, J., Baxter, A.J., Ferrari, A.J., Erskine, H.E., Charlson, F.J., Norman, R.E., Flaxman, A.D., Johns, N., Burstein, R., Murray, C.J., Vos, T., 2013. Global burden of disease attributable to mental and substance use disorders: findings from the Global Burden of Disease Study 2010. Lancet 382 (9904), 1575–1586.

Wilens, T.E., 2008. Effects of methylphenidate on the catecholaminergic system in attention-deficit/hyperactivity disorder. J. Clin. Psychopharmacol. 28, S46–S53.

Winterer, G., 2010. Why do patients with schizophrenia smoke? Curr. Opin. Psychiatry 23, 112–119.

Yehuda, R., Harvey, H., 1997. Relevance of neuroendocrine alterations in PTSD to cognitive impairments of trauma survivors. In: Read, D., Lindsay, S. (Eds.), Recollections of Trauma. Plenum Press, New York, pp. 221–252.

Yehuda, R., McFarlane, A.C., Shalev, A.Y., 1998. Predicting the development of posttraumatic stress disorder from the acute response to a traumatic event. Biol. Psychiatry 44 (12), 1305–1313.

Young, A.H., Gallagher, P., Watson, S., Del-Estal, D., Owen, B.M., Ferrier, I.N., 2004. Improvements in neurocognitive function and mood following adjunctive treatment with mifepristone (RU-486) in bipolar disorder. Neuropsychopharmacol 29, 1538–1545.

Yurgelun-Todd, D.A., Ross, A.J., 2006. Functional magnetic resonance imaging studies in bipolar disorder. CNS Spectr. 11 (4), 287–297.

Zarate Jr., C.A., Singh, J.B., Carlson, P.J., et al., 2006. A randomized trial of an N-methyl-D-aspartate antagonist in treatment-resistant major depression. Arch. Gen. Psychiatry 63 (8), 856–864.

Zarate Jr., C.A., Payne, J.L., Quiroz, J., Sporn, J., Denicoff, K.K., Luckenbaugh, D., et al., 2004. An open-label trial of riluzole in patients with treatment-resistant major depression. Am. J. Psychiatry 161, 171–174.

Zobel, A.W., Schulze-Rauschenbach, S., von Widdern, O.C., et al., 2004. Improvement of working but not declarative memory is correlated with HPA normalization during antidepressant treatment. J. Psychiatr. Res. 38, 377–383.

Zohar, J., Yahalom, H., Kozlovsky, N., Cwikel-Hamzany, S., Matar, M.A., Kaplan, Z., et al., 2011. High dose hydrocortisone immediately after trauma may alter the trajectory of PTSD: Interplay between clinical and animal studies. Eur. Neuropsychopharmacol. 21, 796–809.

Chapter 11

Cognitive Enhancement in Humans

Martin Dresler[1,2] and Dimitris Repantis[3]
[1]Max Planck Institute of Psychiatry, Munich, Germany; [2]Donders Institute for Brain, Cognition and Behaviour, Radboud University Medical Centre, Nijmegen, Netherlands; [3]Charité Universitätsmedizin, Department of Psychiatry, Berlin, Germany

INTRODUCTION

Cognitive enhancement has become a trending topic in both academic and public debate. However, the discussants bring a very diverse background and motivation to this debate: The aim of many empirical researchers of cognitive enhancement is to understand the neurobiological and psychological mechanisms underlying cognitive capacities (McGaugh and Roozendaal, 2009), whereas theorists are rather more interested in their social and ethical implications (Savulescu and Bostrom, 2009). Whereas in basic research very specific mechanisms are studied (mostly in animal models), many theoretical discussions start from the counterfactual idea of a highly effective drug that makes its consumer super smart. In contrast to these thought experiments and to a plethora of data from animal studies, there is a surprising paucity of research that evaluates the effects of currently existing cognitive enhancers in healthy humans. A widely cited definition characterizes cognitive enhancement as interventions in humans that aim to improve mental functioning beyond what is necessary to sustain or restore good health (Juengst, 1998). While the current bioethical debate on cognitive enhancement shows a strong focus on pharmacological ways of enhancement, according to the given characterization, enhancement of mental capabilities also by nonpharmacological means has to be seen as proper for cognitive enhancement. In this chapter we aim to draw attention to several nonpharmacological cognitive enhancement strategies that have been largely neglected in the debate so far. We first summarize studies of the efficacy of psychopharmacological enhancers and then present data on the cognition-enhancing effects of a number of nonpharmacological methods. We start with broadly used interventions that are not commonly recognized as enhancement strategies, such as nutrition, physical exercise, and sleep, and then go over more specific methods such as meditation, mnemonic strategies, computer training,

Cognitive Enhancement. http://dx.doi.org/10.1016/B978-0-12-417042-1.00011-5

and brain stimulation technologies. We limit our review to methods that currently exist and do not speculate on future technologies.

PHARMACEUTICALS

Current debates on cognitive enhancement mainly concentrate on psychopharmaceuticals. In particular, psychostimulants are supposed to be widely used as cognitive enhancers (Talbot, 2009; Smith and Farah, 2011). Prescription stimulants such as amphetamines, modafinil, or methylphenidate (MPH) are thought to be the most frequently consumed "smart drugs," especially on college campuses, where, depending on the survey, 5–35% of healthy students report having consumed them for cognition enhancement purposes in the past year (for a meta-analysis see Wilens et al., 2008). In addition to use among students, MPH also is used in professions involving high cognitive performance and long periods of wakefulness, such as surgeons (Franke et al., 2013). While placebo-controlled trials support some of the claimed benefits for cognitive enhancers, it is worth noting that most of the claims have not been systematically tested. In addition to sparse evidence for efficacy, major concerns include adverse effects, toxicity, and the potential for addiction, especially because these drugs are often consumed without medical follow-up and in some cases over the long-term. Pharmacological cognitive enhancement has the potential to become a major public health concern. Recent publications on pharmacological cognitive enhancement focus mostly on the ethical debate rather than proof of effectiveness. On this background, some authors argue that research on efficacy and safety is or should be the rate-limiting step when considering the ethics of cognitive enhancement (Forlini et al., 2013). In the following, we briefly review data on the most common cognition enhancement drugs used in humans (see Table 11.1; for systematic reviews and meta-analyses see, e.g., Heishman et al., 2010; Repantis et al., 2010a,b).

Amphetamines. Amphetamines such Dexedrine® or Adderall® are sympathomimetic amines with central nervous system stimulant activity that have therapeutic properties and a long history of both medical and nonmedical use and abuse. The pharmacological effects of amphetamines have been attributed to their effects on central catecholamine neurotransmission, where they block reuptake from the synapse, inhibit the action of monoamine oxidase, and facilitate the release of dopamine and norepinephrine (Karoum et al., 1994; Wallace, 2012). Although it was thought that amphetamine use for nonmedical reasons was more widespread in the United States but less so in Europe (mainly because of the higher rates of prescriptions for attention deficit hyperactivity disorder treatment), a recent cross-sectional study suggested that in France amphetamines were used as frequently as MPH by medicine and pharmacology students for neuroenhancement purposes (Micoulaud-Franchi et al., 2014). The first review of the effects of amphetamines on the performance of healthy individuals was published in 1962 and concluded that 10 mg D-amphetamine

TABLE 11.1 Prescription Drugs Commonly Discussed as Cognitive Enhancers in Humans

	Indication/Off-label Use	Enhancement Efficacy	Common Side Effects	Addiction Potential
Amphetamines	Attention deficit hyperactivity disorder/narcolepsy, hypersomnolence, depression	Strong positive effects on verbal learning, delayed memory, vigilance and inhibitory control.	Dizziness, nervousness, headache, weight loss, hair loss, benign tachycardia, decreased libido; psychosis, severe cardiovascular adverse effects also possible	High
Methylphenidate	Attention deficit hyperactivity disorder/narcolepsy, hypersomnolence, depression	Evidence strongest for working memory; weaker for other memory domains and attention; some evidence for subjectively, but not objectively, measured vigilance.	Increased heart rate, headache, anxiety, nervousness, dizziness, drowsiness, insomnia; psychosis, severe cardiovascular adverse effects also possible	High
Modafinil	Narcolepy/hypersomnolence, depression	Moderate positive effect on attention; no evidence for memory or mood; positive effects after moderate sleep deprivation; after prolonged sleep deprivation positive effects on wakefulness but not cognitive functions	Headache, dizziness, gastrointestinal complaints, increased diuresis, palpitations, nervousness, restlessness, and sleep disturbances such as insomnia; psychosis, severe cardiovascular adverse effects also possible	Unclear; most likely high
Acetylcholinesterase inhibitors	Mild to moderate dementia due to Alzheimer's disease	Sparse data and only on donepezil; controversial results, even (transient) negative effects found	Common first dose side effects: Bradycardia, nausea, diarrhea, decreased appetite, abdominal pain, vivid dreams, insomnia	Low
Memantine	Moderate to severe dementia due to Alzheimer's disease	No data from repeated dose trials available	Confusion, dizziness, drowsiness, headache, insomnia, agitation, and/ or hallucinations	Low

may hasten conditioning, increase the rate at which subjects may acquire proficiency in a motor skill, decrease discriminative reaction time (although more in fatigued subjects than in others), and improve coordination performances but do not improve intellectual performance in a more strict sense (Weiss and Laties, 1962). Since this work, several randomized controlled trials (RCTs) assessing cognitive performance of healthy adults after amphetamine administration have been conducted. Surprisingly, no meta-analysis of this data has been carried out to date. A large number of studies found a large positive effect of a D-amphetamine single-dose administration on verbal memory tasks, vigilance, learning, inhibitory control, and delayed memory rather than immediate/short-term memory. Conflicting results for the role of catecholamine-O-methyl-transferase polymorphism in amphetamine effects were found (Ilieva et al., 2013). However, studies with no effect can also be found, whereas a further concern should be the fact that in some of the studies with null findings the participants nevertheless believed their performance was better after taking an amphetamine than after taking a placebo, although the study was conducted in a double-blind manner (see, e.g., Ilieva et al., 2013). Common side effects of amphetamines include dizziness, nervousness, headache, weight loss, alopecia, benign tachycardia, and decreased libido. Psychosis can occur at therapeutic doses during chronic therapy as a treatment-emergent side effect (Berman et al., 2009). A US Food and Drug Administration warning on the packets of these drugs draws awareness to the risk of drug dependence, sudden death, and cardiovascular adverse effects (FDA, 2013). These serious potential side effects of these drugs make their use for enhancement purposes highly problematic.

Methylphenidate. MPH is a dopamine reuptake blocker that also enhances dopamine and norepinephrine release through pharmacologic mechanisms similar to those of amphetamines (Sulzer et al., 2005). A systematic review of the effects of these stimulants on healthy individuals showed that there is a lack of studies addressing this issue (Repantis et al., 2010b). The analysis of the few existing studies provided no consistent evidence for a general cognition-enhancing effect, though evidence for a positive effect on memory (mainly spatial working memory) was found. While such memory benefits seem to be in the large effect size range, the popular opinion that MPH enhances attention was not verified (Repantis et al., 2010b). Some studies even reported negative effects, such as a disruption of attentional control (Rogers et al., 1999). Further studies conducted after the publication of this systematic review provided some further positive results; however, it remains debatable whether these results are enough to support the far-fetched enthusiasm for MPH as cognitive-enhancing drug. Side effects in the majority of the trials of healthy individuals were rare and mostly benign, such as slightly increased heart rate, headache, anxiety, nervousness, dizziness, drowsiness, and insomnia. The long-term effects of MPH consumption on healthy adults, as well as on individuals previously treated for attention deficit hyperactivity disorder, are unknown, but no long-term neuronal toxicity has been described to date (Advokat, 2009).

Modafinil. The mechanisms of action of modafinil are not well understood but are believed to differ from those of MPH and amphetamines. Although there is mounting evidence that the drug's effects on dopamine and norepinephrine are primary, effects on γ-aminobutyric acid, glutamate, histamine, and orexin/hypocretin also are theorized (Volkow et al., 2009; Minzenberg and Carter, 2008; Ballon and Feifel, 2006). In a systematic review, modafinil was found to have mainly moderate enhancing effects, specifically on attention, among individuals who were not sleep deprived (Repantis et al., 2010b). No effect on memory, mood, or motivation was found in the few studies that examined these domains, but the results of the studies were not unequivocal. Newer studies seem to confirm these results. Moreover, there is evidence that the effect of modafinil depends to some extent on the individual's baseline performance (Randall et al., 2005). Adverse reactions to modafinil have been observed in very few cases in these trials of healthy individuals, primarily headache, dizziness, gastrointestinal complains (e.g., nausea, abdominal pain, dry mouth), increased diuresis, palpitations, nervousness, restlessness, and sleep disturbances and, especially in studies with non-sleep-deprived individuals, insomnia. Finally, because the majority of the studies that have been performed are short-term and single-dose studies, no conclusion on the reinforcing effects of, development of dependence on, and tolerance to modafinil in healthy individuals can be drawn.

Antidementia drugs. Prescription drugs currently available for the treatment of dementia provide a further possibility for cognitive enhancement in healthy individuals. Of interest are the drugs used for the treatment of dementia due to Alzheimer's disease, namely acetylcholinesterase inhibitors and memantine. The first category comprises three substances—donepezil, galantamine, and rivastigmine—that are recommended for clinical use for the treatment of patients with mild to moderate Alzheimer's disease (Racchi et al., 2004). Memantine is an N-methyl-D-aspartate receptor antagonist and is registered for the treatment of moderate to severe Alzheimer's disease (Sonkusare et al., 2005). Studies of antidementia drugs used for enhancement purposes in healthy individuals are sparse. In a systematic review (Repantis et al., 2010a), only 10 trials with donepezil, 1 with rivastigmine, and 7 with memantine have been reported. No RCTs examining the effects of galantamine in healthy individuals were found. Antidementia drugs show their effect in clinical populations after intake for several weeks; however, all the memantine and the one galantamine trial were single-dose trials. Repeated trials have been conducted only with donepezil. These were 6 small-scale trials lasting 14–42 days. Of these, only two had older persons as participants (Beglinger et al., 2005; Fitzgerald et al., 2008). The rest of the trials included young healthy participants. This factor complicates comparisons of the results and makes it difficult to generalize the results of the latter studies for the main population of interest, namely the growing elderly population. These few existing studies provide no consistent evidence for a cognitive enhancement effect. One study found that donepezil improved the retention of training on complex aviation tasks

(Yesavage et al., 2002). In another case, verbal memory for semantically processed words was improved (Fitzgerald et al., 2008). Donepezil might also improve episodic memory (Gron et al., 2005), but, interestingly, two studies reported transient negative effects on episodic memory (Beglinger et al., 2004, 2005). A newer study also found impaired working memory in older healthy participants taking donepezil for 6 weeks (Balsters et al., 2011). In a sleep deprivation study, donepezil had no effect when participants were well rested. Nevertheless, the memory and attention deficits resulting from 24 h of sleep deprivation were attenuated after donepezil intake. This effect, however, was seen only in individuals whose performance declined the most after sleep deprivation (Chuah and Chee, 2008; Chuah et al., 2009) and could not be confirmed in a recent study (Dodds et al., 2011). Of note, in most of the studies a large neuropsychological test battery was applied; however, an effect was shown using only one or few of the tests applied. This could speak either to a selective effect of donepezil or for small effects that in these relatively underpowered studies could be revealed in only one (maybe the most difficult) task. Another possible explanation could be that acetylcholinesterase inhibitors require pathologically diminished cholinergic transmission to show their effects; therefore, it is not possible to optimize performance in healthy individuals who already have an optimal concentration of acetylcholine. In conclusion, evidence for cognition-enhancing effects of currently available antidementia drugs in healthy subjects is sparse. In the majority of the trials, donepezil was well tolerated; however, some authors warn that sleep disturbances might become apparent in larger populations (Yesavage et al., 2002). Reported side effects were benign and led to dropouts only in a few cases. The adverse reactions were mainly gastrointestinal complaints (e.g., nausea) but also headache, dizziness, nightmares, and insomnia. For a comprehensive review of available treatment for Alzheimer's disease, please refer to Chapter 9 in this book.

NUTRITION

It has long been known that besides mere nourishment, some foods benefit our health more than others. In addition, in most cultures certain foods or dietary supplements are claimed to benefit cognitive capabilities. During recent years, an increasing number of studies have tested such claims for "functional foods" or isolated "nutraceuticals," and they indeed found cognition-enhancing effects of herbal products such as ginseng or bacopa (Neale et al., 2013), of ingredients such as omega-3 fatty acids (Luchtman and Song, 2013), or even of candies such as chocolate (Scholey and Owen, 2013) and chewing gum (although, in the latter, probably not because of its nutritional ingredients but because of the effects of chewing activity on enhancing alertness; see Scholey, 2004). The enhancing effects of two of the most common dietary constituents, namely caffeine and glucose, have been extensively studied and are briefly reviewed here.

Caffeine exerts its stimulating effects within less than an hour after administration. Caffeine is an adenosine receptor antagonist; it reduces inhibition of neural firing largely through increased turnover of noradrenaline in the brain (Smith et al., 2003; Ferre, 2008). Typical behavioral effects of caffeine include elevated mood, increased alertness, and increased sustained attention (Smith et al., 1991, 2005; Hewlett and Smith, 2007). It improves attention and reaction times (Warburton et al., 2001) and motor-skill performance on tasks that are impaired when arousal is low, for example, during driving simulations (Reyner and Horne, 1997). The effects of caffeine on more complex and cognitively demanding tasks are, however, controversial; both enhancing and impairing effects have been reported and probably depend on the dose administered (Kaplan et al., 1997; Rogers and Dernoncourt, 1998; Heatherley et al., 2005). The effects of caffeine on memory and learning are particularly disputed, and positive effects have been attributed to indirect effects from elevated arousal, mood, and concentration during encoding (Nehlig, 2010). However, it has recently been demonstrated that postencoding caffeine intake might also enhance certain aspects of memory (Borota et al., 2014).

It is debated whether and to what extent differences in prior caffeine consumption and their lack of experimental control contribute to the conflicting observations of cognition-enhancing effects of caffeine. Stronger enhancing effects of caffeine after short-term abstinence have been demonstrated during caffeine abstinence in some tasks for subjects with high versus low habitual caffeine intake (Smit and Rogers, 2000; Addicott and Laurienti, 2009). Caffeine tolerance has been demonstrated (Evans and Griffiths, 1992), and caffeine withdrawal in strong habitual consumers has been associated with headaches, increased subjectively perceived stress, feelings of fatigue, and reduced alertness (Ratcliff-Crain et al., 1989; Schuh and Griffiths, 1997; Dews et al., 2002; Juliano and Griffiths, 2004). Hence, positive effects of caffeine in studies with acutely abstinent habitual caffeine consumers might be explained, at least in part, through the reversal of withdrawal effects rather than the actual enhancement potential of caffeine. However, withdrawal effects also have been suggested to rely on psychological rather than pharmacological factors of reduced caffeine intake (Dews et al., 2002), and it has been shown that expectancy mimics effects of caffeine when consumers believe they consume a caffeinated beverage (Fillmore, 1994), thus further corroborating a psychological component of the caffeine effect following both consumption and withdrawal. In contrast, several studies demonstrate that caffeine yields similar effects when administered in a coffee, in a tea, or as a capsule, supporting a pharmacological rather than a psychological mechanism when participants' expectations are controlled for (Smith, 2002).

Glucose is the primary energy source for most organisms. Within minutes after glucose administration, a subjective increase in mental energy associated with higher glucose metabolism in the brain has been reported (Posner et al., 1988; Reivih and Alavi, 1983). Objective measures of cognitive performance demonstrate that glucose improves attention (Benton et al., 1994), reaction times (Owens and Benton, 1994), and working memory (Scholey et al., 2001), the latter occurring under conditions of high as well as under low glucose depletion (Owen et al., 2012; Jones et al., 2012). In contrast to caffeine, the most pronounced effects of glucose on cognition are found for declarative memory (Messier, 2004; Smith et al., 2011), where large effect sizes over a large range have been demonstrated, in particular for demanding tasks (e.g., Sünram-Lea et al., 2001, 2002a, 2002b; Meikle et al., 2004). High blood glucose concentrations are associated with improved memory function (Benton and Owens, 1993), and glucose administration before and after learning similarly improves memory performance, indicating that attentional or other non-memory-specific processes during encoding alone cannot be responsible for the memory-enhancing effects of glucose (Sünram-Lea et al., 2002a). Memory effects are more pronounced in elderly compared to young adults, and glucose tolerance was predictive for declarative memory performance (Manning et al., 1990; Meikle et al., 2004; Messier, 2004). On a neural level, the hippocampus has been proposed as the main brain region mediating the memory-enhancing effects of glucose; more specific mechanisms involve glucose effects on cerebral insulin, acetylcholine synthesis, potassium adenosine triphosphate channel function, and extracellular glucose availability in the brain (Smith et al., 2011).

In conclusion, there is evidence that caffeine and glucose enhance mood, subjectively perceived energy, vigilance, attention, and some aspects of memory and may even exert their effects in a synergistic fashion if administered together (Adan and Serra-Grabulosa, 2010). However, individual differences, for example, in glucose tolerance or nutritional habits such as caffeine consumption, influence the extent and direction of these effects.

PHYSICAL EXERCISE

It is common knowledge that regular physical activity is a highly beneficial factor for preventing cardiovascular diseases and staying healthy in general. In the first half of the twentieth century it was demonstrated that athletes outperform physically inactive individuals in cognitive functions as well (Burpee and Stroll, 1936), and an emerging body of evidence suggests that regular aerobic exercise indeed has beneficial effects on brain function and cognition (Hillman et al., 2008). Many studies of the effects of physical exercise on cognition focus on developmental issues, examining either children of different age groups or elderly adults. In school-age children, physical exercise was demonstrated to benefit, for example, academic achievement, intelligence, perceptual skills, and verbal and mathematical ability (Sibley and Etnier, 2002). In older adults with and without pathological cognitive decline, beneficial effects of various physical exercise programs on different aspects of cognition were observed (Richards et al., 2003; van Uffelen et al., 2008). A recent meta-analysis of RCTs demonstrated that aerobic exercise training improves attention, processing speed, executive function, and memory, whereas effects on working memory were less consistent (Smith et al., 2010). Even if methodological issues in measuring the effect of exercise on cognition, in particular for studies with elderly subject populations, remain (Miller et al., 2012; Hötting and Röder, 2013), the conclusion that physical activity helps to preserve mental abilities throughout aging seems to be warranted.

In contrast to research in children and older adults, there are fewer studies of the effects of physical exercise on the cognition of younger and middle-aged adults. Most data on these age groups can be found in studies of older adults, in which they were examined as control groups for comparison with the elderly. An exception to this pattern constitutes studies focusing not on the chronic effects of regular physical activity but on the acute effects of exercise. For example, brief bouts of physical exercise improved long-term memory in young adults (Coles and Tomporowski, 2008). Intense exercise in the form of high-impact anaerobic running was shown to strongly enhance learning speed in a vocabulary memorizing task (Winter et al., 2007). A recent meta-analysis demonstrated that mental speed in particular and memory processes are consistently enhanced after acute exercise, whereas the effects during acute exercise seem to depend on the specific exercise mode and cognitive domain; attention and certain memory and executive function tasks show the strongest effects (Chang et al., 2012). In general, however, cognition-enhancing effects of acute exercise seem to be in the small to medium range (Lambourne and Tomporowski, 2010; Chang et al., 2012). In addition to motivational factors, an increase in general arousal level related to physical exertion has been hypothesized as a potential mechanism (Brisswalter et al., 2002); however, increased oxygenation of the frontal cortex also has been discussed as a mechanism underlying the cognition-enhancing effects of acute exercise (Yanagisawa et al., 2010; Ando et al., 2011; Endo et al., 2013).

Data on specific neural mechanisms underlying the effects of physical exercise on human cognition are rather sparse. Regular physical exercise training improved resting functional efficiency in higher-level cognitive networks including the frontal, posterior, and temporal cortices of older training participants compared a control group (Voss et al., 2010). In particular, greater task-related activity in frontoparietal networks is associated with effects of both general cardiovascular fitness and exercise training on cognition (Colcombe et al., 2004). In addition, hippocampal cerebral blood flow and hippocampal connectivity exhibited significant increases through physical exercise (Burdette et al., 2010). Structurally, cardiovascular fitness within the healthy elderly correlates with areas of preserved gray matter that typically show age-related decline (Gordon et al., 2008); in particular, hippocampal volume was found to be positively correlated with physical fitness in older adults (Erickson et al., 2009) as well as in children (Chaddock et al., 2010). Significant brain volume increases in both gray and white matter regions also were demonstrated to be associated with aerobic exercise training (Colcombe et al., 2006). In particular, the size of the anterior hippocampus was shown to increase through physical exercise; this increase was related to enhanced spatial memory and increased serum concentrations of brain-derived neurotrophic factor (BDNF), a mediator of hippocampal neurogenesis in the dentate gyrus (Ericksson et al., 2011). This is in line with data derived from animal models, showing that physical exercise increases BDNF gene expression in the hippocampus (Neeper et al., 1995) and that hippocampal BDNF indeed mediates the effects of physical exercise on cognition (Vaynman et al., 2004; Gomez-Pinilla et al., 2008). Also, the enhancing effects of intense acute exercise seem to be mediated by BDNF increases (Winter et al., 2007). Finally, parallel studies of mice and humans demonstrated that cerebral blood volume measurements provide an imaging correlate to neurogenesis in the dentate gyrus and that physical exercise had a primary effect on cerebral blood volume in the dentate gyrus that correlated with cognitive function (Pereira et al., 2007). In conclusion, there is converging evidence at several levels of observation that physical exercise enhances cognitive function throughout the lifespan; however, acute and long-term physical exercise might exert differential effects on different cognitive functions (Roig et al., 2013).

SLEEP

Humans spend a third of their lifetime asleep. From an evolutionary standpoint, this phenomenon helps to save energy—but it also leaves the sleeper in a potentially dangerous state of inattention. Sleep, therefore, has to provide the organism with important advantages to compensate for this disadvantage. A rapidly growing body of literature suggests that an important function of sleep is to enhance cognitive capacities, in particular memory (Diekelmann and Born, 2010) and creativity (Dresler, 2012).

The first empirical reports of the positive effects of postlearning sleep on memory consolidation were published almost a century ago: Jenkins and Dallenbach (1924) demonstrated that over retention periods including sleep, nonsense syllables are less prone to being forgotten compared to an equivalent period of wakefulness. Since then, hundreds of studies testing different memory systems have confirmed the positive effects of sleep on memory consolidation (Diekelmann and Born, 2010). It might be argued that regular sleep is just a general biological prerequisite to ensure cognitive functioning, and therefore sleep trivially favors memory consolidation compared to sleep deprivation. However, in experimental designs without sleep deprivation as a control condition, sleep positively affects memory consolidation compared to wakefulness, for example, when retention intervals during the day are compared with nocturnal retention intervals of similar length (Fischer et al., 2002; Walker et al., 2002). Furthermore, a growing number of studies demonstrates that additional sleep in the form of daytime naps also benefits memory function in non-sleep-deprived subjects (e.g., Mednick et al., 2003; Korman et al., 2007). Of note, even a nap as short as 6 min has been shown to be sufficient to promote memory performance

(Lahl et al., 2008), and for some memory systems the benefit of a daytime nap is comparable to a whole night of sleep (Mednick et al., 2003). In general, the size of the sleep effect on memory consolidation seems to depend on the involved memory system: whereas for declarative learning, effect sizes of sleep are in the medium range (e.g., Gais et al., 2006), sleep effects on procedural or perceptual learning are large (Fischer et al., 2002) or very large (Karni et al., 1994). In addition to its stabilizing function, sleep boosts certain kinds of memories even above the level of initial acquisition; procedural memories such as motor skills typically reach a plateau after some time of training, but after a night of sleep motor performance starts from a higher level despite the absence of further training (Walker et al., 2002). Interestingly, the sleep–memory relationship is specifically influenced by personal factors such as gender, hormonal status, or mental health (Dresler et al., 2010; Genzel et al., 2012).

The neural mechanisms underlying the effects of sleep on memory consolidation are still poorly understood. A major point of discussion is the question of whether newly formed memories profit from rather passive homeostatic processes (Tononi and Cirelli, 2003) or are actively consolidated during sleep. While several animal studies demonstrated a neuronal replay of activation patterns during sleep that were associated with recent memories (Wilson and McNaughton, 1994; Ji and Wilson, 2007), a study of humans using memory-related odor cues during sleep could demonstrate a causal role of sleep for memory consolidation (Rasch et al., 2007). For several years it was thought that rapid eye movement (REM) sleep supports the consolidation of procedural memories, whereas non-REM sleep supports declarative memories such as verbal information; however, recent studies suggest that this model was too simplistic (Genzel et al., 2009; Rasch et al., 2009; Dresler et al., 2011). Instead of global sleep stages, the role of physiological microprocesses during sleep gained attention. In particular, the interaction of hippocampal sharp wave ripples, thalamocortical sleep spindles, and cortical slow oscillations is thought to play a key physiological role in the consolidation of memories (Genzel et al., 2014).

Anecdotal reports of scientific discovery, inventive originality, and artistic productivity suggest that creativity can also be triggered or enhanced by sleep. Several studies confirm these anecdotes, showing that sleep promotes creative problem solving compared with wakefulness. For example, when subjects performed a cognitive task that could be solved much faster by applying a hidden rule, after a night of sleep more than twice as many subjects gained insight into the hidden rule when compared with a control group that stayed awake (Wagner et al., 2004). Like sleep-related memory enhancement, active processes during sleep seem to promote creativity. If applied during sleep, olfactory stimuli that were associated with creativity tasks before sleep trigger insights overnight (Ritter et al., 2012). In particular, REM sleep, the sleep stage most strongly associated with intense dreaming, enhances the formation of associative networks in creative problem solving (Cai et al., 2009). Selective deprivation of REM sleep but not of other sleep stages impairs postsleep performance on creativity tasks that are presented to the subjects before sleep (Cartwright and Ratzel, 1972; Glaubman et al., 1978). Subjects show greater cognitive flexibility in creativity tasks immediately after awakening from REM sleep compared with awakening from other sleep stages (Walker et al., 2002). However, slow-wave sleep also has recently been related to creative problem solving (Beijamini et al., 2014).

Both theoretical models and empirical research of creativity suggest that sleep is a highly effective creativity enhancer (Dresler, 2012). The historical standard model proposes a passive incubation phase as an essential step to creative insights (Helmholtz, 1896). Psychoanalytical models emphasize primary process thinking for creative cognitions that is explicitly conceptualized as dream-like (Kris, 1952). Cognitive models propose that flat association hierarchies and a state of defocused attention facilitate creativity (Mednick, 1962). Hyperassociativity and defocused attention are phenomenal features of most dreams and physiologically are probably caused by deactivation of the prefrontal cortex (Hobson and Pace-Schott, 2002). Physiological models suggest high variability in cortical arousal levels as beneficial for creativity (Martindale, 1999), and the sleep cycle can be considered a prime example of such arousal variability. The chaotic activation of the cortex during REM sleep through brain stem regions in the absence of external sense data leads to a much more radical renunciation from unsuccessful problem-solving attempts, leading to coactivation of cognitive data that are highly remote during waking life. These coactivations, woven into a dream narrative in a self-organizing manner, repeatedly receive further innervations by the brain stem, leading to bizarre sequences of loosely associated dream topics that might eventually activate particular problem-relevant cognitions or creative cognitions in general (Hobson and Wohl, 2005). In conclusion, the phenomenological and neural correlates of sleep provide ideal incubation conditions for the genesis of creative ideas and insights.

MEDITATION

Meditation has been conceptualized as a family of complex emotional and attentional regulatory training regimes (Lutz et al., 2008). Such approaches include ancient Buddhist mindfulness meditations such as Vipassana and Zen meditations, as well as several modern group-based standardized meditations (Chiesa and Malinowski, 2011). Two rather traditional approaches are the focus of current research: focused attention meditation and open monitoring meditation, which involve voluntary focusing of attention on a chosen object or nonreactive monitoring of the content of experience from moment to moment (Lutz et al., 2008). During recent years, the effects of meditation practice also were systematically studied in western laboratories, and a rapidly growing body of evidence demonstrates that meditation training enhances attention and other cognitive capacities. For example, in comparisons of experienced meditators with meditation-naive control subjects, meditation practice has been associated with increased attentional performance and cognitive flexibility (Moore and Malinowski, 2009; Hodgins and Adair, 2010). In longitudinal studies, 3 months of meditation training could be shown to enhance attentional capacity (Lutz et al., 2009), perception, and vigilance (MacLean et al., 2010). Even a brief training of just four meditation sessions was sufficient to significantly improve visuospatial processing, working memory, and executive functioning (Zeidan et al., 2010). A recent systematic review associated early phases mindfulness meditation training with significant improvements in selective and executive attention, whereas later phases were associated with improved sustained attention abilities. In addition, meditation training was proposed to enhance working memory capacity and some executive functions (Chiesa et al., 2011). A recent meta-analysis of the effects of meditation training reported medium to large effect sizes for changes in emotionality and relationship issues, medium effect sizes for measures of attention, and smaller effects on memory and several other cognitive capacities (Sedlmeier et al., 2012).

The neurophysiological mechanisms underlying meditation practice and its relation to cognition also have been addressed. Electroencephalographic (EEG) studies revealed a significant increase in alpha and theta activity of subjects who underwent a meditation session (Kasamatsu and Hirai, 1966; Murata et al., 1994). Neuroimaging studies showed that meditation practice activates or deactivates brain areas comprising the prefrontal cortex and the anterior cingulate cortex (Hölzel et al., 2007), the basal ganglia (Ritskes et al., 2003), the hippocampus, the pre- and postcentral gyri, as well as the dorsolateral prefrontal and parietal cortices (Lazar et al., 2000). Focusing on attention studies, it has been demonstrated that long-term meditation supports enhanced activation of specific brain areas while also promoting attention sustainability (Davidson et al., 2003). Different studies also emphasized the role of meditation as a mental process that modulates plasticity in neural circuits commonly associated with attention (Davidson and Lutz, 2008). Functional magnetic resonance imaging studies also demonstrated a reduction of neural responses in widespread brain regions that are linked to conceptual processing, which suggests enhanced neural efficiency, probably via improved sustained attention and impulse control (Pagnoni et al., 2008; Kozasa et al., 2012). Moreover, positron emission tomography studies demonstrated increased dopamine release in the ventral striatum as a result of yoga meditation, which in turn suggests regulation of conscious states at the synaptic level (Kjaer et al., 2002). In addition, some studies have suggested that meditation practice is associated with structural brain changes. Compared with meditation-naive control subjects, long-term meditators showed significantly larger volumes of the right hippocampus and orbitofrontal cortex (Luders et al., 2009) and significantly greater cortical thickness in brain regions associated with attention, interoception, and sensory processing, including the prefrontal cortex and right anterior insula (Lazar et al., 2005). In a longitudinal study with meditation-naive subjects undergoing an 8-week meditation program, gray matter increases in the hippocampus and other brains regions could be observed (Hölzel et al., 2011).

MNEMONIC STRATEGIES

In modern society, the ability to cope with verbal or numerical information becomes increasingly important. However, our learning skills evolved to handle concrete visuospatial rather than abstract information. While we can easily remember our last birthday party in great detail and typically do not have any problems recalling a once-walked route including dozens or even hundreds of single sights and branches, most of us have a very hard time memorizing telephone numbers, foreign vocabularies, or shopping lists. The most common way to memorize such information is rote learning: We take up the information to be remembered into our short-term memory and repeat it over and over again. However, such a procedure is slow and inefficient, in particular because of a severe limitation of short-term memory capacity. As Miller (1956) observed more than half a century ago, an average human can hold seven (plus or minus two) chunks of arbitrary information in short-term memory. In contrast, a few individuals show memory skills far beyond this normal range. A century ago some case reports mention exceptional memorizers with memory spans of several dozen digits (Brown and Deffenbacher, 1975). In a seminal case study, a normal college student was trained over the course of 2 years, eventually reaching a memory span of 82 digits read at the pace of one digit per second (Ericsson et al., 1980). Since the early 1990s, the top participants of the annual World Memory Championships regularly prove memory spans of hundreds of digits (Konrad and Dresler, 2010). However, such superior memorizers do not seem to exhibit structural brain changes or superior cognitive abilities in general; they acquired their skills by deliberate training in the use of mnemonic techniques (Brown and Deffenbacher, 1988; Maguire et al., 2003; Ericsson, 2009; Dresler and Konrad, 2013).

To cope with the limitations of natural memory, humans have always used external remembering cues (D'Errico, 2001). The term *mnemonics* is typically used to denote internal cognitive strategies aimed at enhancing memory. Parallel to their success in memory artistry and memory sports, several mnemonics have been shown to strongly enhance memory capacity in scientific studies (Bellezza, 1981; Worthen and Hunt, 2011a,b). The most prominent is probably the so-called method of loci, an ancient technique used extensively by Greek and Roman orators (Yates, 1966). It uses well-established memories of spatial routes: during encoding, to-be-remembered information items are visualized at salient points along such a route, which in turn is mentally retraced during retrieval. A second powerful mnemonic is the phonetic system, which is designed to aid the memorization of numbers: single digits are converted to letters, which are then combined to form words. Both the method of loci and the phonetic system have been shown to be very effective and even increase their efficacy over time, that is, at delayed recall after several days compared to immediate recall (Bower, 1970; Roediger, 1980; Bellezza et al., 1992; Hill et al., 1997; Higbee, 1997; Wang and Thomas, 2000). A third mnemonic that has been shown to be effective is the keyword method, designed specifically to enhance the acquisition of foreign vocabulary (Raugh and Atkinson, 1975) but also helps with learning scientific terminology (Rosenheck et al., 1989; Brigham and Brigham, 1998; Balch, 2005; Carney and Levin, 1998). It associates the meaning of a to-be-remembered term with what the term sounds like in the first language of the learner.

A recently published broad overview of mnemonics demonstrates that research into these techniques has lost attention since 1980 (Worthen and Hunt, 2011b). In particular, neurophysiological data on mnemonics is sparse. A seminal study of expert mnemonics users found that during mnemonic encoding brain regions that are critical for spatial memory—in particular parietal, retrosplenial, and right posterior hippocampal areas—are engaged (Maguire et al., 2003). Likewise, the superior digit memory of abacus experts was associated specifically with brain regions that process visuospatial information(Tanaka et al., 2002). Here, abacus skill can be interpreted as a mnemonic for memorizing digits. In two studies with novices taught in the method of loci, mnemonic encoding led to increases in the activation of prefrontal and occipitoparietal areas in particular, whereas mnemonic-guided recall led to increases in the activation of left-sided areas in particular, including the parahippocampal gyrus, retrosplenial cortex, and precuneus (Nyberg et al., 2003; Kondo et al., 2005).

Another strategic method to enhance memory retention that has gained attention in recent years is retrieval practice. While retrieval of learned information in testing situations is traditionally thought to simply assess learning success, repeated retrieval itself has been shown to be a powerful mnemonic enhancer, producing large gains in long-term retention compared with repeated studying (Roediger and Butler, 2011). For example, when students have to learn foreign vocabulary words, repeated studying after the first learning trial had no effect on delayed recall after 1 week, whereas repeated testing produced a surprisingly large effect on long-term retention (Karpicke and Roediger, 2008). In addition to learning vocabulary, text materials also profit from repeated retrieval (Roediger and Karpicke, 2006; Karpicke and Roediger, 2010). Interestingly, study participants seem to be unaware of this effect, overestimating the value of repeated study and underestimating that of repeated retrieval (Roediger and Karpicke, 2006; Karpicke and Roediger, 2008). Effects of retrieval practice were even shown to produce greater success in meaningful learning than elaborative studying strategies, which are designed to lead to deeper learning and therefore hold a central place in contemporary education (Karpicke and Blunt, 2011). On the neural level, repeated retrieval leads to higher brain activity in the anterior cingulate cortex during retest, which was interpreted as an enhanced consolidation of memory representations at the systems level (Eriksson et al., 2011).

In conclusion, mnemonics strategies can be seen as strong and reliable enhancers of learning and memory capacity. While their immediate benefits for easy-to-learn material seem to be have a small to medium effect size, the effectiveness of mnemonics strikingly grows with task difficulty or retention time and can reach effect sizes in terms of Cohen's d of larger than 3 or 4 (e.g., Higbee, 1997; Karpicke and Roediger, 2008). Of note, the benefits of mnemonics in population groups with particular cognitive training needs, as, for example, in age-related cognitive decline, seem to be less pronounced (Verhaeghen et al., 1992), but they still can reach large effect sizes if memory is assessed after prolonged retention time (Hill et al., 1997).

COMPUTER TRAINING

In addition to the acquisition of mnemonic strategies, the ubiquitous availability of modern computer technology has prompted more straightforward training of cognitive capabilities: cognition-enhancing effects of both recreational and experimental use of computer games and brain training programs have gained increasing attention in recent years. Computer programs allow repeated and highly controlled training of various cognitive capabilities; their game-like nature often is experienced as intrinsically rewarding by the participants. Because enhanced performance on the specific computer program is rather unsurprising, the main goal of many scientific studies of computerized cognitive training is to investigate a potential transfer of effects to other tasks and cognitive domains.

Whereas potential societal effects of the popularity of video games have generated concern among parents, practitioners, and politicians (Anderson et al., 2010), their potential to train perceptual skills also has been emphasized (Achtman et al., 2008; Hubert-Wallander et al., 2011). Compared to nongamers, regular video gamers show improvements in cognitive flexibility (Colzato et al., 2010), enumeration ability (Green and Bavelier, 2006), visual search (Castel et al., 2005), visual attention (Green and Bavelier, 2003), and psychomotor skills (Kennedy et al., 2011). While several video games have been found to improve mental rotation (Okagaki and Frensch, 1994), contrast sensitivity (Li et al., 2009), spatial visual resolution (Green and Bavelier, 2007), and task-switching abilities (Strobach et al., 2012) among nongamers, other studies with naive subjects found no training improvement of cognitive capabilities in which video gamers excelled (Boot et al., 2008).

In addition to recreational video games, a rapidly increasing number of studies tests computerized training programs specifically targeting certain cognitive domains such as memory (Mahncke et al., 2006; Schmiedek et al., 2010; Zelinski et al., 2011), attention (Smith et al., 2009), executive function, and processing speed (Nouchi et al., 2012) in different age groups. Working memory is a cognitive domain that has garnered particular attention in recent years. Measures of working memory correlate strongly with intelligence, and both capabilities have been considered very stable. In recent years, however, several studies of children (Thorell et al., 2009; Nutley et al., 2011) and adults (Jaeggi et al., 2008, 2010) found that training with adaptive versions of working memory tasks such as the n-back task not only improves working memory but also shows transfer to fluid intelligence measures. However, replication of such transfer effects has proved difficult (Dahlin et al., 2008; Holmes et al., 2010; Redick et al., 2013) and hence has been questioned by some authors (Shipstead et al., 2010). Explanations for these inconsistent findings include individual differences in training performance (Jaeggi et al., 2011) and different types of training (strategy versus "core" working memory training) potentially having different transfer effects (Morrison and Chein, 2011). In general, the problem of transfer to tasks and cognitive domains not directly trained is a major issue in cognitive training programs (Fuyuno, 2007; Ackerman et al., 2010). For example, 6-week online study with a very large sample size did not find any evidence for transfer to nontrained tasks (Owen et al., 2010). A video game designed for the training of multitasking performance was recently demonstrated to have the potential to prompt transfer effects to untrained cognitive control abilities such as sustained attention and working memory (Anguera et al., 2013).

Even though commercial offers often overhype their efficacy, video games and computerized training programs are promising tools for cognitive enhancement because of their broad availability and self-motivating nature. Effect sizes of computerized training strongly depend on the cognitive domain trained and tested; processing speed and perceptual measures show medium to large effect sizes, whereas effects for different memory domains are only in the small or medium range (Mahncke et al., 2006; Smith et al., 2009; Schmiedek et al., 2010; Zelinski et al., 2011). Which forms of training produce reliable and strong transfer effects to relevant cognitive domains remains to be determined in future studies.

BRAIN STIMULATION

Since the introduction of electroconvulsive therapy for psychiatric disorders in the 1930s, several forms of invasive and noninvasive brain stimulation have been developed as a tool for enhancing brain function in health and disease (Hoy and Fitzgerald, 2010; McKinley et al., 2012; Guleyupoglu et al., 2013). Invasive methods for brain stimulation include deep-brain stimulation (DBS) and direct vagus nerve stimulation (dVNS). In DBS electrodes are implanted in deep-brain structures and used to modulate their activity through high-frequency stimulation. DBS of the hypothalamus (Hamani et al., 2008) and of the entorhinal area, but not of the hippocampus directly, have been demonstrated to enhance declarative learning (Suthana et al., 2012; Suthana and Fried, 2014). dVNS shows that stimulation of afferent vagal fibers seems to modulate the central nervous system, perhaps by stimulating brain stem structures (Krahl et al., 1998; Groves and Brown, 2005). dVNS has been shown to increase memory function (Clark et al., 1999), specifically memory consolidation (Ghacibeh et al., 2006). Devices for invasive brain stimulation require surgery (Kuhn et al., 2010; Ben-Menachem, 2001), and a significant number of patients with long-term DBS have hardware-related complications (Oh et al., 2002) in addition to complications from the initial surgery.

Since the 1990s, noninvasive brain stimulation techniques have become increasingly popular for the modulation and enhancement of cognitive capabilities in healthy subjects (Dayan et al., 2013). Transcranial magnetic stimulation (TMS) applies brief magnetic pulses through a coil to the scalp, thereby inducing electric currents in the brain. Different protocols including single-pulse, paired-pulse, and high- and low-frequency repetitive TMS have different cognitive effects, either interfering with or enhancing cognitive processes (Rossi and Rossini, 2004). TMS has been demonstrated to speed up encoding and retrieval by stimulating the left or right dorsolateral prefrontal cortex, respectively (Gagnon et al., 2010). TMS over the prefrontal cortex also sped up analogic reasoning but did not change the error rate (Boroojerdi et al., 2001). Furthermore, TMS delivered to the frontal or parietal lobe improved accuracy on the mental rotation task (Klimesch et al., 2003). Also, for procedural skills, an enhancement through TMS has been demonstrated, mainly by reducing intrahemispherical "rivalry" by inhibiting contralateral brain areas (Kobayashi et al., 2004; Bütefisch et al., 2004). Such disinhibition effects also have been used for phonological memory enhancement by reducing interference between similar-sounding words in phonological memory (Kirschen et al., 2006) and visuospatial attention enhancement on one side by impairing the other (Hilgetag et al., 2001; Thut et al., 2004). It has been suggested that TMS inhibition of frontotemporal regions induces savant-like abilities in drawing, mathematics, calendar calculating, number estimation, and proofreading (Young et al., 2004; Snyder et al., 2003, 2006).

In addition to TMS, several methods for transcranial electrical stimulation that change the voltage across neuronal membranes exist (for recent reviews see Paulus, 2011; Ruffini et al., 2013; Guleyupoglu et al., 2013). Transcranial direct current stimulation (tDCS) (for a comprehensive review see Chapter 12) sends a small electric current (typically 1–2 mA) between two electrodes placed on the scalp (Been et al., 2007). The technique seems to work by changing the likelihood of neural firing in superficial parts of the cortex; neurons under the anode neurons become depolarized and more excitable, while neurons under the cathode become hyperpolarized and less excitable. tDCS induces different effects depending on polarity and electrode placement, which can outlast the stimulation by more than an hour (Nitsche et al., 2005). tDCS has frequently been reported to enhance learning and memory (Chi et al., 2010; Clark et al., 2012; Javadi et al., 2011; Kincses et al., 2003; Reis et al., 2008). For example, tDCS of the left dorsolateral prefrontal cortex enhanced verbal learning (Javadi and Walsh, 2011; Javadi et al., 2011), whereas tDCS of the motor areas enhanced motor learning (Reis et al., 2009). tDCS during slow-wave sleep enhanced memory consolidation (Marshall et al., 2004), probably by boosting slow-wave oscillations (Marshall et al., 2006). Performance on working memory tasks also was found to be enhanced by tDCS (Fregni et al., 2005; Luber et al., 2007; Teo et al., 2011; Ohn et al., 2008). In addition to learning and memory, other cognitive capacities also were enhanced by tDCS, such as verbal fluency (Iyer et al., 2005), mathematical abilities (Cohen Kadosh et al., 2010; Iuculano and Cohen Kadosh, 2013), and reasoning in matchstick problems (Chi and Snyder, 2011). For a comprehensive review of tDCS please refer to Chapter 12 in this book.

In contrast to tDCS, transcranial alternating current stimulation (tACS) works with oscillating electrical currents. While sinusoidal stimulation is most common, other waveforms such as rectangular current shapes can also be applied in tACS (Antal and Paulus, 2013). In direct comparison, 10-Hz tACS was suggested to generate more focused fields than tDCS (Manoli et al., 2012), thus enabling more specific modulation of brain regions. tACS over parietal areas was found to increase working memory storage (Jaušovec et al., 2014; Jaušovec and Jaušovec, 2014), whereas tACS over prefrontal areas enhanced fluid reasoning specifically for complex tasks involving logical reasoning (Santarnecchi et al., 2013). A special form of tACS is transcranial random noise stimulation (tRNS), which applies a random electrical oscillation spectrum over the scalp, inducing increases in excitability lasting 60 min after stimulation (Terney et al., 2008). tRNS has been demonstrated to induce long-term enhancement of learning and subsequent performance on complex arithmetic tasks (Snowball et al., 2013). Compared with tDCS, tRNS led to a stronger enhancement of perceptual learning processes (Fertonani et al., 2011), which is in line with a better efficacy of tRNS compared with tDCS or tACS in clinical applications (Vanneste et al., 2013).

As an alternative to applying electrical stimulation, transcranial focused ultrasound was recently used to modulate brain function, enhancing performance on sensory discrimination tasks when applied to the primary somatosensory cortex (Legon et al., 2012, 2014). Whether transcranial focused ultrasound is capable of enhancing other higher cognitive functions still has to be determined.

Effect sizes of cognitive enhancement through brain stimulation seem to be small to modest; however, single studies also report larger effects (e.g., Chi et al., 2010). From a risk perspective, the use of noninvasive brain stimulation in research settings is largely considered unproblematic (Poreisc et al., 2007; Rossi et al., 2009). Reported side effects in healthy subjects include headaches or local pain; the most serious risk is the occurrence of seizure, often caused by incorrect stimulation parameters or the use of medications that lower the seizure threshold. However, long-term effects of noninvasive brain stimulation are currently unknown. Of particular concern are risks of premature use of the technology by lay users based on hype or speculation (Cohen Kadosh et al., 2012). Furthermore, enhancement of one cognitive function by brain stimulation might be associated with impairment of a different function (Iuculano and Cohen Kadosh, 2013).

CONCLUSIONS

Humans have always strived to increase their mental capacities. From symbolic language, writing, and the printing press to mathematics, calculators, and computers—mankind has devised and used tools to record, store, and exchange thoughts and hence enhance cognitive processes and products. In addition to such purely external devices that were designed to aid cognition, a number of tools with a more direct effect on cognitive and neural processes exist. Some behavioral cognitive enhancement strategies such as sleep or physical exercise are, to a different extent, part of our natural lives. Other behavioral techniques such as mnemonics or meditation have a long cultural tradition but must be explicitly learned. Certain psychoactive chemical enhancers such as caffeine, glucose, or other nutritional supplements also have a long history of consumption and are deeply embedded in our culture. In contrast, more modern enhancements strategies such as pharmaceuticals, computer training, or brain stimulation have raised considerable social and medical concern—not always solely based on their potential side effects and health risks. While many ethical arguments brought forward in the debate on pharmacological enhancers can also be applied to nonpharmacological enhancement strategies (Dresler et al., 2013), some arguments require a reliable comparison of the efficacy and risks of different cognitive enhancers. However, surprisingly few data that would allow comparative evaluations of different enhancement interventions exist. When comparing typical effect sizes between studies of different cognitive enhancement tools, many pharmaceuticals currently used for cognitive enhancement show rather modest effects compared with several nonpharmacological strategies. The purpose of ethical debates is not only to build possible future scenarios in which side effect–free smart pills are available to boost any cognitive capacity but also to evaluate current possibilities and constraints of cognitive enhancement. Differential and comparative research on the variety of existing cognitive enhancers is strongly needed to inform the public debate on cognitive enhancement.

ACKNOWLEDGMENTS

This work was funded by a grant from the Volkswagen Foundation, Germany. We thank Anders Sandberg, Kathrin Ohla, Christoph Bublitz, Carlos Trenados, Aleksandra Mroczko-Wąsowicz, and Simone Kühn for their contributions to earlier versions of this chapter.

REFERENCES

Achtman, R., Green, C., Bavelier, D., 2008. Video games as a tool to train visual skills. Restor. Neurol. Neurosci. 26, 435–446.

Ackerman, P., Kanfer, R., Calderwood, C., 2010. Use it or lose it? Wii brain exercise practice and Reading for domain knowledge. Psychol. Aging 25, 753–766.

Adan, A., Serra-Grabulosa, J.M., 2010. Effects of caffeine and glucose, alone and combined, on cognitive performance. Hum. Psychopharmacol. 25, 310–317.

Addicott, M.A., Laurienti, P.J., 2009. A comparison of the effects of caffeine following abstinence and normal caffeine use. Psychopharmacology 207, 423–431.

Advokat, C.J., 2009. What exactly are the benefits of stimulants for ADHD? Atten. Disord. 12, 495–498.

Anderson, C.A., Shibuya, A., Ihori, N., Swing, E.L., Bushman, B.J., Sakamoto, A., Rothstein, H.R., Saleem, M., 2010. Violent video game effects on aggression, empathy, and prosocial behavior in eastern and western countries: a meta-analytic review. Psychol. Bull. 136, 151–173.

Ando, S., Kokubu, M., Yamada, Y., Kimura, M., 2011. Does cerebral oxygenation affect cognitive function during exercise? Eur. J. Appl. Physiol. 111, 1973–1982.

Anguera, J.A., Boccanfuso, J., Rintoul, J.L., Al-Hashimi, O., Faraji, F., Janowich, J., Kong, E., Larraburo, Y., Rolle, C., Johnston, E., Gazzaley, A., 2013. Video game training enhances cognitive control in older adults. Nature 501, 97–101.

Antal, A., Paulus, W., 2013. Transcranial alternating current stimulation (tACS). Front. Hum. Neurosci. 7, 317.

Balch, W.R., 2005. Elaborations of introductory psychology terms: effects of test performance and subjective ratings. Teach. Psychol. 32, 29–34.

Ballon, J.S., Feifel, D., 2006. A systematic review of modafinil: potential clinical uses and mechanisms of action. J. Clin. Psychiatry 67, 554–566.

Balsters, J.H., O'Connell, R.G., Martin, M.P., Galli, A., Cassidy, S.M., Kilcullen, S.M., et al., 2011. Donepezil impairs memory in healthy older subjects: behavioural, EEG and simultaneous EEG/fMRI biomarkers. PLoS One 6, e24126.

Been, G., Ngo, T.T., Miller, S.M., Fizgerald, P.B., 2007. The use of tDCS and CVS as methods of non-invasive brain stimulation. Brain Res. Rev. 56, 346–361.

Beglinger, L.J., Gaydos, B.L., Kareken, D.A., Tangphao-Daniels, O., Siemers, E.R., Mohs, R.C., 2004. Neuropsychological test performance in healthy volunteers before and after donepezil administration. J. Psychopharmacol. 18, 102–108.

Beglinger, L.J., Tangphao-Daniels, O., Kareken, D.A., Zhang, L., Mohs, R., Siemers, E.R., 2005. Neuropsychological test performance in healthy elderly volunteers before and after donepezil administration: a randomized, controlled study. J. Clin. Psychopharmacol. 25, 159–165.

Beijamini, F., Ribeiro, S.I., Cini, F.A., Louzada, F.M., 2014. After being challenged by a video game problem, sleep increases the chance to solve it. PLoS One 9, e84342.

Bellezza, F.S., 1981. Mnemonic Devices: classification, characteristics, and criteria. Rev. Educ. Res. 51, 247–275.

Bellezza, F.S., Six, L.S., Phillips, D.S., 1992. A mnemonic for remembering long strings of digits. Bull. Psychon. Soc. 30, 271–274.

Ben-Menachem, E., 2001. Vagus nerve stimulation, side effects, and long-term safety. J. Clin. Neurophysiol. 18, 415–418.

Benton, D., Owens, D.S., 1993. Blood glucose and human memory. Psychopharmacology (Berl) 113, 83–88.

Benton, D., Owens, D.S., Parker, P.Y., 1994. Blood glucose influences memory and attention in young adults. Neuropsychologia 32, 595–607.

Berman, S.M., Kuczenski, R., McCracken, J.T., London, E.D., 2009. Potential adverse effects of amphetamine treatment on brain and behavior: a review. Mol. Psychiatry 14, 123–142.

Boot, W.R., Kramer, A.F., Simons, D.J., Fabiani, M., Gratton, G., 2008. The effects of video game playing on attention, memory, and executive control. Acta Psychol. 129, 387–398.

Boroojerdi, B., Phipps, M., Kopylev, L., Wharton, C.M., Cohen, L.G., Grafman, J., 2001. Enhancing analogic reasoning with rTMS over the left prefrontal cortex. Neurology, 526–528.

Borota, D., Murray, E., Keceli, G., Chang, A., Watabe, J.M., Ly, M., Toscano, J.P., Yassa, M.A., 2014. Post-study caffeine administration enhances memory consolidation in humans. Nat. Neurosci. 17, 201–203.

Bower, G.H., 1970. Analysis of a mnemonic device. Am. Sci. 58, 496–510.

Bray, C.L., Cahill, K.S., Oshier, J.T., Peden, C.S., Theriaque, D.W., Flotte, T.R., Stacpoole, P.W., 2004. Methylphenidate does not improve cognitive function in healthy sleep-deprived young adults. J. Investig. Med. 52, 192–201.

Brigham, F.J., Brigham, M.M., 1998. Using mnemonic keywords in general music classes: music history meets cognitive psychology. J. Res. Dev. Educ. 31, 205–213.

Brisswalter, J., Collardeau, M., René, A., 2002. Effects of acute physical exercise characteristics on cognitive performance. Sports Med. 32, 555–566.

Brown, E., Deffenbacher, K., 1975. Forgotten mnemonists. J. Hist. Behav. Sci. 11, 342–349.

Brown, E., Deffenbacher, K., 1988. Superior memory performance and mnemonic encoding. In: Obler, L.K., Fein, D. (Eds.), The Exceptional Brain. Guilford, New York.

Burdette, J.H., Laurienti, P.J., Espeland, M.A., Morgan, A., Telesford, Q., Vechlekar, C.D., Hayasaka, S., Jennings, J.M., Katula, J.A., Kraft, R.A., Rejeski, W.J., 2010. Using network science to evaluate exercise-associated brain changes in older adults. Front. Aging Neurosci. 2, 23.

Burpee, R.H., Stroll, W., 1936. Measuring reaction time of athletes. Res. Q. 7, 110–118.

Bütefisch, C.M., Khurana, V., Kopylev, L., Cohen, L.G., 2004. Enhancing encoding of a motor memory in the primary motor cortex by cortical stimulation. J. Neurophysiol. 2110–2116.

Cai, D.J., Mednick, S.A., Harrison, E.M., Kanady, J.C., Mednick, S.C., 2009. REM, not incubation, improves creativity by priming associative networks. PNAS 106, 10130–10134.

Carney, R.N., Levin, J.R., 1998. Coming to terms with keyword method in introductory psychology: a neuromnemonic example. Teach. Psychol. 25, 132–134.

Cartwright, R.D., Ratzel, R.W., 1972. Effects of dream loss on waking behaviors. Arch. Gen. Psychiatry 27, 277–280.

Castel, A.D., Pratt, J., Drummond, E., 2005. The effects of action video game experience on the time course of inhibition of return and the efficiency of visual search. Acta Psychol. 119 (2), 217–230.

Chaddock, L., Erickson, K.I., Prakash, R.S., Kim, J.S., Voss, M.W., Vanpatter, M., et al., 2010. A neuroimaging investigation of the association between aerobic fitness, hippocampal volume, and memory performance in preadolescent children. Brain Res. 1358, 172–183.

Chang, Y.K., Labban, J.D., Gapin, J.I., Etnier, J.L., 2012. The effects of acute exercise on cognitive performance: a meta-analysis. Brain Res. 1453, 87–101.

Chi, P.R., Fregni, F., Snyder, A.W., 2010. Visual memory improved by non-invasive brain stimulation. Brain Res. 1353, 168–175.

Chi, R.P., Snyder, A.W., 2011. Facilitate insight by non-invasive brain stimulation. PLoS One 6 (2), e16655.

Chiesa, A., Calati, R., Serretti, A., 2011. Does mindfulness training improve cognitive abilities? A systematic review of neuropsychological findings. Clin. Psychol. Rev. 31, 449–464.

Chiesa, A., Malinowski, P., 2011. Mindfulness-based approaches: are they all the same? J. Clin. Psychol. 67, 404–424.

Chuah, L.Y., Chee, M.W., 2008. Cholinergic augmentation modulates visual task performance in sleep-deprived young adults. J. Neurosci. 28, 11369–11377.

Chuah, L.Y., Chong, D.L., Chen, A.K., Rekshan III, W.R., Tan, J.C., Zheng, H., et al., 2009. Donepezil improves episodic memory in young individuals vulnerable to the effects of sleep deprivation. Sleep 32, 999–1010.

Clark, K.B., Naritoku, D.K., Smith, D.C., Browning, R.A., Jensen, R.A., 1999. Enhanced recognition memory following vagus nerve stimulation in human subjects. Nat. Neurosci. 2 (1), 94–98.

Clark, V.P., Coffman, B.A., Mayer, A.R., Weisend, M.P., Lane, T.D., Calhoun, V.D., et al., 2012. TDCS guided using fMRI significantly accelerates learning to identify concealed objects. Neuroimage 59 (1), 117–128.

Cohen Kadosh, R., Levy, N., O'Shea, J., Shea, N., Savulescu, J., 2012. The neuroethics of non-invasive brain stimulation. Curr. Biol. 22, R108–R111.

Cohen Kadosh, R., Soskic, S., Iuculano, T., Kanai, R., Walsh, V., 2010. Modulating neuronal activity produces specific and long-lasting changes in numerical competence. Curr. Biol. 20, 2016–2020.

Colcombe, S.J., Kramer, A.F., Erickson, K.I., Scalf, P., McAuley, E., Cohen, N.J., Webb, A., Jerome, G.J., Marquez, D.X., Elavsky, S., 2004. Cardiovascular fitness, cortical plasticity, and aging. PNAS 101, 3316–3321.

Colcombe, S.J., Erickson, K.I., Scalf, P.E., Kim, J.S., Prakash, R., McAuley, E., et al., 2006. Aerobic exercise training increases brain volume in aging humans. J. Gerontol. A Biol. Sci. Med. Sci. 61, 1166–1170.

Coles, K., Tomporowski, P.D., 2008. Effects of acute exercise on executive processing, short-term and long-term memory. J. Sports Sci. 26, 333–344.

Colzato, L.S., Leeuwen, P.J., Wildenberg, W.P., Hommel, B., 2010. DOOM'd to Switch: superior cognitive flexibility in players of first person shooter games. Front. Psychol. 1 (8).

Dahlin, E., Neely, A.S., Larsson, A., Bäckman, L., Nyberg, L., 2008. Transfer of learning after updating training mediated by the striatum. Science 320, 1510–1512.

Davidson, R.J., Kabat-Zinn, J., Schumacher, J., Rosenkranz, M., Muller, D., Santorelli, S.F., et al., 2003. Alterations in brain and immune function produced by mindfulness meditation. Psychosom. Med. 65, 564–570.

Davidson, R.J., Lutz, A., 2008. Buddha's brain: neuroplasticity and meditation. IEEE Signal Proc. Mag. 25. 176–174.

Dayan, E., Censor, N., Buch, E.R., Sandrini, M., Cohen, L.G., 2013. Noninvasive brain stimulation: from physiology to network dynamics and back. Nat. Neurosci. 16, 838–844.

D'Errico, F., 2001. Memories out of mind: the archaeology of the oldest memory systems. In: Nowell, A. (Ed.), In the Mind's Eye. International Monographs in Prehistory, Ann Arbor, MI.

Dews, P.B., O' Brian, C.P., Bergman, J., 2002. Caffeine: behavioral effects of withdrawal and related issues. Food Chem. Toxicol. 40, 1257–1261.

Diekelmann, S., Born, J., 2010. The memory function of sleep. Nat. Rev. Neurosci. 11, 114–126.

Dodds, C.M., Bullmore, E.T., Henson, R.N., Christensen, S., Miller, S., Smith, M., et al., 2011. Effects of donepezil on cognitive performance after sleep deprivation. Hum. Psychopharmacol. 26, 578–587.

Dresler, M., Kluge, M., Genzel, L., Schüssler, P., Steiger, A., 2010. Impaired off-line memory consolidation in depression. Eur. Neuropsychopharmacol. 20, 553–561.

Dresler, M., Kluge, M., Pawlowski, M., Schüssler, P., Steiger, A., Genzel, L., 2011. A double dissociation of memory impairments in major depression. J. Psychiatr. Res. 45, 1593–1599.

Dresler, M., 2012. Sleep and creativity: theoretical models and neural basis. In: Barrett, D., McNamara, P. (Eds.), Santa Barbara. Encyclopedia of Sleep and Dreams, Vol. II. Praeger, pp. 768–770.

Dresler, M., Konrad, B.N., 2013. Mnemonic expertise during wakefulness and sleep. Behav. Brain Sci. 36, 616–617.

Dresler, M., Sandberg, A., Ohla, K., Bublitz, C., Trenado, C., Mroczko-Wasowicz, A., Kühn, S., Repantis, S., 2013. Non-pharmacological cognitive enhancement. Neuropharmacology 64, 529–543.

Endo, K., Matsukawa, K., Liang, N., Nakatsuka, C., Tsuchimochi, H., Okamura, H., Hamaoka, T., 2013. Dynamic exercise improves cognitive function in association with increased prefrontal oxygenation. J. Physiol. Sci. 63, 287–298.

Ericsson, K.A., Chase, W.G., Faloon, S., 1980. Acquisition of a memory skill. Science 208, 1181–1182.

Ericsson, K.A., 2009. Toward a science of exceptional achievement. Ann. N. Y. Acad. Sci. 1172, 199–217.

Erickson, K.I., Prakash, R.S., Voss, M.W., Chaddock, L., Hu, L., Morris, K.S., et al., 2009. Aerobic fitness is associated with hippocampal volume in elderly humans. Hippocampus 19, 1030–1039.

Eriksson, J., Kalpouzos, G., Nyberg, L., 2011. Rewiring the brain with repeated retrieval: a parametric fMRI study of the testing effect. Neurosci. Lett. 505, 36–40.

Evans, S.M., Griffiths, R.R., 1992. Caffeine tolerance and choice in humans. Psychopharmacology 108, 51–59.

Ferre, S., 2008. An update on the mechanisms of the psychostimulant effects of caffeine. J. Neurochem. 105, 1067–1079.

Fertonani, A., Pirulli, C., Miniussi, C., 2011. Random noise stimulation improves neuroplasticity in perceptual learning. J. Neurosci. 31, 15416–15423.

Fillmore, M.T., 1994. Investigating the behavioral effects of caffeine: the contribution of drug-related expectancies. Pharmacopsychoecologia 7 (2), 63–73.

Fischer, S., Hallschmid, M., Elsner, A.L., Born, J., 2002. Sleep forms memory for finger skills. PNAS 99, 11987–11991.

Fitzgerald, D.B., Crucian, G.P., Mielke, J.B., Shenal, B.V., Burks, D., Womack, K.B., et al., 2008. Effects of donepezil on verbal memory after semantic processing in healthy older adults. Cogn. Behav. Neurol. 21, 57–64.

Forlini, C., Hall, W., Maxwell, B., Outram, S.M., Reiner, P.B., Repantis, D., Schermer, M., Racine, E., 2013. Navigating the enhancement landscape. Ethical issues in research on cognitive enhancers for healthy individuals. EMBO Rep. 14, 123–128.

Franke, A.G., Bagusat, C., Dietz, P., Hoffmann, I., Simon, P., Ulrich, R., Lieb, K., 2013. Use of illicit and prescription drugs for cognitive or mood enhancement among surgeons. BMC Med. 11, 102.

Fregni, F., Boggio, P.S., Nitsche, M., Bermpohl, F., Antal, A., Feredoes, E., et al., 2005. Anodal transcranial direct current stimulation of prefrontal cortex enhances working memory. Exp. Brain Res. 166 (1), 23–30.

Fuyuno, I., 2007. Brain craze. Nature 448 (7151), 250–251.

Gagnon, G., Schneider, C., Grondin, S., Blanchet, S., 2010. Enhancement of episodic memory in young and healthy adults: a paired-pulse TMS study on encoding and retrieval performance. Neurosci. Lett. 488 (2), 138–142.

Gais, S., Lucas, B., Born, J., 2006. Sleep after learning aids memory recall. Learn. Mem. 13, 259–262.

Genzel, L., Dresler, M., Wehrle, R., Grözinger, M., Steiger, A., 2009. Slow wave sleep and REM sleep awakenings do not affect sleep dependent memory consolidation. Sleep 32, 302–310.

Genzel, L., Kiefer, T., Renner, L., Wehrle, R., Kluge, M., Grözinger, M., Steiger, A., Dresler, M., 2012. Sex and modulatory menstrual cycle effects on sleep related memory consolidation. Psychoneuroendocrinology 37, 987–998.

Genzel, L., Kroes, M.C., Dresler, M., Battaglia, F.P., 2014. Light sleep versus slow wave sleep in memory consolidation: a question of global versus local processes? Trends Neurosci. 2014 (37), 10–19.

Ghacibeh, G.A., Shenker, J.I., Shenal, B., Uthman, B.M., Heilman, K.M., 2006. The influence of vagus nerve stimulation on memory. Cogn. Behav. Neurol. 19, 119–122.

Glaubman, H., Orbach, I., Aviram, O., Frieder, I., Frieman, M., Pelled, O., Glaubman, R., 1978. REM deprivation and divergent thinking. Psychophysiology 15, 75–79.

Gomez-Pinilla, F., Vaynman, S., Ying, Z., 2008. Brain-derived neurotrophic factor functions as a metabotrophin to mediate the effects of exercise on cognition. Eur. J. Neurosci. 28, 2278–2287.

Gordon, B.A., Rykhlevskaia, E.I., Brumback, C.R., Lee, Y., Elavsky, S., Konopack, J.F., et al., 2008. Neuroanatomical correlates of aging, cardiopulmonary fitness level, and education. Psychophysiology 45, 825–838.

Green, C., Bavelier, D., 2003. Action video game modifies visual selective attention. Nature 423 (6939), 534–537.

Green, C., Bavelier, D., 2006. Enumeration versus multiple object tracking: the case of action video game players. Cognition 101 (1), 217–245.

Green, C.S., Bavelier, D., 2007. Action-video-game experience alters the spatial resolution of vision. Psychol. Sci. 18, 88–94.

Groves, D.A., Brown, V.J., 2005. Vagalnervestimulation: a review of its applications and potential mechanisms that mediate its clinical effects. Neurosci. Biobehav. Rev. 29 (3), 493–500.

Gron, G., Kirstein, M., Thielscher, A., Riepe, M.W., Spitzer, M., 2005. Cholinergic enhancement of episodic memory in healthy young adults. Psychopharmacology 182, 170–179.

Guleyupoglu, B., Schestatsky, P., Edwards, D., Fregni, F., Bikson, M., 2013. Classification of methods in transcranial electrical stimulation (tES) and evolving strategy from historical approaches to contemporary innovations. J. Neurosci. Methods 219, 297–311.

Hamani, C., McAndrews, M.P., Cohn, M., Oh, M., Zumsteg, D., Shapiro, C.M., et al., 2008. Memory enhancement induced by hypothalamic/fornix deep brain stimulation. Ann. Neurol. 63 (1), 119–123.

Heatherley, S.V., Hayward, R.C., Seers, H.E., Rogers, P.J., 2005. Cognitive and psychomotor performance, mood, and pressor effects of caffeine after 4, 6 and 8 h caffeine abstinence. Psychopharmacology 178 (4), 461–470.

Heishman, S.J., Kleykamp, B.A., Singleton, E.G., 2010. Meta-analysis of the acute effects of nicotine and smoking on human performance. Psychopharmacol. (Berl.) 210, 453–469.

Helmholtz, H., 1896. Voträge und Reden. Vieweg, Braunschweig.

Hewlett, P., Smith, A., 2007. Effects of repeated doses of caffeine on performance and alertness: new data and secondary analyses. Hum. Psychopharmacol. Clin. Exp. 22, 339–350.

Higbee, K.L., 1997. Novices, apprentices, and mnemonists: acquiring expertise with the phonetic mnemonic. Appl. Cogn. Psychol. 11, 147–161.

Hilgetag, C.C., Theoret, H., Pascual-Leone, A., 2001. Enhanced visual spatial attention ipsilateral to rTMS-induced "virtual lesons" of human parietal cortex. Nat. Neurosci. 4, 953–957.

Hill, R.D., Campbell, B.W., Foxley, D., Lindsay, S., 1997. Effectiveness of the number-consonant mnemonic for retention of numeric material in community-dwelling older adults. Exp. Aging Res. 23, 275–286.

Hillman, C.H., Erickson, K.I., Kramer, A.F., 2008. Be smart, exercise your heart: exercise effects on brain and cognition. Nat. Rev. Neurosci. 9, 58–65.

Hobson, J.A., Pace-Schott, E.F., 2002. The cognitive neuroscience of sleep: neuronal systems, consciousness and learning. Nat. Rev. Neurosci. 3, 679–693.

Hobson, J.A., Wohl, H., 2005. From Angels to Neurones. Art and the New Science of Dreaming. Mattioli, Fidenza.

Hodgins, H.S., Adair, K.C., 2010. Attentional processes and meditation. Conscious Cogn. 19, 872–878.

Holmes, J., Gathercole, S.E., Place, M., Dunning, D.L., Hilton, K.A., Elliott, J.G., 2010. Working memory deficits can be Overcome: impacts of training and medication on working memory in children with ADHD. Appl. Cogn. Psychol. 24, 827–836.

Hölzel, B.K., Carmody, J., Vangel, M., Congleton, C., Yerramsetti, S.M., Gard, T., Lazar, S.W., 2011. Mindfulness practice leads to increases in regional brain gray matter density. Psychiatry Res. 191, 36–43.

Hölzel, B.K., Ott, U., Hempel, H., Hackl, A., Wolf, K., Stark, R., Vaitl, D., 2007. Differential engagement of anterior cingulate and adjacent medial frontal cortex in adept meditators and non-meditators. Neurosci. Lett. 421, 16–21.

Hötting, K., Röder, B., 2013. Beneficial effects of physical exercise on neuroplasticity and cognition. Neurosci. Biobehav. Rev. 37, 2243–2257.

Hoy, K.E., Fitzgerald, P.B., 2010. Brain stimulation in psychiatry and its effects on cognition. Nat. Rev. Neurol. 6, 267–275.

http://www.fda.org. (accessed 2013).

Hubert-Wallander, B., Green, C., Bavelier, D., 2011. Stretching the limits of visual attention: the case of action video games. Wiley interdisciplinary reviews. Cogn. Sci. 2 (2), 222–230.

Ilieva, I., Boland, J., Farah, M.J., 2013. Objective and subjective cognitive enhancing effects of mixed amphetamine salts in healthy people. Neuropharmacology 64, 496–505.

Iuculano, T., Cohen Kadosh, R., 2013. The mental cost of cognitive enhancement. J. Neurosci. 33, 4482–4486.

Iyer, M.B., Mattu, U., Grafman, J., Lomarev, M., Sato, S., Wassermann, E.M., 2005. Safety and cognitive effect of frontal DC brain polarization in healthy individuals. Neurology 64 (5), 872–875.

Jaušovec, N., Jaušovec, K., 2014. Increasing working memory capacity with theta transcranial alternating current stimulation (tACS). Biol. Psychol. 96, 42–47.

Jaušovec, N., Jaušovec, K., Pahor, A., 2014. The influence of theta transcranial alternating current stimulation (tACS) on working memory storage and processing functions. Acta Psychol. (Amst.) 146, 1–6.

Jaeggi, S.M., Buschkuehl, M., Jonides, J., Perrig, W.J., 2008. Improving fluid intelligence with training on working memory. PNAS 105 (19), 6829–6833.

Jaeggi, S.M., Studer-Luethi, B., Buschkuehl, M., Su, Y.-F., Jonides, J., Perrig, W.J., 2010. The relationship between n-back performance and matrix reasoning – implications for training and transfer. Intelligence 28 (6), 625–635.

Jaeggi, S.M., Buschkuehl, M., Jonides, J., Shah, P., 2011. Short- and long-term benefits of cognitive training. PNAS 108 (25), 10081–10086.

Javadi, A.H., Walsh, V., 2011. Transcranial direct current stimulation, (tDCS) of the left dorsolateral prefrontal cortex modulates declarative memory. Brain Stimul.

Javadi, A.H., Cheng, P., Walsh, V., 2011. Short duration transcranial direct current stimulation, (tDCS) modulates verbal memory. Brain Stimul.

Jenkins, J.K., Dallenbach, K.M., 1924. Obliviscence during sleep and waking. Am. J. Psychol. 35, 605–612.

Ji, D., Wilson, M.A., 2007. Coordinated memory repla in the visual cortex and hippocampus during sleep. Nat. Neurosci. 0, 100–107.

Jones, E.K., Sünram-Lea, S.I., Wesnes, K.A., 2012. Acute ingestion of different macronutrients differentially enhances aspects of memory and attention in healthy young adults. Biol. Psychol. 89, 477–486.

Juengst, E.T., 1998. What does enhancement mean? In: Parens, E. (Ed.), Enhancing Human Traits: Ethical and Social Implications. Georgetown University Press, Washington.

Juliano, L.M., Griffiths, R.R., 2004. A critical review of caffeine withdrawal: empirical validation of symptoms and signs, incidence, severity, and associated features. Psychopharmacology 176, 1–29.

Kjaer, T.W., Bertelsen, C., Piccini, P., Brooks, D., Alving, J., Lou, H.C., 2002. Increased dopamine tone during meditation-induced change of consciousness. Brain Res Cogn Brain Res 13, 255–259.

Kaplan, G.B., Greenblatt, D.J., Ehrenberg, B.L., Goddard, J.E., Cotreau, M.M., Harmatz, J.S., Shader, R.I., 1997. Dose-dependent pharmacokinetics and psychomotor effects of caffeine in humans. J. Clin. Pharmacol. 37, 693–703.

Karni, A., Tanne, D., Rubenstein, B.S., Askenasy, J.J.M., Sagi, D., 1994. Dependence on REM sleep of overnight improvement of a perceptual skill. Science 265, 679–682.

Karoum, F., Chrapusta, S.J., Brinjak, R., Hitri, A., Wyatt, R.J., 1994. Regional effects of amphetamine, cocaine, nomifensine and GBR 12909 on the dynamics of dopamine release and metabolism in the rat brain. Br. J. Pharmacol. 113, 1391–1399.

Karpicke, J.D., Roediger, H.L., 2008. The critical importance of retrieval for learning. Science 319, 966–968.

Karpicke, J.D., Roediger, H.L., 2010. Is expanding retrieval a superior method for learning text materials? Mem. Cognit. 38, 116–124.

Karpicke, J.D., Blunt, J.R., 2011. Retrieval practice produces more learning than elaborative studying with concept mapping. Science 331, 772–775.

Kasamatsu, A., Hirai, T., 1966. An electroencephalographic study on the zen meditation. Zazen. Folia Psychiatrica Neurol. Japonica 20, 315–336.

Kennedy, A., Boyle, E., Traynor, O., Walsh, T., Hill, A., 2011. Video gaming enhances psychomotor skills but not visuospatial and perceptual abilities in surgical trainees. J. Surg. Educ. 68 (5), 414–420.

Kincses, T.Z., Antal, A., Nitsche, M.A., Bartfati, O., Paulus, W., 2003. Facilitation of probabilistic classification learning by transcranial direct current stimulation of the prefrontal cortex in the human. Neuropsychologia 42, 113–117.

Kirschen, M., Davis-Ratner, M., TE, J., Schraedley-Desmond, P., Desmond, J., 2006. Enhancement of phonological memory following transcranial magnetic stimulation, TMS. Behav. Neurol. 17 (3–4), 187–194.

Kjaer, T.W., Bertelsen, C., Piccini, P., Brooks, D., Alving, J., Lou, H.C., April 2002. Increased dopamine tone during meditation-induced change of consciousness. Brain Res. Cogn. Brain Res. 13, 255–259.

Klimesch, W., Sauseng, P., Gerloff, C., 2003. Enhancing cognitive performance with repetitive transcranial magnetic stimulation at human individual alpha frequency. Eur. J. Neurosci. 17 (5), 1129–1233.

Korman, M., Doyon, J., Doljansky, J., Carrier, J., Dagan, Y., Karni, A., 2007. Daytime sleep condenses the time course of motor memory consolidation. Nat. Neurosci. 10, 1206–1213.

Kobayashi, M., Hutchinson, S., Théoret, H., Schlaug, G., Pascual-Leone, A., 2004. Repetitive TMS of the motor cortex improves ipsilateral sequential simple finger movements. Neurology 62 (1), 91–98.

Kondo, Y., Suzuki, M., Mugikura, S., et al., 2005. Changes in brain activation associated with use of a memory strategy: a functional MRI study. NeuroImage 24, 1154–1163.

Konrad, B.N., Dresler, M., 2010. Grenzen menschlicher Gedächtnisleistungen. In: Baudson, T.G., Seemüller, A., Dresler, M. (Eds.), Grenzen Unseres Geistes. Hirzel, Stuttgart.

Kozasa, E.H., Sato, J.R., Lacerda, S.S., Barreiros, M.A., Radvany, J., Russell, T.A., et al., 2012. Meditation training increases brain efficiency in an attention task. Neuroimage 59, 745–749.

Krahl, S.E., Clark, K.B., Smith, D.C., Browning, R.A., 1998. Locus coeruleus lesions suppress the seizure-attenuating effects of vagus nerve stimulation. Epilepsia 39 (7), 709–714.

Kris, E., 1952. Psychoanalytic Explorations in Art. International Universities Press, New York.

Kuhn, J., Gründler, T.O.J., Lenartz, D., Sturm, V., Klosterkötter, J., Huff, W., 2010. Deep brain stimulation for psychiatric disorders. Deutsches Ärzteblatt Int. 107, 105–113.

Lahl, O., Wispel, C., Willigens, B., Pietrowsky, R., 2008. An ultra short episode of sleep is sufficient to promote declarative memory performance. J. Sleep Res. 17, 3–10.

Lambourne, K., Tomporowski, P., 2010. The effect of exercise-induced arousal on cognitive task performance: a meta-regression analysis. Brain Res. 1341, 12–24.

Lazar, S.W., Bush, G., Gollub, R.L., Fricchione, G.L., Khalsa, G., Benson, H., 2000. Function brain mapping of the relaxation response meditation. Neuroreport 11, 1581–1585.

Lazar, S.W., Kerr, C.E., Wasserman, R.H., Gray, J.R., Greve, D.N., Treadway, M.T., et al., 2005. Meditation experience is associated with increased cortical thickness. Neuroreport 16, 1893–1897.

Legon, W., Rowlands, A., Opitz, A., Sato, T.F., Tyler, W.J., 2012. Pulsed ultrasound differentially stimulates somatosensory circuits in humans as indicated by EEG and FMRI. PLoS One 7, e51177.

Legon, W., Sato, T.F., Opitz, A., Mueller, J., Barbour, A., Williams, A., Tyler, W.J., 2014. Transcranial focused ultrasound modulates the activity of primary somatosensory cortex in humans. Nat. Neurosci. 17, 322–329.

Li, R., Polat, U., Makous, W., Bavelier, D., 2009. Enhancing the contrast sensitivity function through action video game training. Nat. Neurosci. 12, 549–551.

Luber, B., Kinnunen, L., Rakitin, B., Ellsassera, R., Stern, Y., Lisanbya, S., 2007. Facilitation of performance in a working memory task with rTMS stimulation of the precuneus: frequency- and time-dependent effects. Brain Res. 1128, 120–129.

Luchtman, D.W., Song, C., 2013. Cognitive enhancement by omega-3 fatty acids from child-hood to old age: findings from animal and clinical studies. Neuropharmacology 64, 550–565.

Luders, E., Toga, A.W., Lepore, N., Gaser, C., 2009. The underlying anatomical correlates of long-term meditation: larger hippocampal and frontal volumes of gray matter. Neuroimage 45, 672–678.

Lutz, A., Slagter, H.A., Rawlings, N.B., Francis, A.D., Greischar, L.L., Davidson, R.J., 2009. Mental training enhances attentional stability: neural and behavioral evidence. J. Neurosci. 29, 13418–13427.

Lutz, A., Slagter, H.A., Dunne, J.D., Davidson, R.J., April 2008. Attention regulation and monitoring in meditation. Trends Cogn. Sci. 12 (4), 163–169.

MacLean, K.A., Ferrer, E., Aichele, S.R., Bridwell, D.A., Zanesco, A.P., Jacobs, T.L., et al., 2010. Intensive meditation training improves perceptual discrimination and sustained attention. Psychol. Sci. 21, 829–839.

Maguire, E.A., Valentine, E.R., Wilding, J.M., et al., 2003. Routes to remembering: the brains behind superior memory. Nat. Neurosci. 6, 90–95.

Mahncke, H.W., Connor, B.B., Appelman, J., Ahsanuddin, O.N., Hardy, J.L., Wood, R.A., et al., 2006. Memory enhancement in healthy older adults using a brain plasticity-based training program: a randomized, controlled study. PNAS 103 (33), 12523–12528.

Manoli, Z., Grossman, N., Samaras, T., 2012. Theoretical investigation of transcranial alternating current stimulation using realistic head model. Conf. Proc. IEEE Eng. Med. Biol. Soc. 4156–4159.

Manning, C.A., Hall, J.L., Gold, P.E., 1990. Glucose effects on memory and other neuropsychological tests in elderly humans. Psychol. Sci. 1, 307–311.

Marshall, L., Mölle, M., Hallschmid, M., Born, J., 2004. Transcranial direct current stimulation during sleep improves declarative memory. J. Neurosci. 24 (44), 9985–9992.

Marshall, L., Helgadóttir, H., Mölle, M., Born, J., 2006. Boosting slow oscillations during sleep potentiates memory. Nature 444, 610–613.

Martindale, C., 1999. Biological bases of creativity. In: Sternberg, R.J. (Ed.), Handbook of Creativity. Cambridge University Press, Cambridge, pp. 137–152.

McGaugh, J.L., Roozendaal, B., 2009. Drug enhancement of memory consolidation: historical perspective and neurobiological implications. Psychopharmacology 202, 3–14.

McKinley, R.A., Bridges, N., Walters, C.M., Nelson, J., 2012. Modulating the brain at work using noninvasive transcranial stimulation. NeuroImage 59 (1), 129–137.

Mednick, S.A., 1962. The associative basis of the creative process. Psychol. Rev. 69, 220–232.

Mednick, S., Nakayama, K., Stickgold, R., 2003. Sleep-dependent learning: a nap is as good as a night. Nat. Neurosci. 6, 697–698.

Meikle, A., Riby, L.M., Stollery, B., 2004. The impact of glucose ingestion and gluco-regulatory control on cognitive performance: a comparison of younger and middle aged adults. Hum. Psychopharmacol. 19, 523–535.

Messier, C., 2004. Glucose improvement of memory: a review. Eur. J. Pharmacol. 490, 33–57.

Micoulaud-Franchi, J.A., MacGregor, A., Fond, G., 2014. A preliminary study on cognitive enhancer consumption behaviors and motives of French Medicine and Pharmacology students. Eur. Rev. Med. Pharmacol. Sci. 18, 1875–1878.

Miller, G.A., 1956. The magical number seven, plus or minus two: some limits on our capacity for processing information. Psychol. Rev. 63, 81–97.

Miller, D.I., Taler, V., Davidson, P.S., Messier, C., 2012. Measuring the impact of exercise on cognitive aging: methodological issues. Neurobiol. Aging 33, 622. e29–43.

Minzenberg, M.J., Carter, C.S., 2008. Modafinil: a review of Neurochemical actions and effects on cognition. Neuropsychopharmacology 33, 1477–1502.

Moore, A., Malinowski, P., 2009. Meditation, mindfulness and cognitive flexibility. Conscious Cogn. 18, 176–186.

Morrison, A.B., Chein, J.M., 2011. Does working memory training work? the promise and challenges of enhancing cognition by training working memory. Psychon. Bull. Rev. 18, 56–60.

Murata, T., Koshino, Y., Omori, M., 1994. Quantitative EEG study on zen meditation, (zaZen). Jpn. J. Psychiatry Neurol. 48, 881–890.

Neale, C., Camfield, D., Reay, J., Stough, C., Scholey, A., 2013. Cognitive effects of two nutraceuticals Ginseng and Bacopa benchmarked against modafinil: a review and comparison of effect sizes. Br. J. Clin. Pharmacol. 75, 728–737.

Neeper, S.A., Gómez-Pinilla, F., Choi, J., Cotman, C., January 12, 1995. Exercise and brain neurotrophins. Nature 373 (6510), 109.

Nehlig, A., 2010. Is caffeine a cognitive enhancer? J. Alzheimer's Dis. 20, S85–S94.

Nitsche, M.A., Seeber, A., Frommann, K., Klein, C.C., Rochford, C., Nitsche, M.S., et al., 2005. Modulating parameters of excitability during and after transcranial direct current stimulation of the human motor cortex. J. Physiol. 568 (1), 291–303.

Nouchi, R., Taki, Y., Takeuchi, H., Hashizume, H., Akitsuki, Y., Shigemune, Y., et al., 2012. Brain training game improves executive functions and processing speed in the elderly: a randomized controlled trial. PLoS One 7 (1), e29676.

Nutley, S.B., Söderqvist, S., Bryde, S., Thorell, L.B., Humphreys, K., Klingberg, T., 2011. Gains in fluid intelligence after training non-verbal reasoning in 4-year old children: a controlled, randomized study. Dev. Sci. 14 (3), 591–601.

Nyberg, L., Sandblom, J., Jones, S., et al., 2003. Neural correlates of training-related memory improvement in adulthood and aging. PNAS 100, 13728–13733.

Oh, M.Y., Abosch, A.M., Kim, S.H., Lang, A.E., Lozano, A.M., 2002. Long-term hardware-related complications of deep brain stimulation. Neurosurgery 50 (6), 1268–1276.

Ohn, S.H., Park, C.-I., Yoo, W.-K., Ko, M.-H., Choi, K.P., Kim, G.-M., et al., 2008. Time-dependent effect of transcranial direct current stimulation on the enhancement of working memory. Neuroreport 19 (1), 43–47.

Okagaki, L., Frensch, P.A., 1994. Effects of video game playing on measures of spatial performance: gender effects in late adolescence. J. Appl. Dev. Psychol. 15 (1), 33–58.

Owen, L., Scholey, A.B., Finnegan, Y., Hu, H., Sünram-Lea, S.I., 2012. The effect of glucose dose and fasting interval on cognitive function: a double-blind, placebo-controlled, six-way crossover study. Psychopharmacology 220, 577–589.

Owen, A.M., Hampshire, A., Grahn, J.A., Stenton, R., Dajani, S., Burns, A.S., et al., 2010. Putting brain training to the test. Nature 465 (7299), 775–778.

Owens, D.S., Benton, D., 1994. The impact of raising blood glucose levels on reaction time. Neuropsychobiology 30, 106–113.

Pagnoni, G., Cekic, M., Guo, Y., 2008. "Thinking about not thinking": neural correlates of conceptual processing during zen meditation. PLoS One 3, e3083.

Pereira, A.C., Huddleston, D.E., Brickman, A.M., Sosunov, A.A., Hen, R., McKhann, G.M., et al., 2007. An in vivo correlate of exercise-induced neurogenesis in the adult dentate gyrus. PNAS 104, 5638–5643.

Paulus, W., 2011. Transcranial electrical stimulation (tES – tDCS; tRNS, tACS) methods. Neuropsychol. Rehabil. 21, 602–617.

Poreisc, C., Boros, K., Antal, A., Paulus, W., 2007. Safety aspects of transcranial direct current stimulation concerning healthy subjects and patients. Brain Res. Bull. 72 (4–6), 208–214.

Posner, M.I., Petersen, S.E., Fox, P.T., Raichle, M.E., 1988. Localization of cognitive operations in the human brain. Science 240, 1627–1631.

Racchi, M., Mazzucchelli, M., Porrello, E., Lanni, C., Govoni, S., 2004. Acetylcholinesterase inhibitors: novel activities of old molecules. Pharmacol. Res. 50, 441–451.

Randall, D.C., Shneerson, J.M., File, S.E., 2005. Cognitive effects of modafinil in student volunteers may depend on IQ. Pharmacol. Biochem. Behav. 82, 133–139.

Rasch, B., Buchel, C., Gais, S., Born, J., 2007. Odor cues during slow-wave sleep prompt declarative memory consolidation. Science 315, 1426–1429.

Rasch, B., Pommer, J., Diekelmann, S., Born, J., 2009. Pharmacological REM sleep suppression paradoxically improes rather than impairs skill memory. Nat. Neurosci. 12, 396–397.

Ratcliff-Crain, J., O' Keefe, M.K., Baum, A., 1989. Cardiovascular reactivity, mood, and task performance in deprived and nondeprived coffee drinkers. Health Psychol. 8 (4), 427–447.

Raugh, M.R., Atkinson, R.C., 1975. A mnemonic method for learning a second-language vocabulary. J. Educ. Psychol. 67, 1–16.

Redick, T.S., Shipstead, Z., Harrison, T.L., Hicks, K.L., Fried, D.E., Hambrick, D.Z., Kane, M.J., Engle, R.W., 2013. No evidence of intelligence improvement after working memory training: a randomized, placebo-controlled study. J. Exp. Psychol. Gen. 142, 359–379.

Reis, J., Robertson, E., Krakauer, J.W., Rothwell, J., Marshall, L., Gerloff, C., et al., 2008. Consensus: can tDCS and TMS enhance motor learning and memory formation? Brain Stimul. 1, 363–369.

Reis, J., Schambra, H.M., Cohen, L.G., Buch, E.R., Fritsch, B., Zarahn, E., et al., 2009. Noninvasive cortical stimulation enhances motor skill acquisition over multiple days through an effect on consolidation. PNAS 106 (5), 1590–1595.

Reivih, M., Alavi, A., 1983. Positron emission tomographic studies of local cerebral glucose metabolism in humans in physiological and pathophysiological conditions. Adv. Metab. Disord. 10, 135–176.

Repantis, D., Laisney, O., Heuser, I., 2010a. Acetylcholinesterase inhibitors and memantine for neuroenhancement in healthy individuals: a systematic review. Pharmacol. Res. 61, 473–481.

Repantis, D., Schlattmann, P., Laisney, O., Heuser, I., 2010b. Modafinil and methylphenidate for neuroenhancement in healthy individuals: a systematic review. Pharmacol. Res. 62, 187–206.

Reyner, L.A., Horne, J.A., 1997. Suppression of sleepiness in drivers: combination of caffeine with a short nap. Psychophysiology 34 (6), 721–725.

Richards, M., Hardy, R., Wadsworth, M.E., 2003. Does active leisure protect cognition? Evidence from a national birth cohort. Soc. Sci. Med. 56, 785–792.

Ritskes, R., Ritskes-Hoitinga, M., Stodkilde-Jorgensen, H., Baeretsen, K., Hartman, T., 2003. MRI scanning during zen meditation: the picture of enlightenment? Constructivism Hum. Sci. 8, 85–90.

Ritter, S.M., Strick, M., Bos, M.W., van Baaren, R.B., Dijksterhuis, A., 2012. Good morning creativity: task reactivation during sleep enhances beneficial effect of sleep on creative performance. J. Sleep Res. 21, 643–647.

Roediger, H.L., 1980. The effectiveness of four mnemonics in ordering recall. J. Exp. Psychol. Hum. Learn. Mem. 6, 558–567.

Roediger, H.L., Butler, A.C., 2011. The critical role of retrieval practive in long-term retention. Trends Cogn. Sci. 15, 20–27.

Roediger, H.L., Karpicke, J.D., 2006. Test-enhanced learning. Psychol. Sci. 17, 249–255.

Rogers, P.J., Dernoncourt, C., 1998. Regular caffeine consumption: a balance of adverse and beneficial effects for mood and psychomotor performance. Pharmacol. Biochem. Behav. 59, 1039–1045.

Rogers, R.D., Blackshaw, A.J., Middleton, H.C., Matthews, K., Hawtin, K., Crowley, C., Hopwood, A., Wallace, C., Deakin, J.F., Sahakian, B.J., et al., 1999. Tryptophan depletion impairs stimulus-reward learning while methylphenidate disrupts attentional control in healthy young adults: implications for the monoaminergic basis of impulsive behaviour. Psychopharmacology 146, 482–491.

Roig, M., Nordbrandt, S., Geertsen, S.S., Nielsen, J.B., 2013. The effects of cardiovascular exercise on human memory: a review with meta-analysis. Neurosci. Biobehav. Rev. 37, 1645–1666.

Rosenheck, M.B., Levin, M.E., Levin, J.R., 1989. Learning botany concepts mnemonically: seeing the forest and the trees. J. Educ. Psychol. 81, 196–203.

Rossi, S., Rossini, P.M., 2004. TMS in cognitive plasticity and the potential for rehabilitation. Trends Cogn. Sci. 8 (6), 273–279.

Rossi, S., Hallett, M., Rossini, P.M., Pascual-Leone, A., Safety of TMS Consensus Group, 2009. Safety, ethical considerations, and application guidelines for the use of transcranial magnetic stimulation in clinical practice and research. Clin. Neurophysiol. 120, 2008–2039.

Ruffini, G., Wendling, F., Merlet, I., Molaee-Ardekani, B., Mekonnen, A., Salvador, R., et al., 2013. Transcranial current brain stimulation (tCS): models and technologies. IEEE Trans. Neural Syst. Rehabil. Eng. 21, 333–345.

Santarnecchi, E., Polizzotto, N.R., Godone, M., Giovannelli, F., Feurra, M., Matzen, L., Rossi, A., Rossi, S., 2013. Frequency-dependent enhancement of fluid intelligence induced by transcranial oscillatory potentials. Curr. Biol. 23, 1449–1453.

Savulescu, J., Bostrom, N. (Eds.), 2009. Human Enhancement. Oxford University Press, Oxford.

Schmiedek, F., Lövdén, M., Lindenberger, U., 2010. Hundred days of cognitive training enhance broad cognitive abilities in adulthood: findings from the COGITO study. Front. Aging Neurosci. 2 (27).

Scholey, A.B., Harper, S., Kennedy, D.O., 2001. Cognitive demand and blood glucose. Physiol. Behav. 73, 585–592.

Scholey, A., 2004. Chewing gum and cognitive performance: a case of a functional food with function but no food? Appetite 43, 215–216.

Scholey, A., Owen, L., 2013. Effects of chocolate on cognitive function and mood: a systematic review. Nutr. Rev. 71, 665–681.

Schuh, K.J., Griffiths, R.R., 1997. Caffeine reinforcement: the role of withdrawal. Psychopharmacology 130 (4), 320–326.

Sedlmeier, P., Eberth, J., Schwarz, M., Zimmermann, D., Haarig, F., Jaeger, S., Kunze, S., 2012. The psychological effects of meditation: a meta-analysis. Psychol. Bull. 138, 1139–1171.

Shipstead, Z., Thomas, S.R., Randall, W., 2010. Does working memory training generalize. Psychol. Belgica 50, 245–276.

Sibley, A., Etnier, J.L., 2002. The effects of physical activity on cognition in children: a meta-analysis. Med. Sci. Sports Exerc. 34, S214.

Smit, H.J., Rogers, P.J., 2000. Effects of low doses of caffeine on cognitive performance, mood and thirst in low and higher caffeine consumers. Psychopharmacology 152 (2), 167–173.

Smith, A., 2002. Effects of caffeine on human behavior. Food Chem. Toxicol. 40, 1243–1255.

Smith, A., Sutherland, D., Christopher, G., 2005. Effects of repeated doses of caffeine on mood and erformance of alert and fatigued volunteers. J. Psychopharmacol. 19, 620–626.

Smith, A.P., Rusted, J.M., Savory, M., Eaton-Williams, P., Hall, S.R., 1991. The effects of caffeine, impulsivity and time of day on performance, mood and cardiovascular function. Psychopharmacology 5, 120–128.

Smith, A., Brice, C., Nash, J., Rich, N., Nutt, D.J., 2003. Caffeine and central noradrenaline: effects on mood, cognitive performance, eye movements and cardiovascular function. J. Psychopharmacol. 17 (3), 283–292.

Smith, G.E., Housen, P., Yaffe, K., Ruff, R., Kennison, R.F., Mahncke, H.W., et al., 2009. A cognitive training program based on principles of brain plasticity: results from the improvement in memory with plasticity-based adaptive cognitive training (IMPACT) study. J. Am. Geriatr. Soc. 57 (4), 594–603.

Smith, M.A., Riby, L.M., Eekelen, J.A., Foster, J.K., 2011. Glucose enhancement of human memory: a comprehensive research review of the glucose memory facilitation effect. Neurosci. Biobehav. Rev. 35, 770–783.

Smith, M.E., Farah, M.J., 2011. Are prescription stimulants "smart pills"? the epidemiology and cognitive neuroscience of prescription stimulant use by normal healthy individuals. Psychol. Bull. 137, 717–741.

Smith, P.J., Blumenthal, J.A., Hoffman, B.M., Cooper, H., Strauman, T.A., Welsh-Bohmer, K., Browndyke, J.N., Sherwood, A., 2010. Aerobic exercise and neurocognitive performance: a meta-analytic review of randomized controlled trials. Psychosom Med. 72, 239–252.

Snowball, A., Tachtsidis, I., Popescu, T., Thompson, J., Delazer, M., Zamarian, L., Zhu, T., Cohen Kadosh, R., 2013. Long-term enhancement of brain function and cognition using cognitive training and brain stimulation. Curr. Biol. 23, 987–992.

Snyder, A., Bahramali, H., Hawker, T., Mitchell, D.J., 2006. Savant-like numerosity skills revealed in normal people by magnetic pulses. Perception 35, 837–845.

Snyder, A., Mulcahy, E., Taylor, J., Mitchell, D., Sachdev, P., Gandevia, S., 2003. Savant-like skills exposed in normal people by suppressing the left fronto-temporal lobe. J. Integr. Neurosci. 2 (2), 149–158.

Sonkusare, S.K., Kaul, C.L., Ramarao, P., 2005. Dementia of Alzheimer's disease and other neuro-degenerative disorders–memantine, a new hope. Pharmacol. Res. 51, 1–17.

Strobach, T., Frensch, P.A., Schubert, T., 2012. Video game practice optimizes executive control skills in dual-task and task switching situations. Acta Psychol. 140 (1), 13–24.

Sulzer, D., Sonders, M.S., Poulsen, N.W., Galli, A., 2005. Mechanisms of neurotransmitter release by amphetamines: a review. Prog. Neurobiol. 75, 406–433.

Sünram-Lea, S.I., Foster, J.K., Durlach, P., Perez, C., 2001. Glucose facilitation of cognitive performance in healthy young adults: examination of the influence of fast-duration, time of day and pre-consumption plasma glucose levels. Psychopharmacology 157, 46–54.

Sünram-Lea, S.I., Foster, J.K., Durlach, P., Perez, C., 2002a. The effects of retrograde and anterograde glucose administration on memory performance in healthy young adults. Behav. Brain Res. 134, 505–516.

Sünram-Lea, S.I., Foster, J.K., Durlach, P., Perez, C., 2002b. Investigation into the significance of task difficulty and divided allocation of resources on the glucose memory facilitation effect. Psychopharmacol. (Berl.) 160, 387–397.

Suthana, N., Haneef, Z., Stern, J., Mukamel, R., Behnke, E., Knowlton, B., et al., 2012. Memory enhancement and deep-brain stimulation of the entorhinal area. New Engl. J. Med. 366 (6), 502–510.

Suthana, N., Fried, I., 2014. Deep brain stimulation for enhancement of learning and memory. Neuroimage 85, 996–1002.

Talbot, M., 2009. Brain Gain. The New Yorker.

Tanaka, S., Michimata, C., Kaminaga, T., Honda, M., Sadato, N., 2002. Superior digit memory of abacus experts: an event-related functional MRI study. NeuroReport 13, 2187–2191.

Teo, F., Hoy, K.E., Daskalakis, Z.J., Fitzgerald, P.B., 2011. Investigating the role of current strength in tDCS modulation of working memory performance in healthy controls. Front. Psychiatry 2 (45).

Terney, D., Chaieb, L., Moliadze, V., Antal, A., Paulus, W., 2008. Increasing human brain excitability by transcranial high-frequency random noise stimulation. J. Neurosci. 28 (52), 14147–14155.

Thorell, L.B., Lindqvist, S., Bergman Nutley, S., Bohlin, G., Klingberg, T., 2009. Training and transfer effects of executive functions in preschool children. Dev. Sci. 12 (1), 106–113.

Thut, G., Nietzel, A., Pascual-Leone, A., 2004. Dorsal posterior parietal rTMS affects voluntary orienting of visuospatial attention. Cereb. Cortex 15 (5), 628–638.

Tononi, G., Cirelli, C., 2003. Sleep and synaptic homoestasis: a hypothesis. Brain Res. Bull. 62, 143–150.

van Uffelen, J.G., Chin, A., Paw, M.J., Hopman-Rock, M., van Mechelen, W., 2008. The effects of exercise on cognition in older adults with and without cognitive decline: a systematic review. Clin. J. Sport Med. 18, 486–500.

Vanneste, S., Fregni, F., De Ridder, D., 2013. Head-to-Head comparison of transcranial random noise stimulation, transcranial AC stimulation, and transcranial DC stimulation for tinnitus. Front. Psychiatry 4, 158.

Vaynman, S., Ying, Z., Gomez-Pinilla, F., 2004. Hippocampal BDNF mediates the efficacy of exercise on synaptic plasticity and cognition. Eur. J. Neurosci. 20, 2580–2590.

Verhaeghen, P., Marcoen, A., Goossens, L., 1992. Improving memory performance in the aged through mnemonic training: a meta-analytic study. Psychol. Aging 7, 242–251.

Volkow, N.D., Fowler, J.S., Logan, J., Alexoff, D., Zhu, W., Telang, F., et al., 2009. Effects of modafinil on dopamine and dopamine transporters in the male human brain: clinical implications. JAMA 301, 1148–1154.

Voss, M.W., Prakash, R.S., Erickson, K.I., Basak, C., Chaddock, L., Kim, J.S., et al., 2010. Plasticity of brain networks in a randomized intervention trial of exercise training in older adults. Front. Aging Neurosci. 2, 32.

Wagner, U., Gais, S., Haider, H., Verleger, R., Born, J., 2004. Sleep inspires insight. Nature 427, 352–355.

Walker, M.P., Brakefield, T., Morgan, A., Hobson, J.A., Stickgold, R., 2002. Practice with sleep makes perfect: sleep-dependent motor skill learning. Neuron 35, 205–211.

Wallace, L.J., 2012. Effects of amphetamine on subcellular distribution of dopamine and DOPAC. Synapse 66, 592–607.

Wang, A.Y., Thomas, M.H., 2000. Looking for long-term mnemonic effects on serial recall: the legacy of Simonides. Am. J. Psychol. 113, 331–340.

Warburton, D.M., Bersellini, E., Sweeney, E., 2001. An evaluation of a caffeinated taurine drink on mood, memory and information processing in healthy volunteers without caffeine abstinence. Psychopharmacology 158 (3), 322–328.

Weiss, B., Laties, V.G., 1962. Enhancement of human performance by caffeine and the amphetamines. Pharmacol. Rev. 14, 1–36.

Wilens, T.E., Adler, L.A., Adams, J., Sgambati, S., Rotrosen, J., Sawtelle, R., et al., 2008. Misuse and diversion of stimulants prescribed for ADHD: a systematic review of the literature. J. Am. Acad. Child Adolesc.Psychiatry 47, 21–31.

Wilson, M.A., McNaughton, B.L., 1994. Reactivation of hippocampal ensemble memories during sleep. Science 265, 676–679.

Winter, B., Breitenstein, C., Mooren, F.C., Voelker, K., Fobker, M., Lechtermann, A., Krueger, K., Fromme, A., Korsukewitz, C., Floel, A., Knecht, S., 2007. High impact running improves learning. Neurobiol. Learn. Mem. 87, 597–609.

Worthen, J.B., Hunt, R.R., 2011a. Mnemonics: underlying processes and practival applications. In: Byrne, J. (Ed.), Concise Learning and Memory. Academic Press, Waltham.

Worthen, J.B., Hunt, R.R., 2011b. Mnemonology. Psychology Press, New York.

Yanagisawa, H.1., Dan, I., Tsuzuki, D., Kato, M., Okamoto, M., Kyutoku, Y., Soya, H., 2010. Acute moderate exercise elicits increased dorsolateral prefrontal activation and improves cognitive performance with stroop test. Neuroimage 50, 1702–1710.

Yates, F.A., 1966. The Art of Memory. Routledge, London.

Yesavage, J.A., Mumenthaler, M.S., Taylor, J.L., Friedman, L., O'Hara, R., Sheikh, J., et al., 2002. Donepezil and flight simulator performance: effects on retention of complex skills. Neurology 59, 123–125.

Young, R.L., Ridding, M.C., Morrell, T.L., 2004. Switching skills on by turning off part of the brain. Neurocase 10 (3), 215–222.

Zeidan, F., Johnson, S.K., Diamond, B.J., David, Z., Goolkasian, P., 2010. Mindfulness meditation improves cognition: evidence of brief mental training. Conscious Cogn. 19, 597–605.

Zelinski, E.M., Spina, L.M., Yaffe, K., Ruff, R., Kennison, R.F., Mahncke, H.W., et al., 2011. Improvement in memory with plasticity-based adaptive cognitive training: results of the 3-month follow-up. J. Am. Geriatr. Soc. 59 (2), 258–265.

Chapter 12

The Use of Transcranial Direct Current Stimulation for Cognitive Enhancement

Chung Yen Looi and Roi Cohen Kadosh

Department of Experimental Psychology, University of Oxford, Oxford, United Kingdom

INTRODUCTION

Transcranial direct current stimulation (tDCS) is a form of noninvasive brain stimulation (NIBS) that is painless, relatively cheap, portable, and safe. This simple technology comprises a battery-driven stimulator that delivers weak currents (0.5–2 mA) typically through saline-soaked sponges. Usually, one electrode is used to stimulate an area of interest, while another is placed close to the circuit and serves as a reference electrode. In most studies, the reference electrode is usually placed on the supraorbital region, but some have positioned it over extracephalic regions (e.g., the shoulder). Contrary to the popular belief of "no pain, no gain," tDCS has been shown to accelerate learning and skill acquisition in complex learning tasks that usually take a long time to master (Clark et al., 2012) and in a range of fundamental human capacities from motor and sensorimotor skills to mathematical cognition, with minimal discomfort or adverse side effects (Cohen Kadosh, 2013; Krause and Cohen Kadosh, 2013; Poreisz et al., 2007). Such positive findings suggest the potential for improving the cognitive functions of clinical and nonclinical populations, whether restoring an impaired function to their former or an average level or raising function to a level "beyond the norm" (Cohen Kadosh, 2013; The Royal Society, 2011), and have promising implications for education (Wlodkowski, 2003), the military (Clark et al., 2012; Nelson et al., 2014), sport (Cohen Kadosh, 2014b; Schermer, 2008), the workplace, and everyday settings (Parasuraman, 2011; Parasuraman et al., 2012).

In this chapter, we review the basic mechanisms and physiological effects associated with tDCS, the effects of tDCS on cognitive processes based on studies of healthy and clinical populations and the limited studies conducted in children and elderly populations. Toward the end, we discuss the parameters

Cognitive Enhancement. http://dx.doi.org/10.1016/B978-0-12-417042-1.00012-7

that contributed to the positive findings observed in the reviewed studies, citing factors that can be optimized for effective cognitive neuroenhancement. Finally, we briefly discuss some open questions on the future use of brain stimulation for cognitive enhancement.

MECHANISMS OF tDCS

Physiological Effects

Animal and human studies suggest that the effects of tDCS are dependent on polarity. Anodal stimulation (A-tDCS) is usually known to facilitate neuronal firing, whereas cathodal stimulation (C-tDCS) usually inhibits neuronal firing beneath the stimulation site (Bikson et al., 2004; Bindman et al., 1964; Nitsche and Paulus, 2000) (Figure 12.1). Through modeling studies, Radman et al. (2009) further showed that specific neurons (the long layer IV and V pyramidal cells) are most affected by tDCS; stimulation has only insignificant or no effects on layer II/III neurons and interneurons. This is consistent with a previous intracranial study of the cat motor region (Creutzfeldt et al., 1962), which revealed that the effects of tDCS are also dependent on the orientation of neurons within cortical regions; neurons in deeper layers are excited by C-tDCS but suppressed by A-tDCS. It also has been proposed that nonsynaptic mechanisms (Ardolino et al., 2005) and glial cells (Ruohonen and Karhu, 2012) could mediate the modulation of brain excitability (for more neurobiological effects of tDCS, see reviews by Medeiros et al. (2012) and the recent collection of reviews in the book *The Stimulated Brain* (Cohen Kadosh, 2014a)).

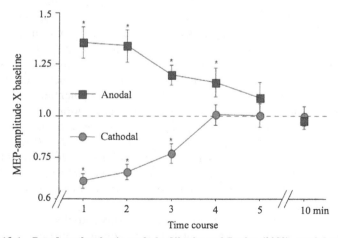

FIGURE 12.1   **Based on the classic study by Nitsche and Paulus (2000), anodal stimulation over the human motor cortex facilitates neuronal firing and cathodal stimulation inhibits neuronal firing up to 5 min after stimulation.** MEP, motor evoked potential. *Figure modified from Nitsche and Paulus (2000), Journal of Physiology, with permission.* (This figure is reproduced in color in the color plate section.)

In contrast, Rothwell (2013) reported that 2-mA A-tDCS over the motor cortex in humans produced the "expected" facilitation only about 60% of the time, whereas cathodal inhibition was observed only 45% of the time. It is also worth highlighting that the meta-analysis by Jacobson et al. (2012) showed that not all studies observed the dual polarity of tDCS; excitation induced by A-tDCS and inhibition by C-tDCS are more consistent in motor studies, but are rare in cognitive studies. Specifically, A-tDCS over a nonmotor area usually produces a measurable excitation-induced effect via cognitive or perceptual tasks, but C-tDCS rarely results in inhibition. The authors postulated that the lack of inhibitory effects by C-tDCS might indicate compensatory processes, which are commonly subserved by rich brain networks.

So far, studies have shown that the effects of tDCS after a few days of basic motor or cognitive training can last for up to 6 months (e.g., Cohen Kadosh et al., 2010; Reis et al., 2009). The mechanisms sustaining such longevity have been proposed to share some features with long-term synaptic plasticity (Stagg et al., 2011) such as protein-dependent processes (Nitsche et al., 2009), protein synthesis (Gartside, 1968a,b), reliance on N-methyl-D-aspartate receptors, which might implicate long-term potentiation and long-term depression (Islam et al., 1995; Liebetanz et al., 2002; Nitsche et al., 2003a), as well as mediation by polymorphisms in the brain-derived neurotrophic factor (*BDNF*) gene at 11p13 (Fritsch et al., 2010).

Pharmacological techniques also have shed light on the possible mechanisms of tDCS in humans (Dayan et al., 2013); for example, ion channel blockers seem to have differential polarity-specific effects on cortical excitability. Application of the voltage-dependent sodium channel blocker carbamazepine (Liebetanz et al., 2002; Nitsche et al., 2003b) or the calcium channel blocker flunarizine (Nitsche et al., 2003b) eradicates only A-tDCS-like plasticity both during and after stimulation. Meanwhile, the introduction of the *N*-methyl-D-aspartate receptor antagonist dextromethorphan prevented the poststimulation effects of tDCS in a non-polarity-specific fashion (Nitsche et al., 2003b).

TDCS also has been associated with modulation of neurotransmitters such as dopamine (Nitsche et al., 2006), decreased concentrations of γ-aminobutyric acid following A-tDCS or C-tDCS, decreased concentrations of glutamate after C-tDCS (Stagg et al., 2011), and increased combined concentrations of glutamate and glutamine after A-tDCS (Clark et al., 2011). It also has been reported that both 1-mA A-tDCS and C-tDCS for 15 min can induce an increase in oxyhemoglobin concentration in the frontal cortex near the electrode (Merzagora et al., 2010) and increased perfusions in regions anatomically well connected to regions stimulated during A-tDCS (Stagg et al., 2013). More recently, Krause et al. (2013) proposed that the excitability/inhibitory balance of γ-aminobutyric acid/glutamate in the stimulated regions could mediate the effects of brain stimulation.

Some also have suggested that tDCS effects could be modulated via cortical oscillatory activity, an index that has been linked to enhancements in cognitive performance (e.g., Hoy et al., 2013; Krause et al., 2000; Meinzer et al.,

2013; Zaehle et al., 2011). Cortical oscillations are the synchronous firing of groups of neurons at specific frequencies, which are thought to be associated with a range of functional processes. For example, theta (4–8 Hz) and alpha (8–13 Hz) oscillations are thought to relate to cognitive and memory performance (Klimesch, 1999). Hoy et al. (2013) suggested that tDCS could improve cognition by directly targeting these intrinsic underlying neuropsychological processes.

The effects of tDCS have recently been shown to operate at the network level (see Hunter et al., 2013). For example, Keeser et al. (2011) found that, compared with sham, 2-mA A-tDCS over the left dorsolateral prefrontal cortex (dlPFC) and C-tDCS over the right supraorbital region induced significant changes in regional brain connectivity for the default mode network and frontal-parietal networks, both of which are proximal to the primary stimulation site. These findings suggest that tDCS can modulate functional connectivity during a resting state in distinct, functional networks in humans. Polania et al. (2011a) also reported changes in functional connectivity between brain regions using electroencephalography (EEG), functional magnetic resonance imaging (fMRI) (Polania et al., 2012), and graph-theoretical approaches (Polania et al., 2011a,b). In another study, Roche et al. (2011) showed that A-tDCS modified not only the cortical circuits involved, but spinal motor circuits as well. They stimulated the motor area representation of the anterior lower leg muscle (tibialis anterior) and observed relaxation of the opposing posterior lower leg. Meinzer et al. (2013) showed that A-tDCS over the left inferior frontal gyrus (IFG) could improve word retrieval, while selectively reducing task-related activations in the left ventral IFG, possibly reflecting an increased efficiency in processing in task-critical regions. Further seed-based, resting-state fMRI showed increased connectivity of the left IFG and core areas overlapping with the bilateral language network. This study suggests that A-tDCS could modulate endogenous low-frequency oscillations (which are thought to reflect underlying anatomic connectivity) in a distributed set of functionally associated brain areas through more efficient processing in key task areas, resulting in improved behavioral performance. Finally, a recent study by Stagg et al. (2013) also showed that A-tDCS to the left dlPFC in healthy participants decreased its coupling with bilateral thalami, showing that behavioral effects of tDCS could arise from modulation at the level of functional connectivity between these regions. To summarize, while there are numerous studies suggesting many possible mechanisms of tDCS, most of the evidence is indirect and thus warrants further investigation.

SAFETY OF tDCS

tDCS is considered as a safe method for brain stimulation. The most common experience is a tingling sensation, although a rare mild burning or pain sensation on the scalp underneath the stimulating electrode(s) can occur, especially when the level of impedance is high. Currently, there are no reports of adverse effects in clinical or healthy adults, children, or elderly populations (Kessler et al., 2013). It also has been consistently shown that stimulation continuously for 20 min (Iyer et al., 2005; Nitsche et al., 2005) and even up to 30 min (Boggio et al., 2012; Lindenberg et al., 2013; Lindenberg et al., 2010) is safe. Furthermore, it was shown that tDCS-induced behavioral and neurophysiological effects in humans were fully reversible (Nitsche et al., 2003c). Based on most published calculations, the maximum electric field in the cortex for the standard M1 tDCS montage is about 0.4 V/m (see Miranda et al., 2013), which is within the occupational limit (between 0.05 and 0.5 V/m) but not the general public exposure limit (between 0.01 and 0.1 V/m), set by the International Commission on Non-Ionizing Radiation Protection (ICNIRP, 2010). It is worth mentioning here that the dosage recommended for general public exposure might be lower than that needed to induce the desired behavioral effects in the laboratory setting (e.g., therapeutic effects, especially within short periods of time); the guideline is intended to regulate safety of exposure/usage in the workplace under the assumption that individuals will be exposed regularly and for long periods of time. Previous studies have shown that tDCS does not alter serum concentrations of human neurone-specific enolase (a sensitive marker of neuronal damage), skin temperature beneath the electrodes, or EEG recordings or induce brain edema or changes in the blood–brain barrier and cerebral tissue that are detectable by magnetic imaging (e.g., Iyer et al., 2005; Nitsche et al., 2003b, 2004; Nitsche and Paulus, 2000). Liebetanz et al. (2009) published one of the few studies that directly explored the safety threshold of tDCS. They investigated the effects of C-tDCS intensity on rats by applying between 1 and 1000 μA for up to 270 min via an epicranial electrode (3.5 mm^2). Through histological evaluations 48 h after stimulation, they found that brain lesions occur at a current density of 142.9 A/m^2 for a duration longer than 10 min. A linear increase in lesion size was observed between current densities of 142.9 and 285.7 A/m^2, with a calculated zero lesion size intercept of 52,400 C/m^2. They noted that there was no tissue damage when stimulated below this current density or charge density threshold, and they showed there was no risk of accumulative tissue damage after 5 days of consecutive stimulation. It is important to note that this threshold estimate is two orders of magnitude higher than the charge density applied in humans (171–480 C/m^2), suggesting that the tDCS dosage used in humans so far is likely to be safe. Overall, although this study does not provide information about long-term morphological modifications or behavioral changes, and hence is of limited value to clinical conditions, it suggests that, with more research, future protocols could be optimized to maximize the effects of tDCS without causing harm.

APPLICATIONS IN COGNITIVE ENHANCEMENT

After discussing the putative physiological mechanisms of tDCS and safety issues in this section, we review studies that have used this stimulation method to assess fundamental, domain-general cognitive processes (such as perception, attention, learning, and memory), as well as domain-specific functions (such as mathematical cognition and language) in both clinical and nonclinical populations.

DOMAIN-GENERAL COGNITIVE PROCESSES

Perception

Visual Perception

Korsakov and Matveeva (1982) explored the effects of tDCS on basic visual perception about three decades ago. They found a reduction in visual perceptual sensitivity with 0.2-mA A-tDCS over the occipital cortex in healthy subjects. This was contradicted by Antal et al. (2001), who applied 1-mA A-tDCS over the same region but did not observe any such effects. Instead, they found that C-tDCS reduced the contrast sensitivity of the occipital cortex. At the neural level, stimulation over the primary visual cortex has been shown to modulate the amplitude of visual evoked potentials and the perception of phosphenes (Antal et al., 2004b), whereas stimulation of V5 modulated motion-detected thresholds and the duration of motion aftereffects (Antal et al., 2004a). In a recent study, Peters et al. (2013) found that A-tDCS to the primary visual cortex could prevent overnight consolidation of visual learning. They suggested that this could be because of inhibitory homeostatic plasticity mechanisms that blocked long-term potentiation. Together, these findings suggest that A-tDCS and C-tDCS can modulate the excitability of the visual cortex (for a review, see Antal and Paulus (2008) and Gall et al. (2012)).

Over the past few years, there has been more research on tDCS and more complex visual perception and its therapeutic potentials. For example, in a study of the perception of facial expressions, Boggio et al. (2009) showed that simultaneous A-tDCS over the temporal cortex and C-tDCS over the right temporal cortex impaired recognition of sad faces in men, but resulted in enhanced recognition of sad faces in female participants. This finding suggests that tDCS-induced effects could be gender dependent. In terms of therapeutic applications, tDCS has been reported to enhance visual functional outcomes in patients with hemianopia, a condition characterized by reduced vision or blindness in half of the visual field of one or both eyes (compared with visual rehabilitation alone) (Plow et al., 2011, 2012), and contributed to long-term improvement in the motion perception in patients with occipital stroke (Olma et al., 2011). These studies suggest that tDCS not only contributes to our understanding of the basics of human visual perception, but also suggests possible opportunities for more effective rehabilitation of visual clinical conditions.

Multisensory Perception

TDCS also has been used in exploring more complex perceptual phenomenon. For example, Bolognini et al. (2011) used a sound-induced flash illusion to

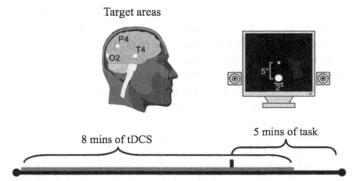

FIGURE 12.2   Design of the study by Bolognini et al. (2011). Each participant underwent five separate sessions, randomized across participants: baseline (without transcranial direct current stimulation (tDCS)), sham tDCS, and temporal, occipital, and parietal tDCS. Top left: targeted brain areas (white); locations following the standard 10–20 EEG system (O2 = right occipital cortex; P4 = right posterior parietal cortex; T4 = right superior temporal gyrus). tDCS was applied 5 min before the experimental task and lasted for 8 min. The experimental task took approximately 5 min. *Figure modified with permission from Elsevier.*

investigate the effects of tDCS on multisensory processing at different scalp locations (Figure 12.2). In this illusion, one to four tones are presented simultaneously with one or two flashes of a visual stimulus. The idea is that the illusion occurs when the presentation of a single visual stimulus is seen as multiple presentations (fission illusion) or when multiple presentations of a visual stimulus are perceived as a single presentation (fusion illusion) when, in both cases, either one or multiple tones also are presented simultaneously. It was found that A-tDCS over the temporal cortex led to an enhancement of the auditory influence on visual perception during the fission illusion, whereas A-tDCS over the occipital cortex suppressed this effect. The authors found the opposite for C-tDCS. This finding suggests that tDCS might modulate sensory perception by biasing competition between brain networks that process conflicting sensory information.

Learning and Memory

The above-mentioned studies relate mostly to online effects (effects of tDCS on task performance during stimulation). However, we believe that the real promise of tDCS is rooted in enhancing learning and memory, with potential long-term effects (Cohen Kadosh, 2013; Krause et al., 2014). We refer to some of these studies in this section.

Implicit Memory (Procedural/Motor Learning)

Procedural learning occurs without our intent or conscious awareness, and it is a major form of learning that shapes our skills, perceptions, and behaviors

(O'Halloran et al., 2012). Blind typing and cycling are two examples of such learning. Ferrucci et al. (2013) explored the effects of sham and A-tDCS (2 mA for 20 min, delivered to the cerebellum) on participants' procedural learning performance. In their study, participants completed a serial reaction time task (SRTT) that involved making key press responses to visual cues, a visual analog scale, and a visual attention task before and 35 min after receiving stimulation. They found that A-tDCS improved performance during procedural learning, but had no observed effects on arousal or alertness.

In another study, Kang et al. (2011) used a randomized crossover experiment and compared the effects of uni-tDCS, bi-tDCS (2 mA for 20 min), and sham stimulation (2 mA for 30 s) on participants' performance on a finger sequence SRTT immediately and 24 h after stimulation. They applied A-tDCS over the left M1 and C-tDCS over the right supraorbital region in both the uni-TDCS and sham conditions, and A-tDCS over the left M1 and C-tDCS over the right M1 in the bi-tDCS condition. Their findings showed that, immediately after the training and tDCS, participants in all conditions showed significantly quicker reaction times, but, most importantly, 24 h later, only those in the uni- and bi-tDCS conditions showed significant decreases in their response times (those in the sham condition showed a marginal decrease). This study suggests that uni- and bi-tDCS led to greater consolidation of implicit motor sequence learning compared with sham, with no significant differences found between these stimulating montages.

In an earlier study, Nitsche et al. (2003d) showed that, compared with sham stimulation, 2 mA of A-tDCS over the primary motor cortex throughout a 15-min SSRT improved participants' performance in the acquisition and early consolidation phase of implicit motor learning. There was a significantly faster decrease in reaction times in the SRTT under A-tDCS compared with sham stimulation during the experiment. Together, these findings highlight the potential of tDCS to affect implicit memory. Moreover, the ability of tDCS to affect the cerebellum opens the possibility of targeting its multiple roles in motor control, cognition, learning, and emotions and modulating its neuroplasticity, with implications for both clinical and healthy populations (for a review see Ferrucci and Priori, 2013).

Explicit Learning

Explicit or declarative learning processes involve memories that can be consciously recalled, accompanying implicit learning processes that are automatic or unconscious (Squire, 1982). For example, when you recall tDCS and cognitive enhancement in a week's time, you will remember that it was achieved by reading this clear and well-written chapter. It is the active acquisition of skills and/or knowledge whereby individuals can explain how they gain such skill and/or knowledge. To date, effects of tDCS have been explored mainly in memory for word lists or objects and memory for spatial location. In studies that used word lists, Marshall et al. (2004) used a unique stimulation protocol that involved a pulsed stimulation technique during sleep: A-tDCS was applied to bilateral dlPFC and pulsed on/off for 15-s intervals during the first 30 min of slow-wave sleep to increase memory of word lists. They found a modest, but significant increase in the number of words recalled from a list that had been learned the day before, but no effects on procedural memory. The authors concluded that tDCS could have modulated neuronal plasticity by generating slow oscillatory neural activity.

Hammer et al. (2011) explored the effects of tDCS over the left dlPFC in two conditions of learning: errorless and errorful learning of new German nouns. After the encoding phase, participants either performed in the errorless or errorful condition. In the errorless condition, they were required to use the word in a sentence, whereas in the errorful condition, they were provided with the first three letters of words in the list and were required to recall from memory the word from the list. The latter task differs from the former because it includes both retrieval and reconsolidation. The authors found a trend toward increased learning from errorful learning with A-tDCS, although the effect was not significant, and significantly decreased learning after C-tDCS in the same condition. They did not observe any effects of tDCS in the errorless learning condition. They concluded that C-tDCS decreased reconsolidation in this type of word list learning task.

In a series of word memorization tasks, Javadi and Walsh (2011) applied sham stimulation, A-tDCS, and C-tDCS over the left dlPFC in healthy participants. They found that, during encoding, A-tDCS improved and C-tDCS impaired later memory recognition. They showed that this effect is site specific: A-tDCS to the M1 had no effect on later recognition. During recognition, C-tDCS impaired recognition compared with sham stimulation, and A-tDCS led to a trend toward improved performance in recognition. Overall, these findings show that the effects of tDCS on verbal memorization and the left dlPFC are polarity- and site-specific.

There are also studies that focus on spatial memory. In addition to the study by Floel et al. (2012) (reviewed in the section "Studies of the Elderly"), Clark et al. (2012) investigated the effects of A-tDCS on object detection in a computerized virtual environment using a camouflaged object detection task of the type performed by military personnel in urban settings (Figure 12.3). They applied either 0.1 or 2 mA of A-tDCS over the right inferior cortex during the first 30 min of an hour-long discovery task. Participants were tested on their performance immediately before and after training and again 1 h later. The authors found that stimulation at a higher current of 2 mA was linked to increased performance for all test stimuli and greater accuracy for target detection sensitivity compared with 0.1 mA. This finding suggests that the effects of tDCS are influenced by current dosage.

Attention

Attention can be defined as the process of selectively concentrating on an aspect of an environment, while ignoring other variables. This important function can be differentiated into multiple components that can be identified using behavioral

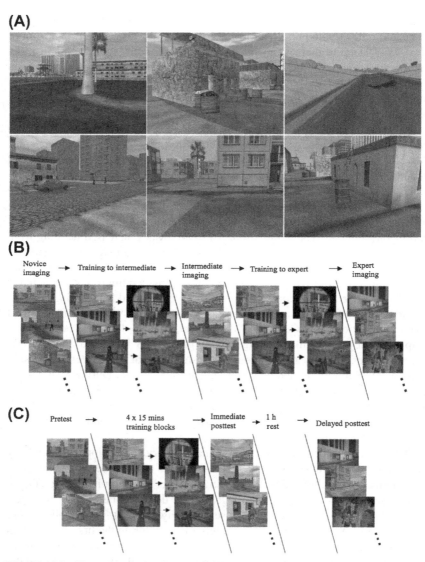

FIGURE 12.3 **Examples of stimuli used by Clark et al. (2012) in functional magnetic resonance imaging (fMRI) and transcranial direct current stimulation (tDCS) learning studies.** (A) Examples of stimuli with and without concealed objects. Only four of the six scenes include hidden objects. Two of these four scenes with concealed objects contain hidden enemy soldiers, and the other two contain hidden bombs. The difficulty of object detection was defined by the size and distinctiveness of objects. (B) The fMRI learning study paradigm followed by 13 participants. Each participant was scanned using fMRI at the novice stage using 100 static scenes without feedback. This was followed by up to 90 min of training per day, whereby participants press a button to indicate whether they observed a concealed image in a series of static images, with each response followed by a short feedback video. Participants trained consecutively until they achieve

and functional neuroimaging measures (Fan et al., 2005; Parasuraman, 1998; Posner and Petersen, 1990). Specific networks that underlie processes of alerting, orienting, and executive control are responsible for the direction and modulation of perception in most, if not all, sensory domains. The activity of these systems is, in turn, linked to function or dysfunction in other cognitive processes including learning and memory (Seitz and Watanabe, 2005) and vigilance and alerting attention (Sturm and Willmes, 2001). The brain regions that have been investigated using tDCS include the dlPFC (vigilance and executive function), the right inferior frontal cortex (alerting), the superior parietal cortex (shifting of attention), the parietal cortex (visuospatial attention), and the right intraparietal sulcus (visuospatial and executive function).

Coffman et al. (2012), for example, reported the effects of tDCS on alerting, orienting, and executive attention. They found that A-tDCS over the right inferior frontal cortex led to an enhancement in the alerting measures of the attentional networks test an hour after training. They did not observe any effects of tDCS on orienting or executive attention in this study, showing that the effects of tDCS are selective and specific to the alerting network of attention when stimulating this brain area.

In a more recent study of vigilance, Nelson et al. (2014) applied 1 mA for 10 min to either the left or right dlPFC either early (10 min) or late (30 min) during a task that requires participants to perform simulated air traffic control, whereby they are asked to detect infrequent collision paths of aircraft (targets) over a prolonged time (40 min). They are not supposed to respond to the more frequent noncollision flight paths (nontargets). Nelson and colleagues also investigated the effects of tDCS on cerebral blood velocity using transcranial Doppler sonography and cerebral oxygenation (using near infrared spectroscopy). They found a significant decrease in vigilance over time on task in the sham condition (15-s ramp up to 1 mA), as indicated by a lower target detection rate, longer reaction times, and a decreased blood flow velocity. In contrast, active tDCS contributed to an improvement in the rate of target detection, reduction in blood flow velocity over time, and greater cerebral oxygenation. This study shows the potential use of tDCS to alleviate decrements in performance resulting from the need for sustained attention over prolonged periods.

---

an intermediate level of performance (>78% correct responses on two consecutive training blocks) and were scanned again. The training continued for seven of these participants until they achieved 95% accuracy, when they were scanned for the last time at the expert level. (C) The paradigm used for behavioral tDCS learning studies; each session was preceded by a pretest involving viewing static scenes without feedback, followed by 4 training blocks of 60 trials each. Participants received tDCS 5 min before their training began for 30 min, followed by additional training without tDCS, for a total of 1 h of training. Immediately after training, a posttest was conducted, followed by an hour break and a final delayed posttest. *Figure adapted with permission from Elsevier.* (This figure is reproduced in color in the color plate section.)

In a double-blind study, Ko et al. (2008) applied 2-mA A-tDCS over the right posterior parietal cortex (PPC) for 20 min in patients with subacute stroke with spatial neglect. They found that only A-tDCS, and not sham stimulation, resulted in an improvement in both figure cancellation and line bisection tasks, indicating the utility of tDCS for remediating the neglect condition.

Sparing et al. (2009) later showed that 1 mA of A-tDCS over the right or left PPC in right-handed healthy participants biased visuospatial attention toward the contralateral hemispace in a visual detection task, whereas C-tDCS over the right or left PPC biased visuospatial attention toward the ipsilateral hemispace. In the same article, they showed that both 1-mA A-tDCS over the lesioned PPC and C-tDCS over the intact homolog in patients with stroke-induced left visuospatial neglect (a clinical condition where patients are unable to attend, respond, or orient voluntarily to people or objects on the side of space opposite to the lesion they suffer from) reduced symptoms of visuospatial neglect based on a line bisection task and the subtest neglect from the attention test battery.

In the first study that showed effects on executive function, Kang et al. (2009) applied A-tDCS over the left dlPFC of participants with decline after stroke during a standard go/no-go task. They found that the response accuracy in this task was enhanced only in patients, not in healthy controls, suggesting that stimulation of the left dlPFC might remediate deficiency in attentional processing. This is an important finding because performance in the go/no-go task is a measure of executive attention network function, which is impaired in many neurodevelopmental disorders such as attention deficit hyperactivity disorder (Castellanos et al., 2006). Together, these studies indicate that tDCS can modulate the different components of attention and show the potential for remediation of attention-related conditions.

Working Memory

The application of tDCS for improving working memory (WM) is a popular area. WM is the ability to hold information for a short period of time for further manipulation. It is strongly correlated with intelligence quotient (Jaeggi et al., 2008) and mathematical ability (Raghubar et al., 2010). Moreover, it is implicated in many higher order cognitive processes such as problem solving, and its improvement has been shown to enhance complex thought and action (Jausovec and Jausovec, 2012). Therefore, improving WM offers implications for a wide range of cognitive capacities. tDCS is traditionally applied over the dlPFC (e.g., Boggio et al., 2006; Fregni et al., 2005; Jo et al., 2009; Marshall et al., 2005; Ohn et al., 2008), and positive effects on WM are consistently reported, especially when delivered to the left (e.g., Andrews et al., 2011; Jacobson et al., 2012; Nitsche et al., 2008), when used in addition to a working memory task such as the n-back and Sternberg visual WM task. In addition, other areas such as the cerebellum and PPC also have been implicated in the functioning in WM (Berryhill et al., 2010; Ferrucci et al., 2008).

Fregni et al. (2005) published one of the earlier studies of the effects of tDCS on WM. They showed that after only 10 min of 1-mA A-tDCS over the left dlPFC, healthy participants showed significantly fewer errors and increased correct responses in a 3-back WM task based letters. No effects were found with C-tDCS or sham stimulation of the same area. Later, Boggio et al. (2006) extended the use of tDCS to enhance WM abilities in patients with Parkinson's disease and were the first to report the use of 2-mA tDCS. They found that patients with Parkinson's disease showed significant improvement in accuracy following only 2-mA and not 1-mA A-tDCS, contrasting the findings in health participants of Fregni et al. and suggesting that the dose response might differ between clinical and healthy populations, possibly because of differences in cortical excitability linked to Parkinson's disease. Nevertheless, the study by Boggio et al. showed the benefits of tDCS for clinical intervention in cognitive dysfunction.

More recently, Hoy et al. (2013) applied 20 min of 1-mA and 2-mA A-tDCS and sham to the left dlPFC of healthy participants over 3 weeks. Participants completed 10 min of the n-back task immediately and 20 and 40 min after receiving stimulation; EEG was recorded concurrently at F3, FZ, and F4 (Figure 12.4). Researchers found that A-tDCS improved efficiency of cognitive processing, with the strongest effects at 1 mA. This finding is similar to the one reported previously by Fregni et al. (2005). This study also supports the view that there is a difference in the tDCS-induced effects between healthy and clinical populations.

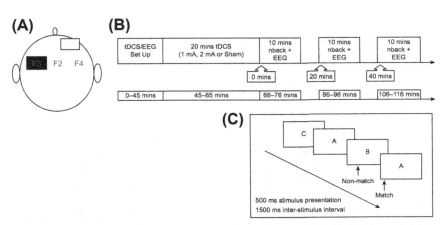

FIGURE 12.4   Setup and protocol used in the study by Hoy et al. (2013). (A) An anodal electrode was positioned over F3 (the left prefrontal cortex) and a cathodal electrode over the right supraorbital space. (B) Each participant completed three experimental sessions with a week. Transcranial direct current stimulation was randomly administered at 1 mA, 2 mA, or sham for 20 min over 3 weeks, followed by 10 min of an n-back task immediately following 20 and 40 min of stimulation with simultaneous electroencephalographic recordings from F3, FZ, and F4. C. The n-back task used. *Figure adapted with permission from Elsevier.*

Meiron and Lavidor (2013) applied A-tDCS over the dlPFC of healthy participants during a modified verbal n-back WM task that is highly sensitive to executive attention. They found significant lateralized "online" WM performance only during the highest WM load condition, whereby male participants benefited from left dlPFC stimulation and female participants benefited from right dlPFC stimulation. This finding highlights the possibility that lateralized stimulation effects in high-load WM maintenance could be sex dependent.

In a unique study targeting the cerebellum (bilaterally), Ferrucci et al. (2008) showed that 2 mA of A-tDCS or C-tDCS could impair reaction time practice effects in a Sternberg visual WM task. This effect was shown to be independent of motor and visual effects, and was the first study to reveal that stimulation of brain regions other than the prefrontal cortex can affect the functioning of WM. Berryhill et al. (2010) showed that C-tDCS over the right inferior PPC reduced recognition, but not recall, in an object recognition and recall WM task. Stimulation (A-tDCS, C-tDCS, and sham) was applied before task performance. They did not find any significant effects with A-tDCS, but instead reported a nonsignificant decrease in performance to a lesser degree than C-tDCS.

These studies and those reviewed by Coffman et al. (2014) and Kuo and Nitsche (2012) suggest that tDCS has the capacity to alter WM performance in healthy and clinical populations, and revealed that factors such as sex and stimulation dosage in mediating the stimulation-induced effects.

Domain-Specific Cognitive Processes

Language Cognition

In recent years, there has been an abundance of research using tDCS in combination with a language-related task to enhance language abilities in word generation (e.g., Iyer et al., 2005), naming (e.g., Sparing et al., 2008), language reacquisition after stroke (e.g., Floel et al., 2008), speech repetition (e.g., Fiori et al., 2014), and improving conditions of anomia (difficulties in recalling words or names) (e.g., Baker et al., 2010; Floel et al., 2012). Current evidence suggests that tDCS can affect language abilities in healthy individuals and enhance linguistic performance in patients with aphasia (a language disorder that involves difficulties from language comprehension to formulation) (for a review, see Monti et al., 2012). More recently, it has been suggested that tDCS could be used as an efficient tool to enhance learning in individuals with congenital developmental dyslexia (Vicario and Nitsche, 2013).

The application of tDCS in this domain is typically over the language-related frontal-temporal network, including the left dlPFC (e.g., Fertonani et al., 2010; Iyer et al., 2005; Wirth et al., 2011), left IFG (e.g., Cattaneo et al., 2011; de Vries et al., 2010), left inferior frontal cortex (e.g., Holland et al., 2011; Marangolo et al., 2011), left posterior perisylvian area (e.g., Fiori et al., 2011; Floel et al., 2008; Sparing et al., 2008), left anterior frontal lobe (e.g., Ross et al., 2010a), and the right IFG (e.g., Jung et al., 2011; Kang et al., 2011; Vines et al.,

2011); for reviews, see Floel (2013) and Monti et al. (2012). Lasting enhancement effects of tDCS were reported for 1 week (Baker et al., 2010), 2 weeks (Floel et al., 2008), 3 weeks (Fiori et al., 2011), and up to 2 months (Marangolo et al., 2011).

In healthy participants, Iyer et al. (2005) showed that A-tDCS over the left prefrontal lobe resulted in significant improvements on a letter cue-word generation task, whereas C-tDCS slightly reduced fluency. However, they observed these effects only at 2 mA, and not 1 mA, showing that the effects of tDCS are dependent on stimulation parameters such as the stimulation dosage.

In a randomized, double-blind study, Floel et al. (2008) combined tDCS with training on a learning task in an attempt to generate long-lasting improvements in language learning when acquiring new vocabulary. They stimulated the posterior part of the left perisylvian area in healthy, young, right-handed adults either with A-tDCS, C-tDCS (1 mA, 20 min each), or sham stimulation while participants trained on acquiring three parallel versions of the miniature lexicon of 30 new object names. They found that participants who received A-tDCS showed quicker and better associative learning compared with those who received sham; more important, there was better transfer of the vocabulary into the participants' native language (A-tDCS group).

Fiori et al. (2011) explored the effects of A-tDCS on associative word learning and word retrieval in both healthy participants and patients with stroke-induced aphasia. In the first study involving healthy subjects, participants were randomized and counterbalanced in a double-blind condition: they received one session of A-tDCS and one sham stimulation over Wernicke's area and A-tDCS over the right occipitoparietal area (stimulation for 20 min at 1 mA once every week over 3 weeks with a 6-day interval). Meanwhile, three aphasic patients took part in a randomized double-blind study involving intensive language training for their anomic difficulties. Those in the A-tDCS group received 1 mA for 20 min over Wernicke's area during a picture-naming task for 5 consecutive days during 2 weeks overall; the results suggest that A-tDCS significantly improved participants' accuracy on the picture-naming task. Compared with sham stimulation, both healthy and aphasic patients showed shorter naming latencies. One and 3 weeks after the study, assessment of 2 aphasic participants revealed that response accuracy and reaction times remained significantly better after A-tDCS compared with sham, indicating long-term improvement.

In clinical populations, the effects of tDCS on naming abilities have been explored in patients with aphasia after stroke, among whom impairment in word retrieval (anomia) is the most common symptom, typically with little or no spontaneous improvement after the first 6 months (Bhogal et al., 2003). Studies of patients who are in the subacute (e.g., Hesse et al., 2011; You et al., 2011) and chronic stages of stroke with mild to moderate aphasia (Baker et al., 2010) and moderate to severe aphasia (Flöel et al., 2011) also have been conducted. These studies all showed positive effects of tDCS on participants' language performance (see reviews by Floel, 2013, and Monti et al., 2012). Some studies also highlighted the influence of the severity of baseline naming deficits on the effect size of tDCS-induced improvements (e.g., Floel et al., 2012; Jung et al., 2011). In terms of language, tDCS has been shown to improve various language abilities such as word acquisition (Floel et al., 2012), production (Iyer et al., 2005), and retrieval (Fiori et al., 2011), depending on stimulation parameters such as stimulation site, dosage, and participants' initial language abilities.

Numerical Cognition

Cohen Kadosh et al. (2010) published the first study highlighting the beneficial effects of tDCS on numerical cognition (Figure 12.5). They showed that 20 min of 1-mA A-tDCS to the right PPC and C-tDCS to the left PPC improved the acquisition of a new number-symbol system over 6 days of training in healthy adults, whereas A-tDCS to the left PPC and C-tDCS to the right PPC resulted in underperformance. The enhancing effects were specific to the learned material rather than to other general functions, and were retained up to 6 months later, suggesting that tDCS could potentially be used as an intervention tool for cases of atypical numerical development or loss of numerical abilities because of stroke or degenerative illness.

In a more recent nontraining study, Hauser et al. (2013) applied tDCS to the left, right, and bilateral PPC of healthy adults to improve numerical magnitude processing and mental arithmetic. They found that only A-tDCS to the left PPC significantly improved performance in a number comparison and subtraction task, but they found no effects in the right and bilateral stimulation conditions compared with sham, suggesting a causal role for left PPC in numerical magnitude processing and mental arithmetic.

Clemens et al. (2013) investigated the effects of tDCS in healthy participants while they solved simple multiplication tasks. The participants were assigned to a real stimulation group (20 min of 2-mA A-tDCS over the right angular gyrus, the main area implicated in arithmetic fact retrieval (Grabner et al., 2009)), sham stimulation (same setting as in the real stimulation group, but turned off after 20 s of stimulation), or a control group (no electrodes attached). They also scanned participants using fMRI before and after tDCS to examine changes in brain activity. At the behavioral level, they did not find significant differences between the performance of the three groups before and after training, although all groups showed a general improvement. At the neural level, however, the fMRI data revealed significantly greater activity in the bilateral angular gyrus for multiplication problems solved during A-tDCS, but not in the control or sham tDCS conditions, providing evidence that tDCS could modulate the neural correlates of arithmetic processing after a single session. These findings might have implications for patients with acalculia (an acquired condition characterized by impaired ability in performing simple mathematical tasks), which comprises about two-thirds of aphasic patients. For example, combining tDCS with functional therapy (e.g., Domahs et al., 2004; Zaunmuller et al., 2009) might further enhance observed improvements within a shorter period of time.

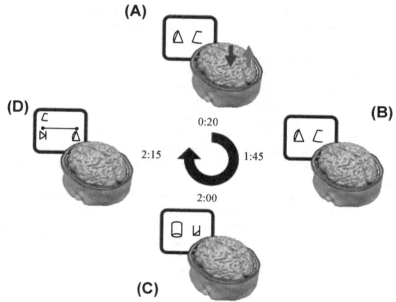

FIGURE 12.5 **The daily training routine of participants in the study by Cohen Kadosh et al. (2010) over six sessions.** (A) Application of transcranial direct current stimulation (tDCS) from the start of an artificial digit learning task for 20 min. Anodal tDCS (A-tDCS) was delivered over the right parietal lobe (red arrow), and cathodal tDCS (C-tDCS) was applied over the left parietal lobe (blue arrow). (B) Training continued after stimulation has stopped. Immediately after training, participants performed the numerical Stroop task (C) and the number-to-space task. (D) The time indicated next to each image shows the time elapsed from the beginning of the daily session until its termination in a cumulative style. *Figure adapted with permission from Cell Press.* (This figure is reproduced in color in the color plate section.)

Klein et al (2013) explored the specificity of bilateral bicephalic tDCS with two active electrodes of the same polarity (i.e., stimulation of homolog structures in both hemispheres with either A-tDCS or C-tDCS instead of the typical bicephalic tDCS with two active electrodes of different polarities) over the intraparietal sulci in a combined between- and within-task approach. They found that bilateral bi-cephalic tDCS modulated performance on a numerical task (mental addition) but not a control task (color word Stroop). This suggests that the effects of tDCS over bilateral intraparietal sulci are specific to numerical rather than domain-general cognitive processes linked to these areas. Specifically, the numerical effect of distractor distance was stronger under C-tDCS compared with A-tDCS. In terms of within-task specificity, only the numerical distractor distance effect, but not target identity, in the mental addition task was affected. This indicates that bilateral bicephalic tDCS influences the recruitment of different processing components (number magnitude processing versus recognition of familiarity) within the same task differently.

Compared to the field of language and tDCS, there is only a small number of studies of numerical cognition, even though it also presents many implications for education, rehabilitation, and the field of numerical cognition. There have been other studies on numerical cognition, but these have mainly used a different form of stimulation—transcranial random noise stimulation (Snowball et al., 2013). Considering that the frontoparietal network subserves numerical cognition, it would be interesting to investigate effects of stimulating the frontal regions involved in numerical processing, such as the dlPFC, to assess the contributions of the frontal network in different numerical processes (Nieder, 2009). Also, because there is a frontoparietal developmental shift in terms of basic numerical processing, tDCS could be a useful tool to test this hypothesis (Rivera et al., 2005).

Overall, there is a large body of research on the effects of tDCS on a range of cognitive functions in healthy adult populations (see the reviews by Coffman et al. (2014), Cohen Kadosh (2013), Krause and Cohen Kadosh (2013) and Kuo and Nitsche (2012)). The following section reviews the limited number of studies on the effects of tDCS on children and elderly populations, providing an overview of the effects of tDCS across ages.

EFFECTS OF tDCS IN DIFFERENT POPULATIONS

Studies of Children

To date, there have been very few studies of children. These have mostly explored tDCS in the context of psychiatric and neurological conditions in small population sizes (from 1 to 12) between the ages of 6–18 years old using doses of 0.65, 1, and 2 mA and ranging from a single session to 10 sessions, for up to 20 min per session.

Mattai et al. (2011) used a double-blind, sham-controlled design in children (aged 10–17 years) with childhood-onset schizophrenia to evaluate the tolerability of tDCS in a pediatric population. Twelve patients received either A-tDCS to the bilateral dlPFC ($n=8$, with an extracephalic cathode) to improve cognitive difficulties, or C-tDCS to the bilateral superior temporal gyrus ($n=4$, with an extracephalic anode) to reduce continued significant hallucinations. This study showed that tDCS at 2 mA, applied for 20 min for 10 sessions over a 2-week period, is easily tolerated, and none of the subjects withdrew because of tDCS effects. Similar to the adult population, there were reports of tingling (37.5%) and itching (50%) during real stimulation; these effects occurred in 20% and 40% of the sham group, respectively (5 of the subjects were randomly chosen to undergo sham stimulation (1 min of 2 mA) during weeks 2 and 3). There was no clinical/symptomatic decompensation or worsening of psychotic/cognitive symptoms. However, as the authors noted, such effects should be monitored on a longitudinal basis, considering the long-term effects of tDCS on cortical excitability.

Another study was published by Varga et al. (2011), who used a sham-controlled, crossover design (5 s of sham stimulation on day 1, and 20 min of 1-mA C-tDCS on day 2 for 20 min) in 5 patients, aged 6–11 years old, with focal epileptic disorder and continuous spikes and waves during slow sleep and at the area of epileptic focus before sleep (a condition marked by strong activation of epileptiform activity in the EEG during sleep, which is found in some encephalopathy syndromes). Although the stimulation did not reduce the spike index (percentage of epileptiform activity during slow-wave sleep), the authors reported that the spikes appeared more focal after C-tDCS in three of the five patients. No adverse effects or evoked seizures were reported, suggesting that tDCS is safe and partially effective in children with epilepsy.

In a case study of an 11-year-old epileptic patient, Yook et al. (2012) applied 2-mA C-tDCS over the epileptogenic zone (an anode over the left supraorbital region and a cathode over the right parietal temporal region) for 20 min for 5 sessions per week over 2 weeks. No adverse effects or evoked seizures were observed, but a decline in the frequency of seizures was reported in the post-treatment period. However, it is important to note that this study did not have a control group, which leaves alternative interpretations open.

Auvichayapat et al. (2013) used tDCS to treat refractory childhood focal epilepsy in children aged 6–15 years old. They applied 1 mA of current for 20 min on presumed epileptogenic regions, and an anode over the contralateral shoulder during a single session as a safety and preliminary efficacy study. They reported a significant decrease in the frequency of epileptiform discharges 24 and 48 h after active stimulation. A small reduction in seizure frequency was detected 4 weeks later. One adverse event was reported: a patient experienced a transient erythema on the shoulder.

In an open-label pilot study, Young et al. (2012) applied C-tDCS to the primary motor cortex to reduce involuntary overflow activity and to control muscle in children with dystonia. Although the outcome of interest was not significant, they found that some children responded to tDCS better than others.

Pinchuk et al. (2012) conducted a retrospective analysis of a comprehensive record of neuropsychological and EEG data from 128 children with learning disorders, 48 children with mild mental retardation who underwent tDCS treatment, 22 healthy children, and 42 children with psychic developmental disorders who had undergone conventional treatments (drug therapy and sessions with psychologists, logopedists, and ergotherapists) as controls. All children were between 8 and 12 years of age at the time of data acquisition. The tDCS treatments received by these children involved the application of 60–120 μA using relatively small stimulating electrodes (2.5–6.25 cm^2) between 25 and 45 min; different electrode positioning was used according to the clinical goals, age of the patient, and severity of the disorder. Each patient underwent 5–9 sessions over 4–5 weeks with 2- to 3-day intervals. Compared with control groups, children who underwent tDCS treatment showed significant improvement in higher mental functions (e.g., attention, memory, working capacity). They found that verbal functions were improved in 80% of children with such disorders, and that children with dysgraphia showed quicker writing and a threefold reduction in their writing mistakes. In addition, improved abilities in visuospatial analysis and synthesis were noted. Overall, no adverse effects or incidences of negative changes in EEG parameters were observed; instead, improvements in the EEG parameters toward the age norms were reported, suggesting that tDCS could be an effective correction technique for children with psychic developmental disorders.

Finally, in a recent computational study, Kessler et al. (2013) suggested that, on average, children are exposed to higher peak electrical fields compared with adults for a given applied current intensity. However, there is likely to be overlap between children and adults with smaller head size. They also highlighted that the amount of exposure is montage specific and that variations in peak electrical fields between individuals depend on neuroanatomical factors and the bioavailable (the sum of current in the brain/cortical area) current dose.

Together, these studies show that tDCS is generally well tolerated in pediatric populations, with few reports of discomfort at the sites of stimulation (e.g., Young et al., 2012). However, there currently are insufficient data to determine the physiological effects in the developing brain and the neurodevelopmental, physiological, and behavioral differences compared with adults. Moreover, it is important to be cautious with the dosage for the developing brain because there children have considerable anatomic differences in terms of head size and skull thickness compared with adults (Kessler et al., 2013). At this time, it is challenging to conduct studies involving pediatric populations because there is a general concern over the effects of tDCS on the developing brain and the lack of measures to monitor any potential side effects. However, it is important to consider that it could also be ethically questionable if such studies are hindered because it might deprive children who require such intervention (Cohen Kadosh et al., 2012).

Studies of the Elderly

Hummel et al. (2010) used a double-blind, crossover design to apply tDCS to the left primary motor cortex in a pseudo-randomized, counterbalanced order (real tDCS: 1 mA for 20 min; sham: 30 s) during two sessions separated by 5 days. The aim was to investigate whether A-tDCS can facilitate performance of right upper extremity tasks required for daily activities. They had 10 subjects between 56 and 87 years old. They found significant improvement in these functions with tDCS relative to sham; this improvement was more prominent among older subjects, suggesting that the effects of tDCS might be modulated by individual differences such as age. There were no reports of undesired side effects, similar to previous findings in younger subjects.

In another study, Floel et al. (2012) applied A-tDCS to the right tempo-roparietal cortex of 20 subjects aged 50–80 years old to modulate learning of object–position relations using an associative learning paradigm. They found that A-tDCS did not alter the learning rates during the task compared with participants in the sham condition, but improved recall performance was observed 1 week after learning in those who received A-tDCS but not sham stimulation. This study suggests that elderly individuals could be assisted to form lasting episodic memories with the aid of exogenous enhancement. Importantly, participants were unable to distinguish reliably whether they received real or sham stimulation.

Berryhill and Jones (2012) applied A-tDCS (1.5 mA for 10 min) or sham stimulation (20 s at the beginning and at the end) to elderly participants (56–80 years old) across 3 testing sessions on left (F3) and right (F4) dlPFC during verbal and visual 2-back WM tasks. They found that tDCS was beneficial across sites, but only among adults with higher education (mean years of education, 16.9). Those in the lower level of education group (mean years of education, 13.5) were generally impaired by tDCS in terms of WM performance; specifically, tDCS to the right prefrontal cortex impaired visual but had no effect verbal WM. It was suggested that the two groups might have used different strategies: the higher education group might have recruited the prefrontal cortex more effectively during WM relative to those in lower education group. This is consistent with previous studies that reported greater benefits of A-tDCS in improvement on recall of proper names among the elderly compared with younger adults (Ross et al., 2010b, 2011) and greater activations in the experts, but not novice, pilots when performing a track-following task (Peres et al., 2000).

In a more recent double-blind, placebo-controlled, randomized, crossover study, Eggert et al. (2013) investigated whether sleep-dependent memory consolidation can be improved, as previously shown in healthy volunteers (Marshall et al., 2006). They applied bifrontal A-tDCS to 26 elderly subjects (69.1 ± 7.7 years old) during early nonrapid eye movement sleep. They found no significant effect of tDCS on sleep-dependent memory consolidation. The authors concluded that, consistent with previous studies, offline consolidation during sleep is less pronounced in elderly compared with younger subjects, and that tDCS did not provide any beneficial effects on memory consolidation in elderly subjects (unlike in healthy adults).

Based on these studies, tDCS seems to be well tolerated, and there have been no reports of physical side effects in elderly individuals. However, further studies are required to examine the cognitive costs in this population, as reported by Berryhill and Jones (2012). Findings by Floel et al. (2012) and Berryhill and Jones (2012) highlight that factors such as age and educational background play a role in mediating the effects of tDCS, and should be taken into account when predicting the effects of tDCS or when considering it as cognitive enhancement in the future. Overall, more tDCS studies using elderly populations are required to fill the knowledge gap on the plasticity of the aging brain and the extent to which it can be modulated based on individual differences in biological profiles and life experiences. Successful cognitive enhancement for the elderly offers not only a higher quality of life at later stages of life, but also promises significant economical benefits at the societal and national levels.

OPTIMIZING THE EFFECTS OF tDCS FOR COGNITIVE ENHANCEMENT

Based on the studies described above, it is clear that there is no standard protocol or a linear dose–response in the use of tDCS for cognitive enhancement. Instead, the effects often depend on many factors that could be further optimized.

It seems that the effects of tDCS are affected by the intensity of the stimulation—for example, Iyer et al. (2005) showed that the effects of interest only emerged at 2 mA but not 1 mA stimulation (Boggio et al., 2006; Hoy et al., 2013), and with respect to duration of stimulation, Ohn et al. (2008) showed that performance on an n-back task was improved after 20 min tDCS and was further enhanced after 30 min of stimulation. Other factors that influence the effects of tDCS include whether they are interleaved or consecutive stimulations (Alonzo et al., 2012; Lin et al., 2011), the type of electrodes used (e.g., EEG electrodes (Marshall et al., 2004)), the distance between stimulation electrodes (e.g., increasing the distance between electrodes might decrease the magnitude of tDCS-induced effects, depending on the specific montage and physiological measure (Bikson et al., 2010; Moliadze et al., 2010)) or sponges (round versus rectangular shape), and the size of sponges (25–35 cm^2) and their arrangement (see Datta et al., 2009; Miranda et al., 2013; Park et al., 2011). The effects of tDCS could also be influenced by the timing of stimulation, that is, before, during, or after a task(s) (Javadi et al., 2012); whether it is applied in combination with pharmacological manipulations (Stagg, 2014) or with a task (Andrews et al., 2011) (which also depends on the type of task used); the sensitivity of measures before and after the stimulation (especially for healthy populations); and the best timing for the interstimulation interval to sustain the achieved enhancement results (Monte-Silva et al., 2010). Further research should work on establishing the optimal number of stimulation sessions for a particular training based on the desired effects, for example, longevity and strength of enhancement.

Some of the studies reviewed above also highlight the importance of considering the brain state of the individual who receives tDCS, such as the baseline state of brain oscillations and their existing brain connectivity. As mentioned earlier, differences in head size and skull thickness, as well as neuroanatomical differences beneath stimulated areas, also affect the distribution of current flow through the cortex (Kessler et al., 2013), raising the question of whether MRI neuronavigation is necessary. There is also an increasing number of studies that suggest that tDCS effects are modulated by age (Floel et al., 2012) and individual differences such as baseline abilities in certain tasks (Tseng et al., 2012), educational background (Berryhill and Jones, 2012), and even personality (Pena-Gomez et al., 2011). Given the observed relationship between brain and behavioral data, future studies could further use multimodal neuroimaging techniques to understand the underlying biochemistry of such interactions. tDCS-induced effects also differ between healthy and clinical populations depending on the intensity and site of stimulation (Boggio et al., 2006; Fregni et al., 2005; Floel et al., 2012; Suzuki et al., 2012). The differential effects of tDCS in clinical compared with healthy patients is thought to be attributable to the presence of dysfunctional synaptic homeostasis (Rodger et al., 2012; Turrigiano, 1999) and synaptic plasticity (Fertonani et al., 2011; Thickbroom and Mastaglia, 2009).

Studies of clinical populations also reveal that the effects of tDCS are affected by the severity of conditions, the presence of other comorbidities, and the time before onset and/or lesion sites of specific conditions such as stroke. For example, Jung et al. (2011) investigated the factors associated with better results when combining tDCS with speech therapy. They found that patients who received C-tDCS over the right IFG improved significantly in terms of the aphasia quotient. This was especially pronounced among those with less severe fluent aphasia who received treatment for fewer than 30 days after the development of stroke. Those with hemorrhagic stroke showed higher likelihood for improvement than those with ischemic stroke. Using logistic regression models, Kang et al. (2011) reported that those with more severe aphasia who were treated early following stroke onset showed the most improvement in naming accuracy under C-tDCS over Broca's homolog area and word retrieval training. Floel et al. (2012) found that A-tDCS to the right temporal-parietal cortex in parallel to 2 h of daily high-frequency anomia training showed significant improvement compared with sham, with more beneficial effects among those with more severe naming deficits.

Finally, it seems that the effects of tDCS might not always occur immediately after stimulation as typically measured by studies, or they might remain consistent during and after stimulation (Auvichayapat et al., 2013; Hoy et al., 2013). These effects could have contributed to the inconsistencies in the findings of replication studies. For example, Penolazzi et al. (2013) investigated the comparative effectiveness of different electrode arrangements (4 different active stimulation arrangements at 2 mA for 20 min and one sham condition) on language production immediately after stimulation (poststimulation test 1) and 18 min after poststimulation test 1. They found that none of the different electrode positions improved fluency immediately after stimulation. Only the left frontal A-tDCS improved fluency 18 min after tDCS, showing that the effects of tDCS might be detected only after a short time interval after stimulation ended. Similarly, the study of elderly participants by Floel et al. (2012), reviewed above, only reported significantly improved memory for object locations after a 1-week delay. These studies suggest that the enhancing effects of tDCS might surface over time, and follow-up measures might be needed to avoid losing important information on the temporal dynamics of tDCS effects.

OPEN QUESTIONS

As the understanding of the use and potential of tDCS continues to expand, so too does the number of unanswered questions. While we do not provide an exhaustive list here (for some open questions see Cohen Kadosh, 2014b), we review some of the important issues.

One of the immediate questions related to tDCS is the debate on the neuroethics of its usage, especially in child population. As discussed by Cohen Kadosh (2014b), stimulating the developing brain could be both a potential benefit as well as a liability. On one hand, one can argue that the developing brain is more plastic than the adult brain (Anderson et al., 2011; Gogtay et al., 2004), and hence tDCS could result in more potent effects. This is especially desirable for the remediation of cognitive abilities of those with atypical neurodevelopment. On the other hand, the greater plasticity of the developing brain could also promote substantial changes that could affect the balance between different brain regions and networks, which could result in impairment in trained and/or nontrained abilities. Considering such dilemmas, we do not recommend studies of children with typical development at this stage. In contrast, we highlight that studies of children with the desperate need to cope with, and eventually alleviate, the outcomes of detrimental atypical development are urgently required. This is of great importance because the negative effects of atypical development extend beyond children's everyday life into their future prospects and affect society as a whole. (To read more on ethical considerations, please refer to Chapter 13.)

In a broad sense, several factors should be taken into account when considering the cost-to-benefit ratio of cognitive enhancement using tDCS (for a detailed review see Levy and Savulescu (2014)). First and foremost, it is important to prioritize the safety of tDCS and the reversibility of its effects and to monitor for any potential side effects (physical or mental) that might arise in parallel to cognitive enhancement. For example, Iuculano and Cohen Kadosh (2013) found that tDCS over the PPC facilitated numerical learning, but automaticity of the learned material was impaired. In contrast, tDCS over the dlPFC impaired numerical learning but enhanced the automaticity of the learned material. This finding is important because it suggest the possibility of cognitive costs for cognitive enhancement in healthy populations and provokes the question of whether tDCS really enhances functions (Brem et al., 2014). Therefore, future studies should assess other cognitive functions besides the main outcome(s) of interest using sensitive tasks that are not time-consuming and cognitively exhausting to detect any unintended side effects. Ideally, follow-up examinations should be conducted to record both the longevity of the enhanced effects and potential side effects, especially after repeated usage. It is also crucial to further investigate whether any resulting side effects could be avoided without reducing the enhanced effects.

Next, it is important to assess the impact and importance of the effects generated by tDCS; in other words, how meaningful are the enhancing effects in messy, everyday settings compared to strictly controlled and methodologically sound experimental and clinical conditions? Although studies have reported significant improvements compared with sham conditions, such improvements are usually faster reaction times in the range of dozens of milliseconds and have been criticized as having restricted ecological validity (Pascual-Leone, 2012). Also, it would be useful to assess the extent to which the gains are generalizable beyond trained tasks to other untrained skills and/or abilities and how such gains differ and compare to other forms or cognitive enhancers such as pharmaceutical-based cognitive enhancement (Repantis et al., 2010), other forms of enhancements (Dresler, 2012), and basic health and nutrition (Lucke and Partridge, 2013). (For more details see Chapter 2.)

Last, it is crucial to consider the moral and social implications of brain stimulation (Brem et al., 2014; Chatterjee, 2004; Cohen Kadosh et al., 2012; Farah et al., 2004; Fox et al., 2005; Hamilton et al., 2011). For example, can cognitive enhancement be afforded only by the rich and/or further increase the function of those with higher baseline abilities, and hence increase existing cognitive inequalities? Is it acceptable to improve certain brain functions at the cost of others? Can we afford the responsibility for its impact on the individual and on society? Will it create pressure to provide cognitive enhancement in the workplace? Is it reasonable to provide cognitive enhancement even if the effects on an individual are predicted to be few? It is important to be aware and consider these questions to guide further inquiries and studies, especially when most studies of cognitive enhancement focus on the positive outcomes of specific functions, but often ignore discussion of the bioethical concerns, possible side effects, and long-term implications on society (Rossi et al., 2009). Considering that such important questions remain to unanswered, amateur use of tDCS by untrained individuals at home could be risky (Bikson et al., 2013; Cohen Kadosh et al., 2012) and we strongly recommend against such use at this stage. It is also important to consider the file-drawer effect (Rosenthal, 1979), where studies that did not find statistically significant effects on the function of interest are not published. Further studies assessing the longevity and the level of impact of brain stimulation on the physiology, cognition, psychology, and everyday performance given the costs invested are needed.

CONCLUSIONS

This chapter provided a comprehensive overview of the current state of the field of tDCS and cognitive enhancement, suggesting that tDCS has the capacity to alter behavioral and brain functions with the potential for further optimization, although the exact mechanisms of action on brain and behavior require further research and clarification. Overall, the use of tDCS for cognitive enhancement is certainly a new and exciting area worthy of further investigation, given its potential to positively impact both individuals and society.

ACKNOWLEDGMENTS

RCK is supported by the Wellcome Trust (WT88378) and filed a patent for an apparatus for improving and/or maintaining numerical ability. We thank Dr. Pedro Miranda for his views on the safety of tDCS and Michael Clayton for his helpful comments.

REFERENCES

Alonzo, A., Brassil, J., Taylor, J.L., Martin, D., Loo, C.K., 2012. Daily transcranial direct current stimulation (tDCS) leads to greater increases in cortical excitability than second daily transcranial direct current stimulation. Brain Stimul. 5 (3), 208–213.

Andrews, S.C., Hoy, K.E., Enticott, P.G., Daskalakis, Z.J., Fitzgerald, P.B., 2011. Improving working memory: the effect of combining cognitive activity and anodal transcranial direct current stimulation to the left dorsolateral prefrontal cortex. Brain Stimul. 4 (2), 84–89.

Antal, A., Nitsche, M.A., Kincses, T.Z., Kruse, W., Hoffmann, K.P., Paulus, W., 2004a. Facilitation of visuo-motor learning by transcranial direct current stimulation of the motor and extrastriate visual areas in humans. Eur. J. Neurosci. 19, 2888–2892.

Antal, A., Nitsche, M.A., Kruse, W., Kincses, T.Z., Hoffmann, K.P., Paulus, W., 2004b. Direct current stimulation over V5 enhances visuomotor coordination by improving motion perception in humans. J. Cogn. Neurosci. 16, 521–527.

Antal, A., Nitsche, M.A., Paulus, W., 2001. External modulation of visual perception in humans. Neuroreport 12 (3553).

Antal, A., Paulus, W., 2008. Transcranial direct current stimulation and visual perception. Perception 37, 367–374.

Anderson, V., Spencer-Smith, M., Wood, A., 2011. Do children really recover better? Neurobehavioural plasticity after early brain insult. Brain 134, 2197–2221.

Ardolino, G., Bossi, B., Barbieri, S., Priori, A., 2005. Non-synaptic mechanisms underlie the after-effects of cathodal transcutaneous direct current stimulation of the human brain. J. Physiol. 568, 653–663.

Auvichayapat, N., Rotenberg, A., Gersner, R., Ngodklang, S., Tiamkao, S., et al., 2013. Transcranial direct current stimulation for treatment of refractory childhood focal epilepsy. Brain Stimul. 6, 696–700.

Baker, J.M., Rorden, C., Fridriksson, J., 2010. Using transcranial direct-current stimulation to treat stroke patients with aphasia. Stroke 41, 1229–1236.

Berryhill, M.E., Jones, K.T., 2012. tDCS selectively improves working memory in older adults with more education. Neurosci. Lett. 521 (2), 148–151.

Berryhill, M.E., Wencil, E.B., Branch Coslett, H., Olson, I.R., 2010. A selective working memory impairment after transcranial direct current stimulation to the right parietal lobe. Neurosci. Lett. 479, 312–316.

Bhogal, S.K., Teasell, R., Speechley, M., 2003. Intensity of aphasia therapy, impact on recovery. Stroke 34, 987–993.

Bikson, M., Bestmann, S., Edwards, D., 2013. Neuroscience: transcranial devices are not playthings. Nature 501, 167.

Bikson, M., Datta, A., Rahman, A., Scaturro, J., 2010. Electrode montages for tDCS and weak transcranial electrical stimulation: role of "return" electrode's position and size. Clin. Neurophysiol. Off. J. Int. Fed. Clin. Neurophysiol. 121 (12), 1976.

Bikson, M., Inoue, M., Akiyama, H., Deans, J.K., Fox, J.E., Miyakawa, H., Jefferys, J.G., 2004. Effects of uniform extracellular DC electric fields on excitability in rat hippocampal slices in vitro. J. Physiol. 557, 175.

Bindman, J.L., Lippold, O.C.J., Redfearm, J.W.T., 1964. The action of brief polarizing currents on the cerebral cortex of the rat (1) during current flow and (2) in the production of long-lasting after-effects. J. Physiol. 172, 369–382.

Boggio, P.S., Ferrucci, R., Mameli, F., Martins, D., Martins, O., Vergari, M., Priori, A., 2012. Prolonged visual memory enhancement after direct current stimulation in Alzheimer's disease. Brain Stimul. 5 (3), 223–230.

Boggio, P.S., Ferrucci, R., Rigonatti, S.P., Covre, P., Nitsche, M.A., Pascual-Leone, A., Fregni, F., 2006. Effects of transcranial direct current stimulation on working memory in patients with Parkinson's disease. J. Neurol. Sci. 249, 31–38.

Boggio, P.S., Khoury, L.P., Martins, D.C.S., Martins, O.E.M.S., De Macedo, E., Fregni, F., 2009. Temporal cortex direct current stimulation enhances performance on a visual recognition memory task in Alzheimer disease. J. Neurol. Neurosurg. Psychiatry 80, 444.

Bolognini, N., Rossetti, A., Casati, C., Mancini, F., Vallar, G., 2011. Neuromodulation of multisensory perception: a tDCS study of the sound-induced flash illusion. Neuropsychologia 49 (2), 231–237.

Brem, A.K., Fried, P.J., Horvath, J.C., Robertson, E.M., Pascual-Leone, A., 2014. Is neuroenhancement by noninvasive brain stimulation a net zero-sum proposition? Neuroimage.

Castellanos, F.X., Sonuga-Barke, E.J., Milham, M.P., Tannock, R., 2006. Characterizing cognition in ADHD: beyond executive dysfunction. Trends Cogn. Sci. 10, 117–123.

Cattaneo, Z., Pisoni, A., Papagno, C., 2011. Transcranial direct current stimulation over Broca's region improves phonemic and semantic fluency in healthy individuals. Neuroscience 183, 64–70.

Chatterjee, A., 2004. Cosmetic neurology: the controversy over enhancing movement, mentation, and mood. Neurology 63, 968–974.

Clark, V.P., Coffman, B.A., Mayer, A.R., Weisend, M.P., Lane, T.D., Calhoun, V.D., Wassermann, E.M., 2012. TDCS guided using fMRI significantly accelerates learning to identify concealed objects. Neuroimage 59, 117–128.

Clark, V.P., Coffman, B.A., Trumbo, M.C., Gasparovic, C., 2011. Transcranial direct current stimulation (tDCS) produces localized and specific alterations in neurochemistry: a 1H magnetic resonance spectroscopy study. Neurosci. Lett. 500, 67–71.

Clemens, B., Jung, S., Zvyagintsev, M., Domahs, F., Willmes, K., 2013. Modulating arithmetic fact retrieval: A single-blind, sham-controlled tDCS study with repeated fMRI measurements. Neuropsychologia 51, 1279–1286.

Coffman, B.A., Clark, V.P., Parasuraman, R., 2014. Battery powered thought: enhancement of attention, learning and memory in healthy adults using transcranial direct current stimulation. NeuroImage 85 (2), 895–908.

Coffman, B.A., Trumbo, M.C., Clark, V.P., 2012. Enhancement of object detection with transcranial direct current stimulation is associated with increased attention. BMC Neurosci. 13 (1), 108.

Cohen Kadosh, R., 2013. Using transcranial electrical stimulation to enhance cognitive functions in the typical and atypical brain. Transl. Neurosci. 4 (1), 20–33.

Cohen Kadosh, R., 2014a. The Stimulated Brain. Elsevier, Amsterdam.

Cohen Kadosh, R., 2014b. The Future Usage and Challenges of Brain Stimulation. In: Cohen Kadosh, R. (Ed.), The Stimulated Brain. Elsevier, Amsterdam.

Cohen Kadosh, R., Levy, N., O'Shea, J., Shea, N., Savulescu, J., 2012. The neuroethics of non-invasive brain stimulation. Curr. Biol. 22 (4), R108–R111.

Cohen Kadosh, R., Soskic, S., Iuculano, T., Kanai, R., Walsh, V., 2010. Modulating neuronal activity produces specific and long lasting changes in numerical competence. Curr. Biol. 20, 2016–2020.

Creutzfeldt, O.D., Fromm, G.H., Kapp, H., 1962. Influence of transcortical dc currents on cortical neuronal activity. Exp. Neurol. 5 (6), 436–452.

Datta, A., Bansal, V., Diaz, J., Patel, J., Reato, D., Bikson, M., 2009. Gyri-precise head model of transcranial direct current stimulation: improved spatial focality using a ring electrode versus conventional rectangular pad. Brain Stimul. 2 (4), 201–207.

Dayan, E., Censor, N., Buch, E.R., Sandrini, M., Cohen, L.G., 2013. Noninvasive brain stimulation: from physiology to network dynamics and back. Nat. Neurosci. 16 (7), 838–844.

de Vries, M.H., Barth, A.C., Maiworm, S., et al., 2010. Electrical stimulation of Broca's area enhances implicit learning of an artificial grammar. J. Cogn. Neurosci. 22, 2427–2436.

Domahs, F., Lochy, A., Eibl, G., Delazer, M., 2004. Adding colour to multiplication: rehabilitation of arithmetic fact retrieval in a case of traumatic brain injury. Neuropsychol. Rehabil. 14, 303–328.

Dresler, M., Sandberg, A., Ohla, K., Bublitz, C., Trenado, C., Mroczko-Wasowicz, A., Kühn, S., Repantis, D., 2012. Non-pharmacological cognitive enhancement. Neuropharmacology 64, 529–543.

Eggert, T., Dorn, H., Sauter, C., Nitsche, M.A., Bajbouj, M., Danker-Hopfe, H., 2013. No effects of slow oscillatory transcranial direct current stimulation (tDCS) on sleep-dependent memory consolidation in healthy elderly subjects. Brain Stimul. 6 (6), 938–945.

Fan, J., McCandliss, B.D., Fossella, J., Flombaum, J.I., Posner, M.I., 2005. The activation of attentional networks. Neuroimage 26, 471–479.

Farah, M.J., Illes, J., Cook-Deegan, R., Gardner, H., Kandel, E., King, P., Wolpe, P.R., 2004. Neurocognitive enhancement: what can we do and what should we do? Nat. Rev. Neurosci. 5, 421–425.

Ferrucci, R., Brunoni, A.R., Parazzini, M., Vergari, M., Rossi, E., Fumagalli, M., et al., 2013. Modulating human procedural learning by cerebellar transcranial direct current stimulation. Cerebellum 12 (4), 485–492.

Ferrucci, R., Marceglia, S., Vergari, M., Cogiamanian, F., Mrakic-Sposta, S., Mameli, F., Priori, A., 2008. Cerebellar transcranial direct current stimulation impairs the practice-dependent proficiency increase in working memory. J. Cogn. Neurosci. 20, 1687–1697.

Ferrucci, R., Priori, A., 2013. Transcranial cerebellar direct current stimulation (tcDCS): motor control, cognition, learning and emotions. Neuroimage 85 (3), 918–923.

Fertonani, A., Pirulli, C., Miniussi, C., 2011. Random noise stimulation improves neuroplasticity in perceptual learning. J. Neurosci. 31, 15416–15423.

Fertonani, A., Rosini, S., Cotelli, M., et al., 2010. Naming facilitation induced by transcranial direct current stimulation. Behav. Brain Res. 208, 311–318.

Fiori, V., Cipollari, S., Caltagirone, C., Marangolo, P., 2014. "If two witches would watch two watches, which witch would watch which watch?" tDCS over the left frontal region modulates tongue twister repetition in healthy subjects. Neuroscience 256, 195–200.

Fiori, V., Coccia, M., Marinelli, C.V., et al., 2011. Transcranial direct current stimulation improves word retrieval in healthy and nonfluent aphasic subjects. J. Cogn. Neurosci. 23, 2309–2323.

Floel, A., 2013. tDCS-enhanced motor and cognitive function in neurological diseases. NeuroImage. Article in press.

Floel, A., Rosser, N., Michka, O., Knecht, S., Breitenstein, C., 2008. Noninvasive brain stimulation improves language learning. J. Cogn. Neurosci. 20, 1415–1422.

Floel, A., Suttorp, W., Kohl, O., Ku¨rten, J., Lohmann, H., Breitenstein, C., Knecht, S., 2012. Noninvasive brain stimulation improves object-location learning in the elderly. Neurobiol. Aging 33 (8), 1682–1689.

Fox, M.D., Snyder, A.Z., Vincent, J.L., Corbetta, M., Van Essen, D.C., Raichle, M.E., 2005. The human brain is intrinsically organized into dynamic, anticorrelated functional networks. Proc. Natl. Acad. Sci. U. S. A. 102, 9673–9678.

Fregni, F., Boggio, P.S., Nitsche, M.A., Bermpohl, F., Antal, A., Feredoes, E., Pascual-Leone, A., 2005. Anodal transcranial direct current stimulation of prefrontal cortex enhances working memory. Exp. Brain Res. 166 (1), 23–30.

Flöel, A., Meinzer, M., Kirstein, R., Nijhof, S., Deppe, M., Knecht, S., Breitenstein, C., 2011. Short-term anomia training and electrical brain stimulation. Stroke 42, 2065–2067.

Fritsch, B., Reis, J., Martinowich, K., Schambra, H.M., Ji, Y., Cohen, L.G., 2010. Direct current stimulation promotes BDNF-dependent synaptic plasticity: potential implications for motor learning. Neuron 66, 198–204.

Gall, C., Antal, A., Sabel, B.A., 2012. Non-invasive electrical brain stimulation induces vision restoration in patients with visual pathway damage. Graefes Arch. Clin. Exp. Ophthalmol.

Gartside, I.B., 1968a. Mechanisms of sustained increases of firing rate of neurones in the rat cerebral cortex after polarization: reverberating circuits or modification of synaptic conductance? Nature 220, 382–383.

Gartside, I.B., 1968b. Mechanisms of sustained increases of firing rate of neurones in the rat cerebral cortex after polarization: role of protein synthesis. Nature 220, 383–384.

Grabner, R.H., Ansari, D., Koschutnig, K., Reishofer, G., Ebner, F., Neuper, C., 2009. To retrieve or to calculate? Left angular gyrus mediates the retrieval of arithmetic facts during problem solving. Neuropsychologia 47 (2), 604–608.

Gogtay, N., Giedd, J.N., Lusk, L., Hayashi, K.M., Greenstein, D., Vaituzis, C.A., Nugent, T.F., Herman, D.H., Clasen, L.S., Toga, A.W., et al., 2004. Dynamic mapping of human cortical development during childhood through early adulthood. Proc. Natl. Acad. Sci. U. S. A. 101, 8174–8179.

Hamilton, R., Messing, S., Chatterjee, A., 2011. Rethinking the thinking cap: ethics of neural enhancement using noninvasive brain stimulation. Neurology 76, 187–193.

Hammer, A., Mohammadi, B., Schmicker, M., Saliger, S., Munte, T., 2011. Errorless and errorful learning modulated by transcranial direct current stimulation. BMC Neurosci. 12, 72.

Hauser, T.U., Rotzer, S., Grabner, R.H., Merillat, S., Janke, L., 2013. Enhancing performance in numerical magnitude processing and mental arithmetic using transcranial direct current stimulation (tDCS). Front. Neurosci. 7 (224), 1–9.

Hesse, S., Waldner, A., Mehrholz, J., Tomerlleri, C., Pohl, M., Werner, C., 2011. Combined transcranial direct current stimulation and robot-assisted arm training in subacute stroke patients: an exploratory, randomized multicenter trial. Neurorehabil. Neural Repair.

Holland, R., Leff, A.P., Josephs, O., et al., 2011. Speech facilitation by left inferior frontal cortex stimulation. Curr. Biol. 21, 1403–1407.

Hoy, K.E., Emonson, M.R.L., Arnold, S.L., Thomson, R.H., Daskalakis, Z.J., Fitzgerald, P.B., 2013. Testing the limits: investigating the effect of tDCS dose on working memory enhancement in healthy controls. Neuropsychologia 51, 1777–1784.

Hummel, F.C., Heise, K., Celnik, P., Floel, A., Gerloff, C., Cohen, L.G., 2010. Facilitating skilled right hand motor function in older subjects by anodal polarization over the left primary motor cortex. Neurobiol. Aging 31 (12), 2160–2168.

Hunter, M., Coffman, B.A., Trumbo, M., Clark, V., 2013. Tracking the neuroplastic changes associated with transcranial direct current stimulation: a push for multimodal imaging. Front. Hum. Neurosci.

ICNIRP, 2010. ICNIRP guidelines for limiting exposure to time-Varying electric and magnetic Fields (1Hz-100kHz). Health Phys. 99 (6), 818–836.

Islam, N., Aftabuddin, M., Moriwaki, A., Hattori, Y., Hori, Y., 1995. Increase in the calcium level following anodal polarization in the rat brain. Brain Res. 684, 206–208.

Iuculano, T., Cohen Kadosh, R., 2013. The mental cost of cognitive enhancement. J. Neurosci. 33 (10), 4482–4486.

Iyer, M.B., Mattu, U., Grafman, J., Lomarev, M., Sato, S., Wassermann, E.M., 2005. Safety and cognitive effect of frontal DC brain polarization in healthy individuals. Neurology 64, 872–875.

Jacobson, L., Goren, N., Lavidor, M., Levy, D.A., 2012. Oppositional transcranial direct current stimulation (tDCS) of parietal substrates of attention during encoding modulates episodic memory. Brain Res. 1439, 66–72.

Jausovec, N., Jausovec, K., 2012. Working memory training: Improving intelligence—Changing brain activity. Brain Cogn. 79, 96–106.

Javadi, A.H., Cheng, P., Walsh, V., 2012. Short duration transcranial direct current stimulation (tDCS) modulates verbal memory. Brain Stimul. 5 (4), 468–474.

Javadi, A.H., Walsh, V., 2011. Transcranial direct current stimulation (tDCS) of the left dorsolateral prefrontal cortex modulates declarative memory. Brain Stimul. Article in press.

Jaeggi, S.M., Buschkuehl, M., Jonides, J., Perrig, W.J., 2008. Improving fluid intelligence with training on working memory. Proc. Natl. Acad. Sci. 105, 6829–6833.

Jo, J.M., Kim, Y.H., Ko, M.H., Ohn, S.H., Joen, B., Lee, K.H., 2009. Enhancing the working memory of stroke patients using tDCS. Am. J. Phys. Med. Rehabil. 88, 404.

Jung, I.Y., Lim, J.Y., Kang, E.K., et al., 2011. The factors associated with good responses to speech therapy combined with transcranial direct current stimulation in post-stroke aphasic patients. Ann. Rehabil. Med. 35, 460–469.

Kang, E.K., Baek, M.J., Kim, S., Paik, N.J., 2009. Non-invasive cortical stimulation improves post-stroke attention decline. Restor. Neurol. Neurosci. 27, 645–650.

Kang, E.K., Kim, Y.K., Sohn, H.M., et al., 2011. Improved picture naming in aphasia patients treated with cathodal tDCS to inhibit the right Broca's homologue area. Restor Neurol. Neurosci. 29, 141–152.

Klein, E., Mann, A., Huber, S., Bloechle, J., Willmes, K., Karim, A.A., Nuerk, H.C., Moeller, K., 2013. Bilateral bi-cephalic tdcs with two active electrodes of the same polarity modulates bilateral cognitive processes differentially. PLoS One 8. e71607.

Keeser, D., Meindl, T., Bor, J., Palm, U., Pogarell, O., Mulert, C., Padberg, F., 2011. Prefrontal transcranial direct current stimulation changes connectivity of resting-state networks during fMRI. J. Neurosci. 31, 15284–15293.

Kessler, S.K., Minhas, P., Woods, A.J., Rosen, A., Gorman, C., Bikson, M., 2013. Dosage considerations for transcranial direct current stimulation in children: a computational modeling study. PLoS One.

Klimesch, W., 1999. EEG alpha and theta oscillations reflect cognitive and memory performance: a review and analysis. Brain Res. Brain Res. Rev. 29, 169–195.

Ko, M.H., Han, S.H., Park, S.H., Seo, J.H., Kim, Y.H., 2008. Improvement of visual scanning after DC brain polarization of parietal cortex in stroke patients with spatial neglect. Neurosci. Lett. 448, 171–174.

Korsakov, I.A., Matveeva, L.V., 1982. Psychophysical characteristics of perception and of brain electrical activity during occipital micropolarization. Hum. Physiol. 8, 259–266.

Krause, B., Cohen Kadosh, R., 2013. Can transcranial electrical stimulation improve learning difficulties in atypical brain development? A future possibility for cognitive training. Dev. Cogn. Neurosci.

Krause, B., Looi, C.Y., Cohen Kadosh, R., 2014. Transcranial Electrical Stimulation to Enhance Cognitive Abilities in the Atypically Developing Brain. In: Cohen Kadosh, R., Dowker, A. (Eds.), The Handbook of Numerical Cognition. Oxford: Oxford University Press.

Krause, B., Márquez-Ruiz, J., Cohen Kadosh, R., 2013. The effect of transcranial direct current stimulation: a role for cortical excitation/inhibition balance? Front. Hum. Neurosci. 7, 602.

Krause, C.M., Sillanmaki, L., Koivisto, M., Saarela, C., Haggqvist, A., Laine, M., 2000. The effects of memory load on event-related EEG desynchronization and synchronization. Clin. Neurophysiol. 111, 2071–2078.

Kuo, M.-F., Nitsche, M.A., 2012. Effects of transcranial electrical stimulation on cognition. Clin. EEG. Neurosci. 43, 192–199.

Levy, N., Savulescu, J., 2014. The Neuroethics of Transcranial Electrical Stimulation. In: Cohen Kadosh, R. (Ed.), The Stimulated Brain. Elsevier, Amsterdam.

Liebetanz, D., Koch, R., Mayenfels, S., König, F., Paulus, W., Nitsche, M.A., 2009. Safety limits of cathodal transcranial direct current stimulation in rats. Clin. Neurophysiol. 120 (6), 1161–1167.

Liebetanz, D., Nitsche, M.A., Tergau, F., Paulus, W., 2002. Pharmacological approach to the mechanisms of transcranial DC-stimulation-induced after effects of human motor cortex excitability. Brain 125, 2238–2247.

Lin, C.H.J., Knowlton, B.J., Chiang, M.C., Iacoboni, M., Udompholkul, P., Wu, A.D., 2011. Brain–behavior correlates of optimizing learning through interleaved practice. Neuroimage 56 (3), 1758–1772.

Lindenberg, R., Nachtigall, L., Meinzer, M., Sieg, M.M., Flo"el, A., 2013. Differential effects of dual and unihemispheric motor cortex stimulation in older adults. J. Neurosci. 21, 9176–9183.

Lindenberg, R., Renga, V., Zhu, L.L., Nair, D., Schlaug, G., 2010. Bihemispheric brain stimulation facilitates motor recovery in chronic stroke patients. Neurology (75), 2176–2184.

Lucke, J., Partridge, B., 2013. Towards a smart population: a public health framework for cognitive enhancement. Neuroethics 6, 419–427.

Marangolo, P., Marinelli, C.V., Bonifazi, S., et al., 2011. Electrical stimulation over the left inferior frontal gyrus (IFG) determines long-term effects in the recovery of speech apraxia in three chronic aphasics. Behav. Brain Res. 225, 498–504.

Marshall, L., Helgadottir, H., Mo"lle, M., Born, J., 2006. Boosting slow oscillations during sleep potentiates memory. Nature 444 (7119), 610–e613.

Marshall, L., Molle, M., Hallschmid, M., Born, J., 2004. Transcranial direct current stimula- tion during sleep improves declarative memory. J. Neurosci. 24, 9985.

Marshall, L., Mo"lle, M., Siebner, H., Born, J., 2005. Bifrontal transcranial direct current stimulation slows reaction time in a working memory task. BMC Neurosci. 6 (1), 23.

Mattai, A., Miller, R., Weisinger, B., Greenstein, D., Bakalar, J., et al., 2011. Tolerability of transcranial direct current stimulation in childhood-onset schizophrenia. Brain Stimul. 4, 275–280.

Meinzer, M., Jahnigen, S., Copland, D.A., Darkow, R., Grittner, U., Avirame, K., Floel, A., 2013. Transcranial direct current stimulation over multiple days improves learning and maintenance of a novel vocabulary. Cortex 33 (30), 12470–12478.

Meiron, O., Lavidor, M., 2013. Prefrontal oscillatory stimulation modulates access to cognitive control references in retrospective metacognitive commentary. Clin. Neurophysiol. 125 (1), 77–82.

Merzagora, A.C., Foffani, G., Panyavin, I., Mordillo-Mateos, L., Aguilar, J., Onaral, B., Levy, D., 2010. Prefrontal hemodynamic changes produced by anodal direct current stimulation. Neuroimage 49, 2304–2310.

Medeiros, L.F., de Souza, I.C.C., Vidor, L.P., de Souza, A., Deitos, A., Volz, M.S., Fregni, F., Caumo, W., Torres, I.L., 2012. Neurobiological effects of transcranial direct current stimulation: a review. Front. Psychiatry 3, 1–11.

Miranda, P.C., Mekonnen, A., Salvador, R., Ruffini, G., 2013. The electric field in the cortex during transcranial current stimulation. Neuroimage 70, 48–58.

Moliadze, V., Antal, A., Paulus, W., 2010. Electrode-distance dependent after-effects of transcranial direct and random noise stimulation with extracephalic reference electrodes. Clin. Neurophysiol. 121 (12), 2165–2171.

Monte-Silva, K., Kuo, M.F., Liebetanz, D., Paulus, W., Nitsche, M.A., 2010. Shaping the optimal repetition interval for cathodal transcranial direct current stimulation (tDCS). J. Neurophysiol. 103 (4), 1735–1740.

Monti, A., Ferrucci, R., Fumagalli, M., Mameli, F., Cogiamanian, F., Ardolino, G., Priori, A., 2012. Transcranial direct current stimulation (tDCS) and language. J. Neurol. Neurosurg. Psychiatry 84, 832–842.

Nelson, J.T., McKinley, R.A., Golob, E.J., Warm, J.S., Parasuraman, R., 2014. Enhancing vigilance in operators with prefrontal cortex transcranial direct current stimulation (tDCS). Neuroimage 85, 911–919.

Nieder, A., 2009. Prefrontal cortex and the evolution of symbolic reference. Curr. Opin. Neurobiol. 19, 99–108.

Nitsche, M.A., Boggio, P.S., Fregni, F., Pascual-Leone, A., 2009. Treatment of depression with transcranial direct current stimulation (tDCS):a review. Exp. Neurol. 1 (219), 14–19.

Nitsche, M.A., Cohen, L.G., Wassermann, E.M., Priori, A., Lang, N., Antal, A., Pascual-Leone, A., 2008. Transcranial direct current stimulation: state of the art 2008. Brain Stimul. 1, 206–223.

Nitsche, M.A., Fricke, K., Henschke, U., Schlitterlau, A., Liebetanz, D., Lang, N., Paulus, W., 2003b. Pharmacological modulation of cortical excitability shifts induced by transcranial DC stimulation. J. Physiol. 553, 293–301.

Nitsche, M.A., Lampe, C., Antal, A., Liebetanz, D., Lang, N., Tergau, F., Paulus, W., 2006. Dopaminergic modulation of long-lasting direct current-induced cortical excitability changes in the human motor cortex. Eur. J. Neurosci. 23, 1651–1657.

Nitsche, M.A., Liebetanz, D., Lang, N., Antal, A., Tergau, F., Paulus, W., 2003c. Safety criteria for transcranial direct current stimulation (tDCS) in humans. Clin. Neurophysiol. 114, 2220–2222.

Nitsche, M.A., Schauenburg, A., Lang, N., Liebetanz, D., Exner, C., Paulus, W., Tergau, F., 2003d. Facilitation of implicit motor learning by weak transcranial direct current stimulation of the primary motor cortex in the human. J. Cogn. Neurosci. 15, 619–626.

Nitsche, M.A., Niehaus, L., Hoffmann, K.T., Hengst, S., Liebetanz, D., Paulus, W., Meyer, B.-U., 2004. MRI study of human brain exposed to weak direct current stimulation of the frontal cortex. Clin. Neurophysiol. 115, 2419–2423.

Nitsche, M.A., Nitsche, M.S., Klein, C.C., Tergau, F., Rothwell, J.C., Paulus, W., Walsh, V., 2003a. Level of action of cathodal DC polarisation induced inhibition of the human motor cortex. Clin. Neurophysiol. 114, 600–604.

Nitsche, M.A., Paulus, W., 2000. Excitability changes induced in the human motor cortex by weak transcranial direct current stimulation. J. Physiol. Lond. 527 (3), 633–639.

Nitsche, M.A., Seeber, A., Frommann, K., et al., 2005. Modulating parameters of excitability during and after transcranial direct current stimulation of the human motor cortex. J. Physiol. 568, 291–303.

O'Halloran, C.J., Kinsella, G.J., Storey, E., 2012. The cerebellum and neuropsychological functioning: a critical review. J. Clin. Exp. Neuropsychol. 34 (1), 35–56.

Ohn, S.H., Park, C.I., Yoo, W.K., Ko, M.H., Choi, K.P., Kim, G.M., Kim, Y.H., 2008. Time-dependent effect of transcranial direct current stimulation on the enhancement of working memory. Neuroreport 19, 43.

Olma, M.C., Kraft, A., Roehmel, J., Irlbacher, K., Brandt, S.A., 2011. Excitability changes in the visual cortex quantified with signal detection analysis. Restor Neurol. Neurosci. 29, 457–466.

Parasuraman, R., 1998. The Attentive Brain. MIT Press, Cambridge, MA.

Parasuraman, R., 2011. Neuroergonomics: brain, cognition, and performance at work. Curr. Dir. Psychol. Sci. 20, 181–186.

Parasuraman, R., Christensen, J., Grafton, S., 2012. Neuroergonomics: the brain in action and at work. Neuroimage 59, 1–3.

Park, J.H., Hong, S.B., Kim, D.W., Suh, M., Im, C.H., 2011. A novel array-type transcranial direct current stimulation (tDCS) system for accurate focusing on targeted brain areas. Magn. IEEE Trans. 47 (5), 882–885.

Pascual-Leone, A., Horvath, J.C., Robertson, E.M., 2012. Enhancement of normal cognitive abilities through noninvasive brain stimulation. In: Rothwell, R.C.J.C. (Ed.), Cortical Connectivity. Springer-Verlag, Berlin, pp. 207–249.

Pena-Gomez, C., Vidal-Piñeiro, D., Clemente, I.C., Pascual-Leone, A., Bartrés-Faz, D., 2011. Down-regulation of negative emotional processing by transcranial direct current stimulation: effects of personality characteristics. PLoS One 6 (7), e22812.

Penolazzi, B., Pastore, M., Mondini, S., 2013. Electrode montage dependent effects of transcranial direct current stimulation on semantic fluency. Behav. Brain Res.

Peres, M., Van de Moortele, P.F., Pierard, C., Lehericy, S., Satabin, P., Le Bihan, D., Guezennec, C.Y., 2000. Functional magnetic resonance imaging of mental strategy in a simulated aviation performance task. Aviat. Space Environ. Med. 71 (12), 1218–1231.

Peters, M.A., Thompson, B., Merabet, L.B., Wu, A.D., Shams, L., 2013. Anodal tDCS to V1 blocks visual perceptual learning consolidation. Neuropsychologia 51, 1234–1239.

Pinchuk, D., Vasserman, M., Sirbiladze, K., Pinchuk, O., 2012. Changes of electrophysiological parameters and neuropsychological characteristics in children with psychic development disorders after transcranial direct current stimulation (tDCS). Polish Ann. Med. 19, 9–14.

Plow, E.B., Obretenova, S.N., Fregni, F., Pascual-Leone, A., Merabet, L.B., 2012. Comparison of visual field training for hemianopia with active versus sham transcranial direct cortical stimulation. Neurorehabil. Neural Repair. 26 (6), 616–626.

Plow, E.B., Obretenova, S.N., Halko, M.A., Kenkel, S., Jackson, M.L., Pascual-Leone, A., Merabet, L.B., 2011. Combining visual rehabilitative training and noninvasive brain stimulation to enhance visual function in patients with hemianopia: a comparative case study. PM R 3, 825–835.

Polania, R., Nitsche, M.A., Paulus, W., 2011b. Modulating functional connectivity patterns and topological functional organization of the human brain with transcranial direct current stimulation. Hum. Brain Mapp. 32, 1236–1249.

Polania, R., Paulus, W., Antal, A., Nitsche, M.A., 2011a. Introducing graph theory to track for neuroplastic alterations in the resting human brain: a transcranial direct current stimulation study. Neuroimage 54, 2287–2296.

Polania, R., Paulus, W., Nitsche, M.A., 2012. Modulating cortico-striatal and thalamo-cortical functional connectivity with transcranial direct current stimulation. Hum. Brain Mapp. 33, 2499–2508.

Poreisz, C., Boros, K., Antal, A., Paulus, W., 2007. Safety aspects of transcranial direct current stimulation concerning healthy subjects and patients. Brain Res. Bull. 72, 208–214.

Posner, M.I., Petersen, S.E., 1990. The attention system of the human brain. Annu. Rev. Neurosci. 13, 25–42.

Radman, T., Datta, A., Ramos, R.L., Brumberg, J.C., Bikson, M., 2009. One-dimensional representation of a neuron in a uniform electric field. Eng. Med. Biol. Soc. EMBC 2009 Annu. Int. Conf. IEEE, 6481–6484.

Raghubar, Kimberly P., Barnes, Marcia A., Hecht, Steven A., 2010. Working memory and mathematics: a review of developmental, individual difference, and cognitive approaches. Learn. Individ. Differ. 20 (2), 110–122.

Reis, J., Schambra, H.M., Cohen, L.G., Buch, E.R., Fritsch, B., Zarahn, E., et al., 2009. Noninvasive cortical stimulation enhances motor skill acquisition over multiple days through an effect on consolidation. Proc. Natl. Acad. Sci. U. S. A. 106, 1590–1595.

Repantis, D., Schlattmann, P., Laisney, O., Heuser, I., 2010. Modafinil and methylphenidate for neuroenhancement in healthy individuals: a systematic review. Pharmacol. Res. 62, 187–206.

Rivera, S.M., Reiss, A.L., Eckert, M.A., Menon, V., 2005. Developmental changes in mental arithmetic: evidence for increased functional specialization in the left inferior parietal cortex. Cereb. Cortex 25, 1779–1790.

Roche, N., Lackmy, A., Achache, V., Bussel, B., Katz, R., 2011. Effects of anodal tDCS on lum- bar propriospinal system in healthy subjects. Clin. Neurophysiol. 589, 2813–2826.

Rodger, J., Mo, C., Wilks, T., Dunlop, S.A., Sherrard, R.M., 2012. Transcranial pulsed magnetic field stimulation facilitates reorganization of abnormal neural circuits and corrects behavioral deficits without disrupting normal connectivity. FASEB (26), 1596–1606.

Rosenthal, R., 1979. The file drawer problem and tolerance for null results. Psychol. Bull. 86, 638–641.

Ross, L.A., McCoy, D., Wolk, D.A., et al., 2010a. Improved proper name recall by electrical stimulation of the anterior temporal lobes. Neuropsychologia 48, 3671–3674.

Ross, L.A., McCoy, D., Wolk, D.A., Coslett, H.B., Olson, I.R., 2010b. Improved proper name recall by electrical stimulation of the anterior temporal lobes. Neuropsychologia 48, 3671–3674.

Ross, L.A., McCoy, D., Wolk, D.A., Coslett, H.B., Olson, I.R., 2011. Improved proper name recall in aging after electrical stimulation of the anterior temporal lobes. Front. Aging Neurosci. 3.

Rossi, S., Hallett, M., Rossini, P.M., Pascual-Leone, A., 2009. Safety, ethical considerations, and application guidelines for the use of transcranial magnetic stimulation in clinical practice and research. Clin. Neurophysiol. 120, 2008–2039.

Rothwell, J., 2013. Variability of the response to brain stimulation plasticity protocols: a concealed problem. Clin. Neurophysiol. 124 (10), e44.

Ruohonen, J., Karhu, J., 2012. tDCS possibly stimulates glial cells. Clin. Neurophysiol. 123, 2006–2009.

Schermer, M., 2008. On the argument that enhancement is "cheating". J. Med. Ethics 34, 85–88.

Seitz, A., Watanabe, T., 2005. A unified model for perceptual learning. Trends Cogn. Sci. 9, 329–334.

Snowball, A., Tachtsidis, I., Popescu, T., Thompson, J., Delazer, M., Zamarian, L., Cohen Kadosh, R., 2013. Long-term enhancement of brain function and cognition using cognitive training and brain stimulation. Curr. Biol. 23 (11), 987–992.

Sparing, R., Dafotakis, M., Meister, I.G., et al., 2008. Enhancing language performance with non-invasive brain stimulation—a transcranial direct current stimulation study in healthy humans. Neuropsychologia 46, 261–268.

Sparing, R., Thimm, M., Hesse, M.D., Kust, J., Karbe, H., Fink, G.R., 2009. Bidirectional al- terations of interhemispheric parietal balance by non-invasive cortical stimulation. Brain 132, 3011–3020.

Squire, L.R., 1982. The neuropsychology of human memory. Annu. Rev. Neurosci. 5 (1), 241–273.

Stagg, C.J., 2014. The Physiological Basis of Brain Stimulation. In: Cohen Kadosh, R. (Ed.), The Stimulated Brain. Elsevier, Amsterdam.

Stagg, C.J., Bachtiar, V., Johansen-Berg, H., 2011. The role of GABA in human motor learning. Curr. Biol. 21, 480–484.

Stagg, C.J., Lin, R.L., Mezue, M., Segerdahl, A., Kong, Y., Xie, J., Tracey, I., 2013. Widespread modulation of cerebral perfusion induced during and after transcranial direct current stimulation applied to the left dorsolateral prefrontal cortex. J. Neurosci. 33, 11425–11431.

Sturm, W., Willmes, K., 2001. On the functional neuroanatomy of intrinsic and phasic alertness. Neuroimage 14, S76–S84.

Suzuki, K., Fujiwara, T., Tanaka, N., Tsuji, T., Masakado, Y., Hase, K., Liu, M., 2012. Comparison of the after-effects of transcranial direct current stimulation over the motor cortex in patients with stroke and healthy volunteers. Int. J. Neurosci. 122 (11), 675–681.

The Royal Society, 2011. Neuroscience: implications for education and lifelong learning. Brain Waves Module 2 (London).

Thickbroom, G., Mastaglia, F., 2009. Plasticity in neurological disorders and challenges for non-invasive brain stimulation. J. NeuroEng. Rehabil. 6 (4).

Tseng, P., Hsu, T.Y., Chang, C.F., Tzeng, O.J., Hung, D.L., Muggleton, N.G., Juan, C.H., 2012. Unleashing potential: transcranial direct current stimulation over the right posterior parietal cortex improves change detection in low-performing individuals. J. Neurosci. 32 (31), 10554–10561.

Turrigiano, G., 1999. Homeostatic plasticity in neuronal networks: the more things change the more they stay the same. Trends Neurosci. 22, 221–227.

Varga, E.T., Terney, D., Atkins, M.D., Nikanorova, M., Jeppesen, D.S., et al., 2011. Transcranial direct current stimulation in refractory continuous spikes and waves during slow sleep: a controlled study. Epilepsy Res. 97, 142–145.

Vicario, C.M., Nitsche, M.A., 2013. Transcranial direct current stimulation: a remediation tool for the treatment of childhood congenital dyslexia? Front. Hum. Neurosci. 7, 139.

Vines, B.W., Norton, A.C., Schlaug, G., 2011. Non-invasive brain stimulation enhances the effects of melodic intonation therapy. Front. Psychol. 2, 230.

Wirth, M., Rahman, R.A., Kuenecke, J., et al., 2011. Effects of transcranial direct current stimulation (tDCS) on behaviour and electrophysiology of language production. Neuropsychologia 49, 3989–3998.

Wlodkowski, R.J., 2003. Accelerated learning in colleges and universities. New Dir. Adult Contin. Educ. 97, 5–16.

Yook, S.W., Park, S.H., Seo, J.H., Kim, S.J., Ko, M.H., 2012. Suppression of seizure by cathodal transcranial direct current stimulation in an epileptic patient – a case report. Ann. Rehabil. Med. 35, 579–582.

You, D.S., Kim, D.Y., Chun, M.H., Jung, S.E., Park, S.J., 2011. Cathodal transcranial direct current stimulation of the right Wernicke's area improves comprehension in subacute stroke patients. Brain Lang. 119, 1–5.

Young, S.J., Bertucco, M., Sheehan-Stross, R., Sanger, T.D., 2012. Cathodal transcranial direct current stimulation in children with dystonia a pilot open-label trial. J. Child Neurol.

Zaehle, T., Sandmann, P., Thorne, J.D., Jancke, L., Herrmann, C.S., 2011. Transcranial direct current stimulation of the prefrontal cortex modulates working memory performance: combined behavioural and electrophysiological evidence. BMC Neurosci. 12 (1), 2.

Zaunmuller, L., Domahs, F., Dressel, K., Lonnemann, J., Klein, E., Ischebeck, A., Willmes, K., 2009. Rehabilitation of arithmetic fact retrieval via extensive practice: a combined fMRI and behavioural case-study. Neuropsychol. Rehabil. 19 (3), 422–443.

Chapter 13

Cognitive Enhancement: Ethical Considerations and a Look into the Future

Veljko Dubljević[1,2,3]
[1]*Neuroethics Research Unit, Institut de Recherches Cliniques de Montréal (IRCM), Montréal, QC, Canada;* [2]*Department of Neurology and Neurosurgery, McGill University, Montréal, QC, Canada;* [3]*International Centre for Ethics in the Sciences and Humanities, University of Tübingen, Germany*

INTRODUCTION

As described in Chapter 1, the term "cognitive enhancement" is associated with a wide range of existing and emerging biomedical technologies. These technologies permit cognition to be enhanced in healthy human beings, thereby offering the promise (or threat) of drastically changing the lives of citizens. Unsurprisingly, this has sparked a considerable amount of debate, with proponents of enhancement enthusiastically in favor, whereas opponents fear widespread social changes will be a turn for the worse. Therefore, the debate on cognitive enhancement is to a large extent a normative one. While many questions relating to specific aspects of existing cognitive enhancers remain unanswered (e.g., drugs such as Ritalin (see Chapter 2) and devices like transcranial direct current stimulation (tDCS; see Chapter 12)), including their properties, prevalence, modalities, reasons for use, and likely future developments, the normative issues surrounding their use are perhaps the most contentious (e.g., should they be used, for what and by whom: see Parens, 2005). By applying different moral theories (consequence-, virtue-, or rights-based), philosophers and neuroethicists reach very different conclusions, even when setting off from the same initial set of facts. Indeed, while the normative debate on cognitive enhancement cannot be resolved solely using empirical data, a lack of reliable information on current trends and future developments has created a gap that had been rapidly filled with thought experiments and fictional scenarios.

Cognitive Enhancement. http://dx.doi.org/10.1016/B978-0-12-417042-1.00013-9

WHAT KINDS OF COGNITIVE ENHANCEMENT ARE RELEVANT TO THE NORMATIVE DISCUSSION AND WHY?

While undoubtedly important, and in some cases urgent, any ethical analysis of cognitive enhancement technologies needs to be grounded on empirical facts regarding the plausibility of the drastic changes that promise or threaten (depending on the comprehensive view to which one subscribes) to alter the lives of citizens in all societies. The sheer number of conflicting opinions and the urgent need for social regulation on the issue of neuroenhancement have led some to conclude that *neuropolicy* will be the main source of political and economic conflict in the decades to come. What is more, some even think that the ferocity of this conflict will surpass that of the conflict over means of production that marked the previous century (Hughes, 2006; Lynch, 2006; Lynch and Laursen, 2009). Yet to what extent is this discussion based on science fiction rather than fact? Since most treatises on this topic begin with fictional scenarios and thought experiments (see Buchanan et al., 2000, for example), the justifiability of scenarios that are used as premises for normative discussions needs to be assessed. Ethicists confront readers with highly unlikely events that are not relevant to the present and this can only be justified if the scenarios are very likely to happen in the future, or if they serve the purpose of dissociating between relevant aspects of the situation at hand to facilitate moral judgment. I will begin by delineating the relevant topics and establishing the appropriate mode of discourse on the subject. For example, consider the two fictional scenarios presented in Box 13.1. The obviously fictional scenarios in Box 13.1 describe circumstances and consequences of a potential conflict between a fictional religiously ordered society from Rawls's influential book *The Law of Peoples* (2002) and an equally fictional post-communist country, Vaziria. It serves the purpose of depicting some of the worst possible ethical, social, and legal issues stemming from new cognitive enhancement technologies. It also presupposes that cognitive enhancements could actually increase cognitive capacities, as opposed to merely the maintaining cognitive capacities in the face of sleep deprivation and fatigue (see the discussions on *cognitive performance augmentation* and *cognitive performance maintenance* in Chapter 1).

Box 13.1 Fictional scenarios depicting potential conflicts in the future

Scenario 1

World news report: Tensions between Kazanistan and Vaziria reach their highest peak to date—Kazanistan threatens preemptive strikes on Enhancement factories in Vaziria.

The dispute between Kazanistan and Vaziria may lead to an armed conflict. Both countries accuse each other of financial and military support of terrorist or insurgent groups. Vaziria warns that if Kazanistan continues to support groups of religious fundamentalists in Vazirian territory, there will be no option left but to prohibit religious practices in Vaziria. The Prime Minister of Kazanistan vows to put an end to

Box 13.1—cont'd

Vaziri's "illicit drug trade" and "support of nonhumane terrorists." He has issued an ultimatum to Vaziria: either they cease production of Ampakines and cancel their asylum policy for enhancement seekers from Kazanistan, or the Kazani army and intelligence will put a stop to it with preemptive and retaliatory strikes. In the meantime, the Post-Human Liberation Army of Kazanistan has taken responsibility for the recent kidnapping of several prominent religious figures in Kazanistan, and unofficial reports state that both countries could potentially produce nuclear weapons.

Scenario 2

Encrypted transmission from the Department of Recruitment and Neural Resources, Hegemony Marine Corps, Military Post VK-72072.

Dear Sub-Lieutenant Pauperson,

Regarding your request No. 13-56 for release from active service and the issuing of a permit to reenter the civilian population, we regret to inform you that your request has been declined.

According to your service and health insurance contract, any and all enhancements that were installed in your body are the property of Hegemony Armed Forces.

Our records show that after you were wounded during the peacekeeping intervention in Vaziria, you received a replacement right arm with retractable blades and built in submachine gun, as well as a titanium skull replacement with ventromedial prefrontal cortex inhibitor and targeting computer, video–neural interface, night vision, and infrared vision. All these enhancements are class M devices that cannot be released into the civilian population or to foreign powers.

You can only be released from service if and when you have paid for the removal of all these military enhancements, are fitted with civilian replacement enhancements and have found gainful employment in a civilian or mercenary corporation.

We are happy to inform you that according to your last monthly medical and neuropsychiatric evaluation, your CNS is in above-average condition, indicating that you could accumulate sufficient funds for such replacements within 5 years and that you would gain promotion to the status of lieutenant if you volunteer for a mission behind enemy lines now.

Kind regards,

Richard Bolyar, MD, MBA

Department of recruitment and neural resources, Hegemony marine core, Military Post VK-72072

TAG: Be the chosen one! Be superhuman! Join us now! Gain employment, health insurance and enhancement!

Although the use of fictional scenarios (utopian or dystopian) can efficiently draw attention to the problems that could be faced by future societies, this approach has fueled some disagreement in the literature on cognitive neuroenhancement. However, it would be erroneous to conclude that the current failure to agree on adequate regulatory options for these technologies is a result of the use of fictional scenarios and thought experiments per se. Rather, it stems from the strong disagreement between irreconcilable comprehensive doctrines (e.g., post-humanism, dignitarianism) endorsed by those who devise such scenarios. It would also be false to conclude that cognitive neuroenhancement is a fictional social problem or that the regulation of these technologies cannot be justified to citizens holding opposing views.

But how real is this problem, and how can the "reality" of cognitive enhancement as a social issue be assessed? Imaginary worst-case scenarios (or not-yet-attained effects) are not the only means available to evaluate the impact that such enhancements will have on society. Based on the assessment of competitiveness and the technology currently available, it is plausible that the pressure to enhance will be most acute in the fields of space research, military and education. However, the most far-reaching effects will most likely be experienced in the business world (in what follows, I draw on Dubljević, 2012b).

Consider the example of logistics companies in a more-or-less laissez-faire market economy. Let's say that the most profitable trucking route is 1250 km long, a run that could be achieved in 1 day, albeit with considerable stress and fatigue. Without enhancement drugs, companies offer delivery in 2 days, with the price including the cost of the truck driver's accommodation. Suppose that Company A decides to assume an employment policy that places a preference on truck drivers who are willing to use modafinil (a medical treatment for narcolepsy) in order to stay alert and to complete the run in just 1 day. The company offers the service for the same price but completes the job in half the time, thereby accruing extra profit. Company B, the chief competitor of Company A, responds by offering the "overnight express" service and accordingly gives current employees the following choice: either they start using modafinil in order to cope with the requirements of the job, or they will be laid off. The effects on the market are not hard to foresee. All other logistics companies would either adopt similar policies or go out of business. The truck drivers would either use drugs or be out of work. Their choice is dictated by market forces completely beyond their control. Thus, enhancement technologies could have profound effects on the everyday lives of most citizens as the workday and deadline expectations change according to social pressures.

This brief and realistic sketch of possible social problems helps to demonstrate why the issue of cognitive enhancement merits ethical debate and requires regulatory oversight. Although the latter is not a matter of a philosophical discussion but of democratic decision-making and policy, a broad and open public debate on cognitive enhancement is essential, and should take reasonable pluralism seriously. Accordingly, public policy on enhancement should not be based on any sectarian values or principles, or on mere compromise. A legitimate public policy on cognitive enhancement needs to be justified in terms of reasonable conceptions of justice.

The moral of the story is that at least some cognitive enhancements may need to be controlled and regulated, and not just at the state level. However, this conclusion is largely contingent on the condition that such events might occur in the future. Whether this takes the shape of drastic scenarios (as described in the literature and presented above), or less drastic market phenomena, is still unclear at this stage (although the other contributions in this volume provide some initial indications based on the state-of-the-art of the science of cognitive enhancement). However, it should be noted that this issue has not been ignored at the government level. The regulation of cognitive enhancement technologies has been deemed important by relevant policy makers in the United States and the European Union, and several reports addressing these issues have been produced (Kass, 2003; EGE, 2005; BMA, 2007; CONTECS, 2008; JASON, 2008; STOA, 2009). These reports analyze the distinction between therapy and enhancement, and they very often present fictional scenarios about the impact of putative future technologies.

Ethical evaluation and public regulation involves several levels of immediacy: (1) several types of cognitive enhancers are currently in use, reflecting the urgency for ethical discussion (see Chapter 11 on Cognitive Enhancers in Use in Humans); (2) other interventions have been proven to enhance cognition but only in animal models (see Warwick, 2008, for example), and it remains unclear whether these effects can be replicated in humans (which limits the ethical discussion to questions of research ethics); and (3) other interventions are still in the hypothetical stage of development, thereby limiting the ethical/policy discussion to issues of responsibility relating to the public and/or private funding of such research. Focusing only on the most immediate ethical concern that existing medical drugs can be used to enhance cognitive function in healthy adults, several questions need to be answered:

1. What are the relevant examples of cognition-enhancing drugs?
2. What are the available options for public policy on such drugs?
3. What are the relevant external considerations for policy regulating pharmacological enhancers?
4. What are the likely future challenges that will need to be tackled by public policy on cognition-enhancing substances?

Scenario 1 in Box 13.1, although entirely fictional, serves as a useful starting point to answer most of these questions. One of the substances that was referred to in the dispute was a new class of drugs named ampakines. So, to address the first question, ampakines need to be included or excluded from the "most immediate" category. But according to what criteria? The most reasonable criterion is one of pragmatic possibility, and the contributions to this volume constitute important additions to this debate. Studies have repeatedly proved that ampakines significantly improve cognitive performance in animal models (see Sententia, 2006, for a review), and in theory, they will do so in humans, making them good candidates for analysis. However, only when sufficient data are available can the social and ethical impact of substances be analyzed (and the regulatory options), whereas the analysis of those that have not yet completed all phases of clinical trials and that are therefore not yet ready for regulation should be restricted to research ethics.

The question of relevant public policy options has not been introduced in Scenario 1, but the options are constrained by that fact that cognition-enhancing drugs have the potential to create serious social problems beyond the boundaries of a single society, which leads us to the third question. Societies do not implement public policies in a vacuum but they are bound by various international conventions and treaties. The 1971 United Nation Convention on Psychotropic Drugs (UN, 1971) is one example, and this lays out the regulatory framework for at least two relevant substances that are commonly mentioned in the literature on cognitive enhancement: amphetamines and methylphenidate (see Dubljević, 2013a). This is precisely because these drugs can cause serious harm and even major international incidents. However, it should be noted that newer drugs, such as modafinil (or ampakines), are not mentioned in relevant international treaties, and so there is no international regulatory framework in place. For example, the regulation of modafinil appears to be arbitrary and haphazard and differs significantly from country to country (see Dubljević, in press).

The final question regarding foreseeable developments also has to be answered. Although it is very easy to err in the assessment of future problems, some guidelines are available. Future challenges refer to issues that have sufficient potential to cause conflict, that could substantially change our social and/or political world, and that are within the limits of practicable possibility. Ampakines are a perfect example; they have proven effects on animal models and their potential societal effects are within the limits of practicable possibility. By significantly enhancing cognitive function, which is extremely important in the knowledge-based economies of postindustrial societies, they have the potential to both substantially change the social (and perhaps political) world, and to create conflicts within and between societies. However, the technology driving cognitive enhancement is not restricted to drugs, and medical and investigative devices that can enhance cognition must also be analyzed thoroughly. Again, to define the appropriate analytical approach, several questions have to be answered:

1. What are relevant examples of cognition-enhancing devices?
2. In what ways can the use of cognition-enhancing devices be regulated?
3. What are the relevant external considerations for policy on cognition-enhancing devices?
4. What are the likely future challenges facing public policy regarding the use of cognition-enhancing devices?

Scenario 2, although obviously fictional, and even unlikely, serves as a good starting point to answer some of these questions. Recall that the futuristic devices mentioned in the scenario are neuroprosthetics, brain stimulation devices, and computers linked directly to the brain. Thus, in answer to the first question, these types of devices need to be classified as currently in use (i.e., urgent ethical and regulatory issues), effective in animal models (research ethics issue), or still in the theoretical stage of development (issues of ethics and research funding policy). Yet again, according to what criteria? The first criterion is the ability to increase cognitive performance in the narrow sense (i.e., even only in principle). The second criterion is the realistic possibility that this will affect society at large, a criterion that might additionally clarify what exactly needs to be regulated (the selling and use of the device as a *product*, or selling *the use* of a device as a commercial *service*). These criteria should be sufficient to keep the discussion within the realm of science fact and steer clear of science fiction, which, unlike legitimate thought experiments, serves no clear purpose.

Unlike cognition-enhancing drugs, international treaties offer no guidance on the issue of regulation of cognition-enhancing devices. This means that all five general regulatory approaches—mandatory use, encouraged use, laissez faire, discouraged use, and prohibition (see Blank, 2010)—are potentially relevant. The exact policy depends on the safety profiles of the devices, which may differ radically depending on their physiological effects. Furthermore, the fact that some of the devices mentioned in the literature (e.g., deep-brain stimulation) may need to be implanted increases the salience of safety issues and social costs, which leads us to the third question: unlike drugs, which are easy to produce, to use, and even to smuggle across borders, some of the cognition-enhancing devices require special conditions or training in order to be used effectively, which limits their "social penetration."

The criteria governing external considerations and future challenges are not as obvious as in the case of cognition-enhancing drugs. As previously mentioned, there are no international treaties addressing this issue and the nature of the topic is strongly prone to utopian and dystopian thinking, increasing the potential for error. However, history does provide some guidance and neuroethics in general, and the cognitive enhancement debate in particular could be enriched by revisiting the self-understanding of the social and political role attributed by neuroscientists and neuroethicists to findings concerning neuromodulatory devices.

In 1963, the neuroscientist Jose Delgado conducted and recorded his famous experiment with a charging bull. By electrically stimulating the caudate nucleus with a "stimociever," a radio-controlled device implanted in the bull's brain, Delgado was able to stop the bull and turn the animal away from a red flag. Delgado subsequently published a book named *Physical Control of the Mind: Toward a Psychocivilized Society* (Delgado, 1969). In Chapter 20 of that book, Delgado explored ethical considerations pertaining to his work and argued that, on the one hand, this kind of research could benefit society by improving methods of clinical practice and social regulation, and on the other hand, while the research itself should not be regulated, the subsequent (mis)use of the technology might need to be so.

Notwithstanding his view of the ability of neuroscience to "civilize" unruly society, Delgado is right to point out that social control of reasonably beneficial research needs to be kept at a necessary minimum, whereas the products of research could and should be regulated and controlled. Thus, the criteria for external considerations and future challenges could be defined as follows: external considerations are based on the reasonableness of allowing public funding for certain neuroscientific interventions (e.g., invasive interventions serving no clear medical purpose could hardly be expected to be financed by public funds), of allowing self-funded neuroscientific interventions (e.g., "cosmetic neurosurgery"), and of offering safe and effective products and services. Furthermore, it is important to differentiate between the political aspects of "neuro-driven" conflicts, and to assess the social penetration of neurostimulation technologies and the likely changes in social practices that these technologies will bring about.

WHAT ARE THE NORMATIVE ISSUES ASSOCIATED WITH COGNITIVE ENHANCEMENT?

The normative debate concerning cognitive enhancement revolves around issues such as authenticity (Parens, 2005), human nature (Kass, 2003), and utility (Levy, 2007). However, one of the most contentious issues is the question of whether cognitive enhancement (drugs or devices) can be defined as "cheating" (in what follows, I draw on Dubljević, Sattler and Racine, 2014). Defining a certain practice as cheating can be viewed as a social process driven by group interests. Such processes happen continually, leading to alterations in such definitions over time. Accordingly, proponents of enhancement claim that the use of stimulant drugs by students is not cheating, as cheating is defined as: (1) breaking formal or informal social norms and (2) attempting to gain an unfair advantage (Harris, 2011, pp. 266–267). Moreover, stimulant drug use is not explicitly banned by all or even the majority of universities, and if stimulant drugs are permitted as "study aids," proponents of cognitive enhancement claim that stimulant use would be an advantage for all and, hence, could not be regarded as cheating (Harris, 2011). Harris uses the analogy with education and goes on to say that cognitive enhancement is comparable to seeking the best, to improving oneself or one's children. Furthermore, the costs of stimulant drugs are relatively low, unlike the costs of university education or specialized training. Moreover, proponents contend that we should use any means of improvement as long as they are effective, and by using examples such as aspirin, literacy, electricity, coffee, and computers, it can be concluded that enhancement is synonymous with evolution and progress (see Harris, 2011; Levy, 2007).

However, those who are skeptical about the claims of enhancement have a markedly different view on the matter (see Selgelid, 2007, for example). Some critics (see Dubljević, 2012a, for example) begin with the premise that rules are put in place when new cheating practices are discovered and draw on influential theories of justice[1] to make the case that cognitive enhancement is unfair. According to this argument, the therapeutic use of drugs or devices that might improve cognition (e.g., in persons with attention-deficit/hyperactivity disorder (ADHD) or narcolepsy) is a means of providing a basic necessity to those who are disadvantaged, restoring them to a position of equal opportunity and liberty. This differs markedly to the use of drugs (or devices) for cognitive enhancement where there is no clear medical need (Dubljević, 2012a). This line of argument is recognized even by authors that occupy the middle ground between opponents and proponents of cognitive enhancement. A prominent position held by this group is that cognitive enhancement has more potential to increase factual inequalities between members of society than to decrease or ameliorate them (see Glannon, 2008, for example).

Dubljević (2012b) goes on to say that cognitive enhancement is currently being used by individuals to obtain undeserved positional advantage. Thus, if a student uses methylphenidate (Ritalin) during an exam because they are diagnosed with ADHD, they are merely competing with other students on an equal footing. However, if it is used as a cognitive enhancer, the user is attempting to gain an advantage over their colleagues while taking a chance with the unknown long-term side effects. Furthermore, it has been argued that cognitive enhancers could affect the competition between those who would prefer to use them and those who would rather not (Sahakian and Morein-Zamir, 2007). Thus, even for nonusers there is an incentive or pressure to use stimulants (Forlini and Racine, 2009; Sattler and Wiegel, 2013; Dubljević, 2013b). Such practices could ultimately lead to a situation whereby all students need to use cognitive enhancers to be able to compete. Similarly, employees in different lines of work might need to use cognitive enhancers in order to retain their jobs (Appel, 2008). Employers would (indirectly) coerce them in order to gain more profit, while employees would have to take the risks of long-term effects because they cannot refuse. They are robbed of the ability to decide for themselves whether they wish to use cognitive enhancers and at the same time are forced to bear the consequences of the use of these drugs (Dubljević, 2012b). In other words, employers that encourage the use of cognitive enhancers could create additional disadvantages and needs for those already lacking basic necessities (i.e., employees) due to the unknown long-term side effects and/or through coercion. In the long run, through competitive

---

1. A theory of justice formulated by John Rawls (1999) is perhaps the most influential position in contemporary political theory. The final formulation of Rawls's principles of justice states that: (1) each person has the same indefeasible claim to a fully adequate scheme of equal basic rights and liberties, which is compatible with the same scheme of liberties for all (the equal liberty principle); and (2) social and economic inequalities are to satisfy two conditions: first, they are to be attached to positions and offices open to all under conditions of fair equality of opportunity (the principle of fair equality of opportunity) and second, they are to be of greatest benefit to the least advantaged members of society (the difference principle). See Rawls (2001), pp. 42–43.

pressure and the desire to gain at the expense of others, contagion processes may start to affect different dimensions of the basic structure of society, leading to an ever-increasing number of people using cognitive enhancement.

From the point of view of the critics, the unfairness of the social practice of cognitive enhancement calls for the introduction of rules and/or justifies the implicit or explicit norms that are in place. Thus, opponents of enhancement argue that there should be rules that at least discourage the use of stimulant drugs or brain stimulation devices as a matter of justice (Dubljević, 2012a,b) and that a similar position is intuitively shared by the majority of people (see the discussion on public attitudes on cognitive enhancement later). However, in his analysis of cognitive enhancement and justice, Julian Savulescu (2006) reaches a drastically different conclusion—that justice *requires* enhancement. According to Savulescu, nature allots advantages and disadvantages with no regard to fairness. Since enhancement might improve people's lives (and indeed, the effects of stimulant drugs might be more pronounced in those at the lower end of the normal distribution of cognitive capacities (see Lieb, 2010), who are in turn the least advantaged), the social distribution of cognitive enhancers should be designed to ensure that everyone, regardless of natural inequality, has a chance of attaining a decent life (Savulescu, 2006). Whether the least advantaged will benefit or be harmed by cognitive enhancers is an empirical issue that could be resolved with new insights into the physiological and social effects of cognitive enhancement, as discussed in the other chapters in this volume. On the normative side however, with the advent of competing theories of justice (e.g., Nozick, 1974; Walzer, 1983; Miller, 1999; Sen, 2009), this issue is unlikely to be resolved at a single stroke.

The empirical evidence available on the social attitudes toward cognitive enhancement is also ambiguous. In one Australian study, 85% of the general population believed that the use of medications for cognitive enhancement was morally unacceptable (Partridge et al., 2012). Similar findings have been reported in other countries and populations (Dodge et al., 2012; Ragan et al., 2013; Dubljević, Sattler and Racine, 2014). When university students were interviewed, the use of cognitive enhancers was typically regarded to be unfair (Bell et al., 2013). However, as in the academic debate on enhancement, a steady minority of respondents in the student and general population feel that use of cognitive enhancers is acceptable and that it does not represent an unfair advantage. This difference in attitudes may be linked to information regarding adverse effects or the context of use. On the one hand, some people may think that adverse effects of cognitive enhancers are minor and as such acceptable, whereas for the majority it is an excessive risk and in the absence of scientific evidence concerning long-term safety, they would choose to avoid and sanction the use of such approaches. On the other hand, the difference between competitive and cooperative contexts (especially in the examples used) might be the relevant feature that guides normative evaluation.

The fact that some students view cognitive enhancement as cheating and some do not may be related to different interpretations of university education—that is, whether it is understood as being dominantly competitive (a zero-sum game) or cooperative (a non-zero-sum game). This explanation is in line with the findings of a study carried out in the United States, which found enhancement of physical performance in sport is viewed as more problematic than enhancement of cognitive capacity in the university context (Dodge et al., 2012). Indeed, sports are more closely associated with zero-sum expectations than university education. However, contrary to the conclusions of the study, promotional activities that describe the use of cognitive enhancers as cheating in educational contexts may be counterproductive. If, as hypothesized here, the use of cognition-enhancing drugs is viewed as cheating in a competitive context but not in a cooperative context, clarification of context in future empirical studies could provide less ambiguous data on public attitudes toward cognitive enhancement.

Thus, future studies could be improved by framing the normative valence of different responses using the context in which cognitive enhancers are taken. Considering the measurement of performance, it could be argued that the use of cognitive enhancement could counteract the aim of tests, such as in cases where memorization is tested but students have used memory enhancers (Schermer, 2008). This problem is similar to the illicit use of calculators (which in itself is not problematic) in tests of mental arithmetic.

TENTATIVE PROPOSAL FOR PUBLIC POLICIES

So what are the specific ethical issues that need to be addressed, and what could be considered plausible policy proposals? While many of the nuances and arguments put forward elsewhere are beyond the scope of this article (see Dubljević, 2012a,b, 2013a,b, in press; Dubljević, Sattler and Racine, 2014, Dubljević, Saigle and Racine, 2014), it is nevertheless helpful to identify the effects and major risks of existing cognitive enhancers, as well as the recommended policy options (see Table 13.1).

Rational choice analysis of cognitive enhancers (see Dubljević, 2013b) has shown that their use could in fact create considerable social pressure and that unqualified prohibition and laissez-faire types of policy would be neither effective nor justified. A moderately liberal public policy shows more promise, although not all approaches within this type of policy would be acceptable from the point of view of a modern pluralist democracy. In the area of permissive regulation, the "gate-keeper" approach is very prominent, as described in many influential neuroethics texts (Glannon, 2008, 2011; Racine 2010; Merkel et al., 2007). However, it is unclear whether such an approach would solve the problem of social pressure (or just create others) and whether it could be justified to citizens that support enhancement as well as those who oppose it as a social practice. Furthermore, analysis of requirements of justice (see Dubljević, 2012a) together with the analysis of the harm profiles of specific stimulants (Dubljević, 2013a, in press) suggests that any model using the gate-keeper approach would be illegitimate and inefficient as policy, as it would lack transparency as well as economic incentives and disincentives for the relevant actors.

TABLE 13.1 Proposed Regulation of Existing Cognition-Enhancing Technologies

Enhancer	Major Risks	Enhancement Effects	Policy
Extended release methylphenidate	Blood pressure increase (BPI)	Maintenance of focus and attention (F & A)	Economic Disincentives Model (EDM)
Instant release methylphenidate	BPI, addiction	Maintenance of F & A	Prohibition of unauthorized production and sale to healthy adults
Amphetamine (all forms)	Addiction, BPI, psychosis	Augmented wakefulness, maintenance of F & A	Prohibition of unauthorized production and sale to healthy adults
Modafinil (all forms)	BPI, stress, shift work, immunity	Augmented wakefulness and working memory	EDM, postmarket monitoring
tDCS (product and service)	Discomfort, inhibitory cognitive "costs"	Augmented working memory and skill learning, reduced reaction time	EDM, moratorium on marketing, postmarket monitoring, service provider model
TMS (service)	Syncope, seizure, hearing loss	Reduced reaction time, savant-like abilities	Service provider model, postmarket monitoring

Note: tDCS, transcranial direct current stimulation; TMS, transcranial magnetic stimulation.

While a "gate-keeper" approach cannot be justified in most instances (and in some specific cases it has to be replaced with the related "service provider model": see later), an approach based on taxation with suitable models might be legitimate and effective. The Economic Disincentives Model (EDM; see Dubljević, 2012b), which would allow legal access to cognitive enhancers with the imposition of taxes, fees, and additional insurance requirements, is the most promising model proposed. This model could ensure state neutrality on personal preferences, protect the best interests of all citizens, provide reliable data on consumption and demand, and promote effective evaluation of long-term health costs among users of cognitive enhancers.

Under the EDM, the prices of cognitive enhancers would be regulated. Standard costs of production and distribution would be incorporated into the price, the profit margin would be limited and an additional tax would be imposed. Companies earning profits from cognitive enhancers could be further taxed and obliged to invest extensively in orphan drugs. The funds collected through such a policy could be used to provide medical necessities for the least well-off and the remaining funds could be allocated to education. Moreover, the use of devices and drugs that enhance cognition could be prohibited in certain instances, such as when sitting exams (see Dubljević, 2012b).

Cognition-enhancing drugs and devices vary in their effectiveness and safety profiles. Case-by-case analyses of the classic stimulants amphetamine (Adderall) and methylphenidate (Ritalin. see Dubljević, 2013a), and the newer atypical stimulant modafinil (Provigil: see Dubljević, in press), found that the use of stimulants by healthy adults to enhance cognitive functions must be distinguished from therapeutic and recreational uses of these drugs. Furthermore, their use as cognitive enhancers needs to be regulated, taking into account the differential safety profiles. On the one hand, extended release formulas of methylphenidate (e.g., Ritalin-SR) could be regulated permissively, since they cannot be recovered by readily applicable means in a quantity liable to abuse, and apparently they do not give rise to public health or social problems. A "discouragement of use with taxation" approach to the regulation of cognition-enhancing drugs could be a good starting point for a moderately liberal public policy, avoiding the pitfalls of both laissez-faire and overly harsh prohibitive policies. However, all models of regulation of stimulants are constrained by the requirements of the UN Convention on Psychotropic drugs (UN, 1971). Although there are several policies that could be used within the broad taxation approach (tobacco model, coffee-shop model, Regulatory Authority for Cognitive Enhancers (RACE) model, and EDM), some of these would not be appropriate or legitimate due to the current framework of international law.

Discouraging use through taxation could take multiple forms (in what follows, I draw on Dubljević, 2013b), and one approach is similar to that used to regulate tobacco in Norway. The aim of government policy in Norway was to decrease an unhealthy but legal habit. The percentage of the population smoking dropped from about 50% in 1973 to 19% in 2010, indicating the relative success of the policy. This decrease was achieved via antismoking measures such as heavy taxation and a ban on the visible display of tobacco products, which together created a negative environment for both users and providers. These measures were designed to create financial burdens and inconveniences for producers, providers, and users. Moreover, when the user finally manages to purchase the discouraged product, the package is adorned with graphic images depicting the potential health hazards associated with use. The rules and regulations in Norway appear to have served as an effective barrier and constitute a legitimate policy to discourage tobacco use. However, it is unclear whether this type of model would be as well suited to cognition-enhancing drugs and devices. The structure of the user population is certainly different and so similar measures could result in a very different outcome. Norwegians with higher levels of income and education tend to abstain from smoking or smoke less. Hard core smokers tend to start earlier, have a lower level of education, live in poorer regions of Norway, and have low incomes. The analysis of cognitive enhancer use (and resulting indirect coercion) assumes a choice based on a competitive advantage, whereas tobacco use offers only health disadvantages. Therefore, a policy that is effective in the case of tobacco could be totally ineffective when applied to cognitive enhancers.

A second option is to apply a model similar to that used to regulate so-called "soft drugs" in the Netherlands. Soft drugs such as cannabis and hallucinogenic mushrooms are legal for personal use, and the use of soft drugs (even in public) is not prosecuted. Sale of these drugs, although technically illegal under the still valid Opium Act, is widely tolerated provided that it takes place in a limited, controlled way. The legal control of sales regulates designated places (coffee shops), product (only soft drugs can be sold, not alcohol), quantity (5 g maximum per transaction), eligible users (only adults, but not limited to citizens), availability of information (advertisement of drugs is prohibited) and the political choice of local residents (the local municipality can give the order to close a coffee shop). The issue of indirect coercion to use cognitive enhancers to acquire a competitive advantage does not apply, as soft drug use offers only recreational benefits. Therefore, a policy that is effective for soft drugs could be totally ineffective if applied to cognitive enhancers. Furthermore, there is the additional potential problem of enhancement tourism, the repercussions of which are unclear.

A third model has been specifically designed for cognitive enhancement. The British Medical Association (BMA, 2007) proposed a permissive system of regulation whereby techniques are permitted under license from a regulatory body, the RACE. This rather sketchy proposal suggests that RACE could approve the use of particular cognitive enhancement techniques and issue guidance. From the few details available about the model, it could be assumed that it would create financial burdens and inconveniences for producers, providers, and users. However, even the BMA envisages drawbacks of such a model: "the establishment of a statutory regulatory body is expensive, bureaucratic, and involves considerable work and time from those regulated" (BMA, 2007, p. 34).

The EDM (see Dubljević, 2012b) explicitly tackles the drawbacks of RACE and seeks to limit the costs for society while optimizing regulatory capacities and demands of justification. Under the EDM, an already existing government agency (e.g., the Food and Drug Administration or the Ministry of Health) would offer a licensing procedure to pharmaceutical companies (or producers of devices) to market cognitive enhancers to healthy adults. This way all citizens could have legal access to cognitive enhancement, but the imposition of taxes, fees, and additional insurance requirements would create financial and regulatory burdens associated with their use.

The EDM envisages an additional licensing procedure for users; in order to use cognitive enhancers, citizens would have to pay to complete a course about the known effects and side effects, and pass an exam as proof of knowledge. Furthermore, additional medical insurance and obligatory annual medical tests would be required to obtain and renew the license to use cognitive enhancers. Although the EDM is designed specifically for the regulation of cognition-enhancing drugs and devices, and thus it may avoid the problems associated with the tobacco and coffee-shop models of regulation, it has yet to be demonstrated whether this approach would resolve the problem of social pressure (or just fill the budget) and whether it could be justified to the proenhancement and antienhancement sectors of the population.

One potential normative problem with taxation approaches is that they presuppose a normative standpoint that could discriminate against those who wish to use cognitive enhancers. Even if there are health costs associated with the use of cognitive enhancers, as is the case with tobacco use, it is not self-evident that taxation would be a legitimate policy. This point merits further elaboration. Modern democratic societies are characterized by a plurality of different views and political theorists have attempted to formulate an impartial standpoint to adjudicate between the conflicting claims of such worldviews. These attempts are perhaps best outlined in Rawls's *Justice as Fairness* (2001) and *Political Liberalism* (2005). Indeed, an analysis of Rawls's principles of justice in the context of cognitive enhancement (see Dubljević, 2012a,b) has been used to justify the general taxation approach and the EDM. However, these principles are far from uncontroversial. For example, the difference principle[1] has come under heavy attack from almost all major political theorists from the 1970s on (e.g., Nozick, 1974; Miller, 1999).

However, from the legal point of view, the EDM explicitly envisages all the measures required by the 1971 UN Convention, making it the most legitimate public policy for the use of safer cognitive enhancement drugs (e.g., extended release methylphenidate and perhaps modafinil: see later) and devices (e.g., tDCS) by healthy adults. On the other hand, the sale of more dangerous stimulants (e.g., instant release formulas of methylphenidate, compounds containing amphetamine or precursors that produce amphetamine via normal metabolism) or stimulation devices (e.g., transcranial magnetic stimulation (TMS)) to healthy adults needs to be prohibited. Although these cognitive enhancers could provide significant benefits if used responsibly, the danger of drug abuse (and the risk of addiction, increased aggression, erratic and violent behavior) and possible seizures induced by devices makes their use a potential social danger.

The safety profile of modafinil, a newer atypical stimulant, is not as clear, because its long term effects are unknown. An analysis of the currently available data (see Dubljević, in press) indicates that more reliable information on the neurophysiological mechanisms of action of modafinil is needed. Even though the physiological profile appears to be beneficial, modafinil could incur additional social and health-related costs if inadequately regulated. Widespread use of modafinil could decrease the range of employment options available and increase the pressure to perform shift work. Apart from increasing stress and decreasing immunity, modafinil can have a plethora of indirect adverse health effects, including increased risk of mortality and even a decrease in the cognitive ability of future generations. The potential beneficial effects of modafinil are therefore accompanied by a significant risk of exploitation, depending on the legal framework used to regulate its use. Hence, regulatory models that provide the missing data on long-term effects are the most normatively and empirically sound, even if the preliminary assumptions turn out to be incorrect in the long term. The EDM is one type of regulatory approach that could generate the data needed for a more reliable assessment, as well as funding to offset the adverse social and health-related costs of modafinil use. However, in poorly regulated regimens with little employee protection, the "nightshift worker syndrome" indication for modafinil could give rise to social problems that would be difficult to detect and resolve. While one solution is to consider revisiting and/ or revoking this indication of modafinil, postmarket monitoring of long-term consumption trends and effects is necessary nevertheless.

An analysis of the ethical challenges of electromagnetic cognitive enhancers has revealed the need to distinguish between the regulation of enhancement devices as products and the use of enhancement devices as a service. Noninvasive brain stimulation devices (e.g., tDCS and TMS) differ in their effectiveness and safety profiles. As tDCS appears to be safe and effective in laboratory settings (see Dubljević, Saigle and Racine, 2014), it is plausible to assume that it is safe and effective in any environment provided that users have been sufficiently well trained. Since tDCS could cause long-term detrimental changes in developing brains, a reasonable precaution might be to set the age requirement at 25. However, there is a lack of information on the effects and mechanisms of action of tDCS. Apart from limiting the availability of tDCS to minors, the regulatory framework needs to fill this gap in the data as soon as possible. The EDM could be used as a first-response policy, as the use of tDCS needs to be regulated urgently. Indeed, tDCS devices can be cheaply and easily built at home and used noncommercially as a do-it-yourself enhancement gadget. Since no data are available on the long-term effects, adverse effects of untrained use (such as temporary respiratory failure) cannot be ruled out. The EDM could quickly, cost-effectively, and objectively generate the data required to fine-tune policy. However, the regulation of the prices of tDCS devices through the EDM may be unnecessary and given the growing risk of home-made tDCS devices, counterproductive. If data on tDCS use generated by the EDM do indicate that trained use of tDCS is reasonably safe, even outside controlled laboratory settings, these requirements, along with additional taxation of providers, could be relaxed. The considerable regulatory burdens placed on those seeking to use cognitive enhancers would limit social penetration until the issue of long-term physiological effects has been fully clarified. Since tDCS would in principle be available to all, this should offset any concerns about fairness. Admittedly, using tDCS in a DIY context defies almost all efforts to regulate the technology. However, having a reasonable legal alternative is enough to promote registered use in most cases. Accordingly, unlicensed use of tDCS on third parties should perhaps be criminalized and a moratorium on direct-to-consumer marketing of tDCS enforced. However, such measures could be dispensed with if postmarket monitoring provided a clear indication that home use of tDCS does not represent a significant danger.

In addition to the regulation of stimulation devices as products, there is a pressing need to regulate the provision of enhancement devices as services. At present, tDCS is offered as a service (see Dubljević, Saigle and Racine, 2014) and the use of TMS as a cognitive enhancer (see Luber and Lisanby, 2013) is only likely to be widespread in the form of service. Due to the considerable costs and training required, it is unlikely that TMS will be readily available as a product or self-administration gadget. Accordingly, a licensing procedure for service providers needs to be defined. For reasons of transparency and fairness, this procedure should not be limited to health professionals but, rather, open to all persons with specialized training in neurology or neuroscience. Given the already high costs (and the need to ensure fair access by affluent citizens and the less well-off), some of the requirements of the EDM that could create additional costs should not be applied to TMS. However, the potential of the EDM to rapidly provide information on the long-term effects, safety, and efficacy of TMS will be very valuable for society. One solution would be to offer a unified policy for enhancement devices, using the licensing of tDCS users for the purpose of restricting TMS availability. Obtaining a license to use enhancement devices could require an individual to pass an exam to demonstrate their knowledge about both tDCS and TMS. An additional medical insurance policy covering both TMS and tDCS could also be required of users. The obligatory annual medical tests necessary to obtain and renew the license would quickly generate the data needed to fine-tune policy on both tDCS and TMS. A unified license to use "enhancement devices" would enable citizens over 25 years of age to purchase and use tDCS devices and to benefit from TMS as a service provided by trained professionals.

FUTURE TECHNOLOGICAL CHALLENGES AND PROACTIVE PUBLIC POLICIES

In the preliminary analysis of both psychopharmacological and electromagnetic enhancers, several substances and devices or techniques were mentioned and deemed nonurgent in terms of the need for public policy. These approaches have been shown to provide enhancement in animal models only, yet it is unclear whether they exert similar effects on humans. Furthermore, some are only at the theoretical stage of development and thus, they do not pose immediate challenges in terms of ethics or public policy. However, as scientific and technological progress will undoubtedly lead to the creation of more cognitive enhancers, I will return briefly to these excluded enhancers and discuss proactive public policy on the research behind future technologies.

Due to the legitimate concerns of citizens opposing cognitive enhancement and the requirements of justice (see Dubljević, 2012a), government funding of enhancement technologies would not be appropriate. However, private and corporate actors would have every right to follow research interests provided that they do so in an ethical manner. Military interest in enhancement technology could well be the driving force behind the development of newer technologies. Indeed, many of the studies on specific extant cognitive enhancers have been conducted for the military, and it stands to reason that ampakines and other drugs will be tested and used by soldiers. In this context, it is important to question the leeway given to the military in spending taxpayers' money and to ensure that the human and civil rights of the soldiers who serve as research subjects are respected (see fictional Scenario 2 in Box 13.1). While it may be naïve to expect complete transparency and civic oversight in military-funded research, military research expenditure on cognitive enhancement could be controlled by a parliamentary body. Furthermore, the informed consent process of military-funded research on cognitive enhancement should be closely examined and the rights of the soldiers to conscientiously object to the use of cognitive enhancers (except in emergency situations) should be publicly asserted and supported. Moreover, the military should guarantee that any long-term medical needs that may arise from the use of these technologies should be covered by the military.

The use of novel cognition-enhancing drugs and devices in the civilian population should be strictly prohibited until sufficient data has been generated to demonstrate that they are safe and effective. Although new technologies such as ampakines and invasive brain–computer interfaces are not yet ready for use in humans, it is reasonable to expect that they will be in the future. The fact that both society and regulatory agencies have had experience and collected reliable data on current cognitive enhancers (e.g., through the provisions of the EDM) should generate sufficient know-how to effectively regulate the use of newer enhancers. Objective measures of the safety profile of specific drugs and devices need to be used, and further perfected, in order to fine-tune the necessary policies. This leads to another important issue that needs to be addressed; the methodology used for establishing the safety profiles of existing drugs. This methodology has been rightly criticized and needs to be examined to identify the shortcomings, and the potential effects these shortcomings may have on proposed public policies.

METHODOLOGICAL WEAKNESSES AND THE FUTURE OF EVIDENCE-BASED POLICY ON COGNITIVE ENHANCEMENT

In the policy analysis of methylphenidate and amphetamines (see Dubljević, 2013a), a key methodological tool used to assess the risk posed is the multicriteria drug harm scale (Nutt et al., 2007, 2010). However, this scale does not take into consideration the differences between prescription amphetamines (the purity of which is controlled) and street amphetamines, to which additional harmful substances are often added. Furthermore, the fact that newer stimulants like modafinil were not rated at all significantly limits the conclusions reached and the resulting policy options (as summarized in Table 13.1). The primary focus of the multicriteria drug harm scale was on illicit drugs, including recreational drugs such as ecstasy and herbal stimulants with amphetamine-like effects, such as khat. The analysis explicitly distinguished between recreational users, users of stimulants, and users of cognitive enhancers. Moreover, khat was not analyzed as an extant cognitive enhancer (compare Table 13.1), as there are insufficient data to suggest that khat has any cognition-enhancing effects and its use is largely limited to certain communities with a cultural tradition of khat use. Although the results of the multicriteria drug harm scale have been interpreted with caution (and it has been noted that the methodology could be improved by soliciting ratings from different stakeholders, in order to guard against expert bias: Dubljević, 2013a), the results are the only available objective measure of the safely profiles of stimulants. However, important criticisms have also been leveled against the multicriteria drug harm scale on methodological grounds, and specific concerns raised in the cases of ecstasy and khat. In an illuminating article, Parrot (2007) offers extensive criticism of the specific ratings of the scale as reflected in the passage presented here in full:

> *Ecstasy users reported an average of eight physical and four psychological problems, which they attributed to Ecstasy use. In many of these Ecstasy/MDMA studies, the non-user control group comprised legal drug users—mostly social drinkers. Hence there is an extensive literature, showing that Ecstasy/MDMA is associated with significantly more functional distress than alcohol used at the same age. … [furthermore] the lowly position attributed to Khat by Nutt et al. (2007) may reflect its infrequent usage in UK, but in societies where it is widely used, the harm score would be much higher.*

> *In parts of Somalia, Kenya and Yemen, Khat (or Qat) is widely used as a social stimulant. The consequences of its use have been extensively researched, and the findings reveal a range of adverse effects: The psychoactive drug is obtained by chewing khat or qat leaves, but this takes considerable time and effort: In an empirical investigation of 1600 users, the authors noted that: 'Subjects in the Qat group chewed leaves for at least 4 hours daily for three successive days'. The leaf residues caused significant gastro-intestinal distress, with epigastric bloating, abdominal distension and genito-urinary problems. Tobacco-leaf chewers tend to develop cancers of the mouth, and qat-leaf chewers similarly develop oral cancers. Cardiac, cerebrovascular and other medical problems also occur. The pharmacodynamic effects of cathinone [the active substance in Khat] are broadly similar to other Central Nervous System (CNS) stimulants, with acute mood gains followed by adverse withdrawal symptoms, insomnia followed by delayed waking, reduced daily work performance, anorexia, drug dependency and increased psychiatric distress.*

> *Khat is also associated with cognitive performance deficits. At one Somali*
> *University, the 25% of students who were khat chewers had significantly lower*
> *academic performance grades, despite coming from higher income families*
> *[...]. The money spent on khat, the time spent chewing and other aspects of drug*
> *dependency can increase psychosocial distress and lead to financial hardship. In*
> *northern Kenya many respondents used more than half of their domestic budgets*
> *on khat, but few perceived this as a waste of resources.*

Parrot's (2007) criticism is not isolated but it is just one example of valid concerns that include situational factors (see Caulkins et al., 2011), value judgments (see Kalant, 2010), and a lack of input from relevant stakeholders (see Forlini et al., 2013). It therefore makes sense to determine how the methodological weaknesses of the multicriteria drug harm scale affect the conclusions drawn from it. As Nutt (2011) rightly notes in his response to critics, the fact that a certain methodology has drawbacks does not mean that this methodology should be abandoned, especially if no alternative has been proposed. Moreover, the most damning criticism concerns stimulant substances that are poorly understood by the experts that made the assessments, whereas amphetamine and methylphenidate have been extensively researched and are well understood. Thus, the way the data is generated in the original multicriteria drug harm scale could provoke the introduction of artifacts. Experts in psychiatry, pharmacology, and addiction used a 4-point scale to rate drugs in three major dimensions of harm (physical health effects, potential for dependence, and social harm), with 0 representing no risk; 1, some risk; 2, moderate risk; and 3, extreme risk (Nutt et al., 2007). The numbers used in the evidence-based analysis of stimulant safety profiles (Dubljević, 2013a) represent mean values from multiple assessments. While I acknowledge that dangers associated with drug use may need to be distinguished from dangers of abuse, for the purposes of this discussion the data are valid. The experts have had plenty of experience with the effects of amphetamine and methylphenidate and the conclusions on the abuse potential were the guiding reason in opting for a more liberal approach to methylphenidate, including the development of extended release formulas, and for a prohibitive response in the case of instant release methylphenidate and all forms of amphetamine. However, concerns about extending the methodology of the multicriteria drug harm scale to cognitive enhancers are legitimate and should be addressed in future studies.

CONCLUSIONS

The term "cognitive enhancement" is associated with use of drugs or devices for non–health-related enhancement of cognition. Most of these technologies have either been established in animal models or through a history of use in humans. While there are many unanswered questions about specific aspects of existing cognitive enhancers (e.g., properties, prevalence, modalities, reasons for use, likely future developments) the normative issues surrounding their use (i.e., should they be used, for what, and by whom) are perhaps the most contentious.

While many normative issues have been analyzed in the literature, this chapter has attempted to provide a general overview of the spectrum of opinions on a key normative issue: whether cognitive enhancement is cheating. Furthermore, the chapter discussed the various options available for the regulation of cognitive enhancers using both fictional and realistic scenarios, as well as public policy options for existing and future cognitive enhancers. In addition, the legal and methodological challenges faced in developing a legitimate, evidence-based policy have been identified.

REFERENCES

Appel, J.M., 2008. When the boss turns pusher: a proposal for employee protections in the age of cosmetic neurology. J. Med. Ethics 34 (8), 616–618.

Bell, S., Partridge, B., Lucke, J., Hall, W., 2013. Australian university students' attitudes towards the acceptability and regulation of pharmaceuticals to improve academic performance. Neuroethics 6 (1), 197–205.

Blank, R., 2010. Globalization: pluralist concerns and contexts. In: Giordano, J., Gordijn, B. (Eds.), Scientific and Philosophical Perspectives in Neuroethics. Cambridge University Press, Cambridge, UK, pp. 321–342.

British Medical Association (BMA), 2007. Boosting Your Brainpower: Ethical Aspects of Cognitive Enhancements. A discussion paper from the British Medical Association. Retrieved from: http://www.bma.org.uk/ap.nsf/AttachmentsByTitle/PDFCognitiveEnhancement2007.

Buchanan, A.E., Brock, D.W., Daniels, N., Wikler, D., 2000. From Chance to Choice: Genetics and Justice. Cambridge University Press, Cambridge, UK.

Caulkins, J.P., Reuter, P., Coulson, C., 2011. Basing drug scheduling decisions on scientific ranking of harmfulness: false promise from false premises. Addiction 106, 1886–1890.

CONTECS, 2008. Converging Technologies and Their Impact on the Social Sciences and Humanities. Frauenhofer Institute, Stuttgart, Germany. Retrieved from: http://www.contecs.fraunhofer.de/images/files/contecs_report_complete.pdf.

Delgado, J., 1969. Physical Control of the Mind: Toward a Psycho-civilized Society. Harper & Row, New York.

Dodge, T., Williams, K.J., Marzell, M., Turrisi, R., 2012. Judging cheaters: is substance misuse viewed similarly in the athletic and academic domains? Psychol. Addict. Behav. 26 (3), 678–682.

Dubljević, V., 2012a. Principles of justice as the basis for public policy on psychopharmacological cognitive enhancement. Law Innovation Technol. 4 (1), 67–83.

Dubljević, V., 2012b. Toward a legitimate public policy on cognition enhancement drugs. Am. J. Bioeth. Neurosci. 3 (3), 29–33.

Dubljević, V., 2013a. Prohibition or coffee-shops: regulation of amphetamine and methylphenidate for enhancement use by healthy adults. Am. J. Bioeth. 13 (7), 23–33.

Dubljević, V., 2013b. Cognitive enhancement, rational choice and justification. Neuroethics 6 (1), 179–187.

Dubljević, V., Sattler, S., Racine, E., 2014. Cognitive enhancement and academic misconduct: a study exploring their frequency and relationship. Ethics Behav. 24 (5), 408–420.

Dubljević, V., Saigle, S., Racine, E., 2014. The rising tide of transcranial direct current stimulation (tDCS) in the media and academic literature. Neuron. 82 (4), 731–736.

Dubljević, V. Enhancement with modafinil: benefiting or harming the society? In: Jotterand, F., Dubljević, V. (Eds.), Cognitive Enhancement: Ethical and Policy Implications in International Perspectives, under Contract at Oxford University Press, in press.

European Group on Ethics in Sciences and New Technologies [EGE], 2005. Opinion on the Ethical Aspects of ICT Implants in the Human Body (16 March 2005.). Opinion of the European Group on Ethics in Sciences and New Technologies to the European Commission, vol. 20, Office for Official Publications of the European Communities, Luxembourg.

Forlini, C., Racine, E., 2009. Autonomy and coercion in academic "cognitive enhancement" using methylphenidate: perspectives of key stakeholders. Neuroethics 2 (3), 163–177.

Forlini, C., et al., 2013. How research on stakeholder perspectives can inform policy on cognitive enhancement. Am. J. Bioeth. 13 (7), 41–43.

Glannon, W., 2008. Psychopharmacological enhancement. Neuroethics 1 (1), 45–54.

Glannon, W., 2011. Brain, Body, and Mind – Neuroethics with a Human Face. Oxford University Press, Oxford.

Harris, J., 2011. Chemical cognitive enhancement: is it unfair, unjust, discriminatory, or cheating for healthy adults to use smart drugs? In: Illes, J., Sahakian, B. (Eds.), Oxford Handbook of Neuroethics. Oxford University Press, Oxford, UK, pp. 265–272.

Hughes, J., 2006. Human enhancement and the emergent technopolitics of the 21st century. In: Bainbridge, W., Roco, M. (Eds.), Managing Nano-bio-info-cogno Innovations: Converging Technologies in Society. Springer, Dordrecht, The Netherlands, pp. 285–307.

JASON (Program for Office of Defense Research and Engineering), 2008. Human Performance. JASON Advisory Group for Department of Defense, Pentagon. JSR-07–625, Available at: www.fas.org/irp/agency/dod/jason/human.pdf.

Kalant, H., 2010. Drug classification: science, politics, both or neither? Addiction 105, 1146–1149.

Kass, L., 2003. Beyond Therapy: Biotechnology and the Pursuit of Happiness; A Report of the President's Council on Bioethics. Dana Press, New York, NY.

Levy, N., 2007. Neuroethics: Challenges for the 21st Century. Cambridge University Press, Cambridge, UK.

Lieb, K., 2010. Hirndoping: Warum Wir Nicht Alles Schlucken Sollten. Artemis & Winkler, Mannheim, Germany.

Luber, B., Lisanby, S.H., 2013. Enhancement of human cognitive performance using transcranial magnetic stimulation (TMS). Neuroimage. 85 (3), 961–970.

Lynch, Z., 2006. Neuropolicy (2005–2035): converging technologies enables neurotechnology creating new ethical dilemmas. In: Bainbridge, W., Roco, M. (Eds.), Managing Nano-bio-info-cogno Innovations: Converging Technologies in Society. Springer, Dordrecht, The Netherlands, pp. 173–192.

Lynch, Z., Laursen, B., 2009. The Neuro Revolution: How the Brain Science Is Changing Our World. St. Martin's Press, New York, NY.

Merkel, R., Boer, G., Fegert, J., et al., 2007. Intervening in the brain: changing psyche and society. Springer, Berlin/Heidelberg, Germany.

Miller, D., 1999. Principles of Social Justice. Harvard University Press, Cambridge, Mass.

Nozick, R., 1974. Anarchy, State, and Utopia. Basic Books, New York, NY.

Nutt, D., 2011. Let not the best be the enemy of the good. Addiction 106, 1892–1893.

Nutt, D., King, L.A., Saulsbury, W., Blakemore, C., 2007. Development of a rational scale to assess the harm of drugs of potential misuse. Lancet 369 (9566), 1047–1053.

Nutt, D.J., King, L.A., Phillips, L.D., 2010. Drug harms in the UK: a multicriteria decision analysis. Lancet 376, 1558–1565.

Parens, E., 2005. Authenticity and ambivalence: toward understanding the enhancement debate. Hastings Center Rep. 35 (3), 34–41.

Parrott, A.C., 2007. Drug-related harm: a complex and difficult concept to scale. Hum. Psychopharmacol. Clin. Exp. 22, 423–425.

Partridge, B., Lucke, J., Hall, W., 2012. A comparison of attitudes toward cognitive enhancement and legalized doping in sport in a community sample of Australian adults. Am. J. Bioeth. Primary Res. 3 (4), 81–86.

Racine, E., 2010. Pragmatic neuroethics: Improving treatment and understanding of the mind-brain. Basic bioethics. In: McGee, G., Caplan, A. (Eds.). MIT Press, Cambridge.

Ragan, C.I., Bard, I., Singh, I., 2013. What should we do about student use of cognitive enhancers? An analysis of current evidence. Neuropharmacology 64, 588–595.

Rawls, J., 1999. A Theory of Justice – Revised Edition. Harvard University Press, Cambridge, Mass.

Rawls, J., 2001. Justice as Fairness: A Restatement. Harvard University Press, Cambridge, Mass.

Rawls, J., 2002. The Law of Peoples with the Idea of Public Reason Revisited. Harvard University Press, Cambridge, Mass.

Rawls, J., 2005. Political liberalism, Expanded ed. Columbia University Press, New York.

Sahakian, B., Morein-Zamir, S., 2007. Professor's little helper. Nature 450 (7173), 1157–1159.

Sattler, S., Wiegel, C., 2013. Test anxiety and cognitive enhancement: the influence of students' worries on their use of performance-enhancing drugs. Subst. Use Misuse 48 (3), 220–232.

Savulescu, J., 2006. Justice, fairness and enhancement. Ann. N.Y. Acad. Sci. 1093, 321–338.

Schermer, M., 2008. On the argument that enhancement is "cheating". J. Med. Ethics 34 (2), 85–88.

Science and Technology Options Assessment (STOA), 2009. Human Enhancement Study. Rathenau Institute, The Hague, The Netherlands.

Selgelid, M.J., 2007. An argument against arguments for enhancement. Stud. Ethics Law Tech. 1 (1) .

Sen, A., 2009. The Idea of Justice. Belknap Press of Harvard University Press, Cambridge, Mass.

Sententia, W., 2006. Cognitive enhancement and the neuroethics of memory drugs. In: Bainbridge, W., Roco, M. (Eds.), Managing Nano-bio-info-cogno Innovations: Converging Technologies in Society. Springer, Dordrecht, The Netherlands, pp. 153–172.

United Nations (UN), 1971. Convention on Psychotropic Substances. United Nations Publications, Herndon, VA. Available at: www.unodc.org/pdf/convention_1971_en.pdf.

Walzer, M., 1983. Spheres of Justice. Basic Books, New York, NY.

Warwick, K., 2008. Cybernetic enhancements. In: Zonneveld, L., Dijstelbloem, H., Ringoir, D. (Eds.), Reshaping the Human Condition. Exploring Human Enhancement. Rathenau Institute, The Hague, The Netherlands, pp. 123–131.

Index

Color Plates

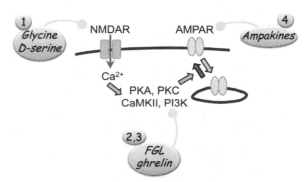

FIGURE 3.1   Schematic representation of three potential sites for cognitive intervention based on the general process of NMDA receptor-dependent synaptic plasticity. (1) Enhancement of NMDA receptor function, based on the availability of the coagonists glycine and/or D-serine. (2, 3) Modulation of the signaling pathways activated during synaptic plasticity downstream from NMDA receptor activation. Of the pathways represented in the figure, only CaMKII is directly sensitive to Ca^{2+} entry from NMDA receptors. Nevertheless, there is significant crosstalk between pathways, and all these kinases have been shown to participate at some level in the process of synaptic plasticity. The pharmacological agent FGL and the natural hormone ghrelin will be presented as modulators of these pathways with potential for cognitive enhancement. (4) To a major extent, these forms of synaptic plasticity are expressed by changes in the number or function of AMPA receptors at synapses. Enhancement of AMPA receptor function by ampakines will be discussed.

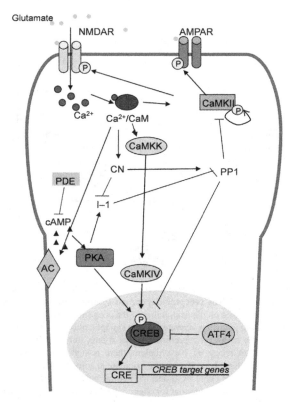

FIGURE 5.2 NMDA receptor–dependent signaling pathways in the postsynaptic neuron.
Ca2+ influx through the N-methyl-D-aspartate (NMDA) receptors (NMDARs) activates a variety of signaling molecules including α-calcium-calmodulin–dependent protein kinase II (αCaMKII) and protein kinase A (PKA). Activations of these signaling cascades eventually turn on the transcription factor, cAMP responsive element binding protein (CREB), in the nucleus. The detailed roles of these molecules in LTP and learning are described in the text. AMPAR, α-amino-3-hydroxy-5-methyl-4-isoxazolepropionic acid receptor; CaM, calmodulin; CaMKK, calcium-calmodulin–dependent protein kinase kinase; CN, calcineurin; I-1, inhibitor-1; PP1, protein phosphatase 1; PDE, phosphodiesterase; AC, adenylyl cyclase; CaMKIV, calcium-calmodulin–dependent protein kinase IV; ATF4, Activating transcription factor 4; CRE, cAMP-responsive element.

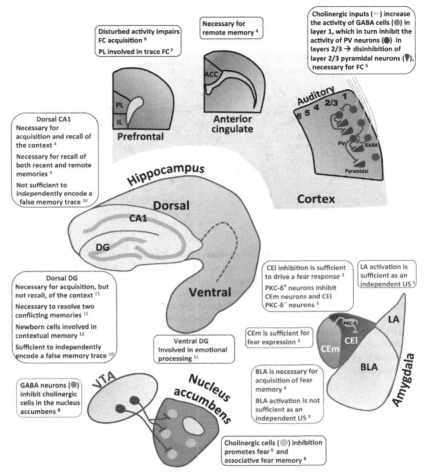

FIGURE 7.2 Optogenetics-based findings in fear memory research. This figure presents the different areas involved in fear memory that were implicated by optogenetics: amygdalar nuclei, primary and high cortical areas, striatum, and hippocampus. Each finding is marked by a number, signifying the corresponding published work, in the order they appear here: (1) Johansen et al. (2010); (2) Jasnow et al. (2013); (3) Ciocchi et al. (2010); (4) Goshen et al. (2011); (5) Letzkus et al. (2011); (6) Yizhar et al. (2011b); (7) Gilmartin et al. (2013); (8) Brown et al. (2012); (9) Witten et al. (2010); (10) Ramirez et al. (2013); (11) Kheirbek et al. (2013); (12) Gu et al. (2012).

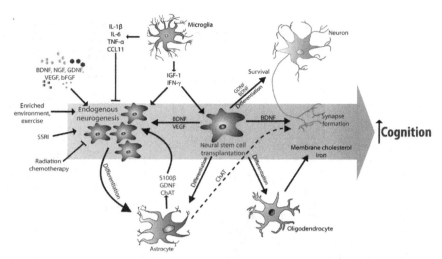

FIGURE 8.2   Stem cells can influence cognition via multiple mechanisms. Considerable evidence supports the notion that both adult neurogenesis and neural stem cell transplantation can contribute to cognition. Factors such as exercise, selective serotonin reuptake inhibitors (SSRIs), and inflammation can modulate adult neurogenesis, leading to enhanced or impaired cognition. Likewise, transplantation of neural stem cells can improve cognition in animal models of aging and neurodegenerative disease. While neurotrophic effects of stem cells are strongly implicated in this process, it is likely that many of the mechanisms shown here interact to modulate cognition. BDNF, brain-derived neurotrophic factor; bFGF, basic fibroblast growth factor; ChAT, choline acetyltransferase; GDNF, glial cell–derived neurotrophic factor; IFN, interferon; IGF, insulin-like growth factor; IL, interleukin; TNF, tumor necrosis factor; NGF, nerve growth factor.

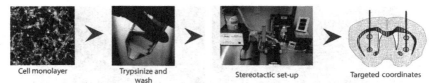

Cell monolayer   Trypsinize and wash   Stereotactic set-up   Targeted coordinates

FIGURE 8.3 **Stem cell preparation and transplantation into the brain.** Neural stem cells (NSCs) are derived at postnatal day 1 (P1) from green fluorescent protein–expressing transgenic mice. NSCs are expanded for 15 passages, at which time cells are dissociated with trypsin and neutralized in antibiotic-free growth media. NSCs then are resuspended and washed twice with transplantation vehicle (Hank's buffered saline solution, 20 ng/mL epidermal growth factor), then counted. Only cell populations with ≥90% viability are used, and concentration is adjusted to yield 50,000 cells/μL. NSCs or vehicle are then transplanted bilaterally into the striatum using a 30-gauge Hamilton microsyringe and stereotaxic apparatus (1 uL/site; anterior/posterior = +0.02; medial/lateral = ±2.00; dorsal/ventral = −3.0 and −3.5).

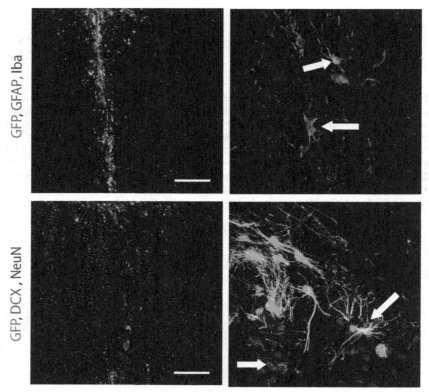

FIGURE 8.4 Neural stem cells engraft and differentiate following transplantation. One month after transplantation, neural stem cells (NSCs) begin to differentiate into astrocytes (GFAP; white arrows, bottom right), neurons (DCX; white arrows, bottom left), or oligodendrocytes (not shown). In recent unpublished studies we found that striatal transplantation of NSCs can improve cognitive function in a transgenic model of Parkinson's disease. Scale bar = 300 μm.

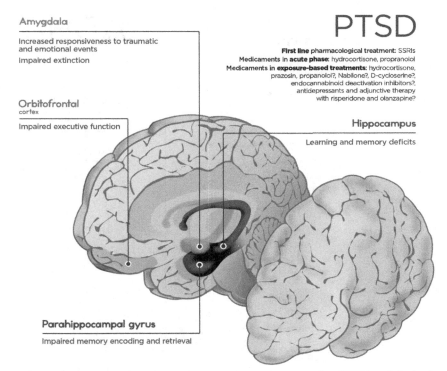

Amygdala

Increased responsiveness to traumatic and emotional events

Impaired extinction

Orbitofrontal
cortex

Impaired executive function

Parahippocampal gyrus

Impaired memory encoding and retrieval

PTSD

First line pharmacological treatment: SSRIs
Medicaments in **acute phase**: hydrocortisone, propranolol
Medicaments in **exposure-based treatments**: hydrocortisone,
prazosin, propanolol?, Nabilone?, D-cycloserine?,
endocannabinoid deactivation inhibitors?,
antidepressants and adjunctive therapy
with risperidone and olanzapine?

Hippocampus

Learning and memory deficits

FIGURE 10.1 **Cognitive symptoms in posttraumatic stress disorder (PTSD) and the brain areas involved.** Medications administered during the acute phase should be given in the initial hours following the traumatic event to prevent the development of PTSD symptoms. The medications used with exposure-based therapies aim to improve the efficacy of such therapies in ameliorating the symptoms of patients suffering from PTSD. SSRI, selective serotonin reuptake inhibitor.

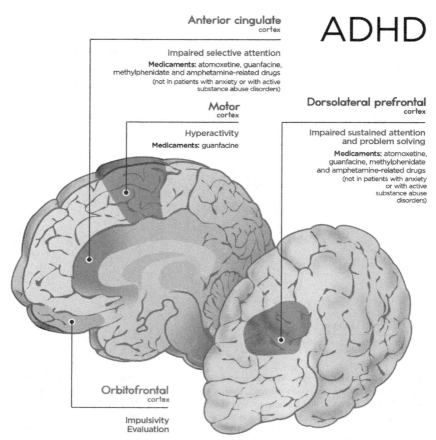

FIGURE 10.2 Pharmacological treatments for attention deficit/hyperactivity disorder (ADHD). Dysfunction in certain frontal brain areas is characteristic of ADHD. The main medications proven to be effective in improving attention and problem solving in patients suffering from ADHD are indicated.

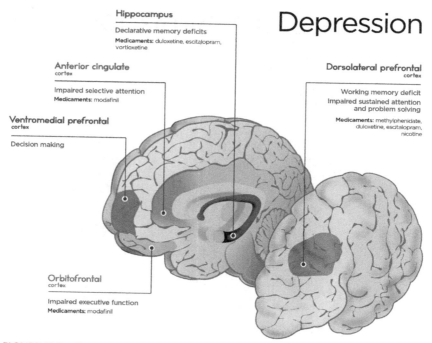

Hippocampus

Declarative memory deficits

Medicaments: duloxetine, escitalopram, vortioxetine

Anterior cingulate cortex

Impaired selective attention

Medicaments: modafinil

Ventromedial prefrontal cortex

Decision making

Orbitofrontal cortex

Impaired executive function

Medicaments: modafinil

Depression

Dorsolateral prefrontal cortex

Working memory deficit

Impaired sustained attention and problem solving

Medicaments: methylphenidate, duloxetine, escitalopram, nicotine

FIGURE 10.3   Cognitive deficits and brain dysfunction in major depressive disorder. The key medications proven to have clinical effects, or that are potentially beneficial, are indicated in each cognitive domain.

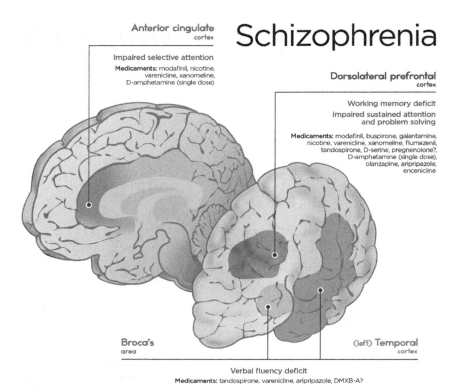

FIGURE 10.4 Brain areas altered in schizophrenia and those involved in cognitive impairment. The adjuvant pharmacotherapy for the different cognitive deficits observed in schizophrenic patients is indicated for each cognitive domain affected. DMXB-A, 3-[2,4-dimethoxybenzylidene] anabaseine.

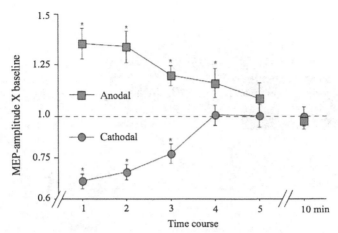

FIGURE 12.1 **Based on the classic study by Nitsche and Paulus (2000), anodal stimulation over the human motor cortex facilitates neuronal firing and cathodal stimulation inhibits neuronal firing up to 5 min after stimulation.** MEP, motor evoked potential. *Figure modified from Nitsche and Paulus (2000), Journal of Physiology, with permission.*

(A)

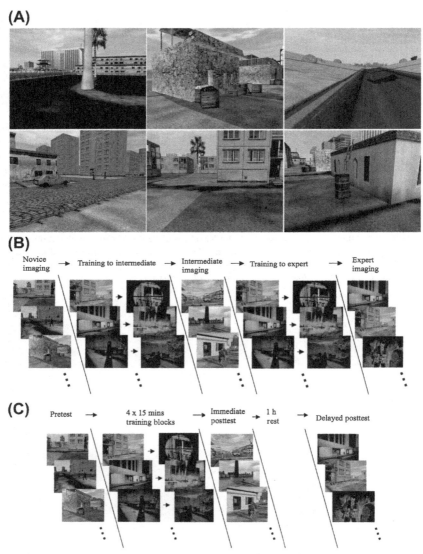

(B)

Novice imaging → Training to intermediate → Intermediate imaging → Training to expert → Expert imaging

(C)

Pretest → 4 x 15 mins training blocks → Immediate posttest → 1 h rest → Delayed posttest

FIGURE 12.3 Examples of stimuli used by Clark et al. (2012) in functional magnetic resonance imaging (fMRI) and transcranial direct current stimulation (tDCS) learning studies. (A) Examples of stimuli with and without concealed objects. Only four of the six scenes include hidden objects. Two of these four scenes with concealed objects contain hidden enemy soldiers, and the other two contain hidden bombs. The difficulty of object detection was defined by the size and distinctiveness of objects. (B) The fMRI learning study paradigm followed by 13 participants. Each participant was scanned using fMRI at the novice stage using 100 static scenes without feedback. This was followed by up to 90 min of training per day, whereby participants press a button to indicate whether they observed a concealed image in a series of static images, with each response followed by a short feedback video. Participants trained consecutively until they achieve

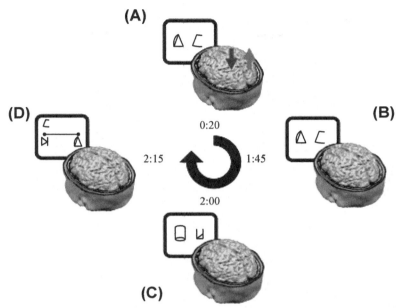

FIGURE 12.5 **The daily training routine of participants in the study by Cohen Kadosh et al. (2010) over six sessions.** (A) Application of transcranial direct current stimulation (tDCS) from the start of an artificial digit learning task for 20 min. Anodal tDCS (A-tDCS) was delivered over the right parietal lobe (red arrow), and cathodal tDCS (C-tDCS) was applied over the left parietal lobe (blue arrow). (B) Training continued after stimulation has stopped. Immediately after training, participants performed the numerical Stroop task (C) and the number-to-space task. (D) The time indicated next to each image shows the time elapsed from the beginning of the daily session until its termination in a cumulative style. *Figure adapted with permission from Cell Press.*

an intermediate level of performance (>78% correct responses on two consecutive training blocks) and were scanned again. The training continued for seven of these participants until they achieved 95% accuracy, when they were scanned for the last time at the expert level. (C) The paradigm used for behavioral tDCS learning studies; each session was preceded by a pretest involving viewing static scenes without feedback, followed by 4 training blocks of 60 trials each. Participants received tDCS 5 min before their training began for 30 min, followed by additional training without tDCS, for a total of 1 h of training. Immediately after training, a posttest was conducted, followed by an hour break and a final delayed posttest.